HEALTH & FITNESS
Fourth Edition
A GUIDE TO A HEALTHY LIFESTYLE

Contains Color Plates

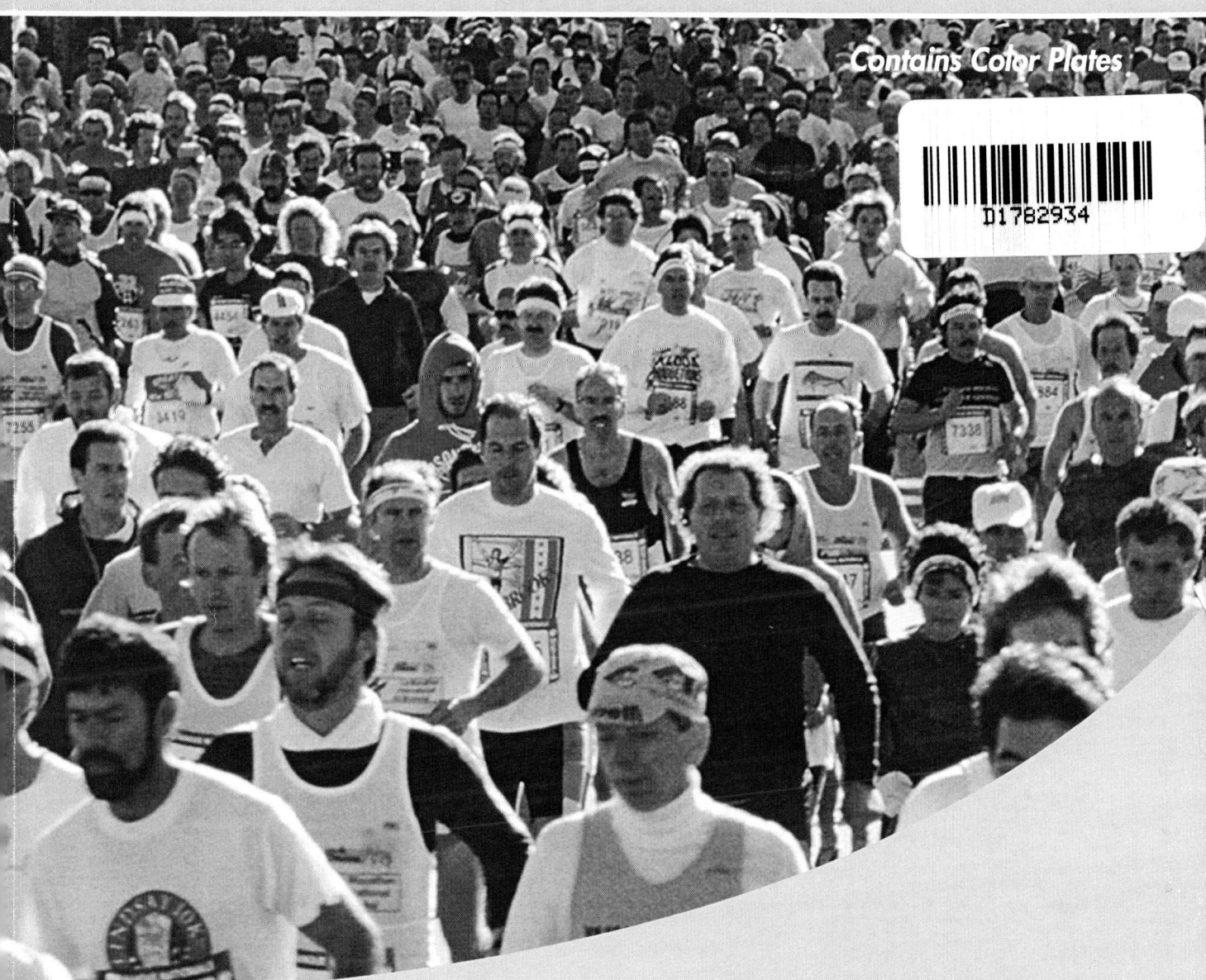

Laura E. Bounds, M.S., CHES
Northern Arizona University

Kirstin Brekken Shea, M.S.

Dottiedee Agnor, M.S.

Gayden S. Darnell, M.S.
Texas A&M University

Kendall Hunt publishing company
4050 Westmark Drive • P O Box 1840 • Dubuque IA 52004-1840

CAUTION: In-class and notebook activity pages contained in this textbook are protected by copyright. Photocopying these pages violates copyright law.

Book Team

Chairman and Chief Executive Officer   Mark C. Falb
President and Chief Operating Officer   Chad M. Chandlee
Vice President, Higher Education   David L. Tart
Director of National Book Program   Paul B. Carty
Editorial Manager   Georgia Botsford
Editor   Denise M. LaBudda
Assistant Vice President, Production Services   Christine E. O'Brien
Senior Production Editor   Mary Melloy
Senior Permissions Editor   Colleen Zelinsky
Cover Designer   Sandy Beck

Cover image © JupiterImages Corporation.

Kendall Hunt
publishing company

www.kendallhunt.com
Send all inquiries to:
4050 Westmark Drive
Dubuque, IA 52004-1840

Copyright © 2000, 2003, 2006, 2009 by Kendall Hunt Publishing Company

ISBN 978-0-7575-6210-5

All rights reserved. No part of this publication may be reproduced, stored in a retrieval system, or transmitted, in any form or by any means, electronic, mechanical, photocopying, recording, or otherwise, without the prior written permission of the copyright owner.

Printed in the United States of America
10 9 8 7 6 5 4 3 2

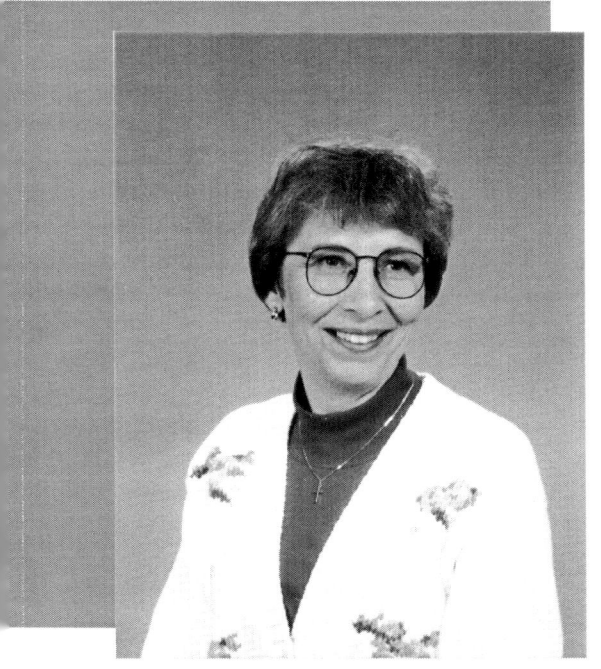

This textbook is dedicated to the memory of Dr. Emma S. Gibbons, who was a valued member of the Department of Health and Kinesiology at Texas A&M University for 25 years. She fought a 12 year battle with breast cancer and passed away on September 7, 2001.

Dr. Gibbons was known for mentoring students, faculty and staff. She had high expectations of herself and others and had the rare quality of making every individual feel appreciated. As the "glue" that held the Department together, she dedicated her life to the betterment of the department through her vision and perseverance. She lived a life of courage and faith in an attempt to give back to the world, and it is through her wisdom and inspiration that we were able to complete this textbook. Texas A&M University is a much better place because she was here.

A portion of the sales proceeds from this textbook benefit The Emma Gibbons Endowed College Scholarship Fund.

"To laugh often and much; to win the respect of intelligent people and the affection of children; to earn the appreciation of honest critics and endure the betrayal of false friends; to appreciate beauty, to find the best in others; to leave the world a little better, whether by a healthy child, a garden patch or a redeemed social condition; to know even one life has breathed easier because you have lived. This is the meaning of success."

—Ralph Waldo Emerson

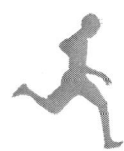

BRIEF CONTENTS

CHAPTER 1
Introduction

CHAPTER 2
Stress and Psychological Health

CHAPTER 3
Personal Fitness

CHAPTER 4
Lifestyle Choices and Hypokinetic Conditions

CHAPTER 5
Nutrition

CHAPTER 6
Lifetime Weight Management

CHAPTER 7
Relationships

CHAPTER 8
Sexuality

CHAPTER 9
Drugs

CHAPTER 10
Safety Awareness

CHAPTER 11
Human Diseases

CHAPTER 12
Alternative and Complementary Medicine

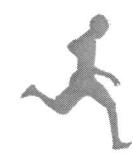

CONTENTS

Acknowledgments	xv
About the Authors	xvii

CHAPTER 1

Introduction	1
Dimensions of Wellness	2
Emotional	2
Intellectual	3
Social	3
Spiritual	3
Physical	3
Occupational	3
Environmental	4
Financial Wellness	4
Factors That Influence Health and Wellness	4
A Wellness Profile	5
Changing Behavior and Setting Goals	6
The Stages of Change	6
Behavior Change and Goal Setting	8
Healthy People 2010	11
Summary	13
References	14
Activities	14
In-Class Activity	15
Notebook Activities	17

CHAPTER 2

Stress and Psychological Health	23
Wellness and Stress	24
Self-Talk Your Way to Reduced Levels of Stress and an Improved Life	28
Stress and Its Impact on Mental Health	30
Who Gets Mental Health Disorders?	30
Depression and Stress	31
Suicidal Behavior and Stress	32
Eating Disorders and Stress	33
Causes of Eating Disorders	37
Ways to Help	40
References	40
Activities	41
Notebook Activities	43

CHAPTER 3

Personal Fitness	53
Why Is Physical Activity Important?	54
Cardiovascular Fitness	58
How Aerobic Exercise Helps Cardiovascular Fitness	59
Aerobic and Anaerobic Exercise	62
Exercise Prescription, or How to Become FITT	63
Frequency	63
Intensity	63
Time	64
Type	65
Components of an Exercise Session	65
Warm-Up	65
Pre-Stretch	66
Activity	66
Cooldown and Stretch	66
Principles of Fitness Training—The Rules	66
Overload and Adaptation	66
Specificity	67
Individual Differences	67
Reversibility	68
Evaluating Cardiovascular Fitness	68
Muscular Fitness	69
Benefits of Muscular Fitness	70
Importance of the Core Musculature in Functional Movement	71
What Makes Up the "Core"?	71
Effective Training	74
Training for the Best Results	74

True or False? Weight Training Myths	76
Flexibility	77
When You Should Not Exercise	79
Injuries	79
Proper Footwear	81
Environmental Conditions	82
Hyponatremia	83
Illness	84
Common Sense Concerns	84
The Biggest Risk to Exercise Is Not Starting!	85
References	86
Contacts	87
Activities	88
Notebook Activities	89

CHAPTER 4

Lifestyle Choices and Hypokinetic Conditions	**103**
Types of Hypokinetic Conditions	108
Cardiovascular Disease (CVD)	108
Arteriosclerosis and Exercise	111
Peripheral Vascular Disease	113
Hypertension	113
Heart Attack	115
Stroke	119
Risk Factors for Cardiovascular Disease	120
Controllable Risk Factors	120
Uncontrollable Risk Factors	121
Contributing Risk Factors	121
Obesity	121
Childhood Obesity	123
Causes of Obesity	124
Physiological Response to Obesity	125
Cancer	125
Who Gets Cancer?	125
Can Cancer Be Prevented?	125
Does Exercise Help?	125
Diabetes	126
Who Gets Diabetes?	127
Can Diabetes Be Prevented?	127
Does Exercise Help?	127
Metabolic Syndrome	127

Low Back Pain	128
Who Suffers from Low Back Pain?	128
Can Low Back Pain Be Prevented?	128
Does Exercise Help?	128
Osteoporosis	129
Who Gets Osteoporosis?	129
Can Osteoporosis Be Prevented?	130
Does Exercise Help?	130
Aging	131
Prevention of Hypokinetic Conditions: Planning Your Activity Program	133
References	134
Contacts	136
Recommended Reading	136
Activities	136
Notebook Activities	137

CHAPTER 5

Nutrition	**145**
Dietary Guidelines for Americans	146
Adequate Nutrients within Calorie Needs	147
Weight Management	147
Physical Activity	148
Food Groups to Encourage	148
Fats	149
Carbohydrates	149
Sodium and Potassium	149
Alcoholic Beverages	150
Food Safety	150
Essential Nutrients	151
Carbohydrates	151
Fats	151
Protein	156
Vitamins	158
Minerals	160
Antioxidants	162
Water	164
The Food Guide Pyramid	165
Grains	165
Vegetables	167
Fruits	167
Milk	168

Meats and Beans	168
Oils	168
Daily Activity	168
What Happened to the "Fat" Group?	168
Other Issues in Nutrition	170
Organic Foods	170
Functional Foods	171
Vegetarianism	171
Reading and Understanding the Nutrition Facts Label	176
References	179
Contacts	180
Activities	180
Notebook Activities	181

CHAPTER 6

Lifetime Weight Management	193
Causes of Obesity and Being Overweight	194
Body Image	197
What Is a Healthy Body Weight?	198
Determining Caloric Needs	199
Obesity	200
Obesity Prevention	200
How Does Activity Help Obesity?	201
How Do I Lose Weight?	201
Weight Loss Guidelines	204
Dietary Supplements	204
Weight Loss Products	205
Healthy Habits	209
Healthy Weight Gain	209
Healthy Food Shopping	210
Fast Foods/Eating Out	215
Fitness or Fatness	215
References	216
Recommended Reading	217
Activities	217
Notebook Activities	219

CHAPTER 7

Relationships	223
Healthy Relationships	224
Positive Self-Worth	224

Open Communication	224
Compromise	225
Trust	226
Types of Relationships	226
Stages of Relationships	229
Dating	230
Ending a Relationship	235
I Do or I Do Not	236
Unhealthy Relationships	238
Abusive Relationships	238
Additional Readings	239
References	239
Contacts	240
Activities	240
In-Class Activity	241
Notebook Activities	243

CHAPTER 8

Sexuality	255
Anatomy	256
Female Sexual Anatomy	256
Male Sexual Anatomy	258
Sexual Orientation	260
Readiness for Sexual Activity	261
Reproduction	263
Menstrual Cycle	263
Ovarian Cycle	264
Endometrial Cycle	264
Pregnancy	265
Emergency Contraception "The Morning After Pill"	278
Unplanned Pregnancy	278
Parenthood	278
Adoption	279
Abortion	279
Sexually Transmitted Infections (STIs)	280
Levels of Risk	281
Bacterial STIs	281
Viral STIs	288
Parasitic STIs	293
STI Prevention	298
References	300

CONTENTS

Contacts	301
Activities	302
In-Class Activities	303
Notebook Activities	309

CHAPTER 9

Drugs	**313**
Tobacco	314
Tobacco Components	314
Types of Tobacco Use	315
Environmental Tobacco Smoke	318
Smoking Cessation	318
Psychoactive Drugs	322
Stimulants	322
Depressants	326
Narcotics	327
Cannabis	328
Hallucinogens	328
Inhalants	329
Club Drugs	330
Anabolic Steroids	332
Prescription Drugs	333
Alcohol	334
Prevalence	334
What Is Alcohol?	334
Physiological Effects	336
Laws Relating to Alcohol	336
Societal Problems	337
Drinking and Driving	337
Alcohol Use in College	340
Binge Drinking	340
Alcohol Poisoning	341
Drinking Problems	342
Alcoholism	343
Chronic Effects	344
References	346
Activities	347
In-Class Activity	349
Notebook Activities	351

CHAPTER 10

Safety Awareness	**363**
Classes of Unintentional Injuries	364
Motor Vehicle Crashes	364
Motorcycles	366
Bicycle Safety	366
Home Accidents	367
Work Accidents	368
Public Accidents	368
Disaster Planning	369
Environmental Safety	369
Reduce, Reuse, Recycle	370
Personal Safety	372
Safety Tips	372
College Campuses	373
Stalking	374
Sexual Assault	375
Acquaintance Rape/Intimate Violence	376
Domestic Violence	377
References	378
Contacts	379
Activities	379
Notebook Activities	381

CHAPTER 11

Human Diseases	**387**
Communicable Diseases	388
HIV/AIDS (Non-Sexual Contraction)	388
Tuberculosis	388
Mononucleosis	389
Hepatitis	390
Meningitis	393
Common Cold	394
Influenza	395
Non-Communicable Diseases	396
Cancer	396
Asthma	407
Diabetes	408

Anemia	411
Lupus	411
Gastrointestinal Disorders	412
References	413
Contacts	414
Activities	414
Notebook Activities	415

CHAPTER 12

Alternative and Complementary Medicine	**419**
Alternative Healthcare Systems	424
Manipulative and Body-Based Therapies	426
Biological-Based Therapies	428
Mind-Body Medicine	431
Energy Therapies	435
Using the Internet for Credible Medical Information	437
References	437
Contacts	439
Recommended Books for Further Reading	440
Appendix	**441**
Glossary	**447**
Index	**457**

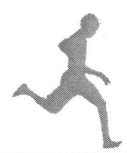

ACKNOWLEDGMENTS

The authors would like to acknowledge the following individuals for their invaluable contributions in the writing of *Health and Fitness: A Guide to a Healthy Lifestyle*:

- Julie Barber, M.S.
- Roger Bounds, Ph.D.
- William Coady, M.S.
- Tamara Franks, M.A.G.
- Melinda Grant, M.S.
- Janet Hardcastle, M.S.
- Sandra Kimbrough, Ph.D.
- Ernie Kirkham, M.S.
- Susan Wagner, M.S.
- Dianne Maddox, M.S.
- Martha Muckleroy, M.Ed.
- Jeremy Nelms, M.S.
- Christine Reeves, M.S.
- Teresa Wenzel, M.S.
- Brian Wigley, M.S.
- Nicole Wilkerson, M.S.

We also acknowledge with appreciation the continuing guidance and support from the expert review panel:

- Robert Armstrong, Ph.D.
- Danny Ballard, Ed.D
- Susan Bloomfield, Ph.D.
- Maurice Dennis, Ph.D.
- Jerry Elledge, Ph.D.
- Margaret Griffith, M.S.
- Linda Mullen, M.D.
- B.E. Pruitt, Ed.D.
- Jack Wilmore, Ph.D.

Special thanks to:
Roger Bounds, Richard Darnell, Kathy Durkin, and Kristin Slagel for their guidance, support, and input.

Without the technical knowledge of Kristin Slagel, M.S., and Beth Netherland, M.S., the development of the Powerpoint presentation and the contribution it makes to the text would not have been possible.

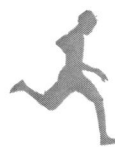

ABOUT THE AUTHORS

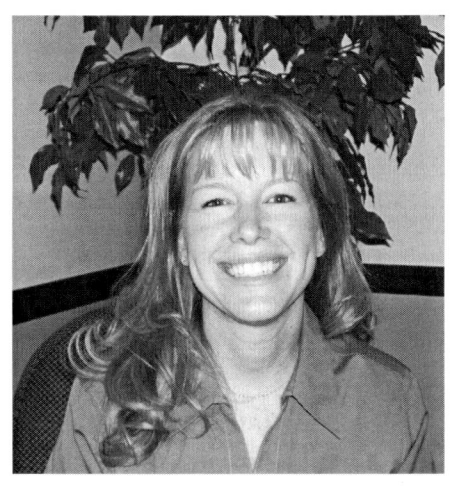

Laura Bounds, M.S., CHES, ACE

Laura Bounds is currently teaching Health Principles, Human Diseases, Theories of Health Behavior, and Emergency Response courses at Northern Arizona University. Prior to her time at NAU she spent fourteen years at Texas A&M University in College Station, where she earned her B.B.A. in Accounting, M.S. in Health Education, taught Health and Fitness courses and coordinated the Health and Fitness program for five years. Outside of the classroom, Laura enjoys spending time with her children, hiking, mountain biking, scuba diving, and snow skiing.

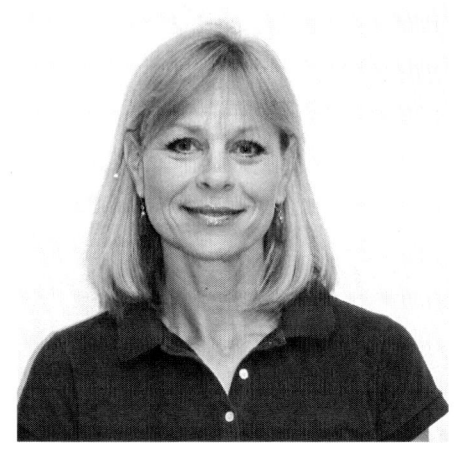

Kirstin Brekken Shea, M.S.

Kirstin is a Senior Lecturer and Coordinator of Group Exercise Activities in the Physical Education and Activity program in the Health and Kinesiology Department at Texas A&M University. Kirstin received her undergraduate degree at Texas Lutheran College in Biology. Kirstin received her Masters in Exercise Physiology in the Health and Kinesiology Department at Texas A&M University. Childhood obesity, stress management through yoga/meditation, and adult fitness/nutrition are her particular areas of interest. She teaches fitness related activities such as step aerobics, cardio-kickboxing, walking, and yoga. Kirstin also teaches Physical Fitness and Motor Assessment to Kinesiology majors as well as two other teacher preparation courses. Kirstin is a soccer mom of three wonderful, active kids. She loves to hang out with her family, cook, garden, and of course attend soccer practices and games.

Dottiedee Agnor, M.S.

Dottiedee has been teaching at Texas A&M University in the Health and Kinesiology Department for the past twelve years. She is coordinator for the areas of Self-Defense, Yoga, Badminton, and Basketball. She also teaches Safety Education courses as well as Alcohol Awareness programs. She received a B.S. in Physical Education and Health and an M.S. in Kinesiology at Texas A&M University. She has also been involved with the National Youth Sports program for the past thirteen years as Director and Project Administrator. Prior to returning to the college setting she was a public school teacher in the Richardson Independent School District, coaching and teaching physical education and health. Her interests are drug and alcohol prevention, personal safety awareness, and underserved youth services.

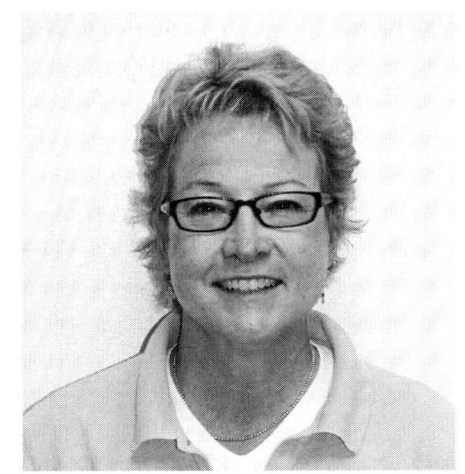

Gayden Darnell, M.S.

Gayden is currently teaching Health and Fitness and Physical Education classes at Texas A&M University. She has taught for the Physical Education Activity program at Texas A&M in College Station since 1997 and has spent several semesters coordinating racquet sports for the department during this time. Prior to teaching at TAMU, she taught and coached in the Bryan, Texas public schools. She attended Millsaps College in Jackson, Mississippi, for two years during which time she played on the varsity tennis and soccer teams. She earned both her B.S. in Kinesiology and M.S. in Health Education from Texas A&M University in College Station. Outside of the classroom, Gayden enjoys spending time with her children, coaching and attending various youth sports, training for half and full marathons, and reading.

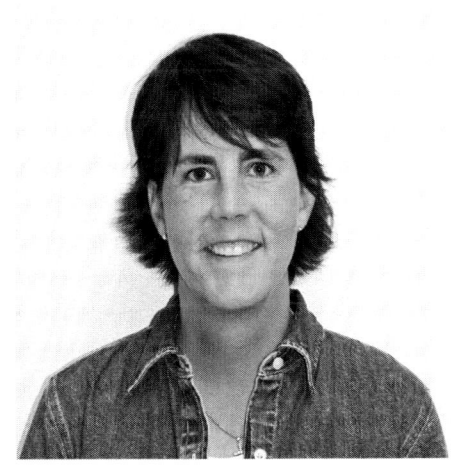

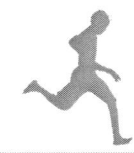

CHAPTER 1

Introduction

"Take care of your body with steadfast fidelity. The soul must see through these eyes alone, and if they are dim, the whole world is clouded."

—Johann Wolfgang Von Goethe

OBJECTIVES

Students will be able to:
- Differentiate between the definitions of health and wellness.
- Describe and discuss the seven components of wellness.
- Identify the link between preventative behaviors and wellness.
- Discuss the health behaviors that increase the quality and longevity of life.
- Identify the significance of *Healthy People 2010*.
- List the five stages of change.
- Describe key elements for a successful behavior change.

Health is a universal trait. The World Health Organization defines **health** as a "state of complete physical, mental, and social well-being and not merely the absence of disease or infirmity." Webster's Dictionary offers "the condition of being sound in body, mind, or spirit; especially: freedom from physical disease or pain . . . the general condition of the body" as a definition of health. However, health also has an individual quality; it is very personal, and unique.

Early on, definitions of health revolved around issues of sanitation and personal hygiene. Today, the definition of health has evolved from a basis of physical health or absence of disease, to a term that encompasses the emotional, mental, social, spiritual, and physical dimensions of an individual. This current, positive approach to health is referred to as wellness. **Wellness** is a process of making informed choices that will lead one, over a period of time, to a healthy lifestyle that should result in a sense of well-being.

Dimensions of Wellness

Wellness emphasizes an individual's potential and responsibility for his or her own health. It is a process in which a person is constantly moving either away from or toward a most favorable level of health. Wellness results from the adoption of low-risk, health-enhancing behaviors. The adoption of a wellness lifestyle requires focusing on choices that will enhance the individual's potential to lead a productive, meaningful, and satisfying life.

It is the complex interaction of each of the seven dimensions of wellness that will lead an individual, over time, to a higher quality of life and better overall health and well-being. Constant, ongoing assessment of one's behaviors in the following dimensions is key to living a balanced life. In addition to the seven dimensions shown in Figure 1.1, there is discussion of other factors that influence wellness.

Emotional

An individual who is emotionally healthy is able to enjoy life despite unexpected challenges and problems. Effectively coping with life's difficulties and unexpected

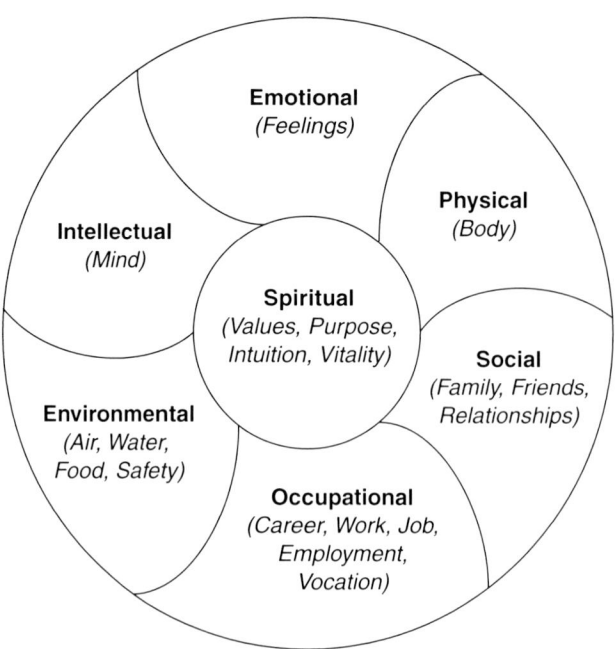

FIGURE 1.1
Seven Dimensions of Wellness

events is essential to maintaining good health. Equally important to good personal wellness is the ability to understand your feelings and express those feelings or emotions outwardly in a positive and constructive manner. "Bottled-up" negative emotions can affect the immune system and result in chronic stress, which in turn can lead to serious illnesses such as high blood pressure and can potentially lead to a premature death.

Intellectual

The mind can have substantial influence over the body. To be intellectually healthy, it is essential to continue to explore new avenues and interests and to regularly engage in new and ongoing learning opportunities and experiences. The more "unknowns" an individual faces or explores, the more opportunities he or she has to learn and grow intellectually.

Social

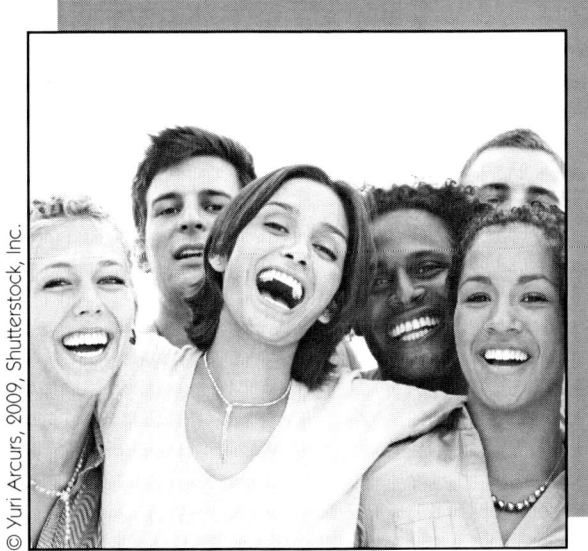

The ability to relate and interact with others is important to a person's overall sense of well-being.

Social health is an individual's ability to relate to and interact with others. Socially healthy people are able to communicate and interact with the other people they come in contact with each day. They are respectful and caring of their family, friends, neighbors, and associates. Although reaching out and communicating with others may be difficult or uncomfortable initially, it is extremely important to a person's social health and their overall sense of well-being.

Spiritual

Spiritual health helps a person achieve a sense of inner peace, satisfaction, and confidence. It can help give the sense that all is right with the world. A person's ethics, values, beliefs, and morals can contribute to their spiritual health. Good spiritual health can help give life meaning and purpose.

Physical

Ensuring good physical health begins with devoting attention and time to attaining healthy levels of cardiovascular fitness, muscular strength and endurance, flexibility, and body composition. When coupled with good nutritional practices, good sleep habits, and the avoidance of risky social behaviors such as drinking and driving or unprotected sexual intercourse, a physically healthy body results. This is the component that is most often associated, at first glance, with a person's health.

Occupational

Attaining occupational wellness begins with determining what roles, activities, and commitments take up a majority of an individual's time. These roles, activities, or commitments could include but are not limited to being a student, parenting, volunteering in an organization, or working at a part-time job while pursuing one's degree. It is when each of these areas are integrated and balanced in a personally and professionally fulfilling way that occupational wellness occurs.

Environmental

An individual's health and wellness can be substantially affected by the quality of their environment. Access to clean air, nutritious food, sanitary water, and adequate clothing and shelter are essential components to being well. An individual's environment should, at the very least, be clean and safe.

Through wellness, an individual manages a wide range of lifestyle choices. How a person chooses to behave and the decisions he or she makes in each of the seven dimensions of wellness will determine their overall quality of life. Making an active effort to combining and constantly trying to balance each of the seven dimensions is key to a long and fulfilling life.

Financial Wellness

There are many different wellness models and most include multidimensional elements. One element which has typically not been included is financial wellness. Financial wellness has an impact on an individual and society as a whole. The first step to gaining financial wellness is financial responsibility. There are numerous ways to be financially responsible, some of which include:

- Have a monthly budget and do not overspend
- Wait for items to go on sale
- Use coupons
- Avoid credit card debt (pay the balance every month)
- Use credit cards only in emergency situations
- Save at least 5 percent of net income in case of an emergency
- Do not get a car loan for more than five years (three- or four-year notes are even better)
- Always pay your bills on time
- Shop and trade at resale stores
- Pay off a mortgage early
- Check out books from a library instead of purchasing them from a bookstore
- Carpool
- Ride your bike
- Eat at home
- Go for a hike instead of going to a movie

Factors That Influence Health and Wellness

In addition to the dimensions of wellness, the factors shown in Figure 1.2 also influence health and wellness, as well as physical fitness. You will see that lifestyle is only one component that works in tandem with other factors to make up good health and wellness.

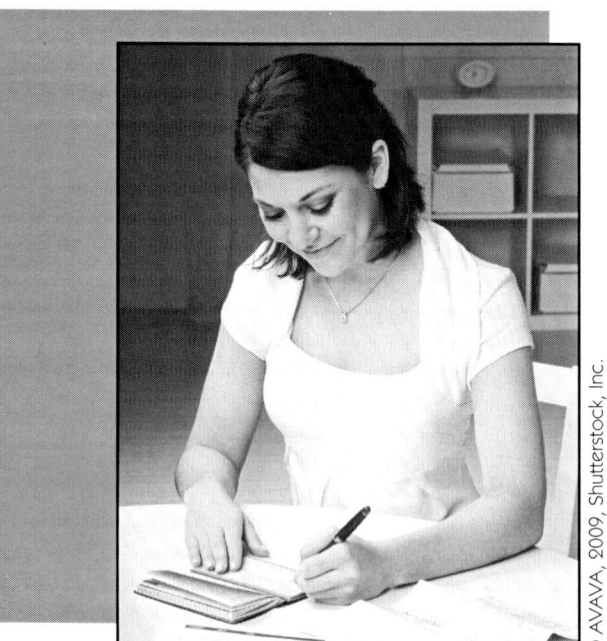

Financial wellness has an impact on an individual and society as a whole.

FIGURE 1.2

Factors Influencing Health, Wellness, and Physical Fitness

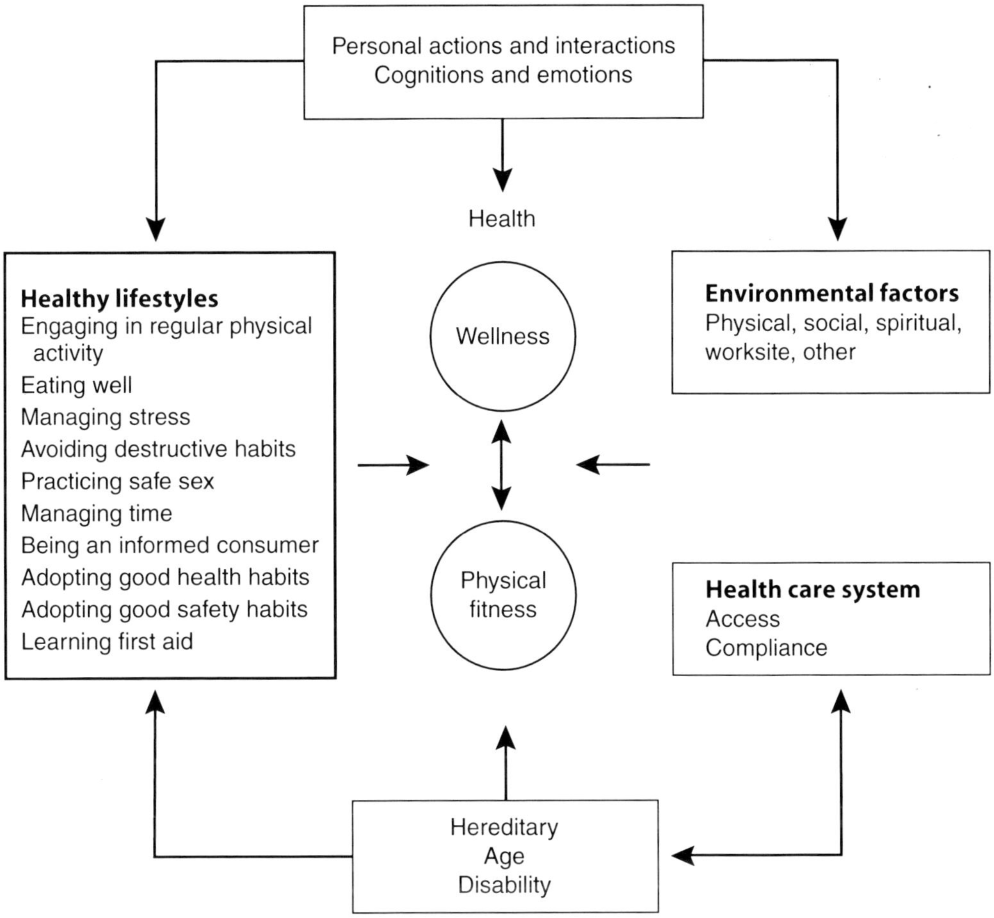

```
                Personal actions and interactions
                Cognitions and emotions
                            │
                         Health
                            
   Healthy lifestyles                    Environmental factors
   Engaging in regular physical          Physical, social, spiritual,
      activity              Wellness     worksite, other
   Eating well
   Managing stress
   Avoiding destructive habits
   Practicing safe sex
   Managing time
   Being an informed consumer
   Adopting good health habits           Health care system
   Adopting good safety habits           Access
   Learning first aid       Physical     Compliance
                            fitness
   
                Hereditary
                Age
                Disability
```

From *Concepts of Physical Fitness* by Corbin et al., 2009. Reprinted by permission of The McGraw-Hill Companies, Inc.

A Wellness Profile

Living well requires constant evaluation and effort on an individual's part. The following list includes important behaviors and habits to include in your daily life:

- Be responsible for your own health and wellness. Take an active role in your life and well-being.
- Learn how to recognize and manage stress effectively.
- Eat nutritious meals, exercise regularly, and maintain a healthy weight.
- Work towards healthy relationships with friends, family, and significant others.
- Avoid tobacco and other drugs; use alcohol responsibly, if at all.
- Know the facts about cardiovascular disease, cancer, infections, sexually transmitted infections, and injuries. Utilize this knowledge to protect yourself.
- Understand how the environment affects your health and take appropriate measures to improve it.

(adapted from Insel & Roth, 2008)

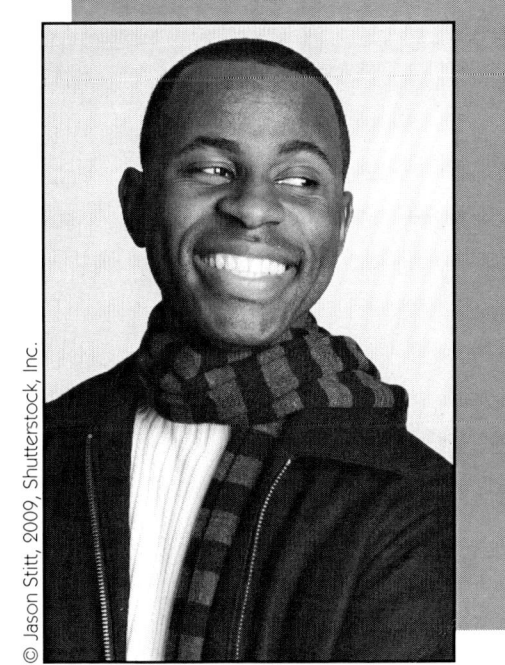

Living well requires constant evaluation and effort.

Changing Behavior and Setting Goals

The Stages of Change

The Stages of Change Model (SCM) was originally developed in the late 1970s and early 1980s by James Prochaska and Carlo DiClemente when they were studying how smokers were able to quit smoking. The SCM model has been applied to many different behavior changes including weight loss, injury prevention, alcohol use, drug abuse, and others. The SCM consists of five stages of change precontemplation, contemplation, preparation, action, and maintenance. The idea behind the SCM is that behavior change does not usually happen all at one time. People tend to progress through the stages until they achieve a successful behavior change or relapse. The progression through each of these stages is different depending upon the individual and the particular behavior being changed. Each person must decide when a stage is complete and when it is time to move on to the next stage.

Precontemplation The stage at which there is no intention to change a specific behavior in the foreseeable future. Many individuals in this stage are unaware of their unhealthy behavior. They are not thinking about change and are not interested in any help. People in this stage tend to defend their current behavior and do not feel it is a problem. They may resent efforts to help them change.

Contemplation The stage at which people are more aware of the consequences of their unhealthy behavior and have spent time thinking about the behavior but have not yet made a commitment to take action. They consider the possibility of changing, but tend to be ambivalent about change. In this stage, people straddle the fence, weighing the pros and cons of changing or modifying their behavior.

Preparation A stage that combines intention and behavioral criteria. In this stage, people have made a commitment to make a change. This can be a research phase where people are taking small steps toward change. They gather information about what they will need to do to change their behavior. Sometimes, people skip this stage and try to move directly from contemplation to action. Many times, this can result in failure because they did not research or accept what it was going to take to make a major lifestyle change.

Action The stage at which individuals actually modify their behavior. This stage requires a considerable commitment of time and energy. The amount of time people spend in the action stage varies. On average, it generally lasts about six months. In this stage, unhealthy people depend on their own willpower. They are making efforts to change the unhealthy behavior and are at greatest risk for relapse. During this stage, support from friends and family can be very helpful.

Along the way to a permanent behavior change, most people experience a relapse. In fact, it is much more common to have at least one setback than not. Relapse is often accompanied by feelings of discouragement. While relapse can be frustrating, the majority of people who successfully change their behavior do not follow a straight path to a lifetime free of unwanted behaviors. Rather, they cycle through the five stages several times before achieving a consistent behavior change. Therefore, the SCM considers relapse to be normal. Relapses can be important opportunities for learning and becoming stronger. This is where a behavior change journal and weekly reflections can help an individual see how much progress has been made, as well as what may trigger relapses. The main thing to remember is

Introduction

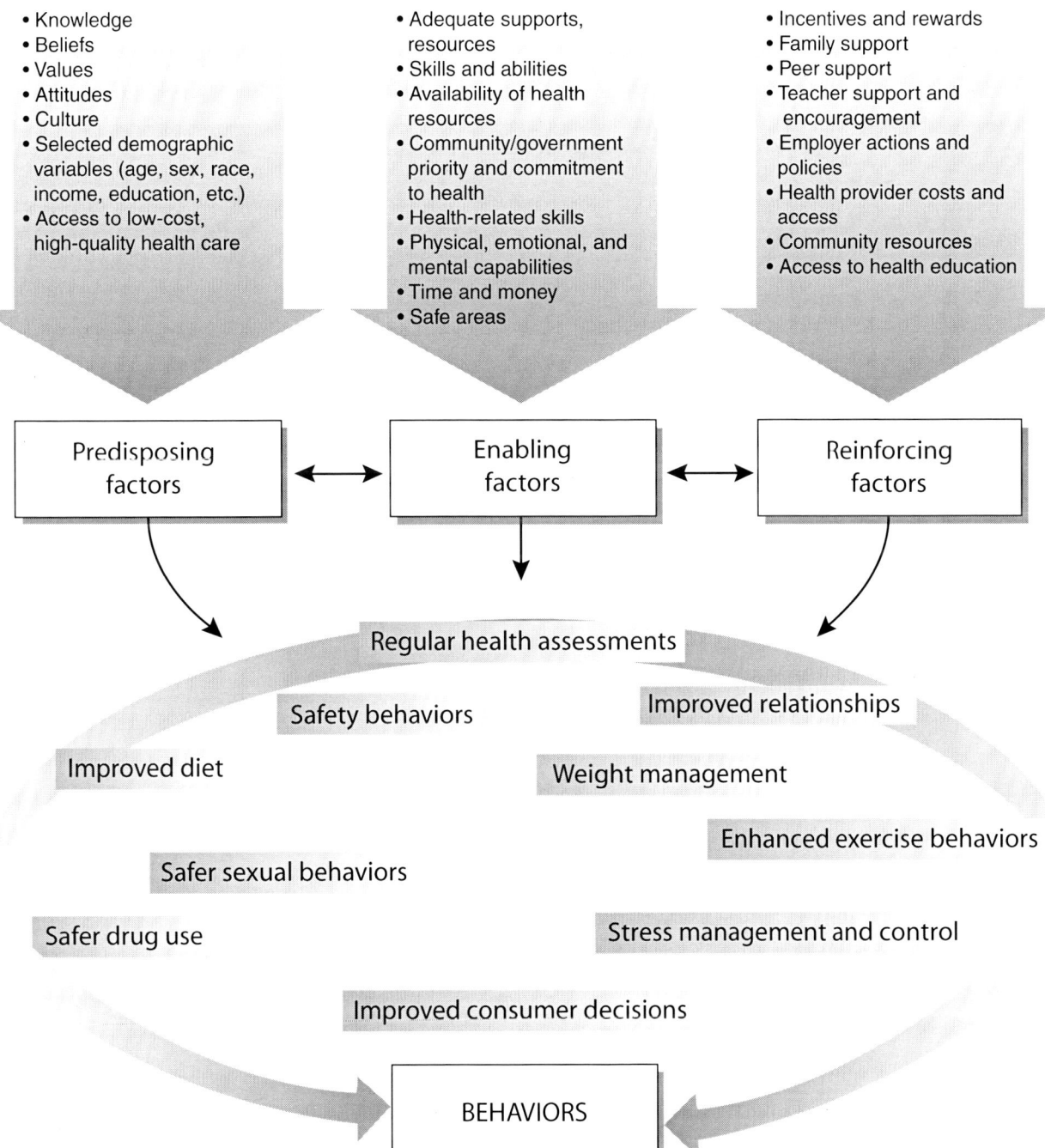

FIGURE 1.3
Factors That Influence Behavior Change Decisions

Fig 1.3, p. 18 from *Access to Health*, 6th edition by Rebecca J. Donatelle and Lorriane G. Davis. Copyright © 2000 by Allyn and Bacon. Reprinted by permission of Pearson Education, Inc.

that the goal is getting closer. Do not get upset by life or setbacks, but keep moving forward and get closer to the end goal.

Maintenance The stage in which people work to prevent relapse and focus on the gains attained during the action stage. Maintenance involves being able to successfully avoid temptations to return to the previous behavior. The goal of the maintenance stage is to continue the new behavior or lack there of without relapse. People are more able to successfully anticipate situations in which a relapse could occur and prepare coping or avoidance strategies in advance.

Behavior Change and Goal Setting

Listed below are some tips for successful behavior change.

Choose a behavior that an individual is really invested in. Utilize the Lifestyle Assessment Inventory at the end of this chapter to see what behavioral areas need the most attention. Ideas for behavior change include: better communication, working on a particular relationship (parent, friend, significant other), increasing exercise, quitting smoking, decreasing procrastination, decreasing or eliminating sodas, eating more fruits and/or vegetables, flossing teeth every day, stretching, and so on.

Only change one behavior at a time. After reviewing lifestyle behaviors, people tend to get excited and want to change several different behaviors. Even if the behaviors are related, it is best to choose only one to focus on at a time. After a specific behavior has become a habit (at least six months in the maintenance stage) the individual can consider working on another behavior.

The goal should be specific and measurable. The more specific the goal and the plan to achieve this goal are, the more likely the behavior change will be successful. If an individual wants to increase fitness, it would be best to be very specific about the short- and long-term goals. For example, the individual should consider their baseline (where they are right now). If someone is not exercising at all, they should not begin working out five times per week the following week. During the first week the individual may want to exercise two times for fifteen minutes each exercise session. The following week the goal could be three times at twenty minutes each exercise session. The final goal may be five days per week for thirty minutes each time. This particular goal should take at least a month or two to achieve. The Behavior Change and Goal Setting notebook activity at the end of the chapter can help outline a plan of change.

Any behavior change target should be realistic. Often, behavior change goals include weight loss. To increase the long-term success rate, the most a person should lose is two pounds per week. One pound is equal to 3,500 calories. In order to lose two pounds per week the caloric deficit would need to be 7,000 calories. This translates to a deficit of 1,000 calories per day, which is not easy to achieve. The best way to achieve this caloric deficit is to include both exercise and limit caloric consumption. For example, an individual could expend part of the needed caloric deficit with exercise (approximately 500 calories per day) as well as consume fewer (approximately 500) calories per day for a total daily caloric deficit of 1,000. Remember, this is the most an individual should lose per week.

Have a reward system. It is nice to have short- and long-term goals that have a small reward when a goal is reached. These rewards should never be counterproductive. For example, if an individual is trying to lose weight, the worst type of reward would be to have a dessert. Some constructive reward ideas could be to go to a movie, go for a specific hike, buy a new pair of shorts, purchase a book or magazine.

Keep a journal. Recording notes on a regular basis is a great way to keep a behavior change project on an individual's mind. It also creates a method to track progress and setbacks. A lot can be learned from looking at what worked and what did not in previous weeks. It is best to journal a minimum of three days per week and include a weekly reflection statement summarizing how the week progressed. This can give the individual critical insight that they may not have had without the journaling process.

Have a support group. Tell friends and family members who will be supportive about a particular behavior change. The more people who know about the behavior change, the more likely the change will be successful.

By regularly evaluating your lifestyle and making small changes, you can maintain a healthy lifestyle. There are significant benefits to choosing healthy behaviors early on. The earlier these healthy behaviors are achieved, the more graceful aging will be. In Figure 1.4 the life expectancy is differentiated between healthy life expectancy and unhealthy years. In Figure 1.5 the number one cause of death is unintentional injury until the age of 44. After age 44, the leading causes of death are cancer and heart disease. These two figures demonstrate how critical it is that healthy behavior choices are made now rather than waiting until an injury or disease has occurred.

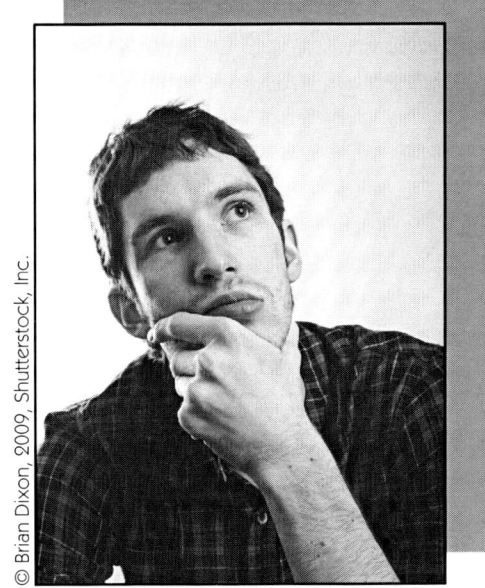

The Stages of Change Model consists of precontemplation, contemplation, preparation, action, and maintenance.

FIGURE 1.4 Healthy Life Expectancy for North America

Country	Healthy life expectancy	Unhealthy years	Total life expectancy
USA			
Females	71.5	8.6	80.1
Males	67.3	7.5	74.8
All	69.5	8.1	77.6
Canada			
Females	74.0	8.5	82.5
Males	70.1	7.1	77.2
All	72.0	8.5	80.5
Mexico			
Females	67.6	9.3	76.9
Males	63.4	8.4	71.8
All	65.5	8.8	74.3

Years

Sources: World Health Organization and National Center for Health Statistics

FIGURE 1.5
10 Leading Causes of Death, United States 2005, All Races, Both Sexes

Age Groups

Rank	<1	1-4	5-9	10-14	15-19	20-24	25-34	35-44	45-54	55-64	65+	All Ages
1	Congenital Anomalies 5,552	Unintentional Injury 1,664	Unintentional Injury 1,072	Unintentional Injury 1,343	Unintentional Injury 6,616	Unintentional Injury 9,137	Unintentional Injury 13,997	Unintentional Injury 16,919	Malignant Neoplasms 50,405	Malignant Neoplasms 99,240	Heart Disease 530,926	Heart Disease 652,091
2	Short Gestation 4,714	Congenital Anomalies 522	Malignant Neoplasms 485	Malignant Neoplasms 515	Homicide 2,076	Homicide 3,390	Suicide 4,990	Malignant Neoplasms 14,566	Heart Disease 38,103	Heart Disease 65,208	Malignant Neoplasms 388,322	Malignant Neoplasms 559,312
3	SIDS 2,230	Malignant Neoplasms 377	Congenital Anomalies 196	Suicide 270	Suicide 1,613	Suicide 2,599	Homicide 4,752	Heart Disease 12,688	Unintentional Injury 18,339	Chronic Low. Respiratory Disease 12,747	Cerebro-vascular 123,881	Cerebro-vascular 143,579
4	Maternal Pregnancy Comp. 1,776	Homicide 375	Homicide 121	Homicide 220	Malignant Neoplasms 731	Malignant Neoplasms 986	Malignant Neoplasms 3,601	Suicide 6,550	Liver Disease 7,517	Diabetes Mellitus 11,301	Chronic Low. Respiratory Disease 112,716	Chronic Low. Respiratory Disease 130,933
5	Placenta Cord Membranes 1,110	Heart Disease 151	Heart Disease 106	Congenital Anomalies 200	Heart Disease 389	Heart Disease 730	Heart Disease 3,249	HIV 4,363	Suicide 6,991	Unintentional Injury 10,853	Alzheimer's Disease 70,858	Unintentional Injury 117,809
6	Unintentional Injury 1,083	Influenza & Pneumonia 110	Cerebro-vascular 52	Chronic Low. Respiratory Disease 55	Cerebro-vascular 76	Congenital Anomalies 251	HIV 1,318	Homicide 3,109	Cerebro-vascular 6,381	Cerebro-vascular 10,028	Influenza & Pneumonia 55,453	Diabetes Mellitus 75,119
7	Respiratory Distress 860	Septicemia 85	Influenza & Pneumonia 51	Influenza & Pneumonia 55	Influenza & Pneumonia 68	Complicated Pregnancy 141	Diabetes Mellitus 617	Liver Disease 2,688	Diabetes Mellitus 5,691	Liver Disease 7,126	Diabetes Mellitus 55,222	Alzheimer's Disease 71,599
8	Bacterial Sepsis 834	Cerebro-vascular 62	Benign Neoplasms 40	Septicemia 45	Diabetes Mellitus 67	Diabetes Mellitus 135	Cerebro-vascular 546	Cerebro-vascular 2,260	HIV 4,516	Suicide 4,210	Unintentional Injury 36,729	Influenza & Pneumonia 63,001
9	Neonatal Hemorrhage 665	Perinatal Period 58	Chronic Low. Respiratory Disease 49	Septicemia 36	Diabetes Mellitus 67	HIV 131	Congenital Anomalies 436	Diabetes Mellitus 2,045	Chronic Low. Respiratory Disease 3,977	Nephritis 4,141	Nephritis 36,416	Nephritis 43,901
10	Necrotizing Enterocolitis 546	Chronic Low. Respiratory Disease 56	Septicemia 36	Cerebro-vascular 43	Septicemia 61	Cerebro-vascular 120	Influenza & Pneumonia 354	Influenza & Pneumonia 934	Viral Hepatitis 2,314	Septicemia 3,912	Septicemia 26,243	Septicemia 34,136

Source: Centers for Disease Control and Prevention

The best way to avoid injuries and disease is through prevention. There are three types of prevention: primary, secondary and tertiary. **Primary prevention** utilizes behaviors to avoid the development of disease. This can include getting immunizations, exercising regularly, eating healthy meals, limiting exposure to sunlight, using sunscreen, having safe drinking water, and guarding against accidents. The focus of this textbook will be primary prevention to help individuals choose behaviors that will prevent disease and premature death.

Secondary prevention is aimed at early detection of disease. This can include blood pressure screenings, mammograms, and annual pap tests to identify and detect disease in its earliest stages. This is before noticeable symptoms develop, when the disease is most likely to be treated successfully. With early detection and diagnosis, it may be possible to cure a disease, slow its progression, prevent or minimize complications, and limit disability. Another goal of secondary prevention is to prevent the spread of communicable diseases. In the community, early identification and treatment of people with communicable diseases, such as sexually transmitted infections, not only provides secondary prevention for those who are infected but also primary prevention for people who come in contact with infected individuals.

Tertiary prevention works to improve the quality of life for individuals with various diseases by limiting complications and disabilities, restoring function, and slowing or stopping the progression of a disease. Tertiary prevention plays a key role for individuals with arthritis, asthma, heart disease, and diabetes.

Healthy People 2010

There are ten major public health issues, which are called leading health indicators. They are:

- Physical activity
- Overweight and obesity
- Tobacco use
- Substance abuse
- Responsible sexual behavior
- Mental health
- Injury and violence
- Environmental quality
- Immunization
- Access to health care

There are four major factors that influence personal health:

1. personal behavior
2. heredity
3. environment
4. access to professional health care personnel

The importance of prevention is made clear in *Healthy People 2010*. *Healthy People 2010* was first developed in 1979 as a *Surgeon General's Report*. It has been reformulated since 1979 as *Healthy People,* and *Healthy People 2000: National Health Promotion and Disease Prevention*. The original efforts of these programs were to establish national health objectives and to serve as a base of knowledge for the development of both state-level and community-level plans and programs to improve the nation's overall health. Much like the programs *Healthy People 2010* is based on, it was developed through broad consultation programs and the best and most current scientific knowledge in the public and private sectors. It is also designed in a way that will allow communities to measure the success rates, over time, of the programs they choose to implement.

Healthy People 2010 has two core concerns. The first concern or goal is to help all individuals to increase not only the quantity of their lives but also to improve the quality of their lives. A second goal of this program is to eliminate health disparities (or health care inequality) among the different segments of the nations' populations. In an attempt to meet these core goals, *Healthy People 2010* has twenty-eight focus areas—each with a concise goal statement that is designed to frame the overall purpose of each of the twenty-eight focus areas. For example:

- Focus Area Three. Cancer

Goal—Reduce the number of new cancer cases as well as the illness, disability, and death caused by cancer.

Each of the chapters in *Health & Fitness: A Guide to a Healthy Lifestyle* corresponds to one or more of the focus areas within *Healthy People 2010*. The chapters of this text and the corresponding focus areas of *Healthy People 2010* are as follows:

Chapter 1—Introduction

- Health Communication

Chapter 2—Stress and Psychological Health

- Mental Health and Mental Disorders

Chapter 3—Personal Fitness

- Physical Activity and Fitness

Chapter 4—Lifestyle Choices and Hypokinetic Conditions

- Arthritis, Osteoporosis, and Chronic Back Conditions
- Diabetes
- Heart Disease and Stroke
- Mental Health and Mental Disorders
- Cancer

Chapter 5—Nutrition

- Mental Health and Mental Disorders
- Nutrition and Overweight

Chapter 6—Lifetime Weight Management

- Physical Activity and Fitness
- Nutrition and Overweight

Chapter 7—Relationships

- Health Communication

Chapter 8—Sexuality

- Family Planning
- Health Communication
- HIV

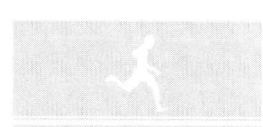

Researchers at the Human Population Laboratory of the California Department of Health published the following list of health-related behaviors that have been associated with good health and a long life. These behaviors include:

1. Regular exercise
2. Adequate sleep
3. A good breakfast
4. Regular meals
5. Weight control
6. Abstinence from smoking and drugs
7. Moderate use of (or abstinence from) alcohol

It was shown that by following six of the seven listed behaviors, not only is an individual's quality of life greatly improved, but also, men could add eleven years to their lives and women could add seven years to their lives.

- Immunization and Infectious Disease
- Maternal, Infant, and Child Health
- Sexually Transmitted Diseases

Chapter 9—Drugs
- Chronic Kidney Disease
- Educational and Community-Based Programs
- Environmental Health
- Oral Health
- Respiratory Diseases
- Substance Abuse
- Tobacco Use

Chapter 10—Safety Awareness
- Injury and Violence Prevention
- Safety and Health

Chapter 11—Human Diseases
- Cancer
- Diabetes
- HIV
- Immunization and Infectious Disease

Chapter 12—Alternative and Complementary Medicine
- Health Communication

The Healthy People 2020 objectives will be released in January 2010. These objectives will be released along with guidance for achieving the new ten-year targets (www.healthypeople.gov/hp2020/).

SUMMARY

Health is "a state of complete physical, mental, and social well-being and not merely the absence of disease or infirmity" according to the World Health Organization. By definition, health is a universal trait. Due to the fact that personal behaviors are one of the four major factors that influence a person's lifespan and quality of life, health also takes on a very individual and unique quality.

The idea of wellness is an individual-based approach to health. Wellness is grounded in behavior modification strategies that result in the adoption of low-risk, health-enhancing behaviors. By balancing the seven components of wellness—emotional, intellectual, social, spiritual, physical, occupational, and environmental—a person can, to some degree, prevent disease and premature death.

Changing behaviors and setting goals to achieve healthy change are major steps to wellness. Using the SCM can be helpful in making behavior changes. The SCM consists of precontemplation, contemplation, preparation, action, and maintenance stages. These stages are very important to recognize when preparing for a behavior change project. The key elements in a successful behavior change include planning, research, and individual willpower. Healthy behaviors chosen early in life affect an individual's wellness now and in the years to come.

Prevention is a fundamental factor in promoting wellness. The three types of prevention include primary, secondary, and tertiary. Primary prevention utilizes behaviors to avoid injuries, the development of diseases, and premature death. Secondary prevention focuses on early detection of disease and tertiary prevention works to improve the quality of life for individuals with various disease processes.

Each decade, since the 1979 *Surgeon General's Report,* the nation has refined its health agenda—first through *Healthy People,* then through *Healthy People 2000: National Health Promotion and Disease Prevention,* and currently through *Healthy People 2010.* When an attempt is made to understand the two goals of *Healthy People 2010:*

- Goal 1—Increasing the quantity and quality of life
- Goal 2—Eliminating health disparities

and connect the focus areas of this program with these goals, the overwhelming importance of prevention in promoting an individual's level of wellness is made clear.

REFERENCES

Corbin, C. B., Welk, G. J., Corbin, W. R. and Welk, K. A. *Concepts of Physical Fitness* (15th ed). McBrown. 2008.

Floyd, P., Mims, S., and Yelding-Howard, C. *Personal Health: Perspectives and Lifestyles* (4th ed). Morton Publishing Co. 2007.

http://ahha.org

http://wellness.ndsu.nodak.edu/education/dimensions.shtml

http://who.int/aboutwho/en/definition.html

http://www.cdc.gov/nchs/data/hp2k99.pdf

http://www.health.gov/healthypeople

http://www.m-w.com/dictionary.htm

http://www.wellnesswise.com/dimensions.htm

Hyman, B., Oden, G., Bacharach, D., and Collins, R. *Fitness for Living* (3rd ed). Kendall-Hunt Publishing Co. 2006.

Insel, P. M. and Roth, W. T. *Core Concepts in Health* (10th ed). McGraw Hill Publishing. 2008.

Payne, W. A., Hahn, D. B., and Lucas, E. B. *Understanding Your Health* (10th ed). McGraw Hill Publishing. 2008.

Pruitt, B.E. and Stein, J. *Health Styles.* Allyn & Bacon. 1999.

ACTIVITIES

In-Class Activities

Human Bingo

Notebook Activities

Lifestyle Assessment Inventory

Behavior Change and Goal Setting

If I Had It to Do Over

Name: _____ Section: _____ Date: _____

IN-CLASS ACTIVITY

Human Bingo

After the leader says "GO!" ask individuals in the group if a statement matches a characteristic of himself or herself or if they have completed an item listed below. If someone answers "yes" to this question, have them sign their initials in that box. An individual can sign no more than two squares per piece of paper. Continue until someone completes a row, column, or diagonal line and yells "BINGO!"

can juggle	has TP'd a house	has colored his or her hair	received 4+ traffic tickets	plays tennis	sings in the shower	watched *Sesame Street*
ever slept in church	never changed a diaper	split their pants in public	has milked a cow	was born out of the country	has been to Hawaii	eats out at restaurants daily
watches reality shows	can touch tongue to nose	has driven a motorcycle	has never ridden a horse	moved twice last year	sleeps in a loft	has a hole in his or her sock
walked in the wrong restroom	loves classical music	ever skipped school	FREE	has broken an arm	has a hot tub	loves eating sushi
has two siblings	loves vegetables	has a 2-inch scar	wears P.J.'s	ever smoked a cigar	has been skinny-dipping	wears size 8 shoes
likes writing poetry	still has their tonsils	can quote a Bible verse	likes bubble gum	has a piercing	doesn't use mouth wash	often watches cartoons
doesn't like fishing	can wiggle their ears	can play the guitar	plays chess regularly	only reads the comics	can touch palms to floor	sleeps with stuffed animals

15

Name: _____ Section: _____ Date: _____

NOTEBOOK ACTIVITY

Lifestyle Assessment Inventory

The purpose of this lifestyle assessment inventory is to increase your awarness of areas in your life that increase your risk of disease, injury, and possibly premature death. A key point to remember is that you have control over each of the lifestyle areas discussed.

Awareness is the first step in making change. After identifying the areas that require modification, you will be able to use the behavior modification techniques presented in Chapter 1 to bring about positive lifestyle changes.

Directions

Put a check by each statement that applies to you. You may select more than one choice per category.

A. Physical Fitness

_____ I exercise for a minimum of twenty to thirty minutes at least three days per week.
_____ I play sports routinely (two to three times per week).
_____ I walk for fifteen to thirty minutes (three to seven days per week).

B. Body Fat

_____ There is no place on my body where I can pinch more than 1 inch of fat.
_____ I am satisfied with the way my body appears.

C. Stress Level

_____ I find it easy to relax.
_____ I rarely feel tense or anxious.
_____ I am able to cope with daily stresses without undue emotional stress.

D. Car Safety

_____ I have not had an auto accident in the past 4 years.
_____ I always use a seat belt when I drive.
_____ I rarely drive above the speed limit.

E. Sleep

_____ I always get seven to nine hours of sleep.
_____ I do not have trouble going to sleep.
_____ I generally do not wake up during the night.

F. Relationships

_____ I have a happy and satisfying relationship with my spouse or boy/girlfriend.
_____ I have a lot of close friends.
_____ I get a great deal of love and support from my family.

G. Diet

_____ I generally eat three balanced meals per day.

_____ I rarely overeat.

_____ I rarely eat large quantities of fatty foods and sweets.

H. Alcohol Use

_____ I consume fewer than two drinks per day.

_____ I never get intoxicated.

_____ I never drink and drive.

I. Tobacco Use

_____ I never smoke (cigarettes, pipe, cigars, etc.).

_____ I am not exposed to second-hand smoke on a regular basis.

_____ I do not use smokeless tobacco.

J. Drug Use

_____ I never use illicit drugs.

_____ I never abuse legal drugs such as diet or sleeping pills.

K. Sexual Practices

_____ I always practice safe sex (e.g., always using condoms or being involved in a monogamous relationship).

Scoring

1. Individual areas: If there are any unchecked areas in categories A through K, you can improve those aspects of your lifestyle.

2. Overall lifestyle: Add up your total number of checks. Scoring can be interpreted as follows:

   23–29   Very healthy lifestyle

   17–22   Average healthy lifestyle

   ≤ 16 Unhealthy lifestyle (needs improvement)

From *Why Weight? A Guide to Ending Compulsive Eating* by Geneen Roth, copyright © 1989 by Geneen Roth. Used by permission of Dutton Signet, a division of Penguin Group (USA) Inc.

Name: _____ Section: _____ Date: _____

NOTEBOOK ACTIVITY

Behavior Change and Goal Setting

In order to make positive changes in your life, you must identify behaviors that need to be modified, and behavior changes that would support your life change goals. This assignment has two parts: (1) Complete this page; (2) Type 1–2 pages reflecting your behavior change at the end of the semester. Besure to address the key elements that contributed to your success or lack thereof. Both parts should be submitted at the end of the semester for credit.

Setting Goals:

1. Make achievable and measurable goals.
2. Establish long-term goals, with weekly or monthly short-term goals that support the long-term goals.
3. Identify behavior changes that will directly support your short-term goals (for example: try to always carry a water bottle, don't keep soda where it is readily available).
4. Identify how you will measure your goals.
5. Set target dates and reasonable rewards for goal achievement.

Rewards:

A reward should be something that you enjoy but might not always get to do. It should be relatively inexpensive and accessible. It should not be anything that would reinforce the behavior you are trying to change. (Don't reward smoking cessation goals with a smoke!)

Goal:

My long-term goal is
_____

My short-term goal in support of my long-term goal is _____
_____

Specific behavior changes that will support my goals are _____,
_____, _____

I will achieve my long-term goal by _____ (date). The reward I will give myself upon completion of my long-term goal is _____
_____.

From *Why Weight? A Guide to Ending Compulsive Eating* by Geneen Roth, copyright © 1989 by Geneen Roth. Used by permission of Dutton Signet, a division of Penguin Group (USA) Inc.

Note:

After achieving your goals, congratulate yourself and then make new goals. If you did not succeed with your goals, examine what behavior changes you were not able to do in order to support your short-term goals. Learn from your mistakes, and try again. Perhaps you made your goals too challenging.

Name: _____ Section: _____ Date: _____

NOTEBOOK ACTIVITY

If I Had It to Do Over

A few years ago I read a piece by Nadine Stair called "If I Had It to Do Over," in which she was looking back on her life as an older woman and remarking about the things she would do differently. Some of the things she said were: "I would wear more purple; I would eat fewer beans and more ice cream; I would go barefoot earlier in spring."

And you? If you were eighty-five years old right now and you were looking back on the life you had lived, what would you want to do differently?

EXAMPLES:
1) I would want to take money less seriously.
2) I would want to tell the people I love that I love them.
3) I would want to take more vacations.

Complete the sentences:
If I had it to do over, I would:

1. _____

2. _____

3. _____

4. _____

5. _____

6. _____

7. _____

Of the seven items you listed, which ones can you begin doing this month?

_____

From *Why Weight? A Guide to Ending Compulsive Eating* by Geneen Roth, copyright © 1989 by Geneen Roth. Used by permission of Dutton Signet, a division of Penguin Group (USA) Inc.

Complete the sentence:
This month, I will:

1. _____

   _____

2. _____

   _____

3. _____

   _____

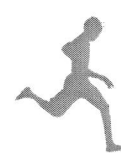

CHAPTER 2

Stress and Psychological Health

"Take care of your body with steadfast fidelity. The soul must see through these eyes alone, and if they are dim, the whole world is clouded."

—Johann Wolfgang Von Goethe

OBJECTIVES

Students will be able to:
- Define stress and describe ways in which stress can manifest itself.
- Introduce general tips to help individuals positively cope with stress.
- Describe the negative health complications that can result from unmanaged stress.
- Establish a link between preventative behaviors and stress.
- List characteristics of good stress managers.
- Establish a link between unmanaged stress and its detrimental effect on psychological health.
- Introduce the concept of self-talk and explain the effects positive and negative self-talk can have on an individual's stress level and its impact on the person's psychological health.
- Show the links between stress, depression and suicidal behaviors.
- Define eating disorders: who is at risk, what are the causes, what are the symptoms, how serious are they, and what can be done to help someone with an eating disorder.

Stress, both positive and negative forms, has always been a part of life. One cannot hope to live and thrive without facing stressful situations daily. Most Americans live a fast-paced, over-booked lifestyle each day in an attempt to make the most of their time and talents. Due to the fact that "working under the gun" has become the rule rather than the exception, stress has become one of the most common detriments to the overall health and well-being of Americans.

Wellness and Stress

Stress was defined by Hans Selye as the nonspecific response to demands placed on the body. "Nonspecific response" alludes to the production of the same physiological reaction by the body regardless of the type of stress placed on the body. Physiologically, when an individual is confronted with a stressor they will experience a surge of adrenaline that causes the discharge of cortisol and the release of endorphins. This, in turn, will increase the person's blood pressure and heart rate, preparing him or her to take immediate action.

While the physiological way in which all people react to stress is the same, the way a person physically, emotionally, or behaviorally reacts to a specific stressor can vary greatly. This is due in part to the fact that when facing the exact same event or circumstance it might be perceived as highly stressful and draining to one person but simply stimulating and exciting to someone else. The ways in which people outwardly react to stressful situations are a personal physical and emotional response to the stimuli. These responses can be either positive or negative.

Eustress is a positive stress that produces a sense of well-being. It is a healthy component of daily life. It can be harnessed to improve health and performance. Examples of activities or events that might initiate a positive stress response include competitive sports, graduation from school, dating, marriage, the birth of a baby, or a long awaited vacation. Eustress can help channel nervous energy into a top-notch performance.

Distress is negative stress. It is a physically and mentally damaging response to the demands placed upon the body. Distress is generally associated with changes that interrupt the natural flow of a person's life. Excessive schoolwork, loss of a job, breaking up with a significant other, or illness or death of a loved one are examples of activities or situations that may produce a negative stress response from an individual. When distress occurs, it is typical to see deterioration in the affected individual's health and performance.

The way each person chooses to manage the stressors that occur in life will, to a large degree, determine overall physical and emotional well-being. An individual's body naturally attempts to maintain a state of homeostasis, or balance, so that it can continue to function in an effective manner. When a stressful situation presents itself, an "alarm" is triggered. Then either the person deals with the situation and the body recovers and returns to a state of homeostasis, or the attempts to avoid or resist the stressor eventually result in exhaustion or illness (see Figure 2.1).

Stress is not the cause of illness, but when it goes on for long periods of time or is particularly irritating, it can become harmful by weakening an individual's immune system. This increases that person's risk of getting sick.

Uncontrolled or unmanaged stress can lead to a variety of negative health consequences such as coronary heart disease, high blood pressure, ulcers, irritable bowel syndrome, migraine headaches, and insomnia.

Certain forms of stress are not only normal but necessary in everyday life. However, the results of continual or inappropriately managed stress can cause disruptions that can be serious or severe to an individual's emotional, intellectual, social, spiritual, physical, occupational, and/or environmental health.

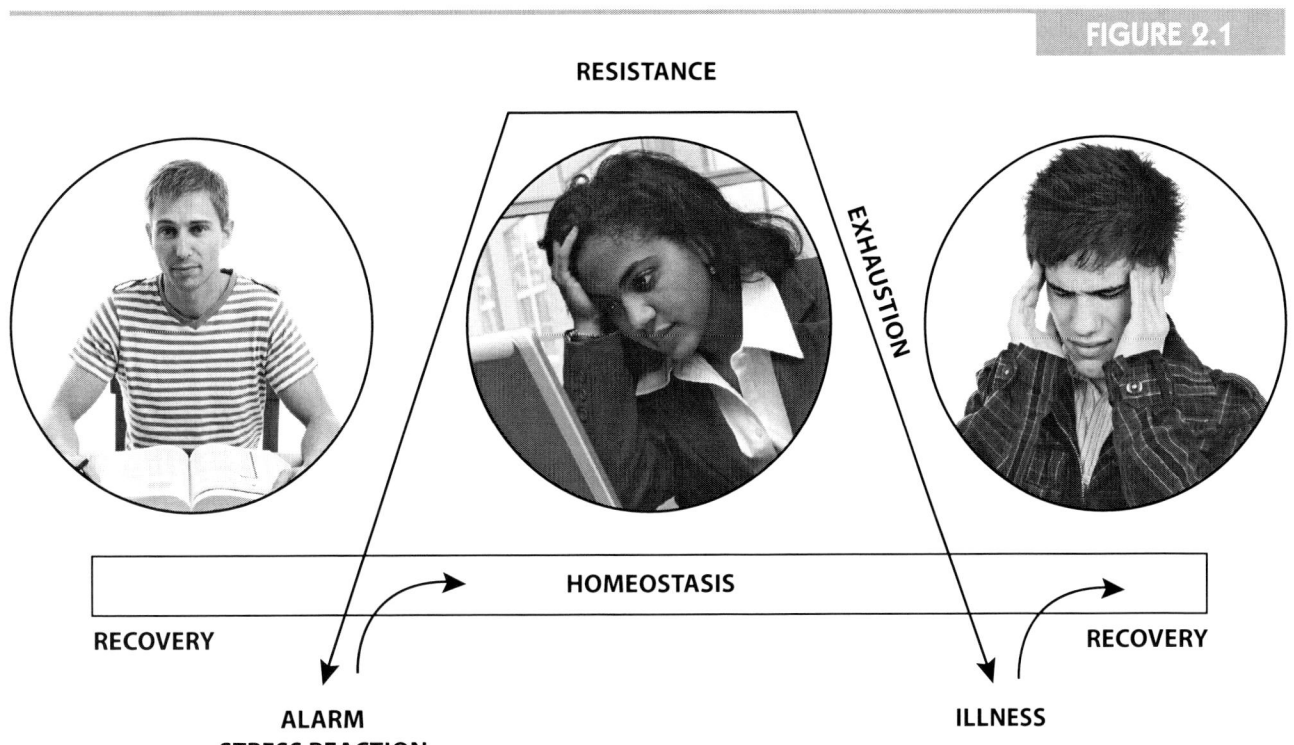

FIGURE 2.1

© Hugo Silveirinha Felix, 2009, Shutterstock, Inc.
© Rob Marmion, 2009, Shutterstock, Inc.
© Rui Vale de Sousa, 2009, Shutterstock, Inc.

It is extremely important for an individual to determine how he or she handles or reacts to stressors, especially if the stress is ongoing. The way stress manifests or "shows itself" is going to vary depending on an individual's personality and past experiences.

There are typically four ways in which stress can manifest itself:

1. Emotionally
   - Do you always feel rushed, without enough time to get all that is needed done well or done at all?
   - Do you find it difficult to relax?
   - Are you irritable and moody, or easily angered?
   - Do you feel helpless or hopeless?
   - Do you want to cry for no apparent reason?
   - Is it difficult for you to listen or pay attention to your friends without being distracted?
   - Is it hard for you to fall asleep even on days when you are exhausted?
   - When you do fall asleep, is it difficult to stay asleep?

2. Mentally
   - Are you indecisive in many areas of your life?
   - Is it difficult for you to concentrate?
   - Do you regularly have bad dreams or nightmares?
   - Do you have negative thoughts, including suicidal thoughts?

3. Behaviorally
   - Has your appetite changed so that you have gained or lost significant amounts of weight?
   - Are you neglecting yourself/your appearance?
   - Have you curtailed social activities?
   - Have you taken to substance abuse, such as cigarette smoking, drug use, or excessive alcohol or coffee intakes?

4. Physically
   - Do you have an increased heart rate or blood pressure?
   - Can you feel your own heart beat?
   - Do you feel out of breath or have tightness in your chest?
   - Do you suffer from frequent headaches or muscle aches due to chronic tension?
   - Is it difficult for you to digest food—leading to nausea or diarrhea?
   - Do you suffer from frequent attacks of infections such as influenza or sore throats?

Recognizing how stress affects their lives allows individuals to recognize stressful situations and to immediately deal with, or cope with, something that has the potential to compromise their overall well-being.

While uncontrolled or unmanaged stress can lead to negative health consequences, there are a number of ways to control stress. What works for one person will not necessarily be helpful to someone else. It is important to recognize the stressor (see Figure 2.2) and determine the most effective way(s) to relieve, reduce, or eliminate that particular stressor. Another key to successfully managing stressors is to use a strategy that produces positive results, rather than a strategy that creates additional stress. Also, to be successful with stress management, give a particular stressor only the amount of energy it warrants—do not give a "10 cent" stressor $10 worth of time or energy. The following are general tips that can help maintain a healthy lifestyle and can prepare an individual to cope with many of the stressors found in everyday life.

1. Deal with the cause:
   Finish the task, talk to the person, fix the tire, write the letter, make the call—do what needs to be done to deal with the situation. The longer a situation gets put off, the more stress it can create.

FIGURE 2.2

Stressors in the Lives of College Students

Stressors in the Lives of College Students

Drug use	Military obligations
Academic competition	Social alienation, anonymity
College red tape	Love/marriage decisions
Religious conflicts	Illness and injury
Choice of major/future job	Lack of privacy
Sexual pressures	Parental conflict
Family responsibilities	Time management
Loneliness, depression, anxiety	Alcohol use
Money troubles	

Source: Adapted from W. W. K. Hoeger, L. W. Turner, and B. Q. Hafen. *Wellness Guidelines for a Healthy Lifestyle.* Wadsworth/Thomson Learning, 2007.

2. Put the situation into perspective: How important is it really? How important will this be tomorrow, in six months? Most situations that tax physical/mental energies will soon be inconsequential and forgotten. Determine if anything can be done about the situation, or if it is a situation that calls for acceptance.

3. Pace yourself:
No one can be in "high gear" all the time. Too often individuals stop to "smell the roses" only after the first accident or heart attack. Set short and intermediate goals—reward yourself upon reaching these goals.

4. Laugh at life and at yourself:
Humor is a wonderful tool. Laughing is internal jogging! She or he who laughs . . . lasts! See the humor in people and the absurdity of situations. Read the "funny pages."

5. Develop quality relationships:
Seek social and emotional support systems—individuals who care, love, and will listen to you. Express feelings constructively. Be there for others and allow others to be there for you in the good times and in the bad times.

6. Time management needs to be life management:
Look at goals and responsibilities from a bigger perspective; this can help with decision making. Streamline activities by breaking big, imposing jobs into small components and list each activity in a daily planner. Seek assistance when it is needed; don't try to do everything yourself—delegate! Avoid common "time killers" (see Figure 2.3).

7. Look at situations and people in a different light—try an attitude adjustment:
Is your perception of the situation, event, or person correct? Is there another way to handle things, or is there another possible way to answer the problem? Go easier on yourself and on others. It is unreasonable to expect perfection from yourself or from others. Perfection is a "moving target" and causes constant stress. Take care of the things you can; don't worry about the things that are beyond your control.

8. Balance fun and responsibility:
Family, society, and community encourage and command constant work and responsibility. It is important to contribute and to meet responsibilities, but it is also important to find enjoyment and fun in life as well. Do something you find enjoyable on a regular basis and don't feel guilty!

9. Exercise and eat sensibly:
Exercise is one of the best stress-busters. Schedule exercise into your life. Walk, bike, swim, stretch, and recreate. Good food in proper proportions is also essential to good health and is an excellent way to reduce the negative effects stress may have on your life.

When an individual is able to identify stress management techniques that work with her or his personality and lifestyle, it can be extremely beneficial to be proactive in recognizing potential sources of stress so that they can be dealt with before they become detrimental to the individual's overall well-being.

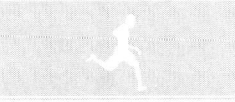

Reduce Stress and Improve Your Life with Positive Self-Talk

Start by following a single, simple rule: If you wouldn't say what you are thinking to someone else, don't "think it" to yourself!!

Try to take time during your day to really think about what is "running, unfiltered through your head."

If you find that you are mentally beating yourself up, stop and try to put a positive angle on your thoughts. For example, if you are thinking "I'll never get better at this," try putting a positive spin on it and change your thinking to, "It never hurts to keep trying!"

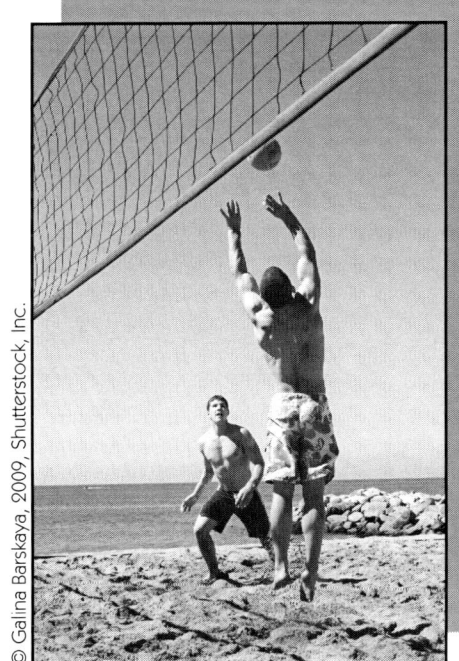

Balance fun and responsibility. Do something you enjoy on a regular basis and don't feel guilty.

FIGURE 2.3

Behavior Modification Planning

COMMON TIME KILLERS

- Watching television
- Listening to radio/music
- Sleeping
- Eating
- Daydreaming
- Shopping
- Socializing/parties
- Recreation
- Talking on the telephone
- Worrying
- Procrastinating
- Drop-in visitors
- Confusion (unclear goals)
- Indecision (what to do next)
- Interruptions
- Perfectionism (every detail must be done)

Source: From HOEGER/HOEGER, *Principles and Labs for Fitness and Wellness* (with Personal Daily Log and CengageNOW,info TracA® Printed Access Card) 9E, © 2008 Brooks/Cole, a part of Cengage Learning, inc. Reproduced by permission. www.cengage.com/permissions

There are several scales or scientific instruments that have been designed in an attempt to measure an individual's level of stress. The Student Stress Scale that is shown in Figure 2.4 has been modified from the Holmes and Rahe's Life Events Scale (1967) to gauge the stress level and corresponding health consequences for college-aged adults.

In the Student Stress Scale, each event, such as beginning or ending school, is given a score that represents the amount of readjustment a person has to make in life as a result of the change. To determine a stress score, add up the number of points corresponding to the events that have happened during the past six months or are likely to occur within the next six months.

People with scores of 300 points or higher have a high health risk. Individuals scoring between 150 and 300 points have about a fifty-fifty chance of developing a serious health condition within the next two years. People scoring below 150 points have a one-in-three chance of developing a serious health condition.

It is imperative that individuals recognize the potential stressors that occur in their lives. However, it is equally important that individuals also acknowledge an overall level of stress. By doing this, a proactive "deal with it" approach can be taken. This lessens the negative impact that stress can have on overall well-being and allows them to become good stress managers (see Figure 2.5 on page 30).

Self-Talk Your Way to Reduced Levels of Stress and an Improved Life

What Is Self-Talk?

Self-talk is the constant interpretation of the different situations that individuals find themselves in throughout each day. It is that "inner voice" that determines one's perception of a situation. Conscious thoughts, as well as subconscious thoughts, are part of a person's inner voice. Negative or positive self-talk begins early in most individuals' lives and can determine the impact stress has on each person's life.

FIGURE 2.4

Student Stress Scale

1. Death of a close family member	☐	100 ☐
2. Death of a close friend	☐	73 ☐
3. Divorce between parents	☐	65 ☐
4. Jail term	☐	63 ☐
5. Major personal injury or illness	☐	63 ☐
6. Marriage	☐	58 ☐
7. Fired from job	☐	50 ☐
8. Failed important course	☐	47 ☐
9. Change in health of a family member	☐	45 ☐
10. Pregnancy	☐	45 ☐
11. Sexual problems	☐	44 ☐
12. Serious argument with close friend	☐	40 ☐
13. Change in financial status	☐	39 ☐
14. Change of major	☐	39 ☐
15. Trouble with parents	☐	39 ☐
16. New girl- or boyfriend	☐	38 ☐
17. Increased workload at school	☐	37 ☐
18. Outstanding personal achievement	☐	36 ☐
19. First quarter/semester in college	☐	35 ☐
20. Change in living conditions	☐	31 ☐
21. Serious argument with instructor	☐	30 ☐
22. Lower grades than expected	☐	29 ☐
23. Change in sleeping habits	☐	29 ☐
24. Change in social activities	☐	29 ☐
25. Change in eating habits	☐	26 ☐
26. Chronic car trouble	☐	26 ☐
27. Change in number of family get-togethers	☐	26 ☐
28. Too many missed classes	☐	25 ☐
29. Change of college	☐	24 ☐
30. Dropped more than one class	☐	23 ☐
31. Minor traffic violations	☐	20 ☐

Source: Adapted from T. H. Holmes and R. H. Rahe, 1967, *Journal of Psychosomatic Research,* 11:213.

Negative or Positive Self-Talk

Negative self-talk such as "I am going to fail my test" or "there is no way I can run that far or fast or perform that move" is self-defeating. Negative interpretation of a situation will often make that situation more stressful than it needs to be.

Replacing negative thoughts or self-talk with positive thoughts can decrease stress levels and improve a person's productivity and overall outlook. There is a line between thinking something and feeling it! People changing the way they think can allow them to change the way they feel.

Some tips for reducing stress and improving your quality of life through the use of positive self-talk are listed in the margin of page 27.

Thinking positively is a habit. Like any other habit, it will take time and practice to master—but health benefits such as decreased negative stress, reduced risk of coronary heart disease, and improved coping skills make it time well spent.

FIGURE 2.5
Behavior Modification Planning

CHARACTERISTICS OF GOOD STRESS MANAGERS

Good stress managers
- are physically active, eat a healthy diet, and get adequate rest every day.
- believe they have control over events in their life (have an internal locus of control).
- understand their own feelings and accept their limitations.
- recognize, anticipate, monitor, and regulate stressors within their capabilities.
- control emotional and physical responses when distressed.
- use appropriate stress management techniques when confronted with stressors.
- recognize warning signs and symptoms of excessive stress.
- schedule daily time to unwind, relax, and evaluate the day's activities.
- control stress when called upon to perform.
- enjoy life despite occasional disappointments and frustrations.
- look success and failure squarely in the face and keep moving along a predetermined course.
- move ahead with optimism and energy and do not spend time and talent worrying about failure.
- learn from previous mistakes and use them as building blocks to prevent similar setbacks in the future.
- give of themselves freely to others.
- have a deep meaning in life.

Source: From HOEGER/HOEGER, *Principles and Labs for Fitness and Wellness* (with Personal Daily Log and CengageNOW,info TracA® Printed Access Card) 9E, © 2008 Brooks/Cole, a part of Cengage Learning, inc. Reproduced by permission. www.cengage.com/permissions

Stress and Its Impact on Mental Health

While stress in general, and specifically unmanaged stress, can have a negative impact on a person's physical health, the detrimental impact it can have on mental health can be equally devastating.

There are many types of mental health disorders. Schizophrenia, depression, general anxiety disorders, bipolar disorders, and panic disorders are just a few of the mental health disorders that can cause havoc in a person's life. These disorders typically include chronic or occasional dysfunctional feelings and/or a lost sense of self worth that may often limit the extent to which an individual participates in life's daily activities.

Who Gets Mental Health Disorders?

According to the 1996 Surgeon General's Report on Physical Activity and Health, one out of two Americans will suffer from some sort of mental health disorder at some point in their lifetime. The many different types of mental health disorders affect 90 million people. Mental health disorders are far-reaching. They affect not only the individual with the disorder but also the people who have intimate and social relationships with them. Mental health disorders have a far-reaching "ripple effect."

Depression and Stress

Depression is a mental health disorder that is prevalent among college populations. One of the reasons college students are particularly vulnerable to depression is that for many students, they face large amounts of unresolved stress. College is a time filled with challenging, new, different, and stressful situations (refer back to Figure 2.2).

It is important to realize that unmanaged stress and depression can quickly become a vicious cycle. The more depressed an individual is, the less day-to-day stress and the fewer activities can be coped with and the more depressed the person becomes.

While stress often plays a major roll in depression, another type of depression also has a biological basis—endogenous depression. In this instance, a person's family mental health history can help determine if a genetic predisposition toward depression exists. This knowledge allows them to take a proactive approach toward diagnosing and battling this mental health condition.

Everyone has occasional feelings of being down or sad at some point. However, when depression results in a person crying a great deal, feeling hopeless, or being unable to take pleasure in life, professional help should be sought so that a life-threatening situation does not occur.

Aside from or along with professional counseling, individual therapy or group therapy can be beneficial to an individual battling with depression. Prescription medications can be another important tool when coping with depression. They may or may not be necessary depending on each individual's situation.

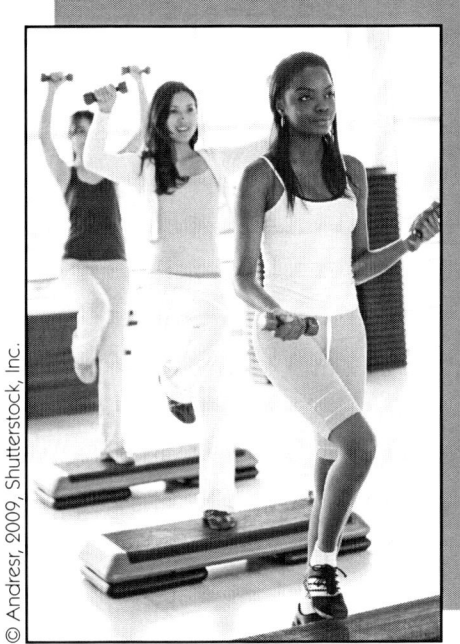

Exercise has been shown to be effective in treating mild to moderate cases of depression.

Exercise has also been shown to be effective in treating mild to moderate cases of depression. Thirty-three percent of all inactive adults consider themselves depressed. "A recent review of more than 20 years of studies found that aerobic exercise and strength training are equally effective in treating depression, can reduce anxiety in patients with panic disorders and can be an important part of treatment for people with schizophrenia" (Payne, 2000).

Jenny's Story

Jenny Smith was diagnosed with bipolar disorder, a condition characterized by severe mood swings from total elation to utter depression. Jenny was hospitalized off and on, and after trying all available drug therapy to no avail, Jenny was told to expect to be in and out of psychiatric hospitals for the rest of her life. Jenny decided to learn hatha yoga. Hatha yoga incorporates breathing, postures, and meditation that relax and strengthen the body. Smith noticed that her panic attacks subsided (a symptom of her bipolar disorder) with her daily yoga practice. Smith now feels better and successfully manages her disorder with the antidepressant Paxil and daily yoga practice. She has taught her 11-year-old daughter relaxation through simple breathing techniques, and now her daughter's panic attacks have also subsided. Some mental health disorders are genetic in nature. Smith's grandmother committed suicide due to depression, and Smith is determined to spread the word that she believes yoga has literally saved her life.

(Weintraub, 2000)

Recently a charity conducted a survey that found that 83 percent of those with mental health problems looked to some form of exercise to help improve their mood or reduce the amount of stress they felt they were under (news.bbc.co.uk). While exercise plays a vital role in reducing the negative impact mental health disorders have on a person's life, it should not be considered a total replacement for other treatments, and patients should always work with and under the close care of a physician.

James Blumenthal, a psychologist at Duke University Medical Center, conducted a study comparing the effects of exercise and drugs on depression. The 156 participants were broken up into three different groups:

1. exercise only,
2. antidepressants only,
3. exercise and antidepressants.

After sixteen weeks, the researchers found that all three groups showed the same amount of improvement on standard measures for depression. An interesting note concerning the participants using exercise as a method of dealing with their depression was that not only did the exercise have a positive impact on their level of depression, but it also improved their cognitive functioning ability (bbc.news.health).

It is critical to realize that for an individual dealing with any type of mental illness, therapy through counseling and/or the use of prescription medications is not a sign of weakness or personal failure. Accepting these means of help requires strength and courage to face the fact that there is a problem and to fight/prevail against a life-draining force. An individual with a mental illness receiving any type of therapy is much the same as a visually impaired person wearing glasses or contacts, or a hearing impaired individual using a hearing aid.

Suicidal Behavior and Stress

Another area in which stress can affect an individual's mental health is thoughts of or attempts at suicide. College students are particularly vulnerable to this problem. Nationwide each year, approximately one in 10,000 college students commits suicide; many more college students have suicidal thoughts.

Most people who contemplate or actually do commit suicide want something in their "world" to change. It may be one thing that will greatly impact their life if it changes or goes away, or it may be a lot of the "little things" that have added up. Often, a suicidal individual does not really want to die; it is just that the person has run out of ways or ideas on how to make that needed change occur.

Intense pressure or stress, along with feelings of depression, alcohol misuse, drug abuse, or a personal loss such as a breakup or lack of academic success, are common causative factors in suicides. Anyone expressing suicidal thoughts should be taken seriously. Friends, roommates, or whoever should seek out help for a suicidal individual immediately.

Typical signs that an individual is contemplating suicide could include:

- skipping classes,
- giving away personal possessions,
- withdrawing from friends,
- withdrawing from "normal" activities,
- engaging in risky behaviors not normal for that person.

An effective tool for helping someone get past suicidal thoughts or desires is counseling to help change the way he or she is thinking and coping. Medications can also be very effective in the prevention of suicidal behaviors. Hospitalization

A Simple Gesture

> Everybody can be great ... because anybody can serve. You don't have to have a college degree to serve. You don't have to make your subject and verb agree to serve. You only need a heart full of grace. A soul generated by love.
>
> Martin Luther King, Jr.

Mark was walking home from school one day when he noticed the boy ahead of him had tripped and dropped all of the books he was carrying, along with two sweaters, a baseball bat, a glove, and a small tape recorder. Mark knelt down and helped the boy pick up the scattered articles. Since they were going the same way, he helped carry part of the burden. As they walked, Mark discovered the boy's name was Bill, that he loved video games, baseball, and history, that he was having a lot of trouble with his other subjects, and that he had just broken up with his girlfriend.

They arrived at Bill's home first, and Mark was invited in for a Coke and to watch some television. The afternoon passed pleasantly with a few laughs and some shared small talk, and then Mark went home. They continued to see each other around school, had lunch together once or twice, and then both graduated from junior high school. They ended up in the same high school where they had brief contacts over the years. Finally the long awaited senior year came, and three weeks before graduation, Bill asked Mark if they could talk.

Bill reminded him of the day years ago when they had first met. "Do you ever wonder why I was carrying so many things home that day?" asked Bill. "You see, I cleaned out my locker because I didn't want to leave a mess for anyone else. I had stored away some of my mother's sleeping pills and I was going home to commit suicide. But after we spent some time together talking and laughing, I realized that if I had killed myself, I would have missed that time and so many others that might follow. So you see, Mark, when you picked up my books that day, you did a lot more. You saved my life."

John W. Schlatter

Source: From *Chicken Soup for the Soul*, © 1992 by John Schlatter. Published by Health Communication, Inc. Permission conveyed by The Permissions Company.

may be needed as well, in order to prevent suicide. The key to helping a suicidal or potentially suicidal individual is for those around them to be aware and actively involved in seeking out help for the person who is at risk

Eating Disorders and Stress

Eating disorders are medically identifiable, potentially life-threatening mental health conditions related to obsessive eating patterns. Eating disorders are not new—descriptions of self-starvation have been found as far back as medieval times.

Even though more men are succumbing to eating disorders each year, the mental health condition is typically thought of as a woman's disease. Unfortunately, even grade school girls can feel pressure to "fit in" or look thin. This can be very troubling and disruptive to young girls struggling to build a positive body image.

Typically, a person with an eating disorder seeks perfection and control over their life. Both anorexics and bulimics tend to suffer from low self-esteem and depression. They often have a conflict between a desire for perfection and feelings of personal inadequacy. Such persons typically have a distorted view of themselves, in that when they look into a mirror, they see themselves differently than others see them. Narcissism, or excessive vanity, can be linked to both anorexia and bulimia. (see Figure 2.6)

FIGURE 2.6

Major Risk Factors for Eating Disorders

Biological
- Dieting
- Obesity/overweight/pubertal weight gain

Psychological
- Body image/dissatisfaction/distortions
- Low self-esteem
- Obsessive-compulsive symptoms
- Childhood sexual abuse

Family
- Parental attitudes and behaviors
- Parental comments regarding appearance
- Eating-disordered mothers
- Misinformation about ideal weight

Sociocultural
- Peer pressure regarding weight/eating
- Media: TV, magazines
- Distorted images: toys
- Elite athletes as at-risk groups

Source: White, Jane. "The Prevention of Eating Disorders: A Review of the Research on Risk Factors with Implications for Practice." *Journal of Child and Adolescent Psychiatric Nursing,* Vol. 13, No. 2, April 2000.

Eating disorders are often accompanied by other psychiatric disorders, such as depression, substance abuse, or anxiety disorders. Eating disorders are very serious and may be life-threatening due to the fact that individuals suffering from these diseases can experience serious heart conditions and/or kidney failure—both of which can result in death. Therefore, it is critically important that eating disorders are recognized as real and treatable diseases.

Anorexia Nervosa

Anorexia nervosa is a state of starvation and emaciation, usually resulting from severe dieting and excessive exercise. An anorexic will literally stop eating in an effort to control body size.

Most, if not all, anorexic individuals suffer from an extremely distorted body image. People with this disease look in a mirror and see themselves as overweight or fat even when they have become dangerously thin.

Major weight loss is the most visible and the most common symptom of anorexia. Anorexic individuals often develop unusual eating habits, such as avoiding food or meals, picking out a few "acceptable" foods and eating them in small quantities, or carefully weighing and portioning foods. Other common symptoms of this disease include absent menstruation, dry skin, excessive hair on the skin, and thinning of scalp hair. Gastrointestinal problems and orthopedic problems resulting from excessive exercise are also specific to this illness.

Anorexic individuals can lose between 15 and 60 percent of their normal body weight, putting their body and their health in severe jeopardy. The medical problems associated with anorexia are numerous and serious. Starvation damages bones, organs, muscles, the immune system, the digestive system, and the nervous system.

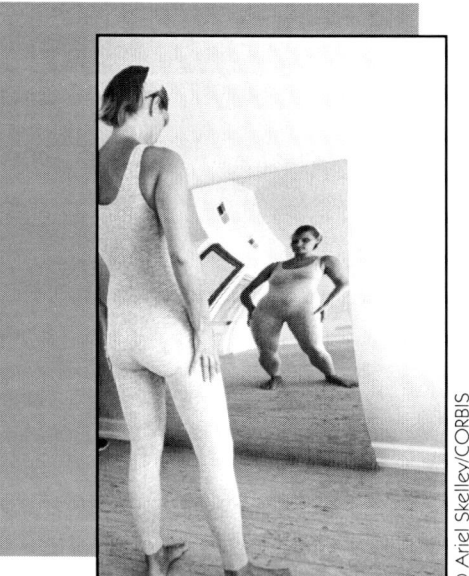

Anorexics and bulimics tend to suffer from low self-esteem and depression and typically have a distorted view of themselves.

> ### Ways to Love Your Body
>
> - Become aware of what your body does each day, as the instrument of your life, not just an ornament for others.
> - Think of your body as a tool. Create a list of all the things you can do with this body.
> - Walk with your head held high, supported by pride and confidence in yourself as a person.
> - Do something that will let you enjoy your body. Stretch, dance, walk, sing, take a bubble bath, get a massage.
> - Wear comfortable styles that you really like and feel good in.
> - Decide what you would rather do with the hours you waste every day criticizing your body.
> - Describe ten positive things about yourself without mentioning your appearance.
> - Say to yourself "Life is too short to waste my time hating my body this way."
> - Don't let your weight or shape keep you from doing things you enjoy.
> - Create a list of people who have contributed to your life, your community, the world. Was their appearance important to their success and accomplishment? If not, why should yours be?
> - If you had only one year to live, how important would your body image and appearance be?
>
> By Margo Maine, Ph.D. and Eating Disorders' Awareness and Prevention

Between 5 and 20 percent of anorexics die due to suicide or other medical complications. Heart disease is the most common medical cause of death for people with severe anorexia.

Long-term irregular or absent menstruation can cause sterility or bone loss. Severe anorexics also suffer nerve damage and may experience seizures. Anemia and gastrointestinal problems are also common to individuals suffering from this illness.

The most severe complication and the most devastating result of anorexia is death.

Bulimia Nervosa

Bulimia nervosa is a process of bingeing and purging. This disorder is more common than anorexia nervosa. The purging is an attempt to control body weight, though bulimics seldom starve themselves as anorexics do. They have an intense fear of becoming overweight, and usually have episodes of secretive binge eating, followed by purging, frequent weight variations, and the inability to stop eating voluntarily. Bulimics often feel hunger, overeat, and then purge to rid themselves of the guilt of overeating.

Bulimic individuals are often secretive and discreet and are, therefore, often hard to identify. Typically, they have a preoccupation with food, fluctuating between fantasies of food and guilt due to overeating. Symptoms of bulimia can include cuts and calluses on the finger joints from a person sticking their fingers or hand down their throat to induce vomiting, broken blood vessels around the eyes from the strain of vomiting, and damage to tooth enamel from stomach acid.

Because purging through vomiting, the abuse of laxatives, or some other compensatory behavior typically follows a binge, bulimics usually weigh within the normal range for their weight and height. However, like individuals with anorexia, they often have a distorted body image and fear gaining weight, want to lose weight, and are intensely dissatisfied with their bodies.

While it is commonly thought that the medical problems resulting from bulimia are not as severe as those resulting from anorexia, the complications are numerous and serious. The medical problems associated with bulimia include tooth erosion, cavities, and gum problems due to the acid in vomit. Abdominal bloating is common in bulimic individuals. The purging process can leave a person dehydrated and with very low potassium levels, which can cause weakness and paralysis. Some of the more severe problems a bulimic can suffer are reproductive problems and heart damage, due to the lack of minerals in the body.

Binge-Eating Disorder

People with binge-eating disorder typically experience frequent (at least two days a week) episodes of out-of-control eating. Binge-eating episodes are associated with at least three of the following characteristics: eating much more rapidly than normal; eating until an individual is uncomfortably full; eating large quantities of food even when not hungry; eating alone to hide the quantity of food being ingested; feeling disgusted, depressed, or guilty after overeating. Not purging their bodies of the excessive calories they have consumed is the characteristic that separates individuals with binge-eating disorder from those with bulimia. Therefore, individuals suffering from this disease are typically overweight for their height and weight.

Fear of Obesity

Fear of obesity is an over-concern with thinness. It is less severe than anorexia, but can also have negative health consequences. This condition is often seen in achievement-oriented teenagers who seek to restrict their weight due to a fear of becoming obese. This condition can be a precursor to anorexia or bulimia if it is not detected and treated early.

Activity Nervosa

Activity nervosa is a condition in which the individual suffers from the ever-present compulsion to exercise, regardless of illness or injury. The desire to exercise excessively may result in poor performance in other areas of that individual's life due to the resulting fatigue, weakness, and unhealthy body weight.

Female Athlete Triad In 1991, a team was formed by the American College of Sports Medicine to educate, initiate a change, and focus on the medical management of a triad of female disorders that included disordered eating, amenorrhea, and osteoporosis (ACSM, 1991). A triangle is used to depict these disorders because the three are interlinked. Disordered eating behaviors result in weight loss and subsequent loss of body fat that halts menstruation. When amenorrhea occurs, calcium is lost and a decline in bone mass occurs. This in turn causes osteoporosis and can easily result in stress fractures. Many times the inactivity necessary to allow stress fractures to heal causes depression that often leads an individual back into disordered eating behaviors, and the cycle continues (see Figure 2.7).

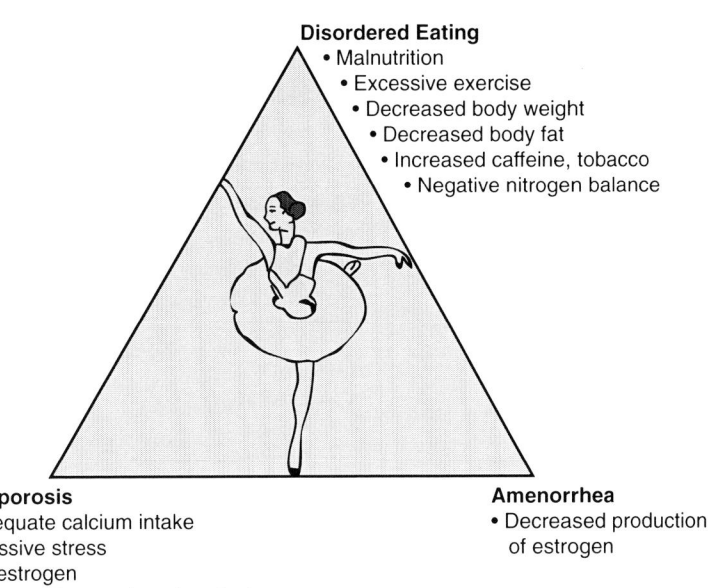

FIGURE 2.7

The Female Athlete Triad

Who Is at Risk?

By far, more women than men succumb to eating disorders; however, the incidence of eating disorders in men is believed to be very underreported.

It is estimated that one in every hundred teenage girls is anorexic. Anorexia usually occurs in adolescent women (90 percent of all reported cases), although all age groups can be affected. It is estimated that one in every five college-bound females is bulimic.

Individuals living in economically developed nations, such as the United States, are much more likely to suffer from an eating disorder, due to the dual factors of an abundance of available food and external, societal pressure. College campuses have a higher incidence of people with eating disorders, and upper-middle-class women who are extremely self-critical are also more likely to become anorexic. Being aware of the groups at risk can be a large step toward prevention.

Activities such as dance and dance team, gymnastics, figure skating, track, and cheerleading tend to have higher instances of eating disorders. An estimate of people suffering from anorexia and bulimia within these populations is 15–60 percent. Male wrestlers and body builders are also at risk due to the unsafe practice of attempting to shed pounds quickly in an attempt to "make weight" before a competition.

Causes of Eating Disorders

The causes of anorexia and bulimia are numerous and complex. Cultural factors, family pressure, psychological factors, emotional disorders, and chemical imbalances can all contribute to eating disorders.

Forty to 80 percent of anorexics suffer from depression, as reduced levels of chemical neurotransmitters in the brain have been found in victims suffering from both eating disorders and depression. Links between hunger and depression have been discovered through research, which contributes to the depression a person with an eating disorder may feel.

I Have Won

One Woman's Recovery from Binge-Eating Disorder

It was a constant nagging voice in my mind, whispering promises of protection, comfort and a life of numbness. I didn't realize it was my enemy, disguised as a savior. This is what my eating disorder was to me. I have been struggling with binge-eating disorder for eight years, and after a year of therapy I am learning how to tell that voice to go away and to love, trust and respect myself and my values.

I have countless memories of daytime binges when my roommates were in class, even digging through the trash to retrieve a half-eaten candy bar or piece of cake. I withdrew from my friends, missed out on beach parties, and felt lonely, scared and completely out of control every waking moment of the day. I became deeply depressed and couldn't face emotional issues that had been with me for a long time. That voice gave soothing promises of a way out, a way to forget, an excuse for any failures or disappointments, and a way to slowly. . . die.

My friends and family were aware there was a problem but I spent years denying the truth. I would tell them I just loved to eat and I just needed to start exercising more. All the while my weight kept slowly growing. I would think constantly about changing, going on a diet, but the diet day would come and I couldn't do it, so I would retreat to the voice and let it take charge. I finally accepted that I had a problem when I was in school completing a Master's Degree in Counseling. I had to constantly analyze myself and my life for projects and papers and could no longer deny the issues at hand.

I entered into therapy and honestly wasn't prepared for the difficulty that lay ahead. I had to confront my demons, that voice, examine every horrible issue that I had suppressed and once again learn how to live life. I learned that I can do other things when I find myself in front of the refrigerator and I am not physically hungry. I can take walks, call my husband, or put together a puzzle. I also had to relearn my body's signals for hunger and fullness and to trust that my body will tell me what I need and when I need it.

Although still in recovery, I can clearly see how far I've come, and I can see the light at the end of the tunnel. I now spend time speaking about eating disorders and volunteering at the Massachusetts Eating Disorder Association. I want people to know that there is hope and that recovery is possible. The voice no longer whispers to me; I now shout at it, "I don't need you anymore. I love myself. I have won!"

by Cathy King, M.S.

A special thanks to the Massachusetts Eating Disorder Association

Source: Courtesy of the Massachusetts Eating Disorder Association

---

For some bulimics, seasonality can adversely affect them, causing the disorder to worsen during the dark, winter months. Another startling statistic is that the onset of anorexia appears to peak in May, which is also the peak month for suicides.

Family factors are also critical. One study showed that 40 percent of all 9- to 10-year-old girls were trying to lose weight, many at the encouragement of their mothers. Mothers of anorexics are often over-involved in their child's life, while mothers of bulimics are many times critical and detached.

It is clear that many people who suffer from eating disorders do not have a healthy body image. From an early age, there is enormous pressure in our culture from society, family, friends, the media, and often from one's self to achieve the unachievable and unnecessary "perfect" body. A woman's self-worth is too often associated with other people's opinions, which in many cases put unrealistic emphasis on physical attractiveness.

Guidelines for Helping a Friend with an Eating Disorder

DO:

- listen with understanding
- appreciate the openness and trust in sharing with you his/her distress
- share your own struggles, be open and real
- learn more about eating disorders
- give support and be available
- give hope that with help and with patience he/she can free themselves from this disorder
- give your friend a list of resources for help

DO NOT:

- tell your friend he/she is crazy
- blame him/her
- gossip about your friend
- follow him/her around to check their eating or purging behavior
- ignore your friend
- reject him/her
- tell him/her to quit this ridiculous behavior
- feel compelled to solve their problem
- make excess comments about being thin

DO heed the signs. Anorexic behavior includes extreme weight loss (often emaciation), obsessive dieting, and distorted body perception (a thin person thinks he/she is fat when they are not). Clues of bulimia are more subtle. Your friend may eat a great deal of food, then rush to the bathroom. She/he may hide laxatives or speak outright about the "magic method" of having the cake and not gaining weight. Anorexics and bulimics tend to be preoccupied with food and many have specific rituals tied to their eating patterns.

DO approach your friend gently, but persistently. Explain that you're worried; listen sympathetically. Don't expect your friend to admit he/she has a problem right away. The first step is realizing there is a problem; therefore, it is important to help your friend realize this.

Source: Student Health Services, Texas A&M University. Guidelines for Helping a Friend with an Eating Disorder, 2002.

DO focus on unhappiness as the reason your friend could benefit from help. Point out how anxious or unhappy he/she has been lately, and emphasize that it does not have to be that way.

DO be supportive, but do not try to analyze or interpret their problem. Being supportive is the most important thing you can do. Show your friend you believe in him/her—it will make a difference in recovery.

DO talk to someone about your own emotions if you feel the need. An objective outsider can emphasize the fact that you are not responsible for your friend; you can only try to help that person help him/herself.

DO be yourself. Be honest in sharing your feelings: i.e., "It's hard for me to watch you destroy yourself."

DO give non-judgmental feedback. For example, "We haven't gone to lunch together in a while, is something wrong?" instead of "You haven't gone to eat with me in a while, do you have a problem?"

DO cooperate with your friend if he/she asks you to keep certain foods out of common storage areas. This may help prevent a binge on such foods.

DON'T keep the "secret" from the family when your friend's health and thinking are impaired.

DON'T forget that denial is a form of selective "deafness."

DON'T be deceived by the excuse: "It's not really bad. I can control myself."

DON'T focus on your friend's weight or appearance. Focus on your concern about his/her health and well-being.

DON'T change your eating habits when you're around your friend. Your "normal" eating is an example to your friend of a more healthy relationship with food.

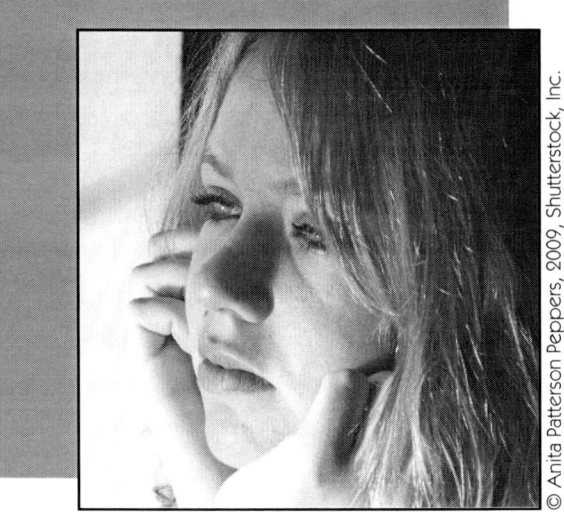

Forty to 80 percent of anorexics suffer from depression.

Ways to Help

The best course of action for a person who suspects they know someone with an eating disorder is to be patient, supportive, and not judge the individual. Learn what you can about the problem by consulting an eating disorder clinic or counseling center (common on college campuses), and offer to help the ill person seek professional help.

Often, individuals suffering from an eating disorder do not realize or will not admit that they are ill. For this reason, seeking help or continuing/completing treatment for the disorder is often difficult.

Medical treatment is often necessary for eating disorders. However, it is extremely encouraging to note that eating disorders can be treated and a healthy weight and relationship with food can be restored. Because of the complexity of eating disorders, the best and most successful treatment is usually a combination of counseling, family therapy, cognitive behavior therapy, nutritional therapy, support groups, and drug therapy. Treatment, many times, includes a hospital stay and is usually resisted by the patient. Support for the anorexic or bulimic person by friends and family and the realization of the severity of the problem is critical to successful treatment of the illness.

REFERENCES

Ballard, D. "A Dozen Ways to Stress-Proof Your Life." 2002.

Corbin, C.B. and Lindsey, R. *Concepts of Physical Fitness.* McBrown. 2008.

Donatelle, R. J. *Access to Health* (9th ed). Allyn & Bacon. Boston. 2006.

Floyd, P., Mims, S., and Yelding-Howard, C. *Personal Health: Perspectives and Lifstyles.* Morton Publishing Co. 2007.

Hahn, D. B. and Payne, W. A. *Understanding Your Health.* McGraw-Hill. 2008.

Hales, D. *An Invitation to Health* (8th ed). New York: Brooks/Cole Publishing Company. 1999.

Hales, D. *An Invitation to Health* (Brief 2nd ed). Belmont, CA: Wadsworth Thomson. 2002.

Hoeger, W. and Hoeger, S. A. *Principles and Labs for Fitness and Wellness* (9th ed). Brooks/Cole Publishing Company. 2008.

Hoeger, W. W. K. and Hoeger, S. A. *Lifetime Physical Fitness and Wellness: A Personalized Program* (8th ed). Belmont, CA: Thomson Wadsworth. 2005.

Holmes, T. H. and Rahe, R. H. Student Stress Scale. *Journal of Psychosomatic Research, 11,* 213.

http://ahha.org

http://healthed.tamu.edu/stress.htm

http://indiana.edu/~health/stress.html

http://stress.about.com/od/optimismspitituality/a/positiveselftalk.html

http://who.int/aboutwho/en/definition.html

http://www.healthdepot.com

http://www.med.nus.edu.sg/pcm/stress

http://www.m-w.com/dictionary.html

http://www.nimh.nih.gov/publicat/eatingdisorder.com

http://www.reachout.com.au/default.asp?ti=2249

http://www.selfcounseling.com/help/depression/suicide.html

http://www.acsm.org

http://www.cdc.gov/nccdphp/sgr/pdf/chap4.pdf

Hyman, B., Oden, G., Bacharach, D., and Collins, R. *Fitness for Living.* Kendall-Hunt Publishing Co. 2006.

Payne, W. A., Hahn, D. B. *Understanding Your Health* (6th ed). St. Louis, MO: Mosby. 2000.

Peterson, M. S. *Eat to Compete* (2nd ed). St. Louis, MO: Mosby. 63146

Powers, S. K., Todd, S. L., and Noland, U. J. *Total Fitness and Wellness* (2nd ed). Boston: Allyn & Bacon. 2005.

Prentice, W. E. *Fitness and Wellness for Life* (6th ed). New York: WCB McGraw-Hill. 1999.

Pruitt, B. E. and Stein, J. *Health Styles.* Boston: Allyn & Bacon. 1999.

Robbins, G., Powers, D., and Burgess, S. *A Wellness Way of Life* (4th ed). New York: WCB McGraw-Hill. 1999.

Rosato, F. *Fitness for Wellness* (3rd ed). Minneapolis: West. 1994.

Roth, G. *Why Weight? A Guide to Compulsive Eating.* New York. Penguin Group. 1989.

Student Health Services, Texas A&M University. *Guidelines for Helping a Friend with an Eating Disorder,* 2002.

Webmaster@noah.cuny.edu

Weinttraub, Amy. Yoga: It's Not Just An Exercise. *Psychology Today,* Nov. 2000.

ACTIVITIES

Notebook Activities

Time Budget Sheet

Stress Journal

Forbidden Foods

Ways I Sneak

What Am I Waiting For?

Name: _____ Section: _____ Date: _____

NOTEBOOK ACTIVITY

Time Budget Sheet

Consider study, classess/labs, church, exercise, personal needs, socializing, and so on.

Time	Monday	Tuesday	Wednesday	Thursday	Friday	Saturday	Sunday
7:00 a.m.							
8:00							
8:30							
9:00							
9:30							
10:00							
10:30							
11:00							
11:30							
12:00 p.m.							
12:30							
1:00							
1:30							
2:00							
2:30							
3:00							
3:30							
4:00							
4:30							
5:00							
5:30							
6:00							
6:30							
7:00							
7:30							
8:00							
8:30							
9:00							
9:30							
10:00							
10:30							
11:00							

Name: _____ Section: _____ Date: _____

NOTEBOOK ACTIVITY

Stress Journal

Directions: To start managing stress, you must first recognize it. Fill in the stress journal entries twice in the morning, twice in the afternoon, and twice in the evening for two weeks. When the two weeks are over, discuss your observations with your classmates. What causes YOU the most stress? (Use as many sheets as necessary to complete the task.)

Date	Time	Situation	Stress Level	Signs
5/29	9:00 a.m.	(Where? With whom? Doing what? At work. . . argued with boss.	(1–100) 85	Heart racing, headache, muscle tension

Source: From *Just for the Health of It* by Patricia Rizzo Toner, Center for Applied Research in Education.

Name: _____ Section: _____ Date: _____

NOTEBOOK ACTIVITY

Forbidden Foods

We usually binge on the foods we won't allow ourselves to eat unless we binge. It is only when we give ourselves permission to eat them that we can choose not to eat them. If, for instance, you allow yourself to eat chocolate any time you are hungry for it, then a "chocolate charge" will not build and you won't feel the need to binge on chocolate at a later time. We forbid and forbid and forbid ourselves to have food that we like, food that brings us pleasure. It should be no surprise to us that when we feel a crack in our steely resolve to restrict ourselves—and make a decision to binge—we immediately run for those foods we have not been allowing ourselves to enjoy.

Make a list of the foods you will not allow yourself to eat freely and without guilt. Let yourself think of the food that you determined years ago to shut out of your life, perhaps as far back as childhood. Are sweets included? Bread? Take your time in making the list, remembering foods that you banished, or attempted to banish, or still berate yourself for eating whenever you "succumb."

My Forbidden Foods Are:

_____

_____

_____

_____

_____

_____

Eating My Forbidden Foods

Using the chart on the back of this page, keep a record of what you discover when you do the following:

1. Look at the list you made and decide which is the first food you would like to eat again without guilt.
2. Bring that food into your house this week. Bring more of it than you could possibly eat at one sitting—and *eat it when you are hungry and until you are satisfied.* Allow yourself the pleasure of good tastes.
3. As you eat it, notice whether you like it as much as you thought you would. Notice how it tastes, how it feels in your throat.
4. Remind yourself that you can have it again any time you are hungry.
5. Do the same next week. And the next.
6. Bring one forbidden food into your house each week, until you have no forbidden foods.

Source: From *Why Weight? A Guide to Ending Compulsive Eating* by Geneen Roth, copyright © 1989 by Geneen Roth. Used by permission of Dutton Signet, a division of Penguin Group (USA) Inc.

Forbidden Foods Chart

Week #	The food I chose from the Forbidden Foods List is	I bought plenty		I ate it when I was hungry		I stopped when I was satisfied		When I ate it, I felt:
		Yes	No	Yes	No	Yes	No	
1								
2								
3								
4								

Name: _____ Section: _____ Date: _____

NOTEBOOK ACTIVITY

Ways I Sneak

"Eating with the intention of being in full view" means not sneaking. If you eat alone, it means not being afraid that someone will walk in the door and see what you're eating. It means telling the truth about the food you eat.

How do you sneak food?

EXAMPLES:

1. By eating modest amounts of food at a party, then coming home and eating a meal.
2. By running back and forth to the kitchen (and eating) while people are in the living room.
3. By ordering a cake at the bakery for yourself and telling the cashier that it is for your kids.

Complete the sentence:

I sneak food by:

1. _____
   _____

2. _____
   _____

3. _____
   _____

4. _____
   _____

5. _____

Source: From *Why Weight? A Guide to Ending Compulsive Eating* by Geneen Roth, copyright © 1989 by Geneen Roth. Used by permission of Dutton Signet, a division of Penguin Group (USA) Inc.

Name: _____ Section: _____ Date: _____

NOTEBOOK ACTIVITY

What Am I Waiting For?

Most compulsive eaters are waiting until they have the "right" body to begin living the kind of life they want to live. You don't have to wait. You deserve to have what you want now. Being thin does not suddenly make you worthy of a job you like, relationships that are meaningful, clothes that you find attractive. Your decision that you are worthy is what makes you worthy.

What are you waiting to get thin to do?

Complete the following list:
I am waiting to get thin so I can:

Example:

1. go to my high school reunion and not be ashamed of myself.
2. be in a relationship.
3. make love with the lights on.

_____

_____

_____

_____

_____

_____

_____

Read over the list. Pick two things on it that you can begin doing this week. Make a commitment to yourself to do them on specific days. You'll find that when you begin acting as if you deserve to treat yourself and to be treated with respect and kindness you will slowly begin believing that you do.

Complete the sentence:
This week I will:

1. _____

2. _____

Source: From *Why Weight? A Guide to Ending Compulsive Eating* by Geneen Roth, copyright © 1989 by Geneen Roth. Used by permission of Dutton Signet, a division of Penguin Group (USA) Inc.

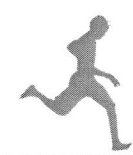

CHAPTER 3

Personal Fitness

"Physical Fitness is not only one of the most important keys to a healthy body, it is the basis of dynamic and creative intellectual activity. The relationship between the soundness of the body and the activities of the mind is subtle and complex. Much is not yet understood. But we do know what the Greeks knew: That intelligence and skill can only function at the peak of their capacity when the body is healthy and strong; that hardy spirits and tough minds usually inhabit sound bodies."

—President John F. Kennedy,
"The Soft American," *Sports Illustrated*,
December 26, 1960

OBJECTIVES

Students will be able to:
- Define key terms related to cardiovascular fitness, muscular fitness, and flexibility.
- Explain the benefits of regular physical activity.
- Explain the relationship between cardiovascular fitness and heart disease.
- Identify the FITT formula components.
- Identify the benefits of resistance training.
- Identify the benefits of flexibility.
- Identify the components of a workout and the importance of each component.
- Identify when the environment is not safe to exercise.

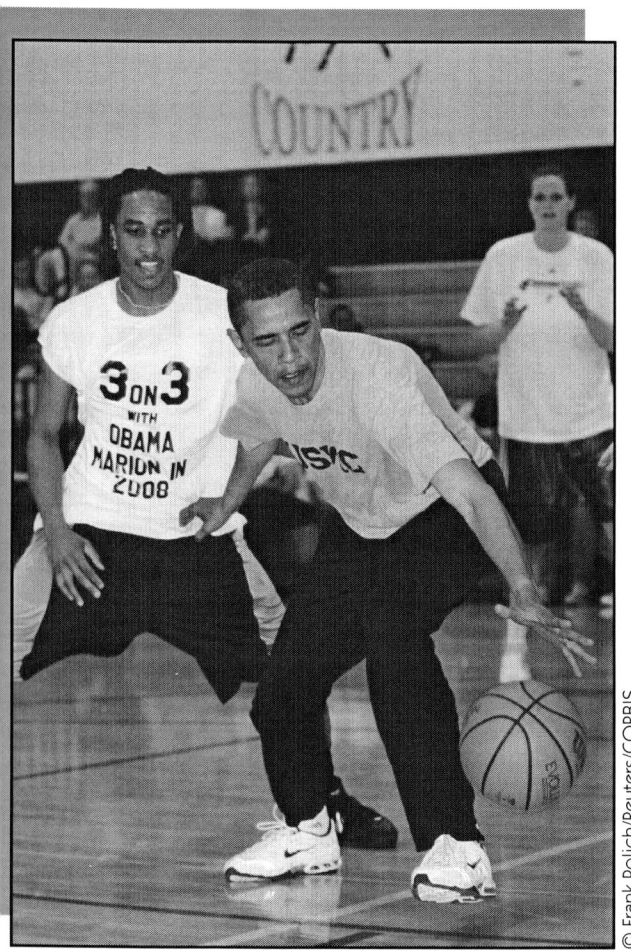

President Obama commits forty-five to ninety minutes, six days a week, for cardio, weights, and basketball.

"It gives you more mental endurance and more energy to think clearly," said President Barack Obama. You might think the president was talking about the newest energy drink on the market, but he was referring to exercise. "He is quietly confident and competitive" was a description of President Barack Obama by U. S. Senator Bob Casey, D-Pa. Although it may sound like the way Mr. Obama ran his marathon election campaign, Senator Casey was actually describing Obama on the basketball court. The president commits forty-five to ninety minutes six days a week for cardio, weights, and basketball. He has good blood pressure and he eats fairly well, so President Obama told *Men's Health* magazine that "The main reason I do it is just to clear my head and relieve me of stress." The Obama children stay active with organized sports like soccer and gymnastics while wife Michelle Obama enjoys hitting the gym at least three days a week for ninety minutes doing cardio and lifting weights. The first lady calls exercise "therapeutic." The president also enjoys healthy snacks of nuts, seeds, and raisins. His vice happens to be an on-again off-again smoking habit. Perhaps the president will not only be a good example of living a fit lifestyle, but he might encourage many who may try to quit the smoking habit alongside him. The White House is, after all, a nonsmoking area.

Before President George W. Bush took office for his first term, President Clinton was known for jogging through the streets of Washington. In his first term President George W. Bush jogged for fitness, but in his second term he traded in his running shoes for a mountain bike. The biking allowed him to work his heart without stressing his knees. President John F. Kennedy wrote in 1960 that hardy minds and tough spirits usually inhabit sound bodies (see quote at the beginning of this chapter). In June 2002, the White House kicked off the "Healthier U.S. Initiative." Members of the Oval Office have a nonpartisan request, which is for Americans to increase their activity to hopefully decrease the increased prevalence of obesity and heart disease in America (see Figure 3.3 on page 58). If the president of the United States finds time to exercise, perhaps our excuse of "I don't have time" is not valid.

Why Is Physical Activity Important?

Regular physical activity decreases cardiovascular risk. Clinical, scientific, and epidemiological studies indicate that physical activity has a positive effect on the delay in development of cardiovascular disease (ACSM, 2007). In a landmark report in 1996, the Surgeon General recommended that all Americans accumulate thirty minutes of activity on most, if not all, days of the week. Recent recommendations state that thirty minutes might not be enough (see Figure 3.5 on page 60). The 2005 dietary guidelines recommend most Americans should bump activity time to sixty minutes daily and up to ninety minutes if a recent significant weight loss is to be maintained. In 2002, the Institute of Medicine issued a statement that all Americans, regardless of age, weight, size, race, and so on, should achieve a total of sixty minutes of moderately intense physical activity daily. In December 2003, the National Sports and Physical Education (NASPE) changed the previous recommendation (1998) to be increased to "at least sixty minutes, and up to several hours of physical activity per day" for children 5 to 12 years of age.

In 2007 the American College of Sports Medicine (ACSM) and the American Heart Association (AHA) together released updated physical activity guidelines that emphasize thirty minutes of moderate activity five times weekly for most Americans. An alternative would be three twenty minute vigorously intense bouts of activity. Strength training is also recommended. Both ACSM and AHA endorse recommendations by the Institute of Medicine that in order to lose weight when these guidelines are already being met, "an increase in activity is a reasonable component of a strategy to lose weight" (ACSM/AHA, 2007). For individuals that are overweight and want to avoid becoming obese, exercise sessions of forty-five to sixty minutes may be prudent. Formerly obese individuals who are trying to avoid regaining weight should consider up to ninety minutes of aerobic activity on most days of the week.

NASPE has released physical activity guidelines for infants and toddlers as well. Infants should interact with parents and caregivers in daily physical activities. They should not be placed in one environment for the whole day, and they should be given opportunities to encourage the development of movement skills. This means play pat-a-cake, peek-a-boo, or other interactive games. Toddlers should accumulate at least thirty minutes of structured activity a day, and at least sixty minutes of unstructured play. "Prevention and treatment of obesity entails changes in lifestyle that promote physical activity and minimize sedentary behavior, said Nazrat Mirza, MD, pediatrician at Children's National Medical Center in Washington, D.C. "Promoting positive behaviors early on in childhood may lead to persistence of these behaviors in to adulthood—helping alleviate the problem of obesity."

In 2008, the U.S. Department of Health and Human Services (DHHS) released new physical activity guidelines for Americans (see Figure 3.1).

How do we define moderate or vigorous activities? Examples of each follow. **Moderate activities** (You can still speak while doing them) are activities like line dancing, biking with no hills, gardening, tennis (doubles), manual wheelchair wheeling, walking briskly, and water aerobics. **Vigorous activities** are aerobic dance or step aerobics, biking hills or going faster than ten miles per hour, dancing vigorously, hiking uphill, jumping rope, martial arts, racewalking, jogging or running, sports with continuous running such as basketball, soccer and hockey, swimming laps, and singles tennis. With vigorous activities it would be difficult to carry on a conversation due to the intensity of the exercise. Try to do all of these activities for a minimum of ten minutes at a time. It is important to recognize that moderate activity is beneficial to everyone, while vigorous activity may not be appropriate for everyone.

FIGURE 3.1

At-A-Glance: A Fact Sheet for Professionals

U.S. Department of Health & Human Services — www.hhs.gov

Physical Activity Guidelines for Americans

These guidelines are needed because of the importance of physical activity to the health of Americans, whose current inactivity puts them at unnecessary risk. The latest information shows that inactivity among American children, adolescents, and adults remains relatively high, and little progress has been made in increasing levels of physical activity among Americans.

Key Guidelines

Substantial health benefits are gained by doing physical activity according to the guidelines presented below for different groups.

Children and Adolescents (aged 6–17)

- Children and adolescents should do one hour (sixty minutes) or more of physical activity every day.
- Most of the one hour or more a day should be either moderate- or vigorous-intensity aerobic physical activity.
- As part of their daily physical activity, children and adolescents should do vigorous-intensity activity on at least three days per week. They also should do muscle-strengthening and bone-strengthening activity on at least three days per week.

Adults (aged 18–64)

- Adults should do two hours and thirty minutes a week of moderate-intensity, or one hour and fifteen minutes (seventy-five minutes) a week of vigorous-intensity aerobic physical activity, or an equivalent combination of moderate- and vigorous-intensity aerobic physical activity. Aerobic activity should be performed in episodes of at least ten minutes, preferably spread throughout the week.
- Additional health benefits are provided by increasing to five hours (three hundred minutes) a week of moderate-intensity aerobic physical activity, or two hours and thirty minutes a week of vigorous-intensity physical activity, or an equivalent combination of both.
- Adults should also do muscle-strengthening activities that involve all major muscle groups performed on two or more days per week.

Older Adults (aged 65 and older)

- Older adults should follow the adult guidelines. If this is not possible due to limiting chronic conditions, older adults should be as physically active as their abilities allow. They should avoid inactivity. Older adults should do exercises that maintain or improve balance if they are at risk of falling.
- For all individuals, some activity is better than none. Physical activity is safe for almost everyone, and the health benefits of physical activity far outweigh the risks. People without diagnosed chronic conditions (such as diabetes, heart disease, or osteoarthritis) and who do not have symptoms (e.g., chest pain or pressure, dizziness, or joint pain) do not need to consult with a healthcare provider about physical activity.

Adults with Disabilities

Follow the adult guidelines. If this is not possible, these persons should be as physically active as their abilities allow. They should avoid inactivity.

Children and Adolescents with Disabilities

Work with the child's healthcare provider to identify the types and amounts of physical activity appropriate for them. When possible, these children should meet the guidelines for children and adolescents—or as much activity as their condition allows. Children and adolescents should avoid being inactive.

Pregnant and Postpartum Women

Healthy women who are not already doing vigorous-intensity physical activity should get at least two hours and thirty minutes (one hundred fifty minutes) of moderate-intensity aerobic activity a week. Preferably, this activity should be spread throughout the week. Women who regularly engage in vigorous-intensity aerobic activity or high amounts of activity can continue their activity provided that their condition remains unchanged and they talk to their healthcare provider about their activity level throughout their pregnancy.

Source: U.S. Department of Health & Human Services

FIGURE 3.2

Health Benefits of Physical Activity—A Review of the Strength of the Scientific Evidence

Adults and Older Adults

Strong Evidence
- Lower risk of:
  - Early death
  - Heart disease
  - Stroke
  - Type 2 diabetes
  - High blood pressure
  - Adverse blood lipid profile
  - Metabolic syndrome
  - Colon and breast cancers
- Prevention of weight gain
- Weight loss when combined with diet
- Improved cardiorespiratory and muscular fitness
- Prevention of falls
- Reduced depression
- Better cognitive function (older adults)

Moderate to Strong Evidence
- Better functional health (older adults)
- Reduced abdominal obesity

Moderate Evidence
- Weight maintenance after weight loss
- Lower risk of hip fracture
- Increased bone density
- Improved sleep quality
- Lower risk of lung and endometrial cancers

Children and Adolescents

Strong Evidence
- Improved cardiorespiratory endurance and muscular fitness
- Favorable body composition
- Improved bone health
- Improved cardiovascular and metabolic health biomarkers

Moderate Evidence
- Reduced symptoms of anxiety and depression

Evidence abounds that everyone, all ages, can benefit from an enhanced quality of life with regular physical activity.

Source: U.S. Department of Health & Human Services.

Regardless of recommendations, children and adults alike benefit from regular, consistent physical activity (see Figure 3.2). Choosing to seek opportunities to move such as walking, biking, swimming, gardening, and other activities can impact risk of disease as well as quality of life. In this chapter, we will discuss why you should exercise and give suggestions to help ensure your success.

Five components of health-related fitness:

1. cardiovascular fitness,
2. muscular strength,
3. muscular endurance,
4. flexibility, and
5. body composition.

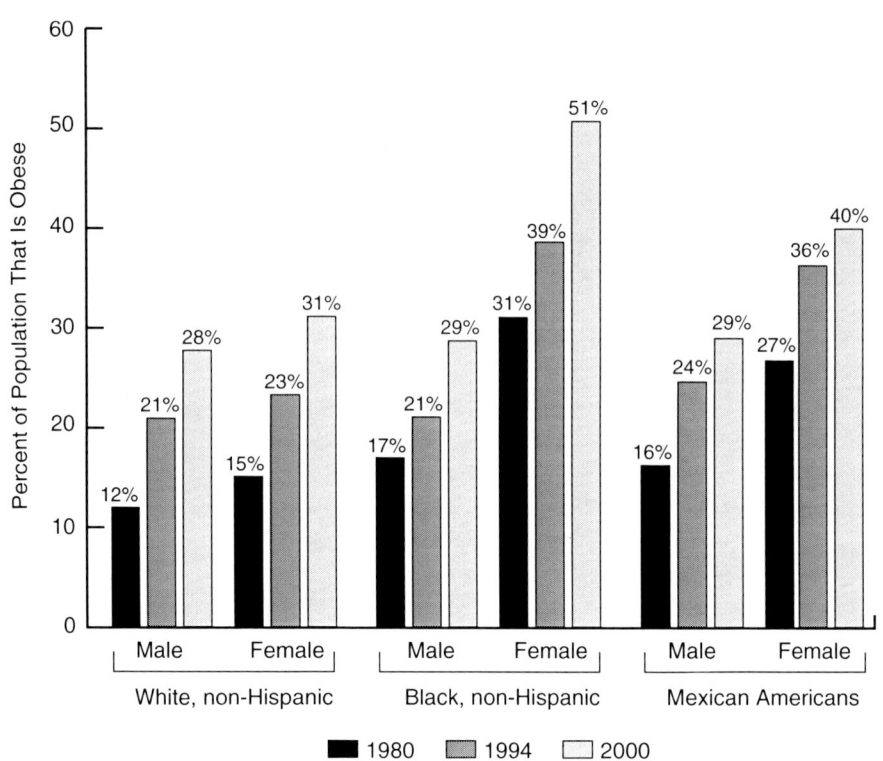

FIGURE 3.3

Prevalence of Obesity by Race and Gender over the Past 20 Years

Source: Center for Disease Control and Prevention

Cardiovascular Fitness

Cardiovascular fitness refers to the ability of the heart, lungs, circulatory system, and energy supply system to perform at optimum levels for extended periods of time. **Cardiovascular endurance** is defined as the ability of the body to perform prolonged, large-muscle, dynamic exercise at moderate to high levels of intensity. The word **aerobic** means "in the presence of oxygen" and is used synonymously with *cardiovascular* as well as *cardiorespiratory* when describing a type of exercise.

Complete fitness is comprised of health-related fitness and skill-related fitness. **Health-related fitness** consists of cardiovascular fitness, muscular strength, muscular endurance, flexibility, and optimal body composition. The components of health-related fitness affect the body's ability to function efficiently and effectively. Optimal health-related fitness is not possible without regular physical activity. Most health clubs and fitness classes focus primarily on the health-related fitness components. **Skill-related fitness** includes agility, balance, coordination, reaction time, speed, and power. These attributes are critical for competitive athletes. Skill-related fitness is not essential in order to have cardiovascular fitness, nor will it necessarily make a person healthier. Balance is, however, important for seniors. Staying active helps seniors maintain strength and balance, which can be critical in avoiding injuries.

Cardiovascular fitness is often referred to as the most important aspect of physical fitness because of its relevance to good health and optimal performance. **Muscular fitness** is important because of its effect on efficiency of human movement and basal metabolic rate. **Flexibility** is important for everyone, athletes and non-athletes alike, especially as a

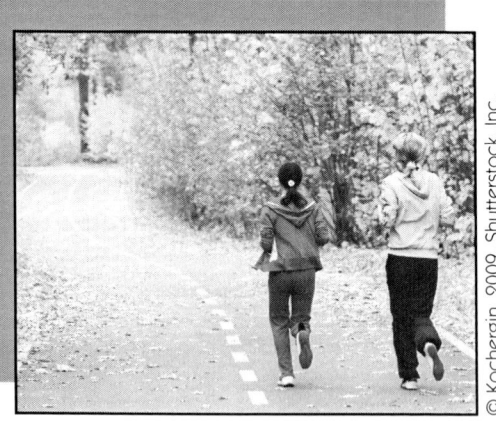

Exercising with friends can be enjoyable and help to keep you motivated and committed to your fitness program.

person ages. Knowing how to exercise correctly for effectiveness and reduced risk of injury is also important. Physically active individuals can expect to experience a positive impact on glucose regulation, blood pressure, blood cholesterol, bone density, body weight, and their outlook on life. Small amounts of activity for sedentary individuals can have an impact on overall health risk. For those who are overweight or obese, a loss of 5 to 10 percent of body weight can have a significant impact on body composition and overall health risk.

How important is participation in physical activity in achieving and maintaining good health? Since 1992, the American Heart Association has considered **inactivity** as important a risk factor for heart disease as high blood cholesterol, high blood pressure, and cigarette smoking. According to the American Heart Association's 2009 statistics, more than 80 million Americans have one or more forms of cardiovascular disease, and coronary heart disease is the single leading cause of death in America today with an estimated economic cost (direct and indirect expenditures) for 2009 of 475.3 billion (AHA, 2009). The U.S. Centers for Disease Control and Prevention (CDC) and the American College of Sports Medicine (ACSM) reported that 300,000 lives are lost each year due to inactivity (AHA, 2006). In 1996 the U.S. Surgeon General's Report made several definitive statements regarding physical activity and its impact on one's health (see Figure 3.4). Evidence is mounting that physical activity is an integral part of good health.

Stress and the Heart
A strong heart will be more efficient than a weak heart when demands are imposed on it through stress. Exercise makes the heart stronger. Sympathetic nerve stimulation is responsible for the *fight-or-flight response* experienced as a result of emotional or physical stress. High fitness levels decrease the impact of this stress on the heart.

How Aerobic Exercise Helps Cardiovascular Fitness

There are many benefits associated with aerobic exercise. When one is aerobically fit, there is an overall reduction in the risk of coronary artery disease, i.e., stroke, blood vessel diseases, and heart diseases. Related to this reduction, there is a decrease in resting heart rate due to the improved efficiency of the heart. There is also an increase in **stroke volume**, which is the amount of blood pumped from the heart with each heartbeat. A decrease in **systolic blood pressure**, which is the highest arterial blood pressure attained during the heart cycle, and a decrease in **diastolic blood pressure**, or lowest arterial pressure attained during the heart cycle, also occurs. There is also an increase in collateral circulation, which refers to the

---

1. Males and females of all ages benefit from regular physical activity.
2. Significant health benefits can be obtained by moderately increasing daily activity on most, if not all, days of the week.
3. Additional health benefits can be gained through greater amounts of physical activity.
4. Physical activity reduces the risk of premature mortality in general, and of coronary heart disease, hypertension, colon cancer, and diabetes mellitus in particular.
5. More than 60 percent of American adults are not regularly physically active.
6. Nearly half of American youth 12 to 21 years of age are not vigorously active on a regular basis.
7. *People of all ages should try to accumulate thirty minutes of activity of moderate intensity (e.g., brisk walking) on most, if not all, days of the week.*

FIGURE 3.4

1996 U.S. Surgeon General's Report: Physical Activity and Health

FIGURE 3.5

Planned exercise is great, but also look for opportunities to move throughout your day. Try new activities occasionally.

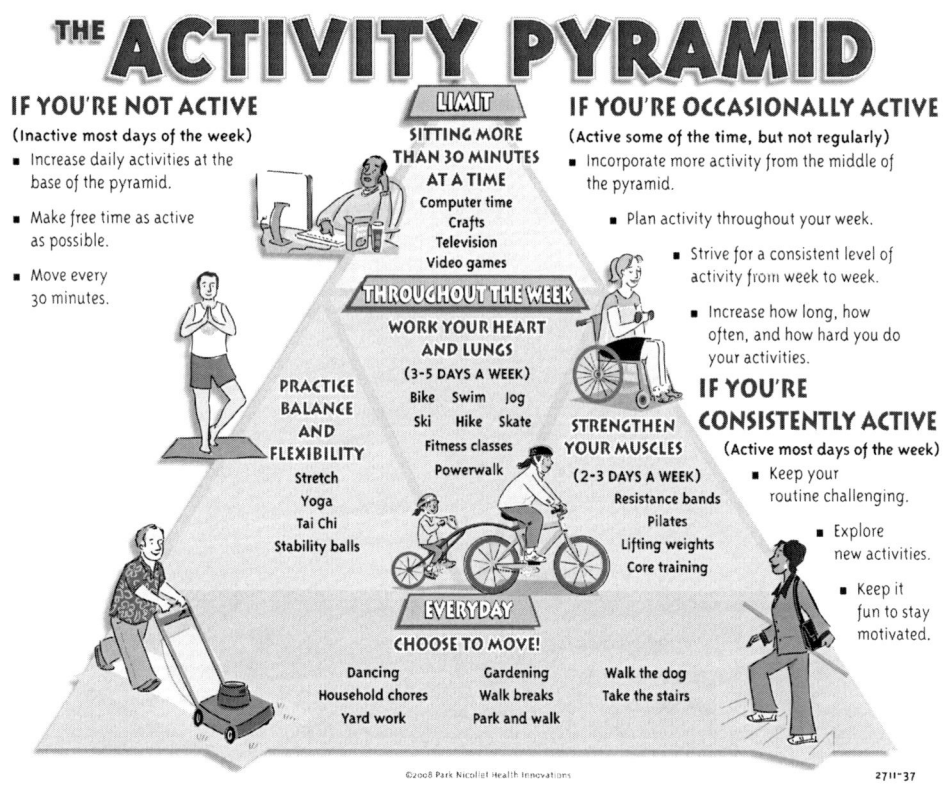

Source: Copyright © 2003 Park Nicollet *HealthSource,* Minneapolis, U.S.A.

number of functioning capillaries both in the heart and throughout the body. Increased capillarization is an adaptation to regular aerobic activity. Delivery of oxygen to the working muscles and removal of metabolic wastes is more efficient with increased collateral circulation. In addition to the specific physiological changes just listed, other benefits of a mental, emotional, and physical nature will increase with regular aerobic exercise. Some of the potential benefits that have been documented when aerobic fitness levels increase are:

- a decrease in percent body fat,
- an increase in strength of connective tissues,
- a reduction in mental anxiety and depression,
- improved sleep patterns,
- a decrease in the speed of the aging process,
- an improvement in stress management,
- an increase in cognitive abilities (Sharkey, 1997).

Heart rate becomes elevated during exercise because of the increase in demand for oxygen in the muscle tissues. Oxygen is attached to hemoglobin molecules and is transported in the blood. The heart pumps at a faster rate to meet the increased demand for oxygen. The heart is a muscle, and like other muscles, it becomes stronger due to the stress of exercise. Through regular exercise, the heart will increase slightly in size and significantly in strength, which results in an increased stroke volume. The primary difference is seen in the increased thickness and strength of the left ventricle wall. As a result of exercise, blood plasma volume increases, which allows stroke volume to increase. These two factors will cause resting heart

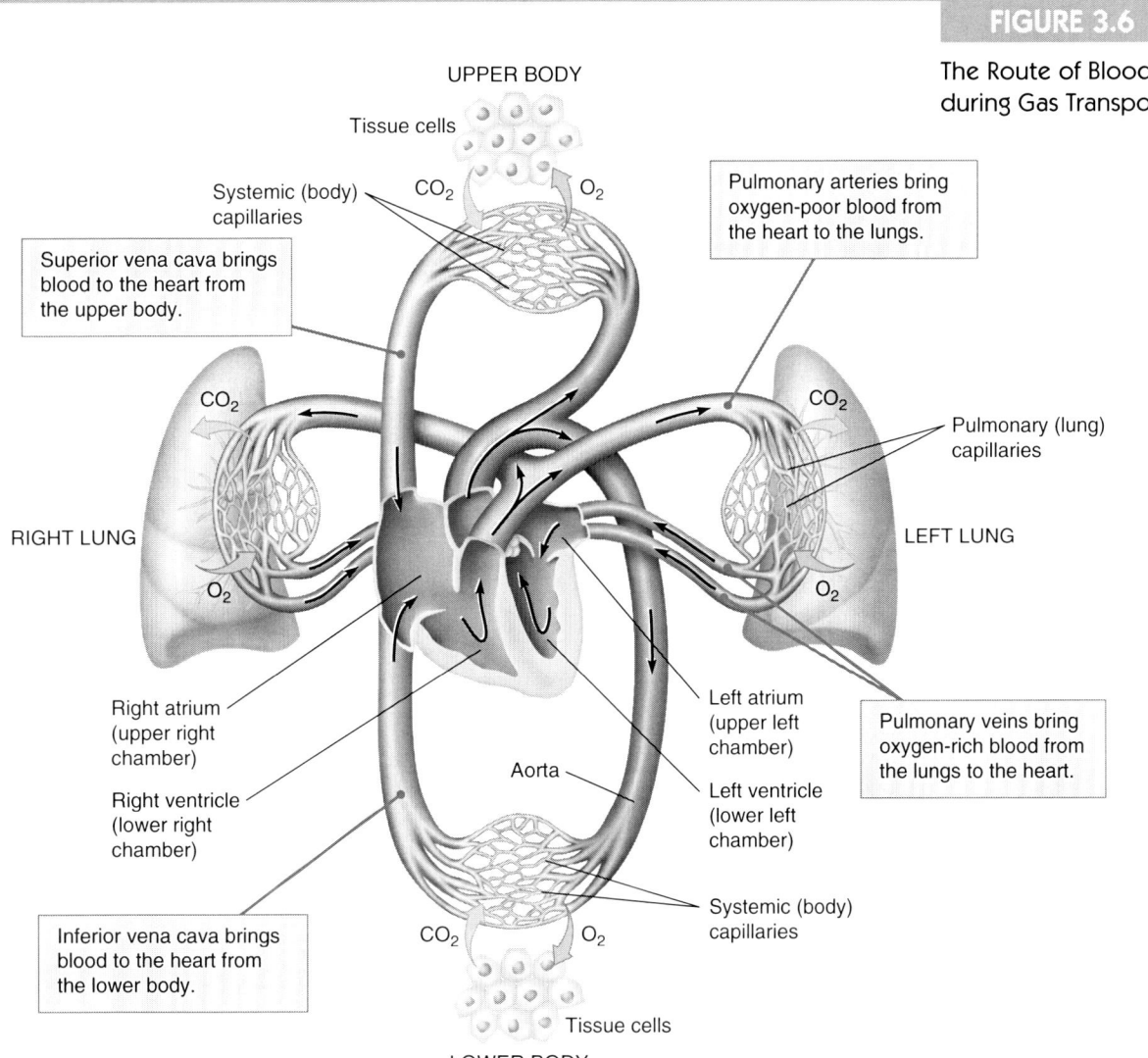

FIGURE 3.6
The Route of Blood during Gas Transport

Source: From *Biology: Understanding Life* by Alters and Alters, © 2006 by Alters and Alters. Reproduced with permission of John Wiley & Sons, Inc.

rate to decrease, exercising heart rate will become more efficient, and there will be a quicker recovery to a resting heart rate after exercise ceases. Lack of exercise can contribute to many cardiovascular diseases and conditions, including **myocardial infarction**, or heart attack; **angina pectoris**, a condition caused by insufficient blood flow to the heart muscle that results in severe chest pain; and **atherosclerosis**, a build-up of fatty deposits causing blockage within the blood vessel.

Closely associated with the function and efficiency of the heart is the function and efficiency of the **circulatory system**. Blood flows from the heart to arteries and capillaries where oxygen is released and waste products are collected and removed from the tissues. The deoxygenated blood then makes the return trip to the heart through the venous system (see Figure 3.6). As a result of aerobic exercise, blood flow to the skeletal muscles improves due to an increase in stroke volume, an increase in the number of capillaries, and an increase in the function of existing capillaries. This provides more efficient circulation both during exercise and during daily activities.

Blood flow to the heart muscle is provided by two coronary arteries that branch off from the aorta and form a series of smaller vessels. With regular aerobic activity, the size of the coronary blood vessels increase and collateral circulation improves.

These small blood vessels can supply oxygen to the cardiac muscle tissue when a sudden block occurs in a major vessel, such as during a heart attack. Often the degree of developed collateral circulation determines one's ability to survive a myocardial infarction, or heart attack. It appears that a regular exerciser might survive a heart attack due to collateral circulation within the heart, as the smaller collateral vessels take over when the primary artery becomes occluded, or blocked.

The lungs, air passages, and muscles involved in breathing that supply oxygen and remove carbon dioxide from the body are known as the respiratory system. During exercise, pulmonary ventilation, which is the movement of gases into and out of the lungs, increases in direct proportion to the body's metabolic needs. At lower exercise intensities, this is accomplished by increases in respiration depth. At higher intensities, the rate of respiration also increases. Although fatigue in strenuous exercise is frequently referred to as feeling "out of breath" or "winded," it appears that the normal capacity for pulmonary ventilation does not limit exercise performance (McArdle, Katch, and Katch, 1999). In a normal environment, one inhales sufficient amounts of oxygen. The breathing limitation is in the efficiency of the oxygen exchange at the cellular level. *The primary benefit of aerobic exercise to the respiratory system is an increase in strength and endurance of the respiratory muscles, not an increase in lung volume.* Maximal pulmonary ventilation volumes are dependent on body size (Wilmore and Costill, 1999). Muscles that elevate the thorax such as the diaphragm are referred to as muscles of inspiration. Muscles of expiration, including the abdominal muscles, depress the thorax. Regular aerobic training will result in an increase in both the strength and endurance of these muscles, and will also result in more efficient respiration.

Aerobic and Anaerobic Exercise

Aerobic exercise is activity that requires the body to supply oxygen to support performance over a period of time. Aerobic exercise is characterized by the use of the large muscle groups in a rhythmic mode with an increase in respiration and heart rate. *Aerobic* literally means "with oxygen." Walking, the most common form of exercise in the United States, is an aerobic activity. Other aerobic exercises include running, swimming, biking, cardiokickboxing, rowing, jump-roping, and any activity that fits the above criteria. As with most exercise, the rate of energy expenditure varies with an individual's skill level and intensity of exercise. Aerobic activities of low intensity are ideal for the beginning or sedentary exerciser because they can be maintained for a longer period of time and have been shown to be effective in promoting weight loss and enhancing cardiovascular health. Many activities are too intense to be maintained more than a few minutes; these activities are considered anaerobic.

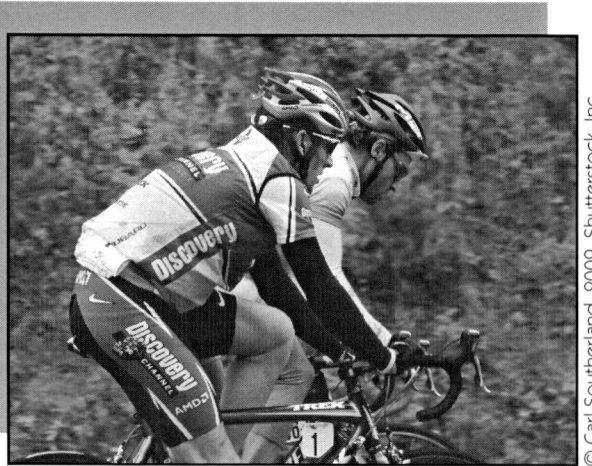

Bicycling is an aerobic exercise that uses the large muscle groups in a rhythmic mode with an increase in respiration and heart rate.

Anaerobic literally means "in the absence of oxygen." **Anaerobic exercise** is exercise performed at intensity levels so great that the body's demand for oxygen exceeds its ability to supply it. Anaerobic activities are usually short in duration, high intensity, and result in the production of blood lactate. The energy for anaerobic activity is primarily from carbohydrates stored within the muscles, called **glycogen**, which is in limited supply. Fatigue rapidly sets in when glycogen stores are depleted. Examples of anaerobic activities include strength training, sprinting, and interval training. Sprinting requires so much energy that the intensity of the activity cannot be maintained for a long period of time. Anaerobic training can enhance the body's ability to cope with the effects of lactic acid and fatigue, thus promoting greater anaerobic fitness. Although it is not recommended for all people, those who are interested in participating in competitive sports would benefit from a high-intensity, anaerobic workout program (Corbin and Lindsey, 2009).

Exercise Prescription, or How to Become FITT

To improve cardiovascular fitness, one must have a well-designed regimen of cardiovascular exercise. In order for improvement to occur, specific guidelines must be adhered to when designing a personal exercise program. As will be discussed later, the following guidelines apply not only to aerobic exercise, but to other components of physical fitness as well. The **FITT** acronym is easy to remember when identifying an appropriate cardiovascular exercise prescription: **frequency**, **intensity**, **time**, and **type**.

Frequency

Frequency refers to the number of exercise sessions per week. The American College of Sports Medicine recommends exercising three to five days per week at a moderate to vigorous level of intensity.

For individuals with a low level of aerobic fitness, beginning an exercise program by working out two times a week will result in an initial increase in aerobic fitness level. However, after some time, frequency and/or intensity will need to be increased for improvement to continue.

Intensity

Intensity refers to how hard one is working, and it can be measured by several techniques. These techniques include measuring the heart rate while exercising, rating of perceived exertion (RPE), and the talk test. To use heart rate as a measure of intensity, one's target heart rate range needs to be calculated before exercising. **Target heart rate range** is the intensity of training necessary to achieve cardiovascular improvement (see Figure 3.7). This target heart rate range indicates what an individual's heart rate should be during exercise. Calculation of target heart rate range is done by multiplying maximum heart rate (220 minus one's age) by a designated intensity percentage. The American College of Sports Medicine guidelines for intensity recommends working between 55 and 90 percent of maximum heart rate, or between 50 and 85 percent of heart rate reserve (maximum heart rate minus resting heart rate). For individuals who are very unfit, the recommended range is 55 to 64 percent of maximum heart rate or 40 to 49 percent of heart rate reserve (Pollock, Gaesser, Butcher, Despres, Dishman, et al., 1998). Use of a heart rate monitor is also useful for specific heart rate and intensity feedback. Programs can be designed using heart rate to alleviate boredom and increase efficiency of the workout.

Another technique for measuring exercise intensity is through subjective self-evaluation of how hard one is working. Gunner Borg designed the **Rating of Perceived Exertion Scale (RPE)** (see Table 3.1) in the early 1950s. It is a numbered scale from 6 to 20, with the lowest numbers being "very, very light" exercise, the highest numbers being "maximal" exercise, and the numbers in between representing a gradual increase in exercise intensity, from low to high. Using this scale, a rating of 10 corresponds roughly to 50 percent of maximal heart rate and a rating of 16 corresponds roughly to 90 percent of maximal heart rate. A person estimates his or her exercise intensity level by taking into consideration or "perceiving" how

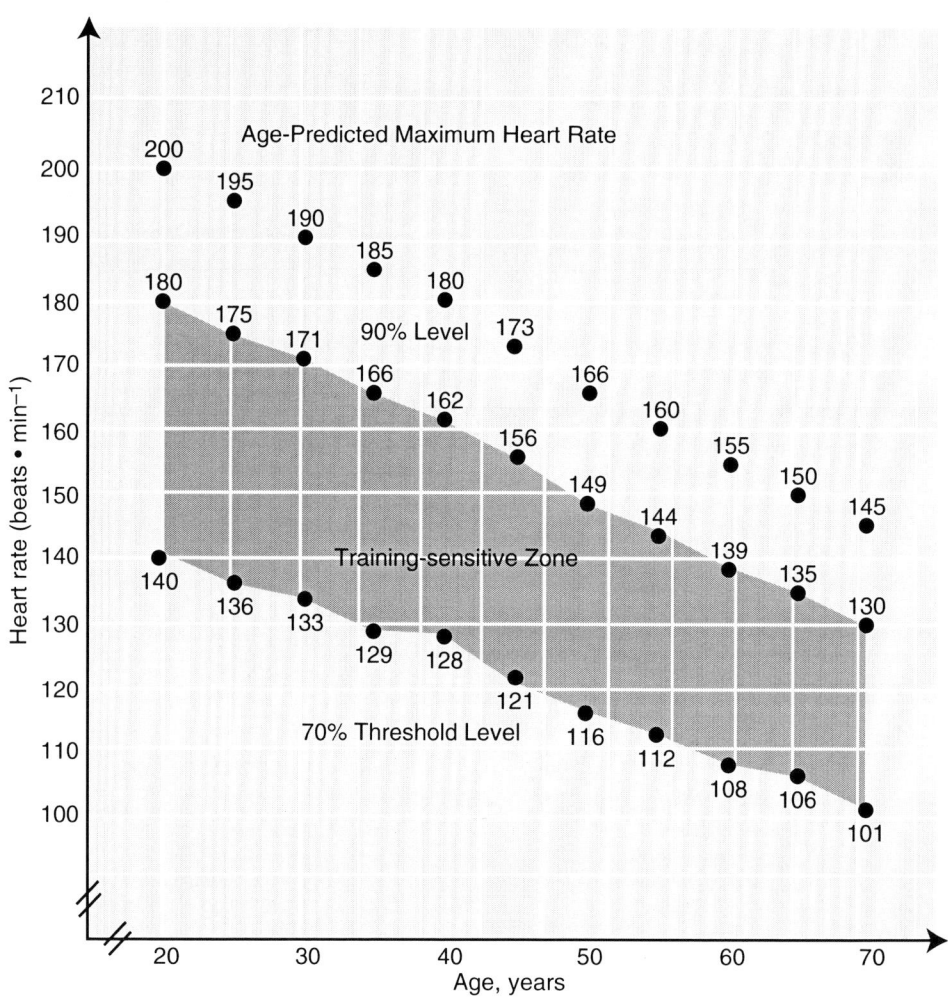

FIGURE 3.7

Target Heart Rate Zones for Individuals of Ages 20 through 70. The zones cover 70–90 percent of maximum heart rate, which is indicated above the zones for selected ages.

Source: From *Total Fitness and Wellness*, 5th Edition, by Powers and Dodd, Pearson Benjamin Cummings Publishers.

Table 3.1
The Borg RPE Scale

Score	Degree of Exertion
6	No exertion at all
7	Extremely light
8	
9	Very light
10	
11	Light
12	
13	Somewhat hard
14	
15	Hard (heavy)
16	
17	Very hard
18	
19	Extremely hard
20	Maximal exertion

Source: © Gunner Borg, 1970, 1985, 1998.

they feel, how much sleep they have had, whether or not they have eaten, whether or not they are ill, and so on. This scale is a useful tool for estimating exercise intensity when exact measures are not needed, and it is often used in a clinical setting as well as fitness classes and health clubs. Perceived exertion is also useful when a person is taking medication that can alter the heart rate.

A third, and probably the easiest, technique to measure exercise intensity is the **talk test.** If you are exercising and must laboriously breathe rather than participate in a conversation, the exercise intensity is too high and training heart rate has probably been exceeded. Exercise at this intensity will be difficult to maintain for long periods of time. On the other hand, if you are able to sing, intensity level is probably insufficient for improvement in your fitness level.

Time

The third factor to be considered when designing a cardiovascular exercise workout is **time**, or duration. For benefits to be accrued in the cardiovascular system, exercise duration should be a minimum of twenty minutes of continuous exercise or several intermittent exercise sessions of a minimum of ten minutes each. Some beginning exercisers may not be capable of exercising continuously for twenty minutes at a prescribed intensity. While a minimum of twenty minutes is recommended, a duration of ten minutes can certainly be beneficial to people who are at a low fitness level and just beginning an exercise program. Duration and exercise intensity are interdependent, having an inverse relationship. As exercise effort increases, duration typically decreases. Distance runners exert a moderate effort for a long period of time, called long slow distance training. Sprinters exert a maximal effort for a brief period of time. Duration at a lower intensity is optimal for beginning exercisers. Exercise intensity levels should remain within recommended guidelines, while maximum duration is only limited by the participant's available fuel for energy and mental determination to keep going.

Type

Another factor that should be considered in determining a cardiovascular exercise prescription is **type**, or mode, of exercise. The choice of exercise modality is up to each individual, but one must keep in mind the specific requirements of cardiovascular exercise: use the large muscle groups via continuous and rhythmic movement, and exercise for a duration of twenty to thirty minutes or more in the target heart rate range a minimum of three to five times per week. Common types of aerobic exercise include running, walking, swimming, step aerobics, cross-country skiing, biking, or using a machine such as a rower, stairstepper, or treadmill. However, these are certainly not the only types of exercise available. Any exercise that meets the requirements of intensity and duration is acceptable. Some sports can provide aerobic exercise, depending on the nature of the sport, the position being played, and the skill level of the player. For example, an indoor soccer player could get an aerobic workout by playing a game, provided there is constant movement and training heart rate was maintained in the target heart rate range. Many sports provide an excellent way for people to expend a lot of energy and burn a significant number of calories, but the "play some and rest some" nature often prevents them from being good aerobic exercise. In order to achieve long-term cardiovascular fitness, it is good to pick a variety of activities, and to find activities that are pleasurable to the individual.

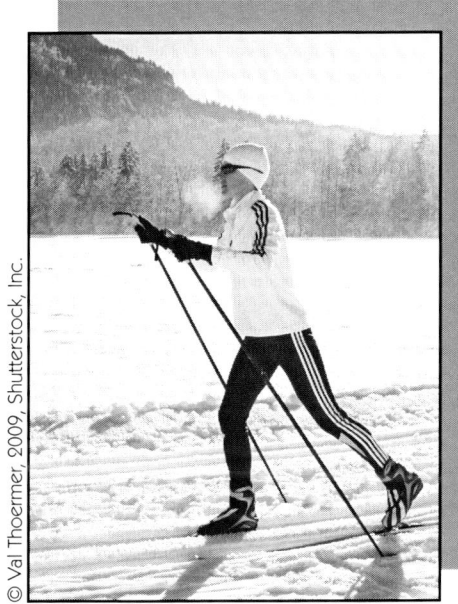

To achieve long-term cardiovascular fitness, select a variety of activities you find pleasureable.

Components of an Exercise Session

The sequence of a cardiovascular workout should be as follows: warm-up, easy optional stretch, workout, cool down, and stretch again with more intensity for increased flexibility.

Warm-Up

A good cardiovascular workout follows a specific sequence of events. First and foremost, to prepare the body and increase the comfort level for a cardiovascular workout, a warm-up is crucial. The purpose of the warm-up is to prepare the body and especially the heart for the more vigorous work to come. The warm-up should increase body temperature, increase heart rate, increase blood flow to the muscles that will be used during the workout, and include some rhythmic movement to loosen muscles that may be cold and/or tight. A warm-up should raise the pulse from a resting level to a rate somewhere near the low end of the

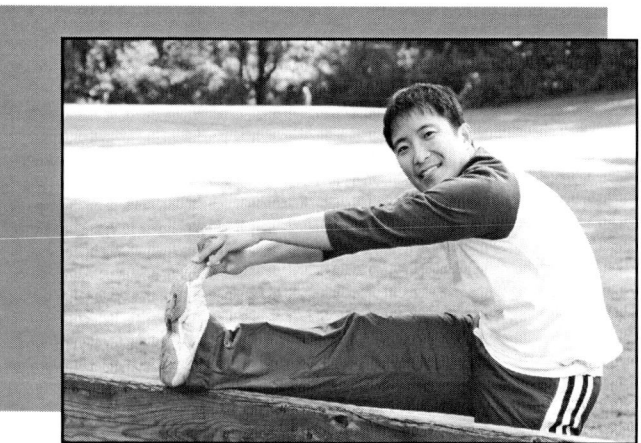

It is important to stretch to warm up muscles that will be used during a workout.

recommended heart rate training zone. Beginning vigorous exercise without some kind of warm-up is not only difficult physically and mentally, but it can also contribute to musculoskeletal injuries.

Pre-Stretch

It is important to warm up the muscles that will be used during the workout. Use caution when stretching prior to the workout, holding the stretches for a brief time and not stretching with much intensity. Stretching prior to the workout is optional. Many athletes choose to go through rhythmic limbering, or focusing on functional movements that will be used in the race, sport, or fitness class rather than holding a static stretch. The time to stretch for increased flexibility seems to be when the muscle is warmest, which is typically after the activity.

Activity

When doing cardiovascular exercise, the aerobic component should be from fifteen minutes to sixty minutes, depending on the individual's fitness level and goals. A gradual increase in intensity and duration is recommended for beginners. It is important to pay attention to your body's signals to slow down or perhaps stop.

Cooldown and Stretch

After an aerobic exercise session, heart rate should be lowered gradually by slowly reducing the intensity of the exercise. Sudden stops are not recommended and can lead to muscle cramps, dizziness, and blood pooling in the legs. After a gradual cooldown such as walking, static stretching of the muscle groups is needed and highly recommended. When muscle core and body core temperature are elevated, it is an optimal time to stretch for increased flexibility. Warmer muscle core temperature increases the pliability of the muscle, allowing it to lengthen better.

Principles of Fitness Training—The Rules

There are specific principles that can be applied to any exercise program. Understanding these exercise principles will increase a person's chance of success with his/her exercise program.

Overload and Adaptation

The principle of overload and adaptation states that in order for a body system to become more efficient or stronger, it must be stressed beyond its normal working level. In other words, it must be overloaded. When this overload occurs, the system will respond by gradually adapting to this new load and increasing its work efficiency until another plateau is reached. When this occurs, additional overload must be applied for gain. The cardiovascular system can be overloaded in more than one way. For example, a person has been running for a few months and is running a distance of three miles in thirty minutes. The runner never goes farther than three miles and never runs faster than a ten-minute per mile pace. For this individual, some techniques of overloading would be: to increase distance, to run the same distance at a faster pace, or to add hills or sprint segments to the run. In

> ## A Complete Physical Activity Program
>
> There are three principle components to a rounded program of physical activity: aerobic exercise, strength training exercise, and flexibility training. It is not essential that all three components be performed during the same workout session. Try to create a pattern that fits into your schedule and one to which you can adhere. *Commitment to a regular physical activity program is more important than intensity of the workouts.* Therefore, choose exercises you are likely to pursue and enjoy.
>
> ACSM/AHA recent position stand *Guideline for adults under 65* states that aerobic training should be moderate intensity for thirty minutes five times per week or three times per week for twenty minutes with vigorous intensity. Remember that *if your schedule is tight, it is better to exercise for a shorter period of time than not at all.* Typical forms of aerobic exercise are walking and running (treadmills), stair climbing, bicycling (bicycle ergometers), rowing, cross-country skiing, and swimming. Many devices contain combinations of these motions.
>
> For general purposes, strength training should be done two or three times per week. Strength training is performed with free weights or weight machines. For the purposes of general training, two or three upper body and lower body exercises should be done. Additionally, abdominal exercises are an important part of strength training.
>
> Flexibility training is important and frequently neglected, resulting in increased tightness as we age and become less active. Stretching is most safely done with sustained gradual movements lasting a minimum of fifteen seconds per stretch. Strive to stretch every day.

terms of weight training, any time a person adds more weight to the bench press or increases the number of repetitions, that person is using the principle of overload. In order for improvements to be realized, overload must occur. The principle of overload and adaptation applies to muscular strength, cardiovascular and muscular endurance, and flexibility training.

Specificity

The principle of specificity refers to training specifically for an activity, or isolating a specific muscle group and/or movement pattern one would like to improve. For example, a 200-m sprinter would not train by running long, slow distances. Likewise, a racewalker would not train for competition by swimming. Workouts must be specific to one's goal with respect to the type of exercise, intensity, and duration. The warm-up should also be specific to a particular activity. Cross training, defined as using several different types of training, has recently increased in popularity. The benefits of cross training are to prevent injury from overuse and to decrease boredom. The principle of specificity does not negate participation in cross training activities; rather, it indicates that the primary training protocol should be in one's chosen activity.

Individual Differences

The principle of individual differences states that individuals will respond differently to the same training protocol. This difference in response is primarily the result of different fitness levels at the beginning of the training process. Age, gender, genetic composition, and previous history will also cause individual responses to specific activities to differ. Coaches, athletic trainers, and personal trainers should be especially aware of this principle when designing workouts in order to achieve maximum performance levels. It is also critical that individuals realize that body type is genetically determined. Body fat distribution and metabolism are individual. Lifestyle and activity can affect one's physique; however, a large-framed person will never be a small-framed person and vice versa. Focusing more on enhanced health rather than trying to change one's body type is prudent.

Reversibility

The inevitable process of losing cardiovascular benefits with cessation of aerobic activity is known as the reversibility principle. The old adage "if you don't use it you lose it" applies here. Physiological changes will occur within the first two weeks of detraining and will continue for several months. Bed rest causes this detraining process to greatly accelerate. Consider the muscle atrophy that occurs with disuse when a cast is removed from a body part that has been immobilized for several weeks. The reversibility principle is clearly the justification for off-season programs for athletes and immediate initiation of physical rehabilitation programs for individuals with limited mobility.

Evaluating Cardiovascular Fitness

There are many ways to measure a person's level of cardiovascular fitness. Over time, the body adapts to regular activity by not working as hard when given the same workload. An example would be running the mile. A person may have a goal of running the mile in eight minutes. At first an eight-minute mile may be a challenge, but with continuous practice, an eight-minute mile can be achieved, and may actually become easier. The body has adapted by allowing the pace to be maintained with less apparent effort. Working heart rate, the heart rate during activity, is lower. Oxygen delivery is increased to the working muscles. Respiration rate is less as the respiratory muscles become stronger. Muscles become stronger with use, creating ease of movement. Body composition typically becomes more favorable, which contributes to efficiency of movement. Powers and Howley have shown that in general twelve to fifteen weeks of endurance exercise results in a 10 percent to 30 percent improvement in VO_2 Max.

VO_2 **Max** is the nomenclature for **maximum oxygen uptake,** the measure of the maximum amount of oxygen that an individual can utilize per minute of physical activity. VO_2 Max is expressed as mililiters of oxygen per kilogram of body weight per minute (ml/kg/min). As aerobic capacity increases, so does VO_2 Max. VO_2 Max is considered the best indicator of cardiovascular fitness. Unfortunately, measurement in a laboratory takes time, equipment, and technicians to administer the tests. Other ways to measure cardiovascular fitness include:

- 1.5-mile run (see 1.5-mile run activity (Notebook Activity on page 101))
- 12-minute run (page 137)
- 1-mile walk (page 69)
- various submaximal tests on cycle ergometers and treadmills

The Rockport one-mile walk test is often used. See Table 3.2 for the Rockport Fitness test. In order to correctly evaluate cardiovascular fitness, walk the distance in the shortest amount of time, find your age and corresponding time and estimated fitness level.

Recovery heart rate is taken after an exercise session is completed, typically for thirty seconds, and multiplied by two for a per minute count. The higher a person's

Table 3.2
Rockport One-Mile Walk Test

Fitness Category	Age (years)			
	13–19	20–29	30–39	40+
Men				
Very Poor	>17:30	>18:00	>19:00	>21:30
Poor	16:01–17:30	16:31–18:00	17:31–19:00	18:31–21:30
Average	14:01–16:00	14:31–16:30	15:31–17:30	16:01–18:30
Good	12:31–14:00	13:01–14:30	13:31–15:30	14:01–16:00
Excellent	<12:30	<13:00	<13:30	<14:00
Women				
Very Poor	>18:01	>18:31	>19:31	>22:01
Poor	16:31–18:00	17:01–18:30	18:01–19:30	19:01–22:00
Average	14:31–16:30	15:01–17:00	16:01–18:00	16:31–19:00
Good	13:01–14:30	13:31–15:00	14:01–16:00	14:31–16:30
Excellent	<13:00	<13:30	<14:00	<14:30

Because the one-mile walk test is designed primarily for older or less conditioned individuals, the fitness categories listed here do not include a "superior" category.

Source: Modified from Rockport Fitness Walking Test.

level of cardiovascular fitness, the less time it will take after exercise for the heart rate to return to a pre-exercise level. One minute after the cessation of exercise, a male heart rate should have returned to below 90, and a female heart rate to below 100 beats per minute. Five minutes post exercise, both male and female heart rates should be below 80 beats per minute. This is an indication not only of one's fitness level, but also of the adequacy of a cooldown period.

Muscular Fitness

Muscular fitness includes two specific components: muscular strength and muscular endurance. Muscular strength is the force or tension a muscle or muscle group can exert against a resistance in one maximal effort. Muscular endurance is the ability or capacity of a muscle group to perform repeated contractions against a load, or to sustain a contraction for an extended period of time. In February 2002 ACSM released a new position stand regarding resistance training progression. The position stand reported that everyone would benefit from resistance training two to three days per week, working eight to ten muscle groups with one to two sets of eight to twelve repetitions. For more information, these statements can be found on the ACSM Web site listed at the end of this chapter.

> "Fitness isn't just for highly skilled athletes. It is for all of us. It's our natural state of being, particularly when we are young. Being out of shape is really being out of sorts with ourselves."
>
> —Kenneth H. Cooper, M.D.,
> The Aerobics Way

Top Ten Reasons to Work Your Muscles

1. *Gain lean body mass and lose body fat.* For each pound of muscle you gain, you'll burn 35 to 50 more calories daily.
2. *Get strong.* Extra strength makes it easier to carry suitcases and accomplish some daily activities, such as lifting children or groceries.
3. *Build denser bones.* Weight training can increase spinal bone mineral density by 13 percent in six months.
4. *Reduce risk of diabetes.* Weight training can boost glucose utilization in the body by 23 percent in four months and lower the likelihood of developing diabetes.
5. *Fight heart disease.* Strength training reduces harmful cholesterol and lowers blood pressure.
6. *Beat back pain.* In a twelve-year study, strengthening the low-back muscles had an 80 percent success rate in eliminating or alleviating low-back pain.
7. *Move easier.* Weight training can ease arthritis pain and strengthen joints, so you feel fewer aches.
8. *Improve athletic ability.* Whatever your sport, strength training may improve proficiency and decrease risk of injury.
9. *Feel younger.* Even men and women in their 80's and 90's can make significant gains in strength and mobility with weight training.
10. *Boost your spirits.* Strength training reduces symptoms of anxiety and depression and instills greater self-confidence.

Benefits of Muscular Fitness

Several physiological adaptations occur as a result of resistance training. Strength gains can be seen within the first six weeks, with little or no change in muscle size, and are attributed to neural changes. These changes include decreased activation of antagonistic muscles, learning how to perform the activity, changes in activation of the motor unit, improved recruitment patterns of muscle fibers, change in the gain of the muscle spindle and Golgi tendon organ, and reduction in the sensitivity of force-producing limiting factors.

As strength training activities continue, hypertrophy, or an increase in the size of the muscle fibers, occurs (see Figure 3.10 on page 76). Another result from training is an increase in the amount of energy available for contraction. Carbohydrates are stored in the form of glycogen in the muscle and can be used as the primary energy source for contraction. These muscle glycogen stores increase as a result of training. Bone and connective tissue also undergo changes with resistance training, including an increase in bone matrix, an increase in bone mineral density, and an increase in mass and tensile strength of ligaments and tendons. These increases help prevent injury and decrease the chance of development of osteoporosis after middle age. More muscle mass increases an individual's basal metabolic rate, which is why weight training is excellent for "dieters," or those wanting to reduce their percentage of body fat. "An increase in one pound of muscle elevates basal metabolic rate by approximately 2–3 percent" (Powers and Dodd, 2009).

Along with the physiological adaptations previously discussed come benefits that improve the quality of one's life. These benefits of muscular fitness include:

- an increase in muscular strength,
- power and endurance,
- a higher percentage of muscle mass,
- improved posture,
- increased metabolic rate,
- improved ease of movement,
- increased resistance to muscle fatigue,
- increased strength of tendons, ligaments, and bones,
- decreased risk of low back pain,
- increased energy and vitality.

Importance of the Core Musculature In Functional Movement

An important new buzzword in the group fitness and personal training field is **functional movement.** Functional movement is exercise based on real-life movement. The actions done by an athlete in his/her sport are functional. Functional movement usually involves gross motor, multi-planar, multi-joint movements which place demand on the body's core—from the hips to the sternum. The core involves the muscles of the abdomen, back, and hips (listed below). Functional exercises (medicine ball warm-up, full squat with military press, wood choppers) attempt to incorporate as many variables as possible (balance, multiple joints, multiple planes of movement). This is in contrast to weight training for a specific muscle group such as the biceps brachai when doing a biceps curl. It is important to stabilize the pelvis, train the core muscles, align the spine, and achieve muscle equity to use functional movement when exercising. A strong core reduces the risk of injury and increases the efficiency of movement. Training the core can lead to an increase in balance and coordination, as well as gains in strength, power, and endurance.

What Makes Up the "Core"?

- *Pelvic floor muscles*—The pelvic floor muscles run collectively from the pubic bone to the tailbone. Contraction of these muscles contributes to spinal stability, which is the foundation from which we move.
- *Abdominal wall*—The rectus abdominus, the internal and external obliques, and the transverse abdominus together are responsible for spinal flexion, extension, and rotation, as well as for assisting in stabilization.
- *Back muscles*—The erector spinae and multifidus produce spine extension, lateral flexion, and rotation. The interconnections of these muscles help contribute to stability of the lower back and pelvis.
- *Hip muscles*—The adductor and abductor muscles of the hip, when in balance, provide optimum stability and mobility to the hip and lumbopelvic area.
- *Lats and glutes*—Both of these muscle groups attach to the spine or pelvis, so each has an important role in the stability and mobility of the trunk.

These muscle groups make up the "core" and play an important role in core stabilization, muscle balance, and proper alignment, as well as strength and flexibility (see Figures 3.8a and 3.8b).

FIGURE 3.8a

Major Anterior Muscles in the Human Body

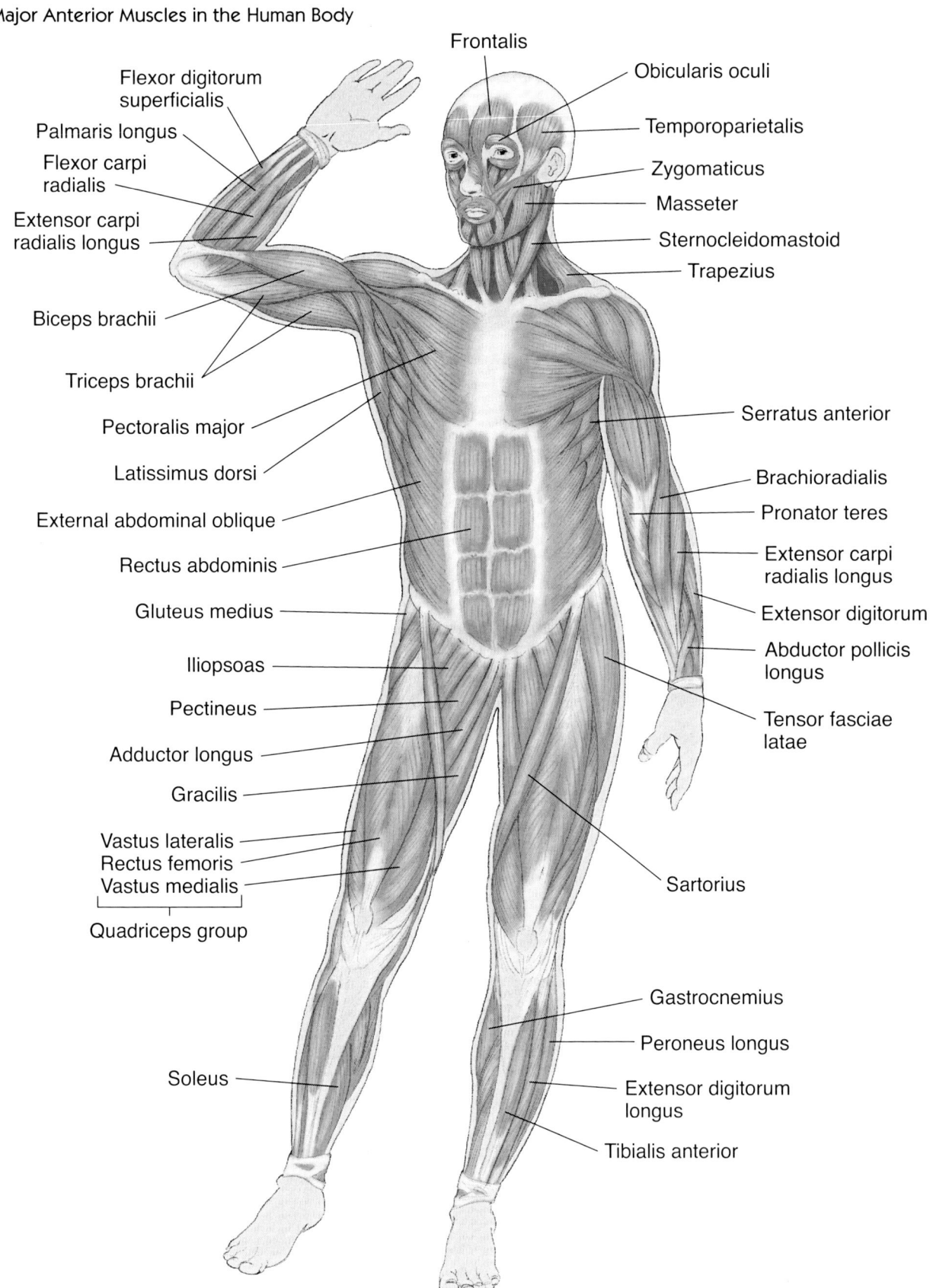

Source: © Kendall/Hunt Publishing Company.

Personal Fitness **73**

FIGURE 3.8b

Major Posterior Muscles in the Human Body

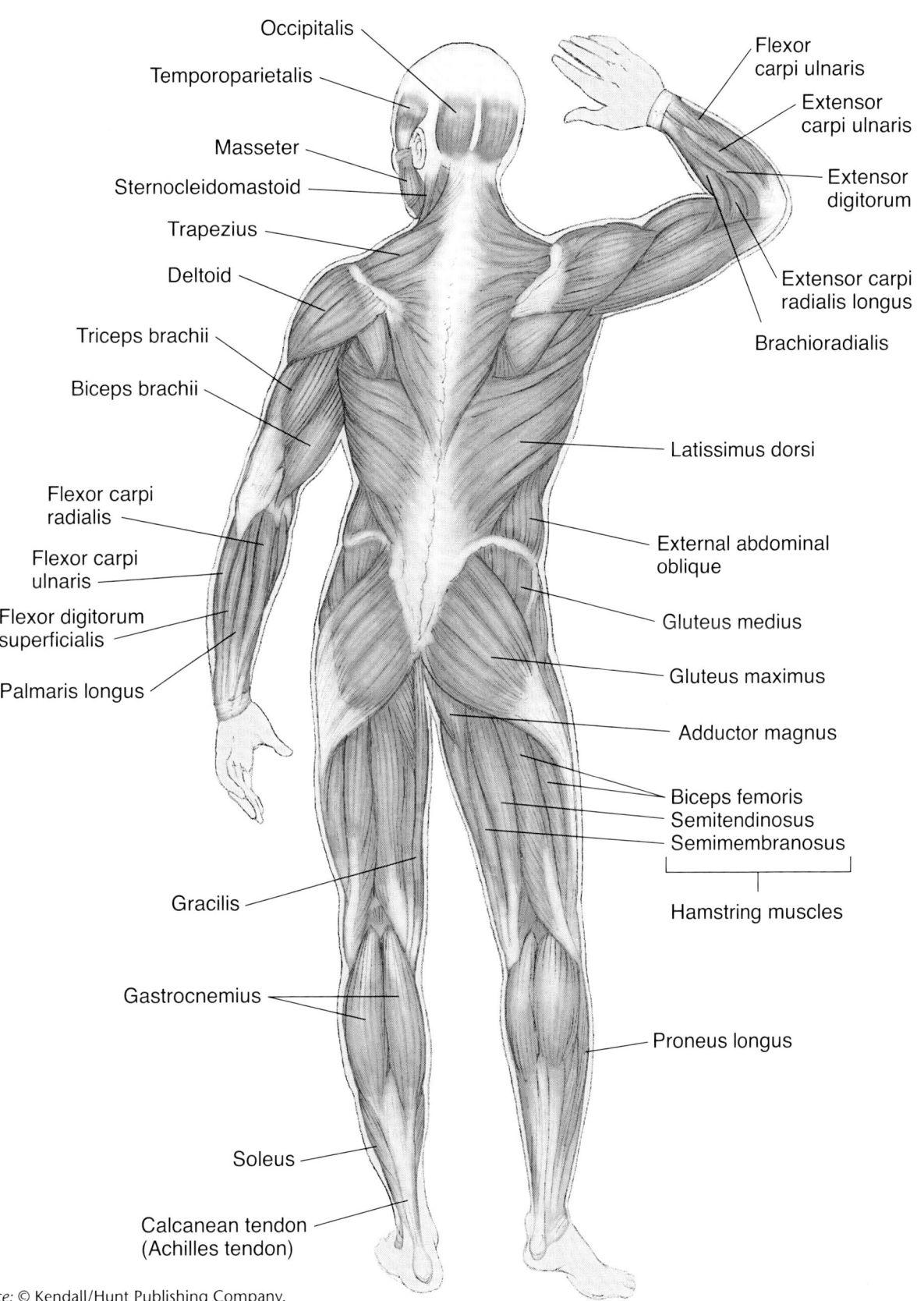

Source: © Kendall/Hunt Publishing Company.

Effective Training

The following are general definitions regarding the use of weight training for developing an exercise protocol to increase muscular endurance (Cissik, 1998).

- **Frequency** refers to how often one should lift, with the recommendation being three nonconsecutive days per week.
- **Load** defines the amount of weight lifted. This will vary with each individual, with the recommended amount being a weight that will allow twelve to fifteen repetitions with good form. If form is compromised, the load should be decreased.
- **Repetition** is simply the performance of a movement from start to finish one time.
- **Set** is the specific number of repetitions performed without resting. Twelve to fifteen repetitions per set are recommended while performing two to three sets of each exercise. Each exercise session should contain eight to ten different exercises, with at least one being a full-body exercise.
- **Recovery** is the amount of time between each set. Thirty seconds is considered the optimum amount; however, taking more time is not detrimental.
- **Repetition-maximum** (also called one rep max) is the maximum amount of weight that can be lifted one time without compromising form.
- **Intensity** is the stress level of the exercise and is expressed as a percent of a one repetition-maximum. The recommended intensity level is less than 70 percent of a one repetition-maximum.

Training for the Best Results

The exercise prescription for developing muscular strength is more intense than for endurance. The number of repetitions decreases from eight to one, with the number of sets increasing from three to five. The percent of the one repetition-maximum that should be lifted increases to 80 to 100 percent. Due to the increase in intensity, the rest period is extended, lasting three to five minutes. Remember the exercise prescription will vary depending on one's goals and objectives for training (see Figure 3.9).

Muscle soreness often accompanies resistance training and will occur at various times during the training process. Muscle soreness that begins late in an exercise session and continues during the immediate recovery period is known as acute muscle soreness. This soreness will last only a brief period of time and is typically gone within twenty-four hours, while **delayed-onset muscle soreness** begins a day or two after the exercise session and can remain for several days. Eccentric contraction seems to be the primary cause of delayed-onset muscle soreness. According to Wilmore and Costill (1999), the causes of delayed-onset muscle soreness include structural damage to muscle cells and inflammatory reactions within the muscles. Muscle soreness can be prevented or minimized by: reducing the eccentric component of muscle action during early training, starting training at a low intensity and gradually increasing it, or beginning with a high-intensity, exhaustive bout, which will cause much soreness initially, but will decrease future pain. During delayed-onset muscle soreness, strength

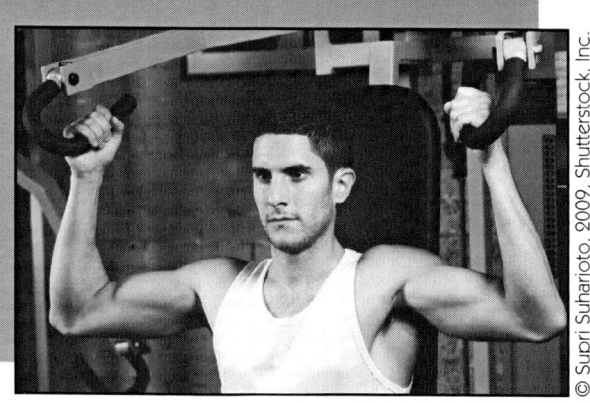

The exercise prescription for developing muscular strength is more intense than for building endurance.

FIGURE 3.9

Beginning Strength Training Guidelines

Preparation:
- Establish goals. Why do you want to weight train? Your goals will affect the way you train.
- Don't train on an empty stomach; fuel your body and brain before working out with a healthy snack.
- Consume a balanced diet daily.
- Stay hydrated with water before, during, and after the workout.
- Dress properly in loose clothing and wear non-slip athletic shoes.
- Commit to a regularly scheduled training time weekly for best results.
- Get instruction in a safe, effective, and balanced program.
- Adjust the weight machine to your body height.

Lifting:
- Always warm up; try ten minutes of cardiovascular activity or calisthenics followed by joint-specific movements for the body parts you will target.
- Progress slowly; use common sense when overloading.
- Work all the major muscle groups; avoid focusing on just one or two areas of the body.
- Consider balance—working opposing muscle groups (biceps-triceps, hamstring-quadriceps, lower back-abdominals).
- Work the larger muscle groups first, progressing to the smaller muscles.
- Complete multi-joint exercises before doing single-joint exercises (squats before leg curls).
- Keep the weights as close to the body as required for proper form and technique.
- Use a full range of motion for each exercise.
- Make sure stretching needs are appropriate to the individual; only stretch the muscle, not the ligaments or joint capsule.
- Maintain good posture throughout each movement.
- Movement should be slow and controlled, with a smooth rhythm.
- Breathe, exhaling on the exertion phase.
- Avoid breath holding during heavy lifting.
- Expect some soreness; excessive muscle soreness may be a sign of overuse or injury.

- Allow forty-eight hours of recovery for a particular body part after heavy lifting; light activity is fine during recovery.
- Get plenty of rest, water, and good nutrition to allow for muscle repair and recovery.
- Enlist a workout buddy to help with technique, motivation, and safety.
- Use a workout log to track your progress, recording weight, sets, and repetitions.

Safety:
- Learn the rules at your facility.
- Don't overtrain; listen to your body.
- Never sacrifice form for additional repetitions or weight.
- When squatting, maintain a natural lordotic curve in your spine; descend until the thighs are parallel to the floor.
- Use collars or other locking devices to keep the plates on the bars when using free weights.
- Use experienced spotters for heavy lifting.
- Always lift free weights with a partner.
- Avoid locking out or hyperextending any joints while lifting.
- Don't lift if you are too fatigued to maintain good form.

Etiquette:
- Practice good weight room etiquette; don't drop or bang the weights.
- Always re-rack free weights.
- Use a towel to wipe equipment when you are done at an exercise station.
- Be considerate of others who are waiting to use the equipment.

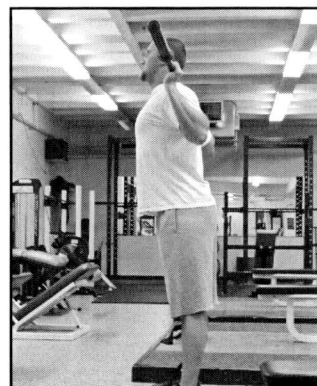
(a) Standing

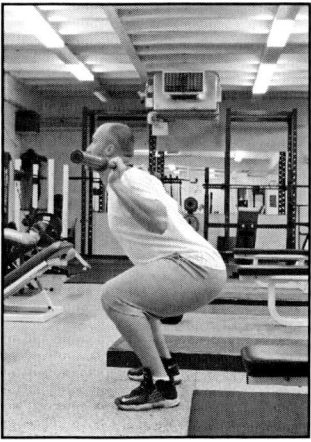
(b) Beginning Squat

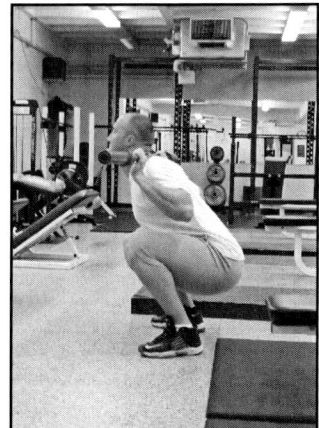
(c) Advanced Full Squat

production is reduced by as much as 50 percent during the first five days and a reduction in strength can occur for as long as fourteen days. The best technique for prevention of delayed-onset muscle soreness is to maintain an appropriate training program. Diet supplements of vitamin E, an antioxidant, may also help to reduce damage to muscle fiber membranes (Evans, 2000).

As with any type of training program, watch for signs of over-training. With muscular fitness training, these indicators include a decrease in physical performance, weight loss, increase in muscle soreness, increase in resting heart rate, sleeplessness, nausea after a workout, constant fatigue, and decreased interest in exercise.

True or False? Weight Training Myths

1. Myth: Weight training causes one to lose flexibility.

   Fact: Resistance training will increase muscle size, but it does not necessarily make one less flexible. In fact, proper strength training can actually increase flexibility when a full range of motion is used.

2. Myth: Resistance training or "spot reducing" is beneficial in reducing deposits of fat from specific areas on the body, such as in the hips, thighs, and waist.

   Fact: Resistance training focuses on the muscles used. Fat is not removed from one area of the body by working the muscles in that area. Creating a caloric deficit consistently, through diet, exercise, or a combination of both, loses fat. The location of fat deposits is determined genetically. The majority of women tend to be "pears" with fat deposits collecting on the hip and thigh region. The majority of men tend to be "apples" with fat deposits collecting around the torso. Abdominal fat has been shown to indicate an increased health risk.

3. Myth: Fat will be converted to muscle with resistance training.
   Fact: Fat is not converted to muscle with exercise, nor is muscle converted to fat through disuse. Muscle cells and fat cells are different entities. The size of muscle cells can be increased with resistance training. Fat cell size is increased with sedentary living combined with a poor diet.

FIGURE 3.10

Changes in Body Composition from Combined Aerobic and Strength Training Program

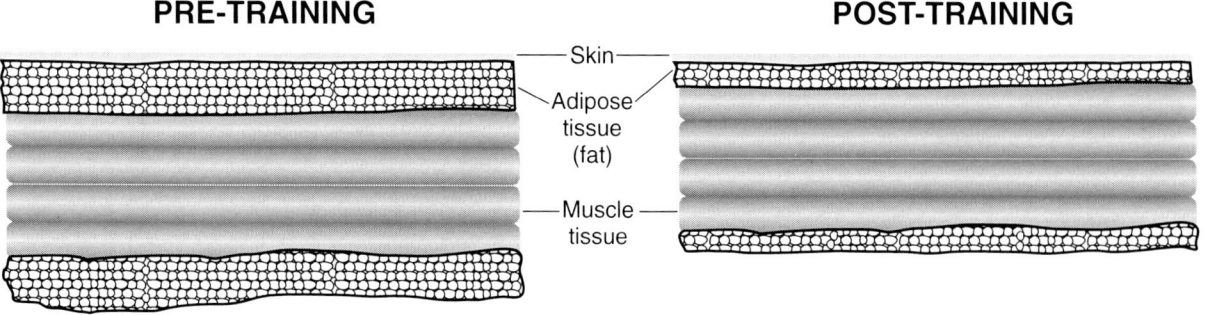

4. Myth: Dietary supplements will make one bigger and stronger.

   Fact: A balanced diet and hard work in the weight room will increase muscle size and strength. Most dietary supplements will only cause the manufacturer's wallet to become bigger. Often when a person spends money on a supplement believing that supplement to work, the placebo effect might result in some apparent short-term improvement.

5. Myth: Performance-enhancing drugs such as steroids, growth hormones, diuretics, and metabolism boosters will help make one fit.

   Fact: These drugs are extremely dangerous and potentially fatal. They can contribute to aesthetic changes, but can also have a negative impact on health. Some fitness enthusiasts have lost their lives searching for a short-cut to health by using supplements.

6. Myth: Women will become masculine in appearance by participating in resistance training activities.

   Fact: Masculinity and femininity are determined through hormones, not through resistance training. Resistance training will cause an increase in muscle tone, which is perceived to increase the attractiveness of both males and females.

7. Myth: Kids should not weight train.

   Fact: Pre-adolescent children can and should use their body as resistance. Swinging on the monkey bars or climbing a tree are good examples of using one's body as resistance; push-ups, sit-ups, and tumbling activities are also great. Teaching 11- to 13-year-olds proper technique and form lifting light weight with proper supervision helps lay a strong foundation for future training. Proper training can improve flexibility, as well as strengthen muscles and the skeletal structure. Body composition and self-esteem are also usually enhanced with a training program, which can be a positive outcome with childhood obesity on the rise.

Flexibility

Can you touch your toes? Think of how much your flexibility has changed in the last ten years. How much more will it change in the next ten years? Truly, if you don't stretch or if you are not active, flexibility will be lost. Why is this a concern? Loss of flexibility with age or injury can greatly affect a person's quality of life. Simple activities such as putting on your socks, or bending to lift a toddler can be painful or worse, impossible. Individuals who are active tend to be more

Yoga is gaining in popularity in the United States. Most forms of yoga encourage the buildup of heat within the body to facilitate movement and internal focus. Relaxation is a common goal of most yoga participants, yet most experience enhanced flexibility and increased strength as a fringe benefit. One style of yoga, Bikram yoga, advocates practicing yoga in rooms with temperatures as high as 105 degrees. The premise is that the heat will allow the tendons, ligaments, and muscles to loosen up more and stretch further. A common yoga truism is that even steel, when heated hot enough, will bend.

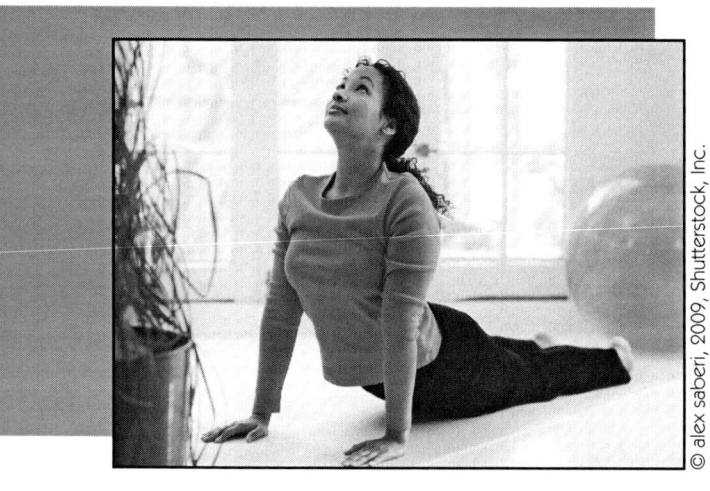

flexible simply because they tend to use a full range of motion in their activity. Active individuals are also more likely to engage in health-enhancing behaviors. Several factors can have an impact on the amount of flexibility a person can achieve, including gender, age, genetic composition, activity level, muscle core temperature, and previous or current injury. Old injuries often hamper flexibility for adults later in life, therefore affecting future activity.

Flexibility and balance are a concern for the aging population. Non-impact activities such as tai chi and yoga are gaining in popularity with all ages, both of which are appropriate to the aging population.

Flexibility is defined as the range of motion around a joint. Flexibility is also specific to individual joints. For instance, an individual may have complete range of motion in the wrist but be very limited or stiff in the shoulder. An individual could be very flexible on the right side of the body, and inflexible on the left side. Flexibility exercises should be included in all exercise programs regardless of the objectives. The benefits of maintaining flexibility include having the ability to perform daily activities without developing muscle strains or tears and being able to participate in sports with enhanced performance. Consider a swimmer who increases shoulder flexibility is able to reach further, pull more water, and thus swim faster.

The athlete, whether serious about competition or a weekend recreator, will have a greater ability to perform particular sports skills with an increased range of motion. Consider a football coach encouraging his receivers to bench press as much as possible. That receiver can be very strong in the weight room; however, if he cannot apply that strength on the football field, he will not be an effective player. Athletes should train for **functional strength.** A wide receiver should train to jump high and extend from his shoulders to catch a pass. Strength without flexibility is limiting. It is especially important to include flexibility exercises in a muscular fitness workout. Flexibility also helps to prevent injuries through a reduction in strains and muscle tears.

Stretching exercises are identified through three specific categories: **ballistic**, **static**, and **PNF**.

Time, Inc reported (Aug. 5, 2002) that tai chi is the perfect exercise for seniors. **Tai chi** is an ancient martial art involving graceful movement performed slowly with great concentration and focus on breathing. The atmosphere is non-competitive, and participants are encouraged to progress at their own pace. The Oregon Research Institute reports that studies show older men and women who are inactive yet relatively healthy attain many benefits from participation in tai chi.

1. **Ballistic** stretching involves dynamic movements, or what is commonly referred to as "bouncing." Ballistic stretching is not recommended for the general population as a means to improve flexibility. An exception is athletes who have ballistic movement in their sport. This type of stretch actually stimulates receptors in the muscle that are designed to help prevent injury due to over-extending the muscle. Thus, the ballistic stretch can cause the muscle to contract rather than relax, and can contribute to muscle soreness. A more appropriate type of muscular stretching for the general population is identified as static stretching.
2. **Static** stretching involves slowly moving the joint to the point of mild discomfort in the muscle and maintaining that angle for approximately thirty seconds before allowing the muscle to relax. The entire procedure should be repeated several times for maximum benefit. As previously noted, a warm-up is highly recommended prior to stretching for injury prevention and to facilitate the stretch. A warm environment and a warm muscle will greatly

enhance the stretch. If the stretch hurts the muscle or the joint, then stop. Learn to distinguish between the mild tensions needed to overload from pain, indicating a potential injury.
3. A third type of stretching activity is called **proprioceptive neuromuscular facilitation** or **PNF**. This activity requires a partner to provide resistance. The basic formula for this activity is to isometrically resist against a partner using the muscle groups surrounding a particular joint, causing contraction, and then relaxing the same muscle group. For example, in stretching the hamstring, both the hamstrings and the quadriceps will be contracted and then relaxed. This contraction and relaxation process will increase the range of motion in the hamstrings. When stretching with a partner, communication is essential to avoid injury to the joint.

When You Should Not Exercise

Injuries

Although injuries do occur during exercise, the benefits of regular exercise far outweigh the risk of injury. In most cases, proper training, clothing, and equipment will prevent injuries. Avoiding injury requires common sense and moderation. One should not attempt to self-diagnose, nor try to "train through the pain." Pain is a signal that something is wrong, and activity should be stopped until the source of the pain is identified and a trained medical professional can advise you. Some common injuries resulting from exercise include joint sprains, muscle strains, and other musculoskeletal problems. Knowing how to treat an acute, or immediate, injury is important (see Table 3.3). **RICE** most injuries, such as a twisted ankle: Rest, Ice, Compression, and Elevation.

Of course, using proper equipment, wearing proper clothing and shoes, and practicing correct technique are essential for injury prevention. Weight-bearing forms of exercise will obviously cause more stress on the joints, but also have benefits that non-weight-bearing activities do not have, such as increasing strength of the bones and other connective tissues.

RICE
R—**Rest** the injured limb, preventing further injury.
I—**Ice** will help reduce swelling by reducing circulation and easing pain. Apply ice in thirty-minute periods several times per day. A Styrofoam cup with frozen water can be used as an ice rub. A bag of frozen peas also works well!
C—**Compression** will help reduce swelling and fluid collection at the injury site. An elastic bandage works well to wrap the injured limb.
E—**Elevating** the injured limb will reduce swelling. Ideally, raise the injured area above the heart. Placing the injured area on pillows on a stool is helpful.

Table 3.3
Reference Guide for Exercise-Related Problems

Injury	Signs/Symptoms	Treatment*
Bruise (contusion)	Pain, swelling, discoloration	Cold application, compression, rest
Dislocations, fractures	Pain, swelling, deformity	Splinting, cold application, seek medical attention
Heat cramps	Cramps, spasms and muscle twitching in the legs, arms, and abdomen	Stop activity, get out of the heat, stretch, massage the painful area, drink plenty of fluids
Heat exhaustion	Fainting, profuse sweating, cold/clammy skin, weak/rapid pulse, weakness, headache	Stop activity, rest in a cool place, loosen clothing, rub body with cool/wet towel, drink plenty of fluids, stay out of heat for two to three days
Heat stroke	Hot/dry skin, no sweating, serious disorientation, rapid/full pulse, vomiting, diarrhea, unconsciousness, high body temperature	Seek immediate medical attention, request help and get out of the sun, bathe in cold water/spray with cold water/rub body with cold towels, drink plenty of cold fluids
Joint sprains	Pain, tenderness, swelling, loss of use, discoloration	Cold application, compression, elevation, rest, heat after thirty-six to forty-eight hours (if no further swelling)
Muscle cramps	Pain, spasms	Stretch muscle(s), use mild exercises for involved area
Muscle soreness and stiffness	Tenderness, pain	Mild stretching, low-intensity exercise, warm bath
Muscle strains	Pain, tenderness, swelling, loss of use	Cold application, compression, elevation, rest, heat after thirty-six to forty-eight hours (if no further swelling)
Shin splints	Pain, tenderness	Cold application prior to and following any physical activity, rest, heat (if no activity is carried out)
Side stitch	Pain on the side of the abdomen below the rib cage	Decrease level of physical activity or stop altogether, gradually increase level of fitness
Tendinitis	Pain, tenderness, loss of use	Rest, cold application, heat after forty-eight hours

*Cold should be applied three or four times a day for fifteen to twenty minutes. Heat should be applied three times a day for fifteen to twenty minutes.

Proper Footwear

It many seem trivial, but proper footwear is critical to success in weight bearing exercise. Shoe technology has come a long way in the past decade. Sport-specific shoes are highly recommended to avoid injury and to enhance performance. Unfortunately, the consumer pays for the research and technology, as well as the logo on the shoes. A good cross trainer shoe is the way to go if you like to do a variety of activities. Cross trainers are not, however, recommended for aerobic dance or running. Running shoes are also not appropriate for "studio activities" such as aerobic dance, step aerobics, BOSU activities, as well as court activities like tennis or racquetball. Running shoes have little lateral support and the higher flared heel can actually cause a person participating

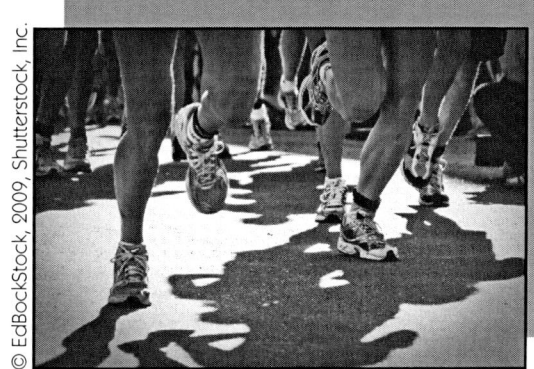

Proper footwear is critical to success in weight bearing exercise. Sport-specific shoes help prevent injury and enhance performance.

How to Buy Athletic Shoes

For many aerobic activities, good shoes are the most important purchase you'll make. Take the time to choose well. Here are some basic guidelines:

- Shop for shoes in the late afternoon, when your feet are most likely to be somewhat swollen—just as they will be after a workout.
- For walking shoes, look for a shoe that's lightweight, flexible, and roomy enough for your toes to wiggle, with a well-cushioned, curved sole; good support at the heel; and an upper made of a material that breathes (allows air in and out).
- For running shoes (see the figure), look for good cushioning, support, and stability. You should be able to wiggle your toes easily, but the front of your foot shouldn't slide from side to side, which could cause blisters. Your toes should not touch the end of the shoes because your feet will swell with activity. Allow about half an inch from the longest toe to the tip of the shoe.
- For racquetball shoes, look for reinforcement at the toe for protection during foot drag. The sole should allow minimal slippage. There should be some heel elevation to lessen strain on the back of the leg and Achilles tendon. The shoe should have a long throat to ensure greater control by the laces.
- For tennis shoes, look for reinforcement at the toe. The sole at the ball of the foot should be well padded because that's where most pressure is exerted. The sides of the shoe should be sturdy, for stability during continuous lateral movements. The toe box should allow ample room and some cushioning at the tips. A long throat ensures greater control by the laces.

What to Look for When You Buy Running Shoes

- Well-molded Achilles pad prevents irritation of Achilles tendon
- Well-padded tongue prevents extensor tendinitis and irritation of dorsum of foot
- Laces not too long so they stay tied longer
- High, rounded toe box (at least 1½" high) prevents subungual hematomas ("black toes")
- Studded sole absorbs shock and provides traction in mud and snow
- Firm heel counter for hindfoot stability
- Flared heel for stability and beveled or rounded heel for quick roll-off
- Soft, raised heel wedge to absorb impact at heel strike
- Flexible midsole helps prevent Achilles tendon problems

Don't wear wet shoes for training. Let wet shoes air dry, because a heater will cause them to stiffen or shrink. Use powder in your shoes to absorb moisture, lessen friction, and prevent fungal infections. Break in new shoes for several days before wearing them for a long-distance run or during competition.

Source: Canadian Podiatric Sports Medicine Academy.

in step aerobics to be more prone to twisting an ankle or knee joint. Some steps also have a rubber top which can grip the waffle sole of the running shoe and increase the risk of injury.

In any athletic shoe, fit and comfort are of the utmost importance. It is worth going to a store staffed by knowledgeable personnel. Often they can give you good insight into the type of shoe that is most appropriate for your foot and your gait.

Environmental Conditions

Take into consideration environmental conditions such as temperature, air pollution, wind-chill, altitude, and humidity that can affect one's health and safety. Dressing appropriately is important when exercising in extreme weather conditions.

When exercising in the cold weather, layering of clothes is advised. There are new fabrics that can wick away moisture from the body better than fabrics such as wool, polypropylene, and cotton. Avoid cotton as a base layer in cold weather because if it gets wet with perspiration it will stay wet and make you colder. The Dupont company pioneered such a fabric called ComfortMax (Powers and Dodd, 2009). This is an advantage because moisture from perspiration can be transferred away (called "wicking") from the body, allowing evaporation to occur. This type of fabric is excellent as a first layer when skiing, jogging, or hiking in cold weather. Outer layers are ideally a waterproof shell that has mesh or zippered compartments to "breathe" and can be peeled off as needed. It is advisable to limit exercise time in extremely cold weather to avoid hypothermia.

Exercising in the heat can be a challenge (see Figure 3.11). It is important to acclimate to the heat and humidity, especially when moving from an area that is cool and arid. Gradually increase duration and intensity when exercising in a new type of environment. Especially in the Southern states, heat injuries are a real concern. Heat cramps, heat exhaustion, and heat stroke can all occur with prolonged exposure to the heat. Heat stroke is a life-threatening condition, and necessitates hospitalization. Heat exhaustion is more common, with individuals typically suffering from dehydration. In order for the body to effectively cool, evaporation of sweat needs to occur. In a humid environment when perspiration drips off of a person, evaporation is not occurring, and therefore cooling is not taking place. A hot and humid environment is especially risky to the very young, the old, and those with low cardiovascular fitness levels.

Heat injuries are much less likely to occur if a person is adequately hydrated. Proper hydration is necessary for the body to function properly. Water aids in controlling body temperature, contributes to the structure and form of the body, and provides the liquid environment for cell processes. When the thirst mechanism is activated, dehydration has already begun. It is important to pre-hydrate, drink before thirst occurs, and especially drink before exercising. The standard recommendation is to drink at least eight eight-ounce glasses of water a day. Exercise increases the body's demand for water due to an increase in metabolic rate and body temperature. Therefore, this amount should be increased. Drinking water every waking hour is a good habit for individuals who exercise on a regular basis. Hydration is very critical in a humid environment. Before, during, and after aerobic exercise, increase the amount of water consumed. Water is necessary for the efficient functioning of the body; thus, the importance of hydration cannot be overstated. Electrolyte levels, especially calcium, sodium, and potassium, are critically important in muscle contraction and should also be carefully maintained. This may be accomplished

Guidelines for Exercising in the Heat

1. Stay hydrated with cool water (cool water is absorbed best in the gut) before, during and after activity.
2. Dress appropriately in clothes that can wick moisture away from the body.
3. Limit exposure time.
4. Exercise with a buddy, or let someone know your plan and stick to it.
5. Wear lightweight sunglasses for eye protection against sun glare, dust and debris in the air. (Important if you exercise near a construction site or near traffic.)
6. Exercise in the coolest time of the day if possible.
7. Stop activity if you experience nausea, dizziness, or extreme headache.
8. Monitor your heart rate, staying within your target heart rate zone.
9. Check the heat index to make sure it is safe to exercise.

Figure 3.11
Heat and Humidity Chart

Air temperature (F°)	Apparent temperature (what it feels like)									
	70°	75°	80°	85°	90°	95°	100°	105°	110°	115°
Relative humidity										
0%	64°	69°	73°	78°	83°	87°	91°	95°	99°	103°
10%	65°	70°	75°	80°	85°	90°	95°	100°	105°	111°
20%	66°	72°	77°	82°	87°	93°	99°	105°	112°	120°
30%	67°	73°	78°	84°	90°	96°	104°	113°	123°	135°
40%	68°	74°	79°	86°	93°	101°	110°	123°	137°	151°
50%	69°	75°	81°	88°	96°	107°	120°	135°	150°	
60%	70°	76°	82°	90°	100°	114°	132°	149°		
70%	70°	77°	85°	93°	106°	124°	144°			
80%	71°	78°	86°	97°	113°	136°				
90%	71°	79°	88°	102°	122°					
100%	72°	80°	91°	108°						

Apparent temperature:	Heat stress risk with exertion:
90°–105°	Heat cramps and heat exhaustion possible.
105°–130°	Heat cramps or heat exhaustion likely; heat stroke possible.
130° and above	Heat stroke highly likely with continued exposure.

To determine the risk of exercising in the heat, locate the outside air temperature on the top horizontal scale and the relative humidity on the left vertical scale. Where these two values intersect is the apparent temperature. For example, on a 90°F day with 70 percent humidity, the apparent temperature is 106°F. Heat cramps or heat exhaustion are likely to occur, and heat stroke is possible during exercise under these conditions.
Source: Adapted from U.S. Department of Commerce, National Oceanic and Atmospheric Administration, Heat index chart, in *Heat wave: A major summer killer.* Washington, D.C.: Government Printing Office, 1992.

through re-hydrating with sports drinks. Sports drinks are useful for glycogen replacement when the duration of an activity is sixty to ninety minutes or longer or if the athlete is in a tournament with multiple events.

Hyponatremia

Avoiding dehydration is critical when exercising, especially in the heat and high humidity. There is, however, a possibility of over-hydration, which can be just as critical. Due to the popularity of longer road races, more people are participating in 10-K races, triathlons, and marathons. There are more marathon walkers than ever before. A walker can be on the course for a much longer time than a runner—perhaps six or seven hours. If the walker is hydrating the entire time, it is possible to over-hydrate. This over-hydration can lead to a condition called hyponatremia, also called water intoxication. Hyponatremia is characterized by a low sodium concentration in the blood. Hyponatremia is seen in some medical conditions such as certain forms of lung cancer. Exercise-associated hyponatremia involves excess ADH (antidiuretic hormone) being secreted from the pituitary gland. The longer a person sweats, the higher the risk of hyponatremia due to lost electrolytes. Hyponatremia can be life-threatening, and unfortunately the hyponatremia symptoms mimic the symptoms of heat illness (fatigue, light headedness, nausea, cramping, headache, dizziness). If you treat a hyponatremia victim the same way you would a heat illness victim, you could accelerate their decline. The best way to

Adverse Effects of Dehydration

Exercise in the heat can be extremely dangerous, depending on exercise intensity, ambient temperature, relative humidity, clothing, and state of hydration (water content of the body). Although some forms of heat injury can occur prior to significant weight loss due to sweating, the table in this box shows how weight loss during exercise can be a predictor of some of the dangers associated with exercise in the heat. The loss of body weight during exercise in the heat is simply due to water loss through sweating. Thus, prolonged, profuse sweating is the first warning signal of impending dehydration.

% Body Weight Loss	Symptoms	% Body Weight Loss	Symptoms
0.5	Thirst	6.0	Impaired temperature regulation, increased heart rate
2.0	Stronger thirst, vague discomfort, loss of appetite	8.0	Dizziness, labored breathing during exercise, confusion
3.0	Concentrated blood, dry mouth, reduced urine output	10.0	Spastic muscles, loss of balance, delirium
4.0	Increased effort required during exercise, flushed skin, apathy	11.0	Circulatory insufficiency, decreased blood volume, kidney failure
5.0	Difficulty in concentrating		

Source: From *Total Fitness and Wellness,* 5th Edition, by Powers and Dodd, Benjamin Cummings Publishers.

avoid hyponatremia, or dehydration for that matter, is to be aware of fluid loss and fluid intake. After approximately sixty minutes of activity, it is best to rehydrate in part with sports drinks that contain electrolytes such as sodium and chloride. It is also prudent to eat a normal diet including salt-containing foods unless you are restricted by your physician from sodium in your diet. When competing in races, avoid ingesting aspirin, ibuprofen, or acetaminophen, which can interfere with kidney functioning. As with other things in life, balance is the key.

Illness

Use common sense when ill. If you have cold symptoms with no fever, then possibly a light workout might make you feel better. If fever is present, you have a headache, extreme fatigue, muscle aches, swollen lymph glands, or if you have flu-like symptoms, then bed rest is recommended. Marathon efforts of high intensity and long duration have been shown to temporarily suppress the immune system. Mild to moderate exercise has been shown to enhance the immune system and to reduce risk of respiratory infections (ACSM, 1989).

Common Sense Concerns

- *Lightning*—DO NOT exercise if there is lightning in the area. Stay indoors.
- *Air pollution*—When the air quality is poor, exercise early in the morning, later in the evening, or preferably indoors, especially for those with lung or heart disease. Pay attention to air pollution alerts. Avoid high traffic areas.

- *Allergens*—Check weather reports for pollen counts, and avoid outdoor vigorous exercise when the pollen count is high.
- *Night exercise*—It is common for some to walk, jog, or bike on the shoulder of roads. Drivers need to use caution; sometimes the glare from oncoming traffic can obscure visibility. However, night exercisers must be responsible and make themselves more visible at night:

1. Use a flashlight.
2. Dress in *white* clothing—there is an amazing difference in visibility between gray and white shirts at night.
3. Wear a reflective vest or reflective arm bands.
4. Walk in a well-lit, safe area if possible.
5. Be safe, be aware of your surroundings, and use common sense.
6. Don't go alone; go with friends or borrow a dog if you don't have your own.
7. Carry ID with you.
8. Do NOT let headphones distract you from traffic or safety concerns.
9. Use flashing lights that can be attached to a belt or arm band.
10. Remember when walking to face the oncoming traffic if possible.
11. Let someone know your route and expected time back.
12. Be aware that drivers may have difficulty seeing you at twilight.

Use common sense when environmental conditions are significant!

The Biggest Risk to Exercise Is Not Starting!

The internal conditions of the body before and during exercise are even more crucial than exercising with the proper external conditions. Eating a regular meal immediately before exercising will usually result in poor performance, stomach cramps, and sometimes even vomiting. The days of a steak and potato pre-game meal are gone. It is important to fuel your body with low fat and high carbohydrate foods prior to competition; however, even more important is fueling your body on a daily basis. Everyday good nutrition will cause an athlete to perform better in practice, thereby optimizing training that may result in a better performance in competition. This is also sound advice for non-athletes trying to stay active. The recommendations for individuals involved in a regular exercise program are: 55 to 60 percent of total calories consumed should be from carbohydrates, 25 to 30 percent from fat, and 12 to 15 percent from protein. Individuals who are involved in a high-intensity muscular training program should consume a higher amount of protein and less fat for muscle growth and maintenance. Adequate hydration is also critical and can make a difference in the quality of exercise and performance.

If you're interested in training for a 5K or 10K fun run, visit Smart Coach at runnersworld.com. You will find a beginning runner's training guide that includes free advice according to your personal fitness and training level.

Staying active has clearly been shown to enhance a person's quality of life. Exercise is for everyone; it is never too early or too late to start. Most people know that they would benefit from participating in an exercise program, but for many it is difficult to get started. Find an activity you enjoy. Make a plan. Write it down. Get a workout buddy. Start slowly, and listen to your body. Pain is usually a signal that something is wrong. The old adage 'no pain, no gain' can cause beginners to become frustrated. Balance activity, leisure time, and rest each week. With consistency, activity can have a positive impact on reducing risk for many conditions associated with too little activity, called hypokinetic conditions. And most importantly, you should experience increased stamina, enthusiasm, and enhanced mental well-being in your daily life.

REFERENCES

American College of Sports Medicine (ACSM). *Exercise and the Common Cold.* 1989.

ACSM/AHA Joint Position Stand "Exercise and Acute Cardiovascular Events: Placing Risks into Perspective." *Medicine and Science in Sports and Exercise.* 2007.

American Heart Association. *Heart and Stroke Statistical Update.* Dallas: American Heart Association. 2009.

Bishop, J. G. and Aldana, S. G. *Step Up to Wellness.* Needham Heights, MA: Allyn & Bacon. 1999.

Cissik, J. M. *The Basics of Strength Training.* New York: McGraw-Hill Companies, Inc. 1998.

Corbin, C. B. and Lindsey, R. *Concepts of Fitness and Wellness: Active Lifestyles for Wellness* (15th ed). McGraw Hill. 2009.

Corbin, C. et al. Physical Activity for Children: A Statement of Guidelines for Children Age 5–12, NASPE. Dec. 2003.

Evans, W. J. Vitamin E, Vitamin C, and Exercise. *American Journal of Clinical Nutrition,* Vol. 72, 647s-652s. August 2000.

Fox, E., Bowers, R., and Merle, F. *The Physiological Basis for Exercise and Sport* (5th ed). Madison, WI: WCB Brown & Benchmark Publishers. 1989.

Haskell, W. L. et al. Physical Activity and Public Health: Updated Recommendations for Adults from the American College of Sports Medicine. *Medicine and Science in Sports and Exercise* 39 (8):1424–1434 Belmont, CA: Wadsworth/Thompson Learning. 2007.

Healthier U.S. Initiative; www.whitehouse.gov

McArdle, W. D., Katch, F. I., and Katch, V. L. *Exercise Physiology: Energy, Nutrition, and Human Performance.* Baltimore: Williams and Wilkins. 1999.

Pate, R., Pratt, M., Blair, S., Haskell, W., Macera, C., et al. Physical Activity and Public Health: A Recommendation from the Centers for Disease Control and Prevention and the American College of Sports Medicine. *Journal of the American Medical Association,* 273: 402–407. 1995.

Payne, W. A. and Hahn, D. B. *Understanding Your Health* (6th ed). St. Louis, MO: Mosby. 2000.

Physical Activity and Health: A Report of the Surgeon General. Atlanta: U.S. Department of Health and Human Services, Centers for Disease Control and Prevention, National Center for Chronic Disease Prevention and Health Promotion. 1996.

Pollock, M. L., Gaesser, G. A., Butcher, J. D., Despres, J-P., Dishman, R. K., et al. ACSM Position Stand on the Recommended Quantity and Quality of Exercise for Developing and Maintaining Cardiorespiratory and Muscular Fitness, and Flexibility in Adults. *Medicine & Science in Sports & Exercise, 30:* 975–991. 1998.

Powers, S. K., and Dodd, S. L. *Total Fitness and Wellness* (5th ed). San Francisco: Pearson Benjamin Cummings. 2009.

Powers, S. K., and Howley, E. T. *Exercise Physiology: Theory and Application to Fitness and Performance* (6th ed). New York: McGraw-Hill Companies, Inc. 2006.

Rosato, F. *Fitness to Wellness: The Physical Connection* (3rd ed.) Minneapolis: West. 1994.

Sabo, E. *Good Exercises for Bad Knees.* www.healthology.com; Retrieved June 14, 2005.

Sharkey, B. J. *Fitness and Health.* Champaign, IL: Human Kinetics Publishing. 1997.

Sieg, K. W., and Adams, S. P. *Illustrated Essentials of Musculoskeletal Anatomy.* Gainesville, FL: Megabooks Inc. 1985.

2005 Dietary Guidelines, www.health.gov.

Why We Are Losing the War on Obesity; Health Annual Editions 05/06, 26th edition, McGraw-Hill/Dushkin.

Wilmore, J. H. and Costill, D. L. *Physiology of Sport and Exercise.* Champaign, IL: Human Kinetics Publishing Company. 1999.

CONTACTS

American College of Sports Medicine (ACSM)
http://www.acsm.org/index.asp

American Council of Exercise
Cardiovascular Fitness Facts
www.acefitness.org/fitfacts/fitfacts_list.cfm#1

American Running Association
http://www.americanrunning.org

American Heart Association
www.americanheart.org/statistics/

American Heart Association Web site for tips, health facts, a personal trainer, and more
www.justmove.org/fitnessnews

American Medical Association
http://www.ama-assn.org

Centers for Disease Control and Prevention
http://www.cdc.gov/nccdphp/sgr/mm.thm

National Institute of Arthritis and Musculoskeletal and Skin Diseases
http://www.healthfinder.gov/

National Institute for Health
Web site for lowering blood pressure.
http://www.nhlbi.nih.gov/hbp/

President's Council on Physical Fitness and Sports
Fitness Fundamentals
http://www.hoptechno.com/book11.htm

President's Council on Physical Fitness and Sports
The Link Between Physical Activity and Morbidity and Mortality
http://www.cdc.gov/nccdphp/sgr/mm.htm

Tucker Center—Women in Sport
http://www.kls.coled.umn.edu/crgws/

Results from the President's Council on Physical Fitness
http://www.girsite.org/Html/nike2.htm

Shape Up America!
http://www.shapeup.org

Excellent current information regarding osteoporosis treatment and prevention.
www.osteo.org/osteo.html

www.nhlbi.nih.gov

www.healthfinder.gov

www.medlineplus.gov

www.nutrition.gov

www.fitness.gov

UCBerkelyWellnessLetter.com

Women's Health womenshealth.gov

ACTIVITIES

Notebook Activities

Safety of Exercise Participation: PAR-Q and YOU

Calculating Your Activity Index

Karvonen Formula

Developing an Exercise Program for Cardiorespiratory Endurance

Assessing Your Current Level of Muscular Endurance

Check Your Physical Activity and Heart Disease I.Q.

Assessing Cardiovascular Fitness: Cooper's 1.5-Mile Run

Name: _____ Section: _____ Date: _____

NOTEBOOK ACTIVITY

Safety of Exercise Participation: PAR-Q and You
(A Questionnaire for People Aged 15 to 69)

Regular physical activity is fun and healthy, and increasingly more people are starting to become more active every day. Being more active is very safe for most people. However, some people should check with their doctor before they start becoming much more physically active.

If you are planning to become much more physically active than you are now, start by answering the seven questions in the box below. If you are between the ages of 15 and 69, the PAR-Q will tell you if you should check with your doctor before you start. If you are over 69 years of age, and you are not used to being very active, check with your doctor.

Common sense is your best guide when you answer these questions. Please read the questions carefully and answer each one honestly: Check YES or NO.

YES	NO	
❏	❏	1. Has your doctor ever said that you have a heart condition and that you should only do physical activity recommended by a doctor?
❏	❏	2. Do you feel pain in your chest when you do physical activity?
❏	❏	3. In the past month, have you had chest pain when you were not doing physical activity?
❏	❏	4. Do you lose your balance because of dizziness, or do you ever lose consciousness?
❏	❏	5. Do you have a bone or joint problem that could be made worse by a change in your physical activity?
❏	❏	6. Is your doctor currently prescribing drugs (for example, water pills) for your blood pressure or heart condition?
❏	❏	7. Do you know of any other reason why you should not do physical activity?

If you answered

YES to one or more questions

Talk with your doctor by phone or in person BEFORE you start becoming much more physically active or BEFORE you have a fitness appraisal. Tell your doctor about the PAR-Q and which questions you answered YES.
- You may be able to do any activity you want—as long as you start slowly and build up gradually. Or, you may need to restrict your activities to those that are safe for you. Talk with your doctor about the kinds of activities you wish to participate in and follow his/her advice.
- Find out which community programs are safe and helpful for you.

NO to all questions

If you answered NO honestly to all PAR-Q questions, you can be reasonably sure that you can:
- start becoming much more physically active—begin slowly and build up gradually. This is the safest and easiest way to go.
- take part in a fitness appraisal—this is an excellent way to determine your basic fitness so that you can plan the best way for you to live actively.

DELAY BECOMING MUCH MORE ACTIVE:

- if you are not feeling well because of a temporary illness such as a cold or a fever—wait until you feel better, or
- if you are or may be pregnant—talk to your doctor before you start becoming more active.

Please note: If your health changes so that you then answer YES to any of the above questions, tell your fitness or health professional. Ask whether you should change your physical activity plan.

Informed Use of the PAR-Q: The Canadian Society for Exercise Physiology, Health Canada, and their agents assume no liability for persons who undertake physical activity, and if in doubt after completing this questionnaire, consult your doctor prior to physical activity.

> You are encouraged to copy the PAR-Q but only if you use the entire form.

Note: If the PAR-Q is being given to a person before he or she participates in a physical activity program or a fitness appraisal, this section may be used for legal or administrative purposes.

I have read, understood and completed this questionnaire. Any questions I had were answered to my full satisfaction.

Name _____
Signature _____ Date _____
Signature of parent _____ Witness _____
or Guardian (for participants under the age of majority)

© *Canadian Society for Exercise Physiology*
Société canadienne de physiologie de l'exercice

Supported by: Health Canada   Santé Canada

Source: PAR-Q: Reprinted from the 1994 revised version of the Physical Activity Readiness Questionnaire (PAR-Q and YOU). The PAR-Q and YOU is a copyrighted, pre-exercise screen owned by the Canadian Society for Exercise Physiology.

Name: _____ Section: _____ Date: _____

NOTEBOOK ACTIVITY

Calculating Your Activity Index

Frequency: How often do you exercise?

If you exercise:	Your frequency score is:
Less than 1 time a week	0
1 time a week	1
2 times a week	2
3 times a week	3
4 times a week	4
5 or more times a week	5

Duration: How long do you exercise?

If your total duration of exercise is:	Your duration score is:
Less than 5 minutes	0
5–14 minutes	1
15–29 minutes	2
30–44 minutes	3
45–59 minutes	4
60 minutes or more	5

Intensity: How hard do you exercise?

If exercise results in:	Your intensity score is:
No change in pulse from resting level	0
Slight increase in pulse from resting level	1
Slight increase in pulse and breathing	2
Moderate increase in pulse and breathing	3
Intermittent heavy breathing and sweating	4
Sustained heavy breathing and sweating	5

Multiply your three scores:

Frequency _____ × Duration _____ × Intensity _____ = Activity index _____

To determine your activity index, refer to the following table:

If your activity index is:	Your estimated level of activity is:
Less than 15	Sedentary
15–24	Low active
25–40	Moderate active
41–60	Active
Over 60	High active

NOTEBOOK ACTIVITY

Karvonen Formula

Determining Target Heart Rate Zone (THRZ)

Take your resting heart rate early in the morning before you rise, counting for sixty seconds. Use your index and middle finger to palpate either your carotid (neck) or radial (wrist) artery. It is best to do this three different times and then average the three resting heart rates.

Finding your target heart rate zone is beneficial so that you can determine at any given time during a workout how hard your heart is working. This gives you feedback that helps you construct a proper workout that matches your goals. Working out with intensity high enough to bring the heart rate above the minimum threshold is important to attain cardiovascular benefits of exercise.

EXAMPLE:
AGE: 20 yr. old RESTING HEART RATE: 68 bpm

Formula for calculating Maximum Heart Rate (Max HR)
220 – age (in years) = Maximum Heart Rate

Example
220 – 20 = 200 beats per minute (bpm)

Formula for calculating Heart Rate Reserve
Max HR – Resting HR = Heart Rate Reserve

Example
200 – 68 = 132 beats per minute

Formula for calculating Threshold of Training HR
HR Reserve × 60%
Plus Resting HR = Threshold of Training HR

Example
132 × .60 = 80 bpm
80 + 68 = 148 bpm

Formula for calculating the Upper Limit of the THRZ
HR Reserve × 85%
Plus Resting HR = Upper Limit for the THRZ

Example
132 × .85 = 112
112 + 68 = 180 bpm

The target zone for this 20-year-old with a resting HR of 68 bpm is 148 – 180 bpm.

Your age: _____   Your Resting HR _____ bpm

Max HR = 220 – _____ = _____

Max HR – RHR = HR Reserve   _____ – _____ = _____

HR Reserve × 60% + RHR = Minimum Threshold
_____ × .60 = _____ + _____ = _____

HR Reserve × 85% + RHR = Upper Limit
_____ × .85 = _____ + _____ = _____

Your target heart rate zone is _____ bpm (60%) to _____ bpm (85%)

Name: _____ Section: _____ Date: _____

NOTEBOOK ACTIVITY

Developing an Exercise Program for Cardiorespiratory Endurance

Goals: Identify three goals you want to accomplish as a result of this program. Goals should be accomplished by the end of the semester.

1. _____

2. _____

3. _____

Activities: Identify three different activities you will perform.

1. _____
2. _____
3. _____

Duration: Fill in an amount of time for each exercise session and activity.

    Activity   Duration

1. _____
2. _____
3. _____

Name: _____ Section: _____ Date: _____

NOTEBOOK ACTIVITY

Assessing Your Current Level of Muscular Endurance

Push-up Test:

Men should use the standard push-up position with hands shoulder-width apart and feet on the floor. Women may modify the standard push-up position by putting their knees on the floor. Complete as many push-ups as possible without stopping, and evaluate your performance according to the following.

MEN				
Age	20s	30s	40s	50s
Good	40	36	30	27
Fair	35	30	25	22
Poor	30	25	21	18

WOMEN				
Age	20s	30s	40s	50s
Good	38	33	27	22
Fair	32	27	22	18
Poor	27	22	18	15

Curl-up Test:

Begin by lying on your back, arms by your sides with palms down and on the floor and fingers straight. Your knees should be bent at about ninety degrees, with your feet twelve inches away from your buttocks. To perform a curl up, curl your head and upper back upward, keeping your arms straight. Slide your fingers forward along the floor until you touch the back of your heels. Then curl back down until your back and head reach the floor. Palms, feet, and buttocks remain on the floor the entire time. Perform as many curl-ups as you can in one minute without stopping to rest, and evaluate your performance according to the following.

MEN				
Age	20s	30s	40s	50s
Good	25	25	25	25
Fair	22	22	21	19
Poor	13	13	11	09

WOMEN				
Age	20s	30s	40s	50s
Good	25	25	25	25
Fair	22	21	20	15
Poor	13	11	06	04

Name: _____ Section: _____ Date: _____

NOTEBOOK ACTIVITY

Check Your Physical Activity and Heart Disease I.Q.

Test how much you know about how physical activity affects your heart. Mark each statement true or false. See how you did by checking the answers on the back of this sheet.

1. Regular physical activity can reduce your chances of getting heart disease.   T   F

2. Most people get enough physical activity from their normal daily routine.   T   F

3. You don't have to train like a marathon runner to become more physically fit.   T   F

4. Exercise programs do not require a lot of time to be very effective.   T   F

5. People who need to lose some weight are the only ones who will benefit from regular physical activity.   T   F

6. All exercises give you the same benefits.   T   F

7. The older you are, the less active you need to be.   T   F

8. It doesn't take a lot of money or expensive equipment to become physically fit.   T   F

9. There are many risks and injuries that can occur with exercise.   T   F

10. You should consult a doctor before starting a physical activity program.   T   F

11. People who have had a heart attack should not start any physical activity program.   T   F

12. To help stay physically active, include a variety of activities.   T   F

Source: Department of Health and Human Services, National Institutes of Health.

Answers to the Check Your Physical Activity and Heart Disease I.Q. Quiz

1. **True.** Heart disease is almost twice as likely to develop in inactive people. Being physically inactive is a risk factor for heart disease along with cigarette smoking, high blood pressure, high blood cholesterol, and being overweight. The more risk factors you have, the greater your chance for heart disease. Regular physical activity (even mild to moderate exercise) can reduce this risk.

2. **False.** Most Americans are very busy but not very active. Every American adult should make a habit of getting thirty minutes of low to moderate levels of physical activity daily. This includes walking, gardening, and walking up stairs. If you are inactive now, begin by doing a few minutes of activity each day. If you only do some activity every once in a while, try to work something into your routine everyday.

3. **True.** Low- to moderate-intensity activities, such as pleasure walking, stair climbing, yardwork, housework, dancing, and home exercises can have both short- and long-term benefits. If you are inactive, the key is to get started. One great way is to take a walk for ten to fifteen minutes during your lunch break, or take your dog for a walk every day. At least thirty minutes of physical activity everyday can help improve your heart health.

4. **True.** It takes only a few minutes a day to become more physically active. If you don't have thirty minutes in your schedule for an exercise break, try to find two fifteen-minute periods or even three ten-minute periods. These exercise breaks will soon become a habit you can't live without.

5. **False.** People who are physically active experience many positive benefits. Regular physical activity gives you more energy, reduces stress, and helps you to sleep better. It helps to lower high blood pressure and improves blood cholesterol levels. Physical activity helps to tone your muscles, burns off calories to help you lose extra pounds or stay at your desirable weight, and helps control your appetite. It can also increase muscle strength, help your heart and lungs work more efficiently, and let you enjoy your life more fully.

6. **False.** Low-intensity activities—if performed daily—can have some long-term health benefits and can lower your risk of heart disease. Regular, brisk, and sustained exercise for at least thirty minutes, three or four times a week, such as brisk walking, jogging, or swimming, is necessary to improve the efficiency of your heart and lungs and burn off extra calories. These activities are called aerobic—meaning the body uses oxygen to produce the energy needed for the activity. Other activities, depending on the type, may give you other benefits such as increased flexibility or muscle strength.

7. **False.** Although we tend to become less active with age, physical activity is still important. In fact, regular physical activity in older persons increases their capacity to do everyday activities. In general, middle-aged and older people benefit from regular physical activity just as young people do. What is important, at any age, is tailoring the activity program to your own fitness level.

8. **True.** Many activities require little or no equipment. For example, brisk walking only requires a comfortable pair of walking shoes. Many communities offer free or inexpensive recreation facilities and physical activity classes. Check your shopping malls, as many of them are open early and late for people who do not wish to walk alone, in the dark, or in bad weather.

9. **False.** The most common risk in exercising is injury to the muscles and joints. Such injuries are usually caused by exercising too hard for too long, particularly if a person has been inactive. To avoid injuries, try to build up your level of activity gradually, listen to your body for warning pains, be aware of possible signs of heart problems (such as pain or pressure in the left or mid-chest area, left neck, shoulder, or arm during or just after exercising, or sudden light-headedness, cold sweat, pallor, or fainting), and be prepared for special weather conditions.

10. **True.** You should ask your doctor before you start (or greatly increase) your physical activity if you have a medical condition such as high blood pressure, have pains or pressure in the chest and shoulder, feel dizzy or faint, get breathless after mild exertion, are middle-aged or older and have not been physically active, or plan a vigorous activity program. If none of these apply, start slow and get moving.

11. **False.** Regular physical activity can help reduce your risk of having another heart attack. People who include regular physical activity in their lives after a heart attack improve their chances of survival and can improve how they feel and look. If you have had a heart attack, consult your doctor to be sure you are following a safe and effective exercise program that will help prevent heart pain and further damage from overexertion.

12. **True.** Pick several different activities that you like doing. You will be more likely to stay with it. Plan short-term and long-term goals. Keep a record of your progress, and check it regularly to see the progress you have made. Get your family and friends to join in. They can help keep you going.

Name: _____ Section: _____ Date: _____

NOTEBOOK ACTIVITY

Assessing Cardiovascular Fitness: Cooper's 1.5-Mile Run

(Please note: If you are not comfortable with the run, use the Rockport Fitness test found in Table 3.2 on page 69.)

This test is optimally done on a track for six laps.

Prior to testing, get a good night's rest, drink water, and try to choose a time of day when the weather is agreeable. If you cannot run the entire test, you may walk-run as best you can. It may be advisable to practice running a 1.5-mile distance prior to testing to determine a reasonable pace for you. Use a stopwatch for accuracy in timing. The objective of this test is to complete the six laps as quickly as possible.

Warm up first.
Run; note time.
Recover, stretch, drink water.

Fitness Categories for Cooper's 1.5-Mile Run Test to Determine Cardiorespiratory Fitness

Fitness Category	Age (years)					
	13–19	20–29	30–39	40–49	50–59	60+
Men						
Very poor	>15:30	>16:00	>16:30	>17:30	>19:00	>20:00
Poor	12:11–15:30	14:01–16:00	14:46–16:30	15:36–17:30	17:01–19:00	19:01–20:00
Average	10:49–12:10	12:01–14:00	12:31–14:45	13:01–15:35	14:31–17:00	16:16–19:00
Good	9:41–10:48	10:46–12:00	11:01–12:30	11:31–13:00	12:31–14:30	14:00–16:15
Excellent	8:37–9:40	9:45–10:45	10:00–11:00	10:30–11:30	11:00–12:30	11:15–13:59
Superior	<8:37	<9:45	<10:00	<10:30	<11:00	<11:15
Women						
Very poor	>18:30	>19:00	>19:30	>20:00	>20:30	>21:00
Poor	16:55–18:30	18:31–19:00	19:01–19:30	19:31–20:00	20:01–20:30	20:31–21:31
Average	14:31–16:54	15:55–18:30	16:31–19:00	17:31–19:30	19:01–20:00	19:31–20:30
Good	12:30–14:30	13:31–1554	14:31–16:30	15:56–17:30	16:31–19:00	17:31–19:30
Excellent	11:50–12:29	12:30–13:30	13:00–14:30	13:45–15:55	14:30–16:30	16:30–18:00
Superior	<11:50	<12:30	<13:00	<13:45	<14:30	<16:30

Times are given in minutes and seconds. (> = greater than; < = less than)
From Cooper, K. *The aerobics program for total well-being.* Bantam Books, New York, 1982.

Date _____ Temperature _____ Relative Humidity _____

Location of test _____

Finish time _____

Fitness category _____

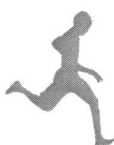

CHAPTER 4

Lifestyle Choices and Hypokinetic Conditions

*"When health is absent
wisdom cannot reveal itself,
art cannot become manifest,
strength cannot be exerted
wealth is useless
and reason is powerless"*

—Herophilies, 300 B.C.

OBJECTIVES

Students will be able to:
- Discuss the major hypokinetic diseases afflicting Americans.
- List the six major cardiac risk factors and the three unalterable cardiac risk factors.
- Know the warning signs for a heart attack.
- Discuss three ways to combat obesity.
- Discuss ways to prevent osteoporosis and achieve a high peak bone mass.
- Explain three ways to prevent low back pain.
- List and discuss four lifestyle choices that prevent hypokinetic conditions.

> Taken from a Report to the President from the Secretary of Health and Human Services and the Secretary of Education
>
> ### Executive Summary: Promoting Better Health for Young People through Physical Activity and Sports
>
> "Our Nation's young people are, in large measure, inactive, unfit, and increasingly overweight. In the long run, this physical inactivity threatens to reverse the decades-long progress we have made in reducing death from cardiovascular diseases and to devastate our national healthcare budget. In the short run, physical inactivity has contributed to an unprecedented epidemic of childhood obesity that is currently plaguing the United States. The percentage of young people who are overweight has doubled since 1980. *Enhancing efforts to promote participation in physical activity and sports among young people is a critical national priority.*"

The life expectancy for someone born at the beginning of the twenty-first century is almost double the life expectancy of those born at the beginning of the twentieth century. Modern medicine has, for the most part, wiped out the threat from infectious diseases. Modern technology has made life easy. Life is so automated that we move less, and therefore we conserve lots of energy. The more sedentary people become, the higher the health risk. It is no longer polio, smallpox, or tuberculosis that are a large-scale threat to survival (see Figure 4.1), it is our own poor lifestyle choices. The Centers for Disease Control and Prevention (CDC) has determined that *lifestyle is the single largest factor affecting longevity of life.* "If exercise could be packed into a pill, it would be the single most widely prescribed, and most beneficial, medicine in the nation" (National Institute on Aging). More than half of the population will die from coronary heart disease—a disease that for many can be prevented with simple healthy lifestyle choices. The choices we make daily determine not only the longevity of our lives but also the quality of our lives—now and in the future.

Daily, we determine whether or not we will eat breakfast, use tobacco, abuse drugs, hold a grudge, or make time for exercise. As Westerners living in an industrialized nation, we are fortunate to have choices. We have the privilege to choose from at least eighteen brands of toothpaste. Toothpaste brands may not have a significant impact on the quality of our life, but other daily decisions do. How we handle ourselves when stressed is a significant factor in whether or not we become ill. Nutrition choices at dinnertime and in between meals . . . Cheetos, Cheerios, or cheese? Choosing to be more active daily, such as gardening, taking the stairs instead of the elevator, walking rather than riding, can make a surprising dent in our energy reserves. The 1996 Surgeon General's Report (Satcher, 1996) encouraged all individuals to try and expend 150 calories extra each day, above and beyond a normal routine. **Lifestyle activity** is searching for opportunities to expend some extra energy, rather than searching for opportunities to conserve energy with convenient devices such as cell phones and electric pencil sharpeners. Students who walk across big campuses between classes rather than take a bus expend more energy. One day might not have a

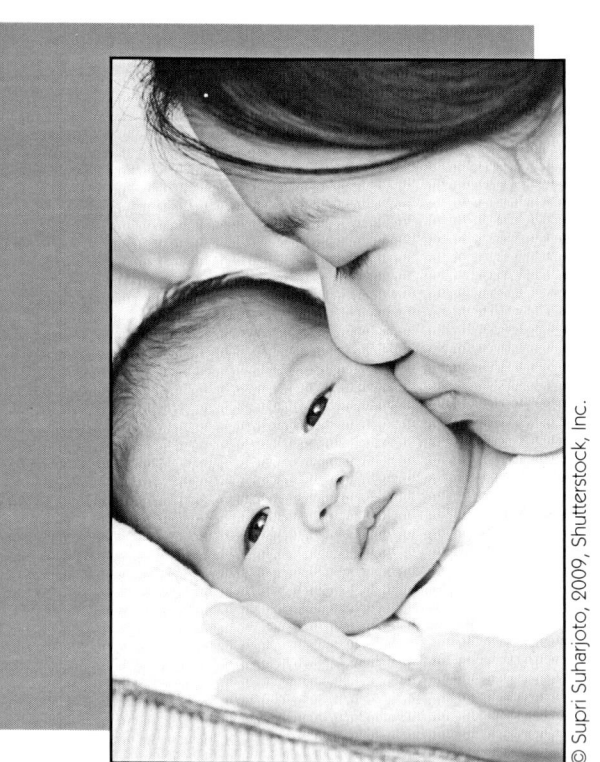

The life expectancy of this baby is almost double that of a baby born one hundred years ago.

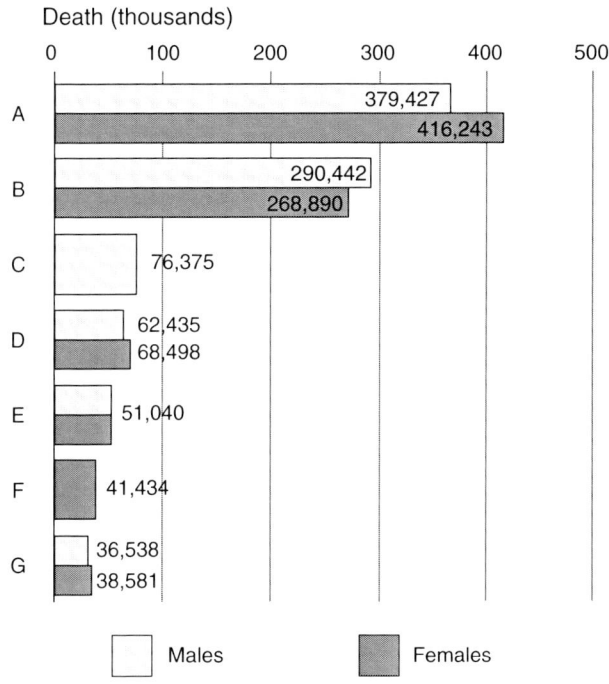

FIGURE 4.1

Leading Causes of Death, United States, 2005

This graph shows that cardiovascular disease is the number one cause of death for both men and women (all races, all ages).

A Total cardiovascular (including cerebrovascular) diseases
B Cancer
C Accidents—males
D Chronic lower respiratory diseases
E Alzheimer's disease
F Accidents—females
G Diabetes mellitus

Source: National Vital Statistics Report 56(10), CDC.

Examples of Lifestyle Activity: Looking for Opportunities to Expend More Calories

- Taking the stairs instead of the elevator.
- Parking farther from your destination to increase walking distance.
- Walking rather than riding.
- Vacuuming with vigor, taking big lunging steps.
- Doing sit-ups during the commercials of your favorite program.
- Playing Frisbee or planting a garden instead of watching TV.

significant impact; however, at the end of the semester the cumulative effects of walking can add up to enhanced health.

Planned exercise is important for fitness benefits. It is important to find an activity that is enjoyable because that will ensure a more sincere commitment—one that may become permanent over a lifetime. Plan it! Don't leave your exercise to chance, because chances are, you won't have time. If you hate to run, don't train for a marathon. Set realistic goals. Research has shown that specific goal setting greatly enhances the chances of achieving said goals. Use the goal activity at the end of Chapter 1. Be reasonable and look for behaviors to change in support of your goals. Enlist the help and support of friends and family. Walking is the most popular activity in the United States, most likely because it is easy and requires no special training or equipment except a good pair of shoes. Choose an activity you enjoy and as the shoe company says "Just do it!"

Lifestyle activity, planned exercise, stress management, and good nutrition choices can make a difference in whether or not an individual suffers from a hypokinetic condition. **Hypokinetic** literally means too little activity. Kraus and Rabb first coined the term hypokinetic in 1961. Hypokinetic diseases include the leading causes of death, such as coronary heart disease and cancer, as well as debilitating conditions such as low back pain, osteoporosis, obesity, diabetes, and mental health disorders. Simply changing an individual's lifestyle to one that includes more physical activity can reduce the incidence of many hypokinetic conditions. Regular consistent activity can decrease the potential of contracting a hypokinetic disease.

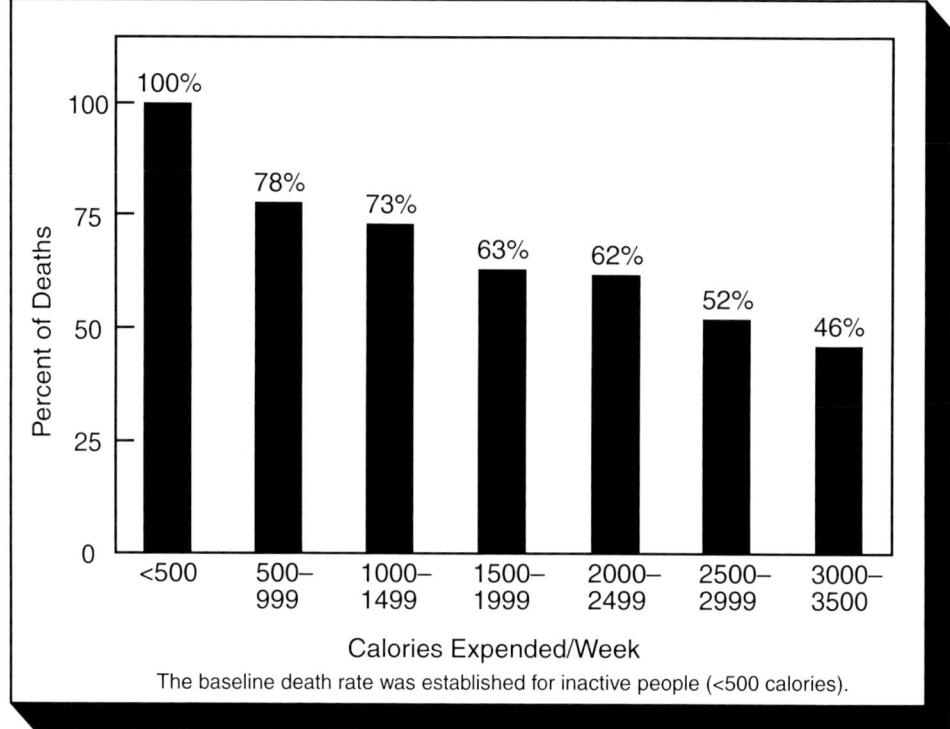

FIGURE 4.2

Deaths Decrease as Caloric Expenditure Increases

Source: Data from C. Bouchard et al. *Exercise Fitness and Health*. Champaign, IL: Human Kinetics Publishers, 1990.

For example, expending an extra 500–1,000 calories per week can decrease health risk (see Figure 4.2). Expending an extra 1,000–2,000 calories per week can decrease overall health risk more and also moderately increase cardiovascular fitness. An expenditure of 2,000–3,500 calories per week can decrease overall health risk, as well as significantly increase cardiovascular fitness over time. Typically expending beyond 3,500 calories can increase risk of musculoskeletal injuries and burnout.

Caloric expenditure from both lifestyle activity and planned exercise has a significant impact on health. Participating in a little extra activity helps by decreasing overall health risk and by enhancing self-confidence. Expending more extra energy does the same as expending a little extra activity with further decreased risk, added fitness benefits, and potential weight loss, particularly if exercise is within the target heart rate zone (see Figure 4.3). However, doing too much activity can cause burn-out, injury, or possibly an obsession with exercise. As in all areas of life, balance and common sense are important.

It has been previously noted that the CDC reported that lifestyle is the single greatest factor affecting longevity of life. This is especially critical to note for future generations as America's children are more sedentary and at higher risk for developing hypokinetic diseases than their parents or grandparents. Childhood obesity is a national epidemic; this is partially due to technology (think energy-saving remote controls and cell phones) and the ease with which tasks are performed. To combat this trend, parents can help plan activities to ensure their children accumulate at least sixty minutes of activity a day. The best way to accomplish this is for parents to be good role models and to lead active lifestyles. Parents

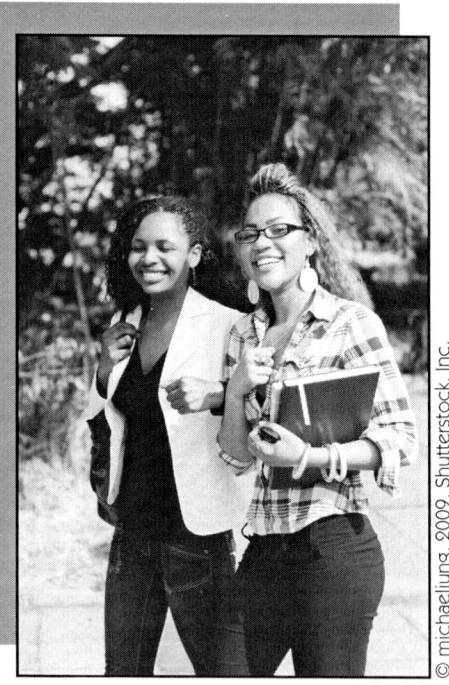

Students who walk to class rather than ride are increasing their lifestyle activity and their metabolic rate.

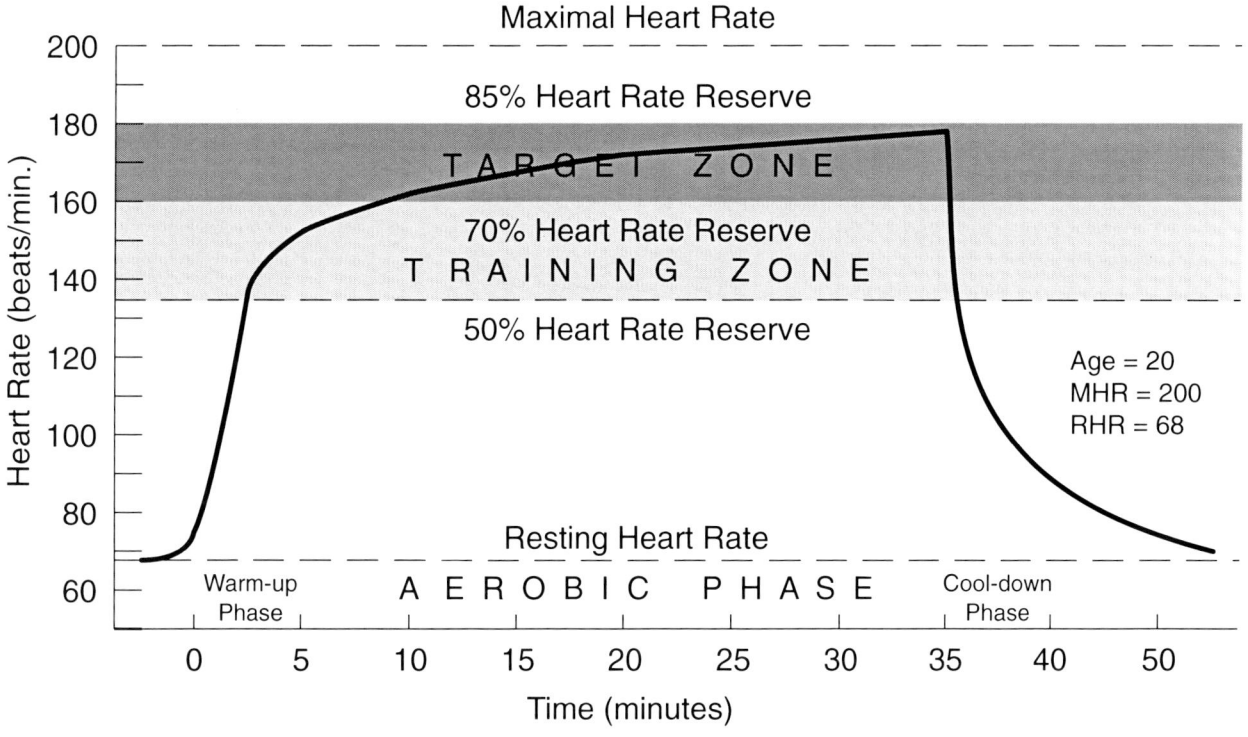

FIGURE 4.3

Cardiovascular Exercise Prescription Guidelines

can plan active family outings and participate with children, as well as limit sedentary activities.

Documentation from many organizations and research facilities supports the benefits of a healthy lifestyle. The following are just some of the significant groups that have contributed to our current knowledge of lifestyle choices related to health.

- The *American Heart Association* (AHA) identified inactivity as a major cardiac risk factor in 1992.

- *Healthy People 2010* (National Health Promotion and Disease Prevention Objectives) developed statements by expert groups representing over 300 national organizations that include realistic health goals to be achieved by the year 2010.

- *Surgeon General's Report (1996)* traced the link between physical activity and good health. This document suggests that a healthy lifestyle is the most critical element for optimal wellness.

- *Centers for Disease Control and Prevention* (CDC) provide scientific and technical leadership and assistance to help states, national organizations, and professional groups reduce major risk factors associated with chronic diseases in the United States.

- The *American College of Sports Medicine* (ACSM) promotes and integrates scientific research, education, and practical applications of sports medicine and exercise science to maintain and enhance physical performance, fitness, health, and quality of life.

- The *U.S. Department of Health and Human Services* (DHHS) released the 2008 Physical Activity Guidelines.

Types of Hypokinetic Conditions

Cardiovascular Disease (CVD)

The cardiovascular system is responsible for delivering oxygen and other nutrients to the body. The major components of the cardiovascular system are the heart, blood, and the vessels that carry the blood. Cardiovascular disease (CVD) is a catch-all term that includes several disease processes including various diseases of the heart, stroke, high blood pressure, congestive heart failure, and atherosclerosis. The heart muscle may become damaged or lose its ability to contract effectively. The vessels that supply the heart with oxygen may become blocked or damaged and subsequently compromise the heart muscle. Finally, the peripheral vascular system (all of the vessels outside the heart) may become damaged and decrease the ability to provide oxygen to other parts of the body.

Who Is At Risk for CVD?

The Surgeon General's Report (Satcher, 1996) placed **physical inactivity** as a significant risk factor for cardiovascular diseases and other health disorders. Most sedentary Americans are at risk as stated previously. There are an estimated 80 million Americans that have some form of CVD. Many factors can predispose a person to be at risk for CVD. Sedentary living, habitual stress, smoking, poor diet, high blood pressure, diabetes, obesity, high cholesterol, and family history can all increase risk. Advancing age increases risk. Males typically have a higher risk than women until women are post-menopausal, then risk evens out. Misconceptions still exist that CVD is not a real problem for women (AHA, 2009). Because more women have heart attacks when they are older, the initial heart attack is more likely to be fatal. It is important for women to realize that CVD is an equal opportunity killer. Just like men, more women die from heart disease than anything else.

Certain populations have an inherently higher risk such as African Americans and Hispanics. Genetic predisposition is a strong factor; familial tendencies toward elevated triglycerides, fat distribution (abdominal fat accumulation denotes a higher health risk than hip/thigh accumulation of fat), and high low-density lipoprotein cholesterol (LDL-C) levels increase risk. LDL-C is a blood lipid that indicates a higher cardiac risk. Saturated fat intake tends to increase LDL cholesterol. Dr. William Franklin of Georgetown University Medical School in Washington claims that anyone who has a close relative who has had a heart attack should begin monitoring his heart with regular

Benefits of Exercise

Consistent physical activity affects cardiovascular disease by one or more of the following mechanisms:

- Improved cardiovascular fitness and health
- Greater lean (fat-free) body mass
- Improved strength and muscular endurance
- Stronger heart muscle
- Lower heart rate
- Increased oxygen to the brain
- Reduced blood fat including low-density-lipoprotein cholesterol (LDL-C)
- Increased protective high-density-lipoprotein cholesterol (HDL-C)
- Delayed development of atherosclerosis
- Increased work capacity
- Improved peripheral circulation
- Improved coronary circulation
- Reduced risk of heart attack
- Reduced risk of stroke
- Reduced risk of hypertension
- Greater chance of surviving a heart attack
- Greater oxygen carrying capacity of the blood

Exercise improves your body and mind more than you might expect.

Claudette's Story

"I consider myself to be relatively healthy and I exercise for about ninety minutes every morning. I started having pain in my chest and face during my exercising, and finally went to the cardiologist. I never thought that the pain in my face could be related to my heart, so I was shocked when the tests showed that I had had a heart attack. I thought I was too young, but my father died of a heart attack when he was only 38, so I had family history as a risk factor. After my second heart attack, I knew that I needed to help get the message out. Women need to know that heart disease is their biggest health threat."

Source: National Heart, Lung and Blood Institute, National Health Institute.

FIGURE 4.4

The Benefits of Exercise

- Increases your respiratory capacity
- Improves your mood and reduces psychological symptoms
- Reduces your risk of heart disease
- Improves your digestion and your fat metabolism
- Lowers your body fat and reduces your weight
- Improves your circulation
- Increases your muscle strength and tone
- Strengthens your bones and increases joint flexibility

stress tests when he is 45. If your father died in his 40's of a heart attack, then you should be concerned a decade earlier in your 30's. Variables such as age, gender, race, and genetic makeup may place you at a higher or lower risk but cannot be changed. These can be termed unalterable risk factors.

CVD Prevention

Since you cannot change your age, your sex, and who your parents are, focus on what you *can* change. These risk factors include but are not limited to: diet, drug use, smoking history, cholesterol levels, obesity, high blood pressure, and last but definitely not least, physical inactivity (see pages 16 and 19). This is a critical point, since activity level is a risk factor that can be easily modified and is often overlooked. Increasing an individual's activity level can prevent many of the diseases discussed in this chapter. Cardiovascular disease is the leading cause of death in the United States. "About every 26 seconds an American will experience a coronary event, and about every minute someone will die from one" (AHA, 2008). With this being the case, consider your own risk. How can you adjust your current lifestyle habits to decrease your risk? Read the Benefits of Exercise (in the margin on page 108) and Figure 4.4 to determine how exercise helps CVD.

Measuring Health Risk

There are two simple measures of overall health risk: waist-to-hip ratio and Body Mass Index (BMI). See Figure 4.5 to determine your waist-to-hip ratio, and see the activity Body Mass Index Calculator in Chapter 6 to determine your BMI. These

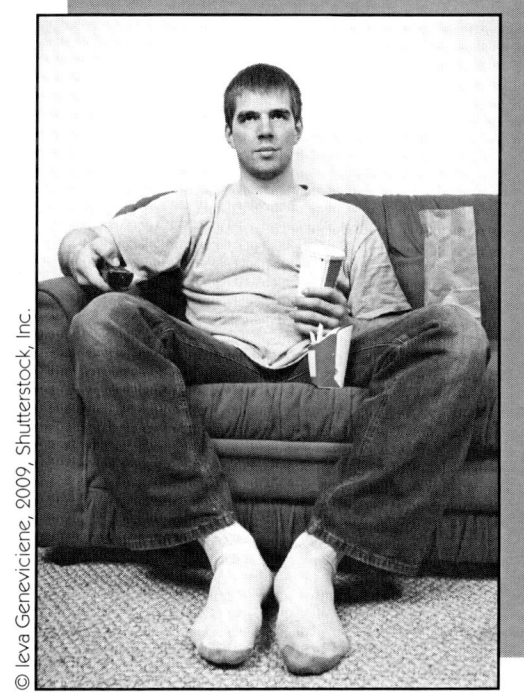

Increasing lifestyle activity by spending less time on the couch and doing something daily will have a positive impact on your health.

FIGURE 4.5

Calculating Waist-to-Hip Circumference Ratio

Equipment
1. Tape measure
2. Partner to take measurements

Preparation
Wear clothes that will not add significantly to your measurements.

Instructions
Stand with your feet together and your arms at your sides. Raise your arms only high enough to allow for taking the measurements. Your partner should make sure that the tape is horizontal around the entire circumference and pulled snugly against your skin. The tape shouldn't be pulled so tight that it causes indentations in your skin. Record measurements to the nearest millimeter or one-sixteenth of an inch.

Waist. Measure at the smallest waist circumference. If you don't have a natural waist, measure at the level of your navel.

Hip. Measure at the largest hip circumference.

Calculating Your Ratio
You can use any unit of measurement (for example, inches or centimeters), as long as you're consistent. Waist-to-hip ratio equals waist measurement divided by hip measurement.

Determine Your Relative Risk
Find the risk category that corresponds to your ratio and age group on the appropriate figure below.

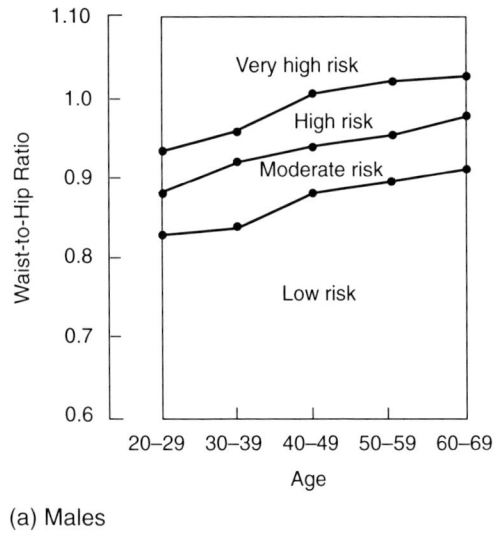

(a) Males

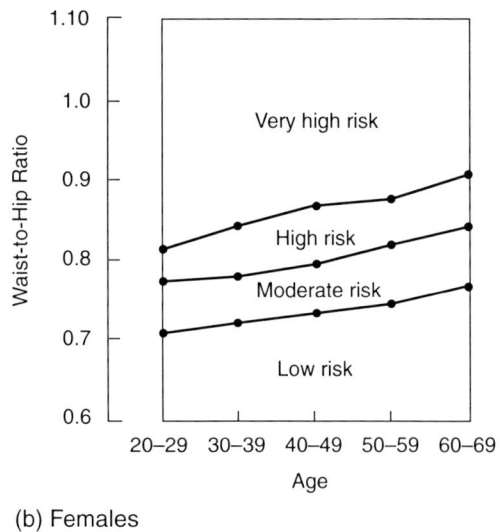

(b) Females

Source: From *Fit & Well* by Fahey, Insel and Roth, Mayfield Publishing.

two measures implicate obesity as increasing health risk. It is true that overweight and obesity are associated with complications and high risk factors such as hypertension, high blood cholesterol, and diabetes. A growing body of evidence, however, indicates physical inactivity is more critical than excess weight in determining health risk. Longitudinal studies such as the ongoing research by epidemiologist Steven Blair at the Cooper Institute in Dallas, Texas, and information from the ongoing Harvard alumni study indicate that lifestyle is more significant than weight. Fitter people have lower death rates regardless of weight (see Figure 4.6). Indeed, the mortality rate for low fit males is more than 20% higher than for those that are high fit. While this effect is smaller for women, the decrease in mortality rate for high fit females is more than 6% compared to those who are low fit. Previously sedentary Harvard alumni (Sesso and Paffenbarger, 1956) who became active reduced their all-cause mortality rate by 23 percent. The alumni who lost weight (but were not active) did not improve their mortality rate. Improvements in metabolic fitness (glucose tolerance, blood pressure, and cholesterol) are often seen with just moderate amounts of physical activity. The good news is that overweight Americans don't need to go on a crash diet, buy a gym membership, or totally give up Twinkies. Increasing lifestyle activity and walking regularly, spending less time on the couch, and doing something daily can have a positive impact on health.

Arteriosclerosis and Exercise

Arteriosclerosis

Arteriosclerosis is a term used to describe the thickening and hardening of the arteries. Healthy arteries are elastic and will dilate and constrict with changes in blood flow, which allows proper maintenance of blood pressure. Hardened, non-elastic arteries do not expand with blood flow and can increase intrarterial pressure causing

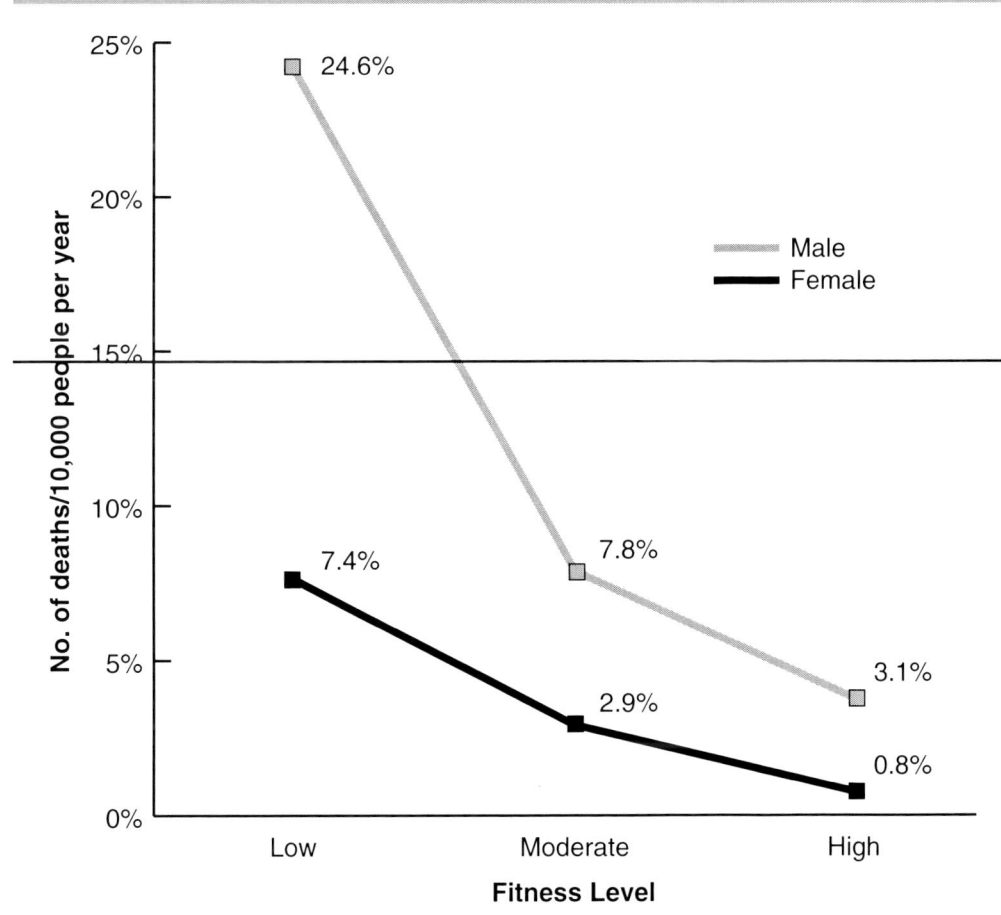

FIGURE 4.6

Relationship between Different Levels of Fitness and Death Due to Cardiovascular Disease among Men and Women

Source: Blair et al., Physical fitness and all-cause mortality: A prospective study of healthy men and women. *Journal of the American Medical Association* 262(17): 2395–2401, 1989. (Adapted from S. N. Blair, H. W. Kohl, III, R. S. Paffenbarger, Jr., D. G. Clark, K. H. Cooper, and L. W. Gibbons. Physical fitness and all-cause mortality: A prospective study of healthy men and women.)

high blood pressure. Both high blood pressure and arteriosclerosis increase the risk of an **aneurysm**. With an aneurysm, the artery loses its integrity and balloons out under the pressure created by the pumping heart, in much the same way as an old garden hose might if placed under pressure. If an aneurysm occurs in the vessels of the brain, a stroke might occur. Aneurysms in the large vessels can place a person at risk of sudden death. Maintaining normal elasticity of the arteries is very important for good health. Exercise helps to manage symptoms and the factors that contribute to cardiac risk.

Atherosclerosis Atherosclerosis is a type of arteriosclerosis. Atherosclerosis is the long-term buildup of fatty deposits and other substances such as cholesterol, cellular waste products, calcium, and fibrin (clotting material in the blood) on the interior walls of arteries (see Figure 4.7). The leading theory states that plaque develops when the endothelium (a thin layer of cells that line the interior vessel wall) is damaged due to major fluctuations in blood pressure, increased levels of blood triglycerides, cholesterol, and cigarette smoking. Conditions such as these accelerate the development of atherosclerosis. Due to this plaque development, the flow of blood within the artery decreases because the diameter of the vessel is decreased. This may create a partial or total blockage (called an occlusion) that may cause high blood pressure, a heart attack, or stroke. This process can occur in any vessel of the body. If it occurs outside of the brain or heart, it is termed peripheral

Waist-to-Hip Ratio

Recent evidence from a study done at the University of Manchester in the United Kingdom indicates that abdominal obesity is a strong independent risk factor for heart disease. "A large waist with large hips is much less worrisome than a large waist with small hips." The conclusion of the study determined that the simple waist-to-hip ratio is a strong predictor of heart disease (AHA, 2007).

FIGURE 4.7

Atherosclerosis

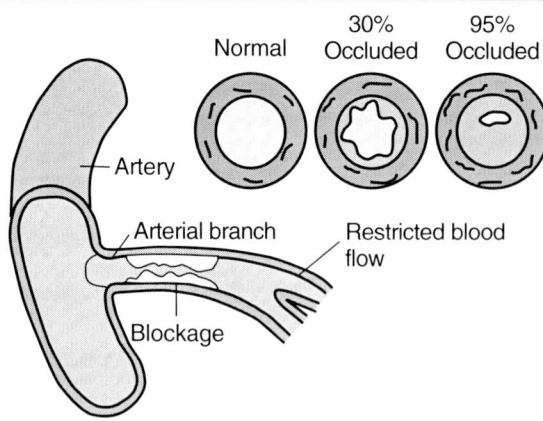

Atherosclerosis occurs in stages. Plaque deposits in a normal "clean" artery can partially block the flow of blood. As the size of the blockage increases, blood supply decreases until tissues downstream from the block fail to receive adequate blood and are damaged.

Source: From *Step Up to Wellness* by Jan Galen Bishop and Steven G. Aldana. Copyright © 1999 by Allyn & Bacon. Reprinted by permission of Pearson Education, Inc.

vascular disease. Within the heart the gradual narrowing of the coronary arteries to the myocardium, or heart muscle, is called coronary artery disease. Atherosclerosis is a disease that can start early in childhood. The rate of progression of the disease depends on family history and lifestyle choices. Exercise helps manage symptoms as well as increase coronary collateral circulation. Collateral arteries are the vessels that form preceding the blockage as an artery slowly becomes occluded. Collateral vessels such as these can help lessen the severity of a heart attack when the artery becomes totally blocked. High cholesterol levels can increase risk of atherosclerosis, and low-density lipoprotein cholesterol is thought to contribute to the arterial occlusion. Triglycerides are another type of blood fat that in high levels is associated with high risk (see Figure 4.8). Regular physical activity has been shown to lower risk by lowering blood lipid (fat) levels.

Peripheral Vascular Disease

Peripheral vascular disease is simply a term attributed to disease of the peripheral vessels. The lack of proper circulation may cause fluids to pool in the extremities. Associated leg pain, cramping, numbness, tingling, coldness, and loss of hair to affected limbs are common signs. The restrictions in blood flow are typically caused by years of arteriosclerosis and atherosclerosis in the vessels of the extremities. The risk factors are the same as those for cardiovascular disease. One difference is that the disease process may progress extensively before the affected person begins to notice any problems. The heart and brain are much more sensitive to compromised blood flow than are the extremities.

Hypertension

Hypertension, or high blood pressure, is often called the "silent killer" because typically there are no symptoms. Because hypertension is asymptomatic, it is important to get your blood pressure checked on a regular basis. In 2005, the estimated prevalence of hypertension (a blood pressure reading of 140/90 mm or higher) was 73 million Americans (see Figure 4.10 on page 115). High blood pressure is associated with a shortened life span. Interestingly, under the age of 45 more males typically have a higher blood pressure, while after age 55, more females tend to have a higher blood pressure (AHA, 2008). High blood pressure causes the heart to work harder. Chronic, untreated hypertension can lead to aneurysms in blood vessels, heart failure from an enlarged heart, kidney failure, atherosclerosis, and blindness.

The top number is the systolic reading, which represents the arterial pressure when the heart is contracting and forcing the blood through the arteries. The bottom number is the diastolic reading, which represents the force of the blood

In the News

A new study finds that teens who get too little sleep or erratic sleep may elevate their blood pressure. "Our study underscores the high rate of poor quality and inadequate sleep in adolescence coupled with the risk of developing high blood pressure and other health problems which may lead to cardiovascular disease," says Susan Redline, M.D., professor of medicine and pediatrics and director of University Hospital's Sleep Center at Case Western Reserve University in Cleveland, Ohio. Researchers say technology in bedrooms (phone, games, computers, music) may be part of the problem (AHA, 2008).

FIGURE 4.8

Cholesterol and Triglyceride Levels and Risk of Heart Disease

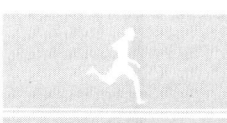

If you don't smoke, don't start. **If you do smoke, get help to quit now!** Many effective programs, nicotine patches, and other medications are available to help you quit. As soon as you stop smoking, your risk of heart disease starts to drop. In time your risk will be about the same as if you'd never smoked.

Total Cholesterol Level	Category
Less than 200 mg/dL	Desirable level that puts you at lower risk for heart disease. A cholesterol level of 200 mg/dL or higher raises your risk.
200–239 mg/dL	Borderline high
240 mg/dL and above	High blood cholesterol. A person with this level has more than twice the risk of heart disease as someone whose cholesterol is below 200 mg/dL.

Cholesterol levels are measured in milligrams (mg) of cholesterol per deciliter (dL) of blood.

LDL Cholesterol Level	Category
Less than 100 mg/dL	Optimal
100–129 mg/dL	Near or above optimal
130–159 mg/dL	Borderline high
160–189 mg/dL	High
190 mg/dL and above	Very High

mg/dL = milligrams per deciliter of blood

HDL Cholesterol Level	Category
Less than 40 mg/dL	A major risk factor for heart disease.
40–59 mg/dL	The higher your HDL level, the better.
60 mg/dL and above	An HDL of 60 mg/dL and above is considered protective against heart disease.

mg/dL = milligrams per deciliter of blood

Triglyceride Level	Category
Less than 150 mg/dL	Normal
150–199 mg/dL	Borderline high
200–499 mg/dL	High
500 mg/dL and above	Very high

mg/dL = milligrams per deciliter of blood

on the arteries while the heart is relaxing between beats. In 2003 new blood pressure guidelines were issued, with a new "prehypertensive" category identified (see Figure 4.9). A blood pressure reading of 115/75 is the new threshold above which cardiovascular complication can occur. The prehypertensive category includes a systolic pressure from 120–139 and a diastolic pressure from 80–89 as a warning zone. If your are considered prehypertensive, it is time to take action by modifying your lifestyle. Any reading consistently over 139/89 mm Hg is

Blood Pressure Category	Systolic (mm Hg)		Diastolic (mm Hg)
Normal	less than 120	and	less than 80
Prehypertension	120–139	or	80–89
Hypertension, Stage 1	140–159	or	90–99
Hypertension, Stage 2	160 or higher	or	100 or higher

*Unusually low readings should be evaluated for clinical significance.

FIGURE 4.9 Blood Pressure Classification for Adults Age 18 and Older

Source: Seventh Report of the Joint National Committee on Prevention, Detection, Evaluation, and Treatment of High Blood Pressure (JNC 7 Express) NIH Publication No. 03-5233, May 2003.

high blood pressure and indicates a high risk. With persons over 50 years old, a systolic reading of 140 or above is a more important CVD risk factor than the diastolic reading (JNC VII, 2003).

Hypertension cannot be cured, but it can be successfully treated and controlled. Most people with hypertension have additional risk factors for cardiovascular disease. Some of the risk factors for high blood pressure include Hispanic or African American heritage, older age, family history, a diet high in fat and sodium, alcoholism, stress, obesity, and inactivity. Exercise has been shown to help symptoms of high blood pressure in mild to moderate hypertension.

Heart Attack

A heart attack or **myocardial infarction** occurs when an artery that provides the heart muscle with oxygen becomes blocked or flow is decreased (see Figure 4.11). The area of the heart muscle served by that artery does not receive adequate oxygen and becomes injured and may eventually die. The heart attack may be so small as to be imperceptible by the victim, or so massive that the victim will die. It is often reported that heart attack victims delay seeking medical help with the onset of symptoms. Every minute counts! In one study, men waited an average of three hours before seeking help. Women waited four hours. It is important to seek medical help at the first sign of a heart attack.

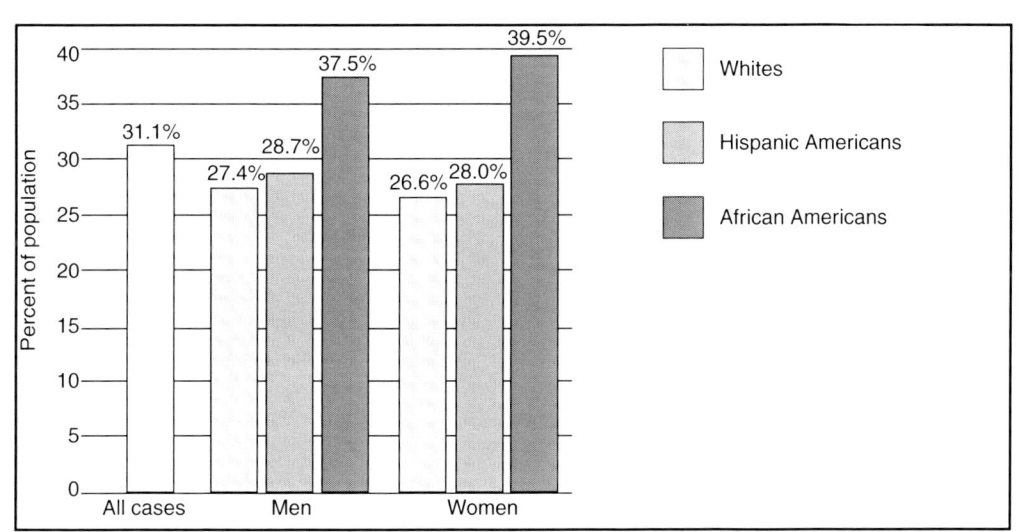

FIGURE 4.10 Incidence of High Blood Pressure in the United States

Source: National Health and Nutrition Examination Study, 2004.

FIGURE 4.11

Narrowed or Blocked Arteries in the Heart Result in a Heart Attack

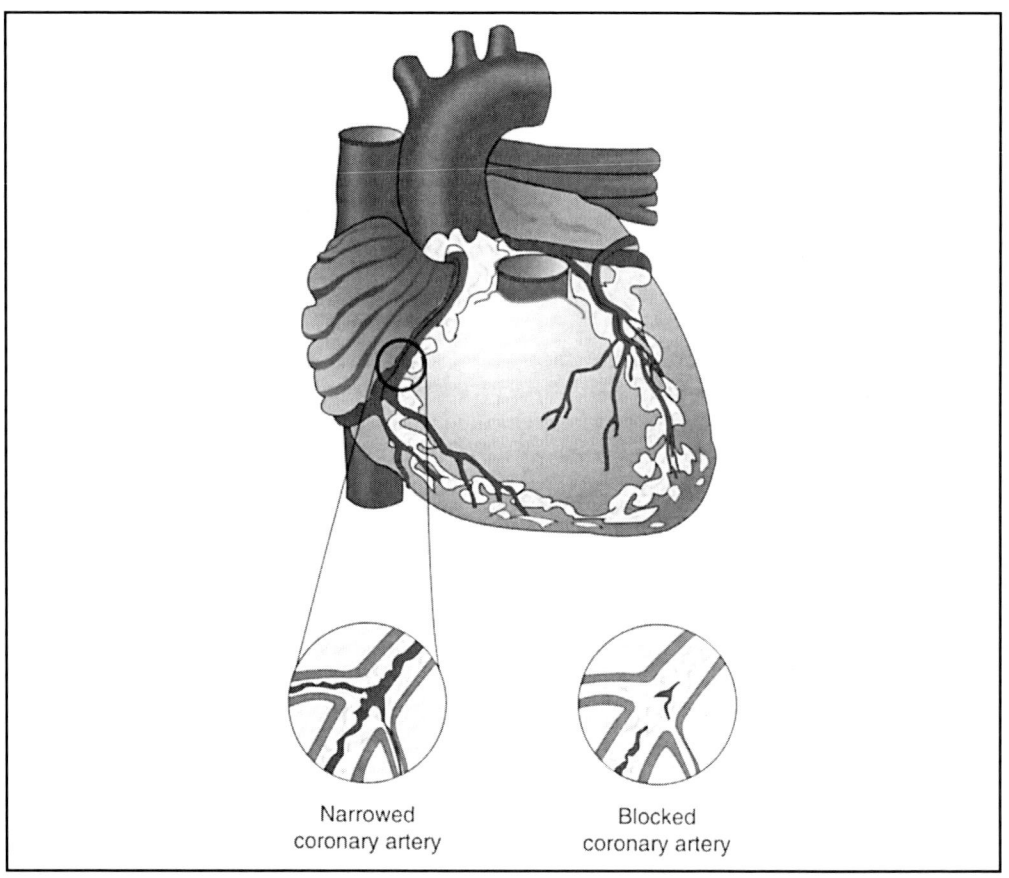

Source: From *Step Up to Wellness* by Jan Galen Bishop and Steven G. Aldana. Copyright © 1999 by Allyn & Bacon. Reprinted by permission of Pearson Education, Inc.

Women who smoke and take oral contraceptives are ten times more likely to have a heart attack (Payne and Hahn, 2000). "Smoking and oral contraceptives (OC) appear to act synergistically in increasing the risk of arterial thrombotic disease, particularly in heavy smokers and with old OC formulations," Ojvind Lidegaard reported in 1998. In addition to the classic symptoms of heart attack listed in the box on page 117, women were more likely than men to report throat discomfort, pressing on the chest, and vomiting.

Exercise is the cornerstone therapy for the primary prevention, treatment, and control of hypertension, according to the Position Stand *Exercise and Hypertension* released from the American College of Sports Medicine (ACSM). Adults with hypertension should seek to gain at least thirty minutes of moderate-intensity physical activity on most, if not all, days of the week, but they should be evaluated, treated, and monitored closely.

Each person may experience heart disease in a different way and unfortunately, a fatal sudden cardiac arrest may be the only symptom. Heart attack symptoms for women may be different than the classic symptoms that are commonly known such as chest, jaw, or left arm pain with shortness of breath and weakness. Women may experience more subtle symptoms such as fatigue, depression, back pain, or pain throughout the chest. Don't wait to get help, as time is critical when experiencing a heart attack.

Some findings suggest that coronary collateral circulation is increased with regular physical activity (Corbin and Welk, 2009). This may decrease the risk of having a heart attack, as well as increase the chances of survival if a heart attack

Heart Attack Symptoms and Warning Signs

If you think you're having a heart attack, call 9-1-1 or your emergency medical system immediately.

Some heart attacks are sudden and intense—the "movie heart attack," where no one doubts what's happening—but most heart attacks start slowly, with mild pain or discomfort. Often people affected aren't sure what's wrong and wait too long before getting help. Here are signs that can mean a heart attack is happening:

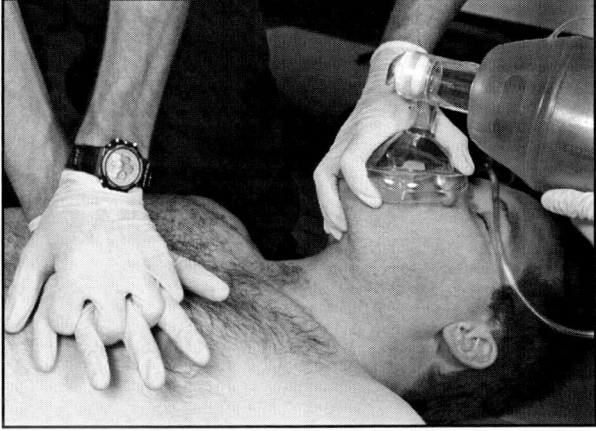

- **Chest discomfort.** Most heart attacks involve discomfort in the center of the chest that lasts more than a few minutes, or that goes away and comes back. It can feel like uncomfortable pressure, squeezing, fullness, or pain.
- **Discomfort in other areas of the upper body.** Symptoms can include pain or discomfort in one or both arms, the back, neck, jaw, or stomach.
- **Shortness of breath.** This feeling often comes along with chest discomfort. But it can occur before the chest discomfort.
- **Other signs:** These may include breaking out in a cold sweat, nausea, or lightheadedness.

If you or someone you're with has chest discomfort, especially with one or more of the other signs, don't wait longer than a few minutes (no more than five) before calling for help. Call 9-1-1... Get to a hospital right away.

Calling 9-1-1 is almost always the fastest way to get lifesaving treatment.

Source: Reproduced with permission. www.americanheart.org © 2009, American Heart Association.

does occur, because the new vessels, which form as a result of exercise, can take over if a major coronary artery is blocked. Since 1951, the death rate from heart attacks has declined by 51 percent, yet more Americans die from coronary artery disease than from any other disease. Both treatment and prevention for heart attacks has increased due to revolutionary new surgical treatments, new drugs, and new information about the etiology of heart disease (see Figure 4.12). Many of the drugs reserved for treating cardiac patients in the past are now used as aggressive

Famed television host David Letterman was not overweight when he had quintuple bypass surgery at age 52 in 2000. Although Mr. Letterman didn't look like the typical person who has a heart attack, he had several risk factors going against him. He had a family history—his father, Harry, died of a heart attack in his 50's. Mr. Letterman had high cholesterol. Most likely his job would be considered high stress. David Letterman credits Dr. Wayne Isom, who operated on his heart, with saving his life. In an interview with another talk show host, Larry King (who coincidentally also was operated on by Dr. Isom for quadruple bypass surgery) asked Dr. Isom what was important in avoiding heart disease. Besides exercise, controlling stress, managing weight, and eating well, Dr. Isom said that attitude is very, very important. Post-heart surgery, the patient must decide for himself that he is going to get well. An important part of cardiac rehabilitation is a positive attitude.

FIGURE 4.12

Estimated Average Reduction in Risk for Heart Attack*

*Estimated risk reductions refer to the independent contribution of each risk factor to heart attack and do not address the wide range of known or hypothesized reactions among them.

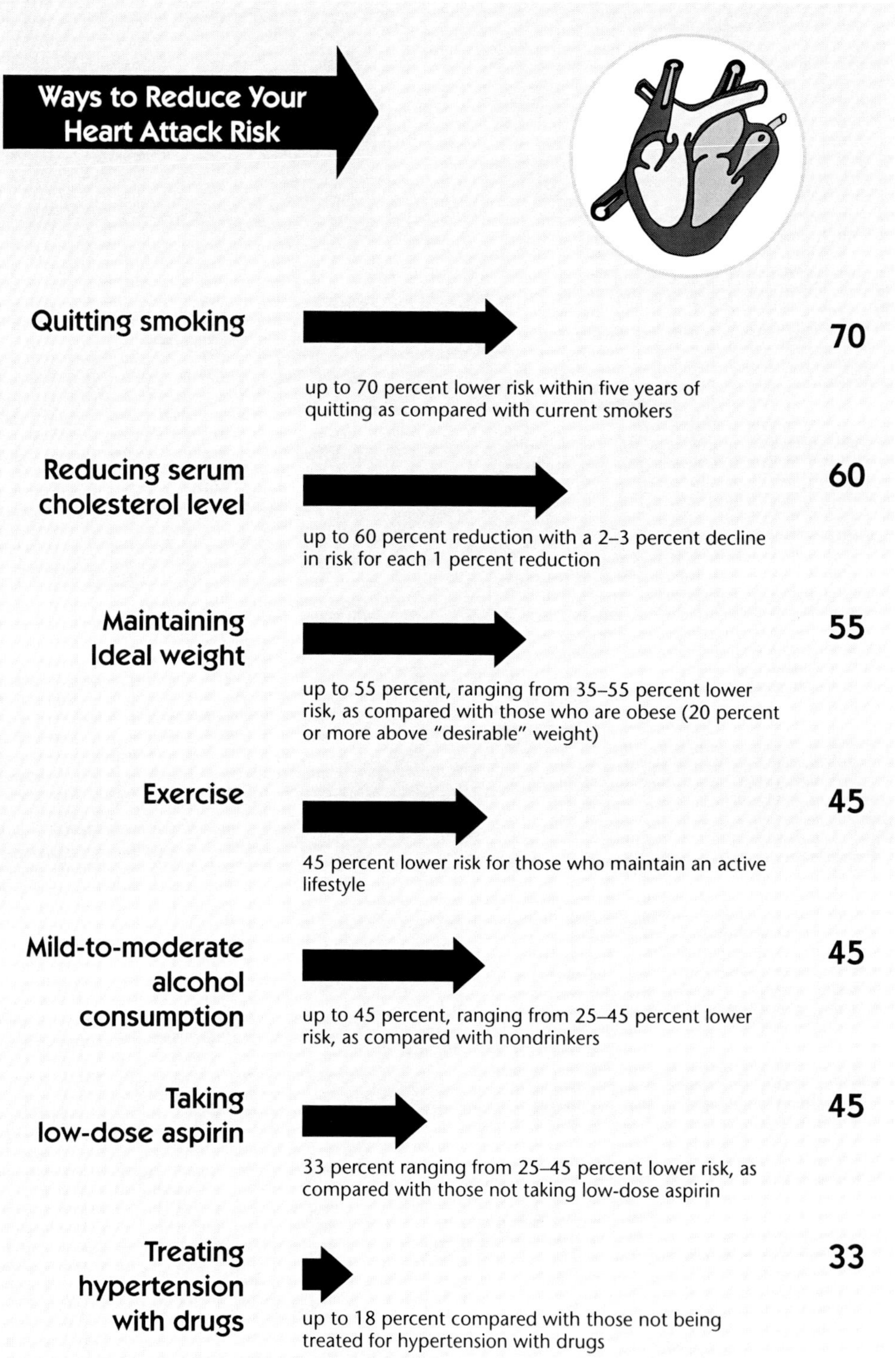

Ways to Reduce Your Heart Attack Risk

Quitting smoking — **70**
up to 70 percent lower risk within five years of quitting as compared with current smokers

Reducing serum cholesterol level — **60**
up to 60 percent reduction with a 2–3 percent decline in risk for each 1 percent reduction

Maintaining Ideal weight — **55**
up to 55 percent, ranging from 35–55 percent lower risk, as compared with those who are obese (20 percent or more above "desirable" weight)

Exercise — **45**
45 percent lower risk for those who maintain an active lifestyle

Mild-to-moderate alcohol consumption — **45**
up to 45 percent, ranging from 25–45 percent lower risk, as compared with nondrinkers

Taking low-dose aspirin — **45**
33 percent ranging from 25–45 percent lower risk, as compared with those not taking low-dose aspirin

Treating hypertension with drugs — **33**
up to 18 percent compared with those not being treated for hypertension with drugs

*Because studies of these lifestyle changes have mostly involved men, the benefits are less clear for women

Source: From R.J. Donatelle and L.G. Davis, *Access to Health,* Tenth Edition. Copyright © 2007. All rights reserved. Reprinted by permission of Benjamin Cummings Publishing.

prevention in high-risk patients. The AHA has developed Heart Attack Symptoms and Warning Signs (see box on previous page).

Stroke

Do you know the warning signs of a stroke? There is a public awareness campaign to increase knowledge of stroke warning signs and symptoms (see box on page 120). Stroke, or more recently called "**brain attack**," is the third leading cause of death affecting 780,000 Americans per year (AHA, 2009). This occurs when the vessels that supply the brain with nutrients become damaged or occluded and the brain tissue dies because of insufficient oxygen (see Figure 4.13). The cerebral artery, the main supply of nutrients to the brain, can be narrowed due to atherosclerosis. The conditions that precipitate stroke may take years to develop. Stroke has the same risk factors as heart disease. Hypertension is the most notable risk factor. Like heart disease, conditions favorable to stroke also respond favorably to exercise. Ischemic (thrombosis and embolism) strokes are the most common form of stroke (87 percent) and occur as a result of a blockage to the cerebral artery (AHA, 2009). The process is similar to that which occurs in a heart attack. Intracerebral hemorrhage, or aneurysm, in which the vessel may rupture and cause bleeding inside the head and result in pressure on the brain, are 10 percent of strokes. Three percent of strokes are caused by hemorrhage. The least common form of stroke results from compression that can occur as a result of a hemorrhage or brain tumor. African Americans have almost twice the risk of a stroke than Caucasians (AHA, 2009). African Americans also have a high incidence of stroke risk factors such as high blood pressure. On the average, someone in the United States has a stroke every forty seconds, and every three to four minutes someone dies of a stroke (AHA, 2009). One-third of all stroke victims die, one-third of stroke victims suffer permanent disability, and one-third of stroke victims gradually return to their normal daily routines (Bishop and Aldana, 1999). Stroke is also a leading cause of serious disability. Various studies have shown significant trends toward lower stroke risk with moderate and high levels of leisure time physical activity.

FIGURE 4.13

Causes of Stroker

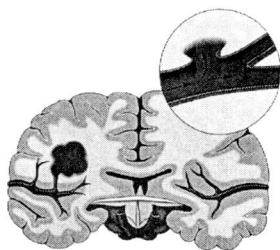
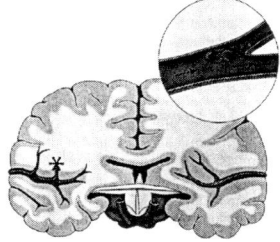
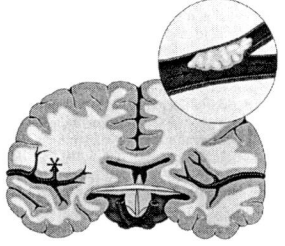
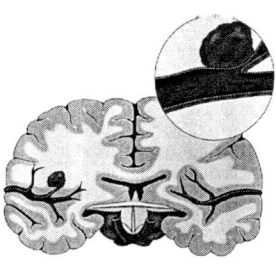

Cerebral Hemorrhage as the Cause of Stroke: A blood vessel in the brain ruptures.

Cerebral Embolism as the Cause of Stroke: A clot or foreign body forms in some other part of the body and travels to the brain.

Cerebral Thrombosis as the Cause of Stroke: There is a blood clot in the brain.

Compression as the Cause of Stroke

Source: From Brent Q. Hafen, Keith J. Karren and Kathryn J. Frandsen, *First Aid for Colleges and Universities,* Seventh Edition. Copyright © 1999 by Allyn and Bacon. Reprinted by permission of Pearson Education, Inc.

Risk Factors for Cardiovascular Disease

Controllable Risk Factors

- ***Cigarette Smoking***—Smokers have two to four times the risk of developing cardiovascular disease than do nonsmokers (AHA, 2009). Cigarette smoking is the most "potent" of the preventable risk factors. Former U.S. Surgeon General C. Everett Koop claims that cigarette smoking is the number one preventable cause of death and disease in the United States and the most important health issue of our time. Smoking accounts for 50 percent of the female deaths due to heart attack before the age of 55 (Rosato, 1994).
- ***Hypertension***—The AHA (2009) reports that approximately 73 million American adults and children have high blood pressure. Reports from the Harvard Alumni Study (1986) show that subjects who did not engage in vigorous sports or activity were 35 percent more likely to develop hypertension than those who were regularly active.
- ***Cholesterol***—Dietary cholesterol contributes to blood serum cholesterol (cholesterol circulating in the blood), which can contribute to heart disease.

Stroke Symptoms / Warning Signs

IF YOU NOTICE ONE OR MORE OF THESE SIGNS, DON'T WAIT. STROKE IS A MEDICAL EMERGENCY. CALL 9-1-1 OR YOUR EMERGENCY MEDICAL SERVICES. GET TO A HOSPITAL RIGHT AWAY!

The American Stroke Association wants you to learn the warning signs of stroke:

- Sudden numbness or weakness of the face, arm, or leg, especially on one side of the body
- Sudden confusion, trouble speaking or understanding
- Sudden trouble seeing in one or both eyes
- Sudden trouble walking, dizziness, loss of balance or coordination
- Sudden, severe headache with no known cause

Be prepared for an emergency.

- Keep a list of emergency rescue service numbers next to the telephone and in your pocket, wallet, or purse.
- Find out which area hospitals are primary stroke centers that have twenty-four-hour emergency stroke care.
- Know (in advance) which hospital or medical facility is nearest your home or office.

Take action in an emergency.

- Not all the warning signs occur in every stroke. Don't ignore signs of stroke, even if they go away!
- Check the time. When did the first warning sign or symptom start? You'll be asked this important question later.
- If you have one or more stroke symptoms that last more than a few minutes, don't delay! Immediately call 9-1-1 or the emergency medical service (EMS) number so an ambulance (ideally with advanced life support) can quickly be sent for you.
- If you're with someone who may be having stroke symptoms, immediately call 9-1-1 or the EMS. Expect the person to protest—denial is common. Don't take "no" for an answer. Insist on taking prompt action.

For stroke information, call the American Stroke Association at 1-888-4-STROKE. For information on life after stroke, ask for the Stroke Family Support Network.

Source: Reproduced with permission, www.americanheart.org © 2009, American Heart Association.

> The Surgeon General Encourages Americans to Know Health History—In the fall of 2008 the acting Surgeon General encouraged all Americans to take advantage of family gatherings to speak with family members to discuss, identify, and make a record of health problems that seem to run in the family. Doing this can offer insight into your health risk. Check out the Web-based tool "My Family Health Portrait" at www.hhs.gov/familyhistory/

Every 1 percent reduction in serum cholesterol can result in a 2–3 percent reduction in the risk of heart disease (AHA, 2009). To lower cholesterol, reduce intake of dietary saturated fat, increase consumption of soluble fiber, maintain a healthy weight, do not smoke, and exercise regularly.

- **Inactivity**—Physical inactivity can be very debilitating to the human body. The changes brought about by the aging process can be simulated in a few weeks of bed rest for a young person. Aerobic exercise on a regular basis can favorably influence the other modifiable risk factors for heart disease. Consistent, moderate amounts of physical activity can promote health and longevity. The Surgeon General's report (Satcher, 1996) states that as few as 150 extra calories expended daily exercising can dramatically decrease CVD risk.
- **Obesity**—Highly correlated to heart disease, mild to moderate obesity is associated with an increase in risk of CVD. Fat distribution can also predict higher risk. A waist-to-hip ratio that is greater than 1.0 for men and greater than 0.8 for women constitutes a higher risk because abdominal fat is more easily mobilized and dispersed into the bloodstream, thereby elevating serum cholesterol levels. A BMI over 30 is considered obese.
- **Diabetes**—At least 65 percent of diabetics die of some form of CVD (CDC, 1999). Exercise is critical to help increase the sensitivity of the body's cells to insulin.

Uncontrollable Risk Factors

- **Age**—Risk of CVD rises as a person ages.
- **Gender**—Men have a higher risk than women until women reach postmenopausal age. Remember that CVD is an equal opportunity killer!
- **Heredity**—A family history of heart disease will increase risk.

Contributing Risk Factors

- **Stress**—Although difficult to measure in concrete form, stress is considered a factor in the development and acceleration of CVD. Without stress-management techniques, constant stress can manifest itself in a physical nature in the human body. Stress contributes to many of today's illnesses.
- **Triglycerides**—Most of the fat in the human body is stored in the form of triglycerides. Elevated triglyceride levels are thought to increase CVD risk by being involved in the plaque formation of atherosclerosis.

Obesity

Since 1979 the World Heath Organization (WHO) has classified obesity as a disease. "Obesity is a complex condition, one with serious social and psychological dimensions, that affects virtually all age and socioeconomic groups and threatens to overwhelm both developed and developing countries. In 1995, there were an estimated

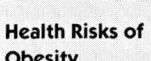

Health Risks of Obesity

Each of the diseases listed below is followed by the percentage of cases that are caused by obesity.

Colon cancer	10%
Breast cancer	11%
Hypertension	33%
Heart disease	70%
Diabetes	90%
(Type II, non-insulin-dependent)	

As these statistics show, being obese greatly increases the risk of many serious and even life-threatening diseases.

Table 4.1
Prevalence of Overweight* among Children and Adolescents

	1963–70	1971–74	1976–80	1988–94	1999–02
Ages 6 to 11	4%	4%	7%	11%	16%
Ages 12 to 19	5%	6%	5%	11%	16%

Source: From the Center for Health and Health Care in Schools, www.healthinschools.org

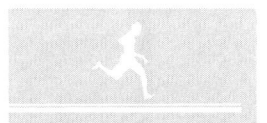

"By promoting healthier eating and encouraging exercise, parents are key in reducing child and adolescent overweight."

Parents Key to Reducing Overweight in Children, 2003

200 million obese adults worldwide and another 18 million under-5 children classified as overweight. As of 2000, the number of obese adults has increased to over 300 million" (WHO, 2008). "Globesity" may be the new term coined for the world's heavy populations. While malnutrition still contributes to an estimated 60 percent of deaths in children ages 5 and under globally, in the United States the excess body weight and physical inactivity that leads to obesity cause more than 112,000 deaths each year, making it the second leading cause of death in our county. In the latest figures available, an estimated 142 million Americans were overweight and 67.3 million were obese in 2005 (Hoeger, Turner, and Hafen, 2009). Overweight has tripled for children and teenagers from 1963 to 2002 (see Table 4.1).

Obesity causes, contributes to, and complicates many of the diseases that afflict Americans. Obesity is associated with a shortened life, serious organ impairment, poor self-concept, and a higher risk of cardiovascular disease and diabetes, as well as colon and breast cancer. The estimated cost of obesity-related diseases in the United States is $132 billion (AHA, 2009). Consumers spend $40 billion yearly in an attempt to combat excess weight.

Fat distribution is related to health risk (Canoy, 2007). "Apples" describe male-fat patterned distribution with fat accumulating mostly around the torso. "Pears" describe female-fat patterned distribution with fat accumulating mostly on the hips and upper thighs (see Figure 4.14). Apples have a higher health risk especially if they have visceral fat located around internal organs.

FIGURE 4.14
Excess Fat Distribution

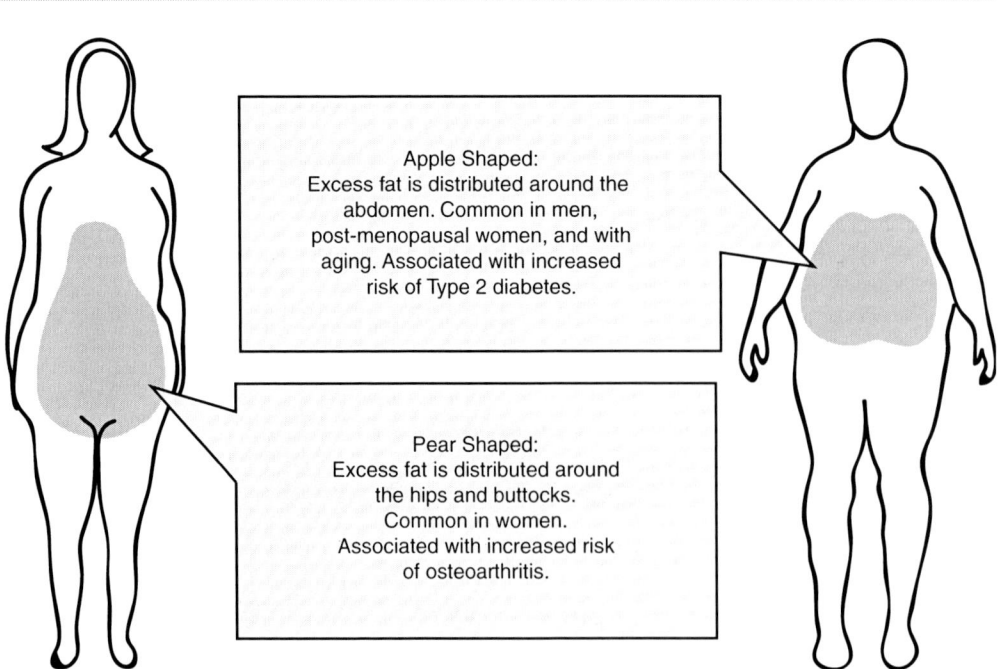

Source: From National Institute of Diabetes and Kidney Disease.

Childhood Obesity

We are a society of excesses. Unfortunately, everyone seems to be getting bigger—all ages, sexes, races independent of socioeconomic status, gender, or locale. The increase in overweight children causes the most concern. Since the 1970s, the prevalence of overweight has doubled for preschoolers ages 2 through 5 and for adolescents ages 12 through 19 (see Figures 4.15 and 4.16). For children ages 6 through 11 the prevalence of overweight has more than tripled (Center for Health and Health Care in Schools, 2007; Frye, 1999).

The causes of **childhood obesity** are complex. As with adult obesity, the bottom line is that if there is a caloric intake surplus, weight will be gained. Infants can be overfed, toddlers can be pacified with candy, and teenagers love soft drinks and junk food. Overweight parents are more likely to have overweight children because the children learn eating and activity patterns from parents. To try to combat childhood obesity, adults should look at their own lifestyle habits: 44 oz sodas several times a day, fast food throughout each week, and lots of time spent playing video games or watching TV will increase the risk of obesity for children and adults alike. These behaviors are not the way to encourage kids to become healthy. Simple things such as eating balanced meals together at home, recreating as a family, and not having junk food always accessible at home are good places to start. Childhood obesity can have a negative impact on overall health risk including psychosocial consequences. Perhaps as individuals, families, schools, communities, and as a nation we should emphasize being more active. Overweight by some arbitrary standard may or may not mean cardiovascular or diabetic risk. Sedentary living, however, almost always predicates poor health in the future, if not sooner. "School aged youth should participate daily in 60 minutes or more of moderate to vigorous physical activity that is developmentally appropriate, enjoyable, and involves a variety of activities" (*Journal of Pediatrics*, 2005). How ironic that we should have to tell our kids to go out and play! Adults would do well to follow this same advice.

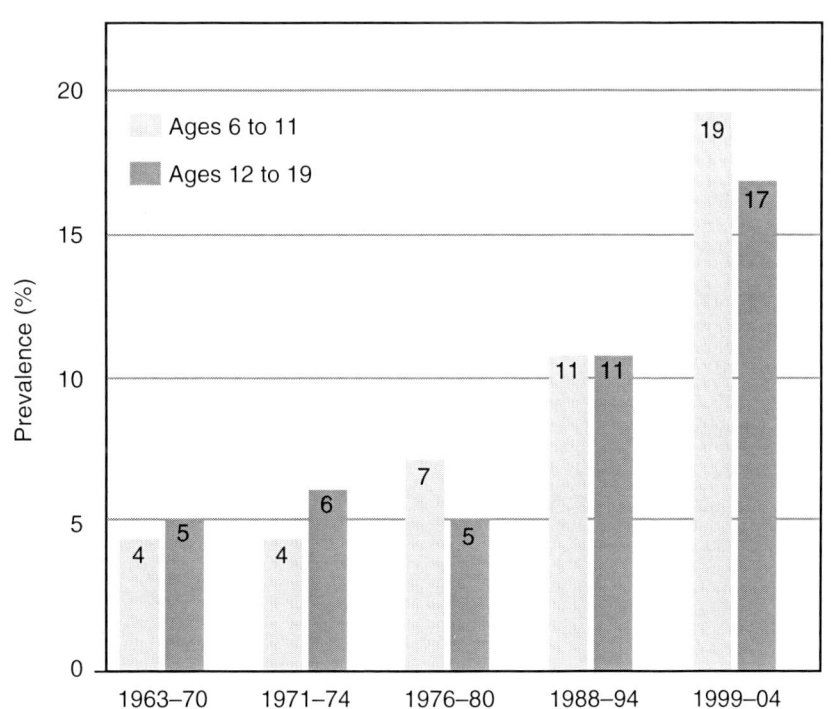

FIGURE 4.15

Prevalence of Overweight* among Children and Adolescents Ages 6–19 Years[1]

*Gender- and age-specific BMI≥ the 95th percentile

Data from NHANES studies for years cited.[1]

Source: National Health and Nutricial Examination Survey, CDC.

FIGURE 4.16

Prevalence of Students in Grades 9–12 Who Met Currently Recommended Levels of Physical Activity during the Past Seven Days by Race/Ethnicity and Sex (YRBS: 2007)

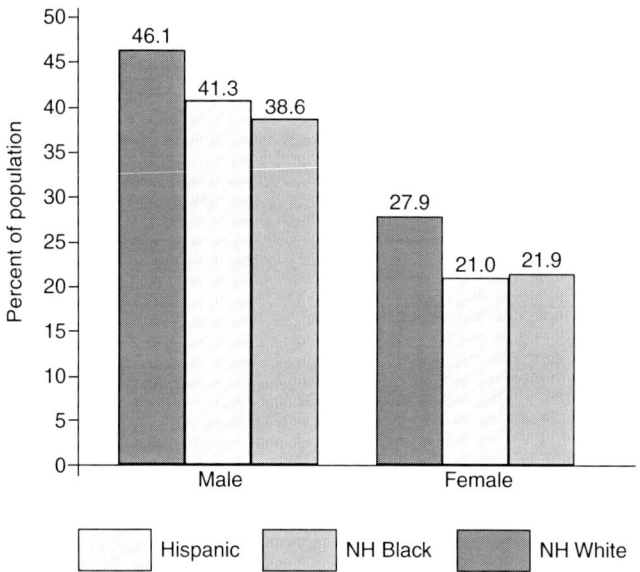

Note: "Currently recommended levels" is defined as activity that increased their heart rate and made them breathe hard some of the time for a total of at least 60 minutes/day on 5 or more of the 7 days preceding the survey.

Source: Morbidity & Mortality Weekly, CDC.gov

Causes of Obesity

Is it your genes or your fast-food lunches every day? Most likely it is both. Since you cannot change who your parents are, change your lifestyle habits. *Physical inactivity is certainly a major, if not the primary, cause of obesity in the United States today* (Wilmore, 1994). Most often caloric intake exceeds caloric expenditure. Glandular disorders affect 2 percent of the obese population which can be treated medically (Corbin, 2009). Genetically we are predisposed to a certain somatotype, fat distribution, size, and weight.

In every person, body weight is the result of many factors; genetic, metabolic, behavioral, environmental, cultural as well as socioeconomic influences (Surgeon General, 2005). An individual's lifestyle choices can help to modify these

Can You Make a Difference?

Get involved in your local school district as an activist for good health. When school budgets are tight, P.E. teachers are often the first to be let go. Often we think one person can't make a difference. Molly Barker didn't let that stop her from forming a grassroots organization that targets the emotional and the mental fitness as well as developing the physical fitness of young girls. The program, called *Girls on the Run*, is a twelve-week program that culminates in the participants running or walking a 5-km road race. The road race is secondary to what the girls experience in the twelve weeks leading up to the race. Positive preteen emotional development is the focus. The girls might warm up by running/walking around a track, and then have focused girl talk. They discuss positive people in their lives. Issues such as pressures to look a certain way, anorexia, bullying, nutrition, the role of women in society, and what makes each girl special are contemplated as a group. *Girls on the Run* is now in over one-hundred cities across Canada and the United States. One person can make a difference. Be a good role model for your kids, your siblings, your relatives, for any children that you come in contact with. Like Molly Barker, choose to be involved not only with your own health, but also with the health of your community.

tendencies. Nineteen out of twenty overweight teenagers will be overweight adults (Texas A&M University Human Nutrition Conference, 1998).

Physiological Response to Obesity

For an obese person, more blood vessels are needed to circulate blood. The heart has to pump harder, therefore increasing blood pressure. Extra weight can be tough on the musculoskeletal joints, causing problems with arthritis, gout, bone and joint diseases, varicose veins, gallbladder disease, as well as complications during pregnancy. Obese individuals often are heat intolerant and experience shortness of breath during heavy exercise. Obesity increases most cancer risks (Bishop and Aldana, 1999).

Fitness or Fatness

Dr. Steven Blair of the Cooper Institute in Dallas is convinced we are too focused on obesity and overweight. Physical activity is much more crucial than a high BMI. People who are active, yet have a high BMI, have lower death rates than those who have a normal BMI but are sedentary. It is clear that if a sedentary person begins an exercise program, blood glucose and cholesterol could improve, yet that person might not loose any weight. *"Fitness is a more important indicator of health outcomes than fatness"* says Steven Ball, University of Missouri exercise physiologist.

Cancer

Cancer is characterized by the uncontrollable growth and spread of abnormal cells. Cancer cells do not follow the normal code of DNA that is encrypted in non-cancerous cells.

Who Gets Cancer?

Possibly in the future people will be able to go to the doctor for a simple blood test to determine whether they will have cancer or not. Unfortunately there seems to be no rhyme or reason for some cancer cases. Lifestyle choices, as well as heredity and also luck, play a big role in a person's risk of developing cancer. Even personality can influence if a person is prone to cancer. With health promotion and prevention, fewer people may develop cancer, and more cancer patients may survive.

Can Cancer Be Prevented?

It is theorized that 80 percent of cancers can be prevented with positive lifestyle choices. Avoiding tobacco and over-exposure to sunlight are two major examples. Eating a varied diet, consuming antioxidants, having a positive attitude, and participating in regular physical activity are simple choices that can have a large impact on cancer prevention. Thirty-five percent of the total cancer death toll is associated with diet (Rosato, 1994), and fit individuals may have a decreased risk of reproductive organ cancers (Bishop and Aldana, 1999). Cancer is the second leading cause of death in the United States, accounting for about 23 percent of all deaths yearly (Hoeger et al., 2009).

Does Exercise Help?

Recognition of the potential of exercise to prevent cancer came in 1985 when the American Cancer Society began recommending exercise to protect against cancer. Regular activity has been shown to reduce risk of colon cancer (see Table 4.2). It is unknown the exact mechanism in exercise that reduces risk of colon cancer, but

"Exercise is a known remedy for the weakness and low spirits that cancer patients experience during their recovery. It boosts energy and endurance, and also builds confidence and optimism. But, within the past five years, several medical investigations have revealed a surprising new fact: Exercise may also help prevent cancer" (Rosato, 1994).

Table 4.2
Physical Activity and Cancer

Cancer Type	Effect of Physical Activity
Colon	Exercise speeds movement of food and cancer-causing substances through the digestive system, and reduces prostaglandins (substances linked to cancer in the colon).
Breast	Exercise decreases the amount of exposure of breast tissue to circulating estrogen. Lower body fat is also associated with lower estrogen levels. Early life activity is deemed important for both reasons. Fatigue from therapy is reduced by exercise.
Rectal	Similar to colon cancer, exercise leads to more regular bowel movements and reduces "transit time."
Prostate	Fatigue from therapy is reduced by exercise.

possibly it is due to the increased transit time of foodstuffs traveling through the gut and intestines due to activity. Active people have lower death rates from cancer than inactive people—50 to 250 percent lower. Colon, breast, rectal, and prostate cancers each have an established link with inactivity.

Exercising early in life also seems to have an impact in reducing risk of breast cancer in post-menopausal women. A study at the USC Norris Cancer Center reported that one to three hours of exercise a week over a woman's reproductive lifetime (between the teens and age 40) may result in a 20 to 30 percent risk reduction for breast cancer. Exercise that averaged four or more hours per week resulted in a 60 percent reduction! A woman starting to exercise in her 20's or 30's can also experience reduced risk. Active females, such as a dancer or track athlete, may put off the age of onset of menstruation, and if they continue to be active, they may experience earlier menopause than their inactive counterparts. This results in a lower lifetime exposure to estrogen, which also reduces cancer risk. Ironically lower estrogen levels may contribute to osteoporosis.

It is also thought that exercise can boost immunity that can help kill abnormal cancer cells (Bishop and Aldana, 1999). Dr. Steven Blair at the Institute for Aerobics Research in Dallas, Texas, has done long-term epidemiological studies that show rate of death due to cancer is significantly lower in patients with elevated levels of fitness. It must also be noted that people who are active tend to also participate in other healthy behaviors, such as eating a varied diet low in fat and high in fiber. These other behaviors may also influence cancer risk and help those with cancer lead more fulfilling and productive lives. The American Cancer Society reports that people with healthy lifestyles (non-smokers, regular physical activity, and sufficient sleep) have the lowest cancer mortality rates.

Diabetes

Diabetes is a disorder that involves high blood sugar levels and inadequate insulin production by the pancreas or inadequate utilization of insulin by the cells (Wilmore, 1994). Type II diabetes will be discussed in this chapter.

> ## Diabetic Walkers Gain Fitness
>
> Diabetics who walked moderately for thirty-eight minutes (4,400 steps or 2.2 miles) did not lose weight; however, they showed significant effects: risk of heart disease decreased; cholesterol improved; triglycerides improved; and they saved $288.00 in health costs per year.
>
>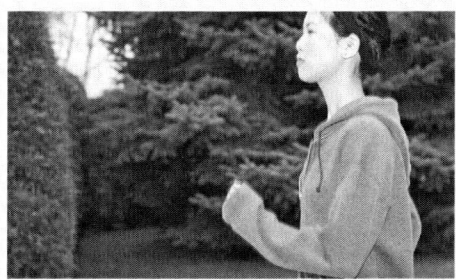
> © 2005 JupiterImages Corporation
>
> Diabetics who walked ninety minutes (10,000 steps or 5 miles) saw bigger benefits: the number of walkers needing insulin therapy decreased by 25 percent; those receiving insulin therapy reduced the dosage by an average of eleven units per day; cholesterol, triglycerides, blood pressure, and heart disease risk decreased; and they saved over $1,200.00 per year.
>
> Diabetics in the control group that did not walk saw health care costs rise $500.00; insulin use, cholesterol, blood pressure, triglycerides, and heart disease risk all increased.
>
> This study was conducted for two years. (Sullivan et al., 2009)

Who Gets Diabetes?

Since 1990 the prevalence of diabetes has increased by 61 percent. Eighty percent of the adults who develop Type II diabetes are obese (Surgeon General, 2005). The mortality rate is greater in diabetics with CVD—two-thirds to three-fourths of people with diabetes die from some form of CVD. Diabetes is the seventh leading cause of death in people over 40 (Corbin and Welk, 2009). Due to the surge in childhood obesity in the decade of the 90's, children are more at risk for diabetes. Diabetes is one of the most important risk factors for stroke in women.

Can Diabetes Be Prevented?

Research shows that changing lifestyle habits to decrease risk for heart disease also decreases risk for diabetes. "According to research, a seven percent loss of body weight and 150 minutes of moderate-intensity physical activity a week can reduce the chance of developing diabetes by 58 percent in those who are at high risk. These lifestyle changes cut the risk of developing type II diabetes regardless of age, ethnicity, gender, or weight" (AHA, 2009). Type II diabetes may account for 90–95 percent of all diagnosed cases of diabetes (AHA, 2009).

Does Exercise Help?

Exercise plays an important role in managing this disease, as exercise helps control body fat and improves insulin sensitivity and glucose tolerance. Exercise does not prevent Type II diabetes; however, exercise does help manage the disorder.

Metabolic Syndrome

Moderate and vigorous activity is associated with a lower risk of developing **metabolic syndrome**. Metabolic syndrome is a "cluster" of cardiovascular risk factors including overweight or obesity (waist circumference above 102 cm for men or above 88 cm for women), high blood pressure (above 130/85 mm Hg or current drug treatment for hypertension), elevated triglycerides (150 mg/dL or higher), low levels of high-density lipoprotein (below 40 mg/dL in men and below 50 mg/dL in women), and high fasting glucose levels (100 mg/dL or higher) (AHA, 2009). Having three or more of these risk factors puts you at higher risk of developing CVD or diabetes. In studies done at the Cooper Institute in Dallas, the risk of metabolic syndrome for men with moderate fitness was 26 percent lower, and for men with high fitness the risk was 53 percent lower compared to their lower fitness counterparts. For women the risk was 20 percent and 63 percent lower, respectively. It is clear that to prevent metabolic syndrome, improving cardiovascular fitness through regular physical activity is critical (AHA, 2005).

Low Back Pain

Low back pain is characterized by chronic discomfort in the lumbar region of the back. Chronic back pain may be the result of an injury; however, back pain is most often due to a lack of fitness. The National Safety Council data indicates that the back is the most frequently injured of all the body parts, with the injury rate double that of other body parts. Intervertebral disks can suffer degeneration from overuse, which is more common in men than in women. Backache is the second leading medical complaint when visiting a physician (Corbin and Welk, 2009).

Who Suffers from Low Back Pain?

More than eight out of ten Americans will suffer some back-related pain at some point in their lifetime (Corbin and Welk, 2009). Low back pain is epidemic throughout the world and is the major cause of disability in people aged 20 through 45 in the United States. Ninety percent of back injuries occur in the lumbar region (Donatelle and Davis, 2007). Thirty to 70 percent of all Americans have recurring back problems; two million Americans cannot hold a job as a result. Back pain is the most frequent cause of inactivity in individuals under the age of 45 (Corbin and Welk, 2009). Improper lifting, faulty work habits, heredity, diseases such as scoliosis, and excess weight are other causes of low back pain. Undue psychological stress can cause back pain via tight muscles and constricted blood vessels (Hoeger et al., 2009).

Can Low Back Pain Be Prevented?

Lack of activity is the most common reason for low back pain, so movement is critical to good back health. Staying active, using common sense regarding lifting heavy objects, and managing weight all are important in low back pain prevention. Decrease occupational risks. Use caution, as it is often employees new to a job who injure their back. Another factor in low back pain is poor posture while sitting, standing, or walking.

Does Exercise Help?

Exercise helps with enhancing posture, balance, strength, and flexibility. Strengthening abdominal muscles, which are the complimentary muscle group to the lower back, helps support the spine. Stretching the hip flexors and the hamstrings are important to help tilt the anterior portion of the pelvis back. Low back pain and tight hamstrings are highly correlated. Excess weight around the torso and abdominal region pulls the pelvis forward, causing potential strain in the lumbar region. In general, strengthening the "core" (all the muscles from the shoulders and the hips) helps prevent back pain. A regular exercise and flexibility program can help to manage weight over a lifetime.

Osteoporosis

Osteoporosis is a disease characterized by low bone density and structural deterioration of bone tissue, which can lead to increased bone fragility and increased risk of fractures to the skeletal structure. Osteoporosis is sometimes called the "silent disease" because there are often no symptoms as bone density decreases. The *Dallas Morning News* (August 26, 2001) describes osteoporosis as an "epidemic of young women with old bones." Many young women delay the onset of menstruation due to high activity levels, which in turn lowers body fat and estrogen levels. Your physician may recommend a bone mineral density test. The test is noninvasive, painless, and safe (Otis and Goldingay, 2000).

How much calcium does a college student need?
1,300 mg daily

- Good sources of calcium: low-fat dairy products, dark green leafy vegetables, tofu, sardines, and salmon.
- Calcium-fortified foods: cereals, breads, orange juice, and some antacids.

Bone is living, growing tissue. With adequate nutrition and activity, bone formation continues to occur throughout a lifetime. Old bone is removed through **resorption**, and new bone is formed through a process called **formation**. Bones need to be fed and cared for just as the rest of our body. Childhood and teenage years are when new bone is developed more quickly than the old bone is resorbed. Bones become stronger and denser until peak bone mass is attained at approximately age 30. Thereafter, bone loss exceeds bone formation. Adequate calcium intake and regular physical activity are critical for young adults because the higher peak bone mass is at age 30, the less likely it is that osteoporosis will develop in later years.

Who Gets Osteoporosis?

For 34 million Americans, osteoporosis is a major public health threat (Surgeon General, 2004). Considered to afflict mostly women, this disease can affect males as well. Of the women with osteoporosis, 80 percent are post-menopausal. One out of two women and one out of eight men over 50 will get osteoporosis in their lifetime.

Risk increases with age. Have you observed older women who seem to slump? Many women with low bone density have kyphosis (also called dowager's hump), or a rounding of the upper back. The head tilts forward because often the cervical vertebrae in the upper spine actually suffer compression fractures. This keeps older women from being able to stand up straight or to get a full breath. Small, thin-boned women are at higher risk, and there may also be a genetic factor. If there are people in a family with weak, thin bones then relatives with the same body type may have an inherently higher risk. Post-menopausal Caucasian and Asian women are at the highest risk. It is unknown why these particular groups are more susceptible to osteoporosis. African Americans have bone that is 10 percent more dense than Caucasians (Greenberg et al., 1998). Others at risk include those with poor diets, especially if calcium and vitamin D are low over a long period of time. It is estimated that 75 percent of adults do not consume enough calcium on a daily basis (Bishop and Aldana, 1999). An inactive lifestyle contributes greatly. A history of excessive use of alcohol or cigarette smoking can also increase risk.

Another growing group of high-risk individuals is the eating disordered. Many active young women suffer stress fractures, which can be a sign of osteoporosis. If a person is extremely active with a low percentage of body fat, then hormone levels may be askew. Prolonged amenorrhea (absence of menstruation) can signal low body fat or an eating disorder. Low estrogen levels characterize amenorrhea and contribute to significant losses in bone density. Estrogen plays a key role in how calcium is used in developing bone density. When a runner, gymnast, or dancer suffers a stress

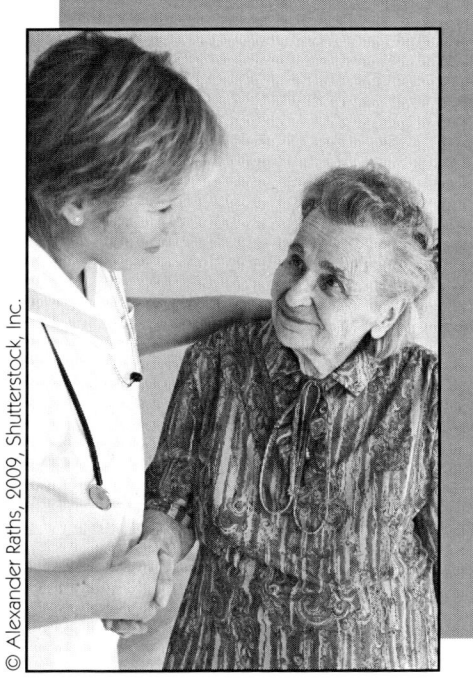

The risk of osteoporosis increases with age and afflicts mostly women.

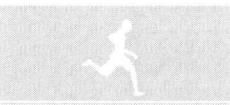

Current Recommendations to Decrease Osteoporosis Risk

- Engage in daily weight-bearing aerobic activity
- Weight training (the ACSM recommends ten–twelve reps, two sets two times weekly)
- Vitamin D (well-balanced diet and adequate exposure to sunlight)
- Estrogen replacement therapy (for some women, especially post-menopausal women)

fracture, it is not typical to administer a bone density test. If other symptoms such as amenorrhea, disordered eating, or abuse of exercise are suspected, then it would be prudent for the physician to order or for the athlete to consider asking for a bone density test.

Can Osteoporosis Be Prevented?

The good news is that osteoporosis can be both prevented and treated. Regular physical activity reduces the risk of developing osteoporosis. A lifetime of low calcium intake is associated with low bone mass (www.osteo.org). Adequate calcium intake is critical for optimal bone mass. Growing children, adolescents, and pregnant and breast-feeding women need more calcium. It is estimated by the National Institutes of Health that less than 10 percent of girls age 10–17 years are getting the calcium they need each day. A varied diet with green leafy vegetables and plenty of dairy will help ensure good calcium intake. Many calcium-fortified foods are now available. A varied diet will also ensure adequate intake of vitamin D, which aids in prevention. It is also advisable to limit caffeine and phosphate-containing soda, which may interfere with calcium absorption. Prolonged high-protein diets may also contribute to calcium loss in bone. A high-sodium diet is thought to increase calcium excretion through the kidneys. For post-menopausal women, some physicians consider hormone replacement therapy to help strengthen bones. Weight-bearing exercise such as walking, running, tennis, and basketball is an excellent way to strengthen bones to help prevent osteoporosis.

Does Exercise Help?

The stress caused by working against gravity during activity strengthens and causes bones to be more dense, just as any other living tissue. Weight training is highly recommended to keep the bones strong and to build bone mass. Consider the muscle atrophy experienced when a person is confined to bed rest, or a limb is in a cast for a period of time. Bones deteriorate just as muscles deteriorate without the stimulation of movement. An interesting current topic of study is the effect of zero gravity in space on bone mass. It appears that even a short duration in space can impact bone density (see Bone Loss during Spaceflight, on page 131).

Physical activity is presented as the only known intervention that can potentially increase bone mass and strength in the early years of life and reduce the risk of falling in older populations according to a new Position Stand from the American

Shape Up America!

If you like gimmicks and gadgets, try a pedometer. A pedometer is a small device that clips on your belt and counts your steps. The average American walks approximately 900–3,000 steps per day in daily normal activities. The former U.S. Surgeon General, C. Everett Koop, developed Shape Up America! in 1994 to highlight health risks of obesity. The extra 150 calories or thirty minutes per day recommended by the Surgeon General's 1996 Report may not be enough for you to reach your fitness or weight loss goals. Studies indicate that a sufficient goal would be to walk 10,000 steps per day. Shape Up America! challenges you to walk 10,000 steps. Without a conscious effort, 10,000 steps would be a difficult task. Be sure and log your steps each day to work up to 10,000. Give it a try; if you like the latest thing, a pedometer is much cheaper than an ab roller or a treadmill!

Bone Loss during Spaceflight

In the 1980's, NASA scientists observed a dramatic spike in calcium excreted by astronauts after the first seven days of spaceflight. Researchers have since confirmed that humans lose bone mineral density during spaceflight at a rate ten-fold faster than does a post-menopausal woman; the lack of gravitational forces, even with daily exercise during space missions, has a very dramatic effect on bone mass. There are also changes in the cross-sectional geometry of long bones, for instance, the femoral neck near the hip joint, that further reduce bone strength and increase risk of a hip fracture should that astronaut fall soon after returning to earth. Some of this bone loss may be due to reduced blood flow to bone with the shifts in body fluids while in microgravity, according to a study by Dr. Michael Delp at Texas A&M University. This reduced blood flow in turn may affect in various ways the activity of bone cells responsible for bone formation and bone resorption, altering the balance in favor of resorption (Colleran et al., 2000). Related studies conducted by Dr. Susan Bloomfield at Texas A&M University demonstrated that this bone loss is not uniform across the skeleton but focused in trabecular ("spongy") bone sites (for instance., in the ends of the long bones) (Bloomfield et al., 2002). This is the same type of bone that is lost first with the development of osteoporosis here on earth. Another potential contributor to bone loss in astronauts might be reduced caloric intake, quite common during busy missions. Restricting caloric intake by 40 percent causes reductions in trabecular bone formation rate similar in magnitude to that observed with the unloading of microgravity (Baek et al., 2008). This finding has important implications for the many Americans who attempt long-term restriction of caloric intake to achieve weight loss.

Colleran, P.N., M.K. Wilkerson, S.A. Bloomfield, L.J. Suva, R.T. Turner, and M.D. Delp. Alterations in skeletal perfusion with simulated microgravity: a possible mechanism for bone remodeling. *J. Appl. Physiol.* 89: 1046–1054, 2000.

Bloomfield, S.A., M.R. Allen, H.A. Hogan, and M.D. Delp. Site- and compartment-specific changes in bone with hindlimb unloading in mature adult rats. *Bone* 31: 149–157, 2002.

Baek, K., A.A. Barlow, M.R. Allen, and S.A. Bloomfield. Food restriction and simulated microgravity: effects on bone and serum leptin. *J. Appl. Physiol.* 104: 1086–1093. 2008.

College of Sports Medicine (ACSM). The official ACSM position stand encourages the adoption of specific exercise prescriptions designed for various ages to best capitalize on the chances to accrue and preserve bone throughout the various stages of life (Surgeon General, 2004).

Aging

Although aging is a completely natural and inevitable process, some people age more gracefully than others. As the typical American's lifespan expands, quality of life for many is compromised due to habits and lifestyle choices made earlier in life. Ensure your independence as you age by choosing how you live your life now. Balancing work, family commitments, and leisure time can be stressful. Stress takes a toll on our bodies, our minds, and our relationships.

Everyone experiences age-related decline in biological functions of the body. Chronological age is our true age in years. Biological age can be different depending on our lifestyle choices. **Biological age** can be younger than chronological age with good nutrition, adequate rest on a regular basis, stress-management techniques,

"Real Age"

Dr. Michael Roizen has developed a "real" age test. Log on to www.realage.com to take the free test. According to Roizen, exercising regularly can make your "real" age as much as nine years younger.

> ## Creativity and Aging
>
> Typically mental processes being to slow down with age; however, some characteristics such as creativity can flourish with age. There are many examples of great creative accomplishments by elderly artists. Michaelangelo completed his final frescoes for the Vatican's Pauline Chapel at 75. Georgia O'Keeffe painted into her 90's despite failing eyesight. Benjamin Franklin invented bifocal glasses at 78 to correct his poor vision. Folks that have lived longer and have had more experience tend to be more comfortable in their own skin. Because mature adults seldom experience the adolescent need to "fit in," they are more likely to have the freedom to express themselves. This may enhance creative endeavors. So look forward to good health and artful aging in your golden years.

and consistent exercise (see Table 4.3). Biological age can be older than chronological age when unhealthy habits are the norm: poor diet, inadequate sleep, excessive alcohol use, smoking, and obesity. You are in charge of your biological age. What will your biological age be in ten, twenty, and thirty years from now? How about fifty years from now? It is interesting to note that physiological changes with aging are similar to those changes seen with inactivity or prolonged weightlessness, such as experienced by the astronauts (Bloomfield et al., 2002). An integrative biology professor at Berkeley, 78-year-old Marian Diamond lists five essentials for staying mentally vigorous:

1. diet,
2. exercise,
3. challenge,
4. novelty,
5. love.

These five essentials seem to be critical to maintain quality of life at retirement age, but perhaps they are essentials for us all, at any age (Springen and Seibert, 2005).

Table 4.3
Effects of Physical Activity and Inactivity on Older Men

	Exercisers	Non-Exercisers
Age (yrs)	68.0	69.8
Weight (lbs)	160.3	186.3
Resting heart rate (bpm)	55.8	66.0
Maximal heart rate (bpm)	157.0	146.0
Heart rate reserve* (bpm)	101.2	80.0
Blood pressure (mm Hg)	120/78	150/90
Maximal oxygen uptake (ml/kg/min)	38.6	20.3

*Heart rate reserve = maximal heart rate – resting heart rate.

Source: From *Principles and Labs for Fitness & Wellness,* 6th edition, Wadsworth Publishing.

It's Never Too Late

He was a world champion. Jesse Coon of College Station, Texas, passed away on July 30, 2005, after a long, full, and active life. He was 94. Coon started swimming competitively at the ripe old age of 64, and he started breaking world records in his early 80's.

The former physics professor at Texas A&M University broke five world records at his last major swim meet in Munich, Germany, in the 90 through 94 age group. His stroke? The butterfly. When competing, Coon worked out in the pool ninety minutes five times per week. Jesse Coon was an active sailor and he mowed his own lawn.

Not all mature Americans need to be world record holders to benefit from a more active lifestyle. Recent studies indicate that regular exercise and physical activity can reduce or slow down the biological process of aging. Older adults can experience increased life satisfaction, happiness, and self-esteem, along with reduced stress with a regular activity. A friend noted that it never occurred to Jesse that he was old. He celebrated life and always had a positive attitude. Coon himself said "the older you get, the more important it is to exercise." Coon is an example not only to others of the gray-haired set, but to all of us of all ages.

Prevention of Hypokinetic Conditions: Planning Your Activity Program

Most adults know that they should be active, and they may be aware that a more active life would make them feel better. The truth is that sometimes it is very difficult to know how to get started and how to incorporate activity into busy lives. The most important thing is to get started. Remember that lifestyle activity is easier to incorporate into a hectic schedule; walk during a coffee break, grab ten minutes to move around while on break, or jump rope for a study break. Planned exercise can be more of a challenge. The following are a few suggestions to help jump-start the new you.

1. Establish why you want to exercise.
2. Write down reasonable long-term goals.
3. Write down short-term goals that support the long-term goals.
4. Record the behaviors that need to change in order to support the goals. (A person wanting to quit smoking may want to quit working at a bar and work in a nonsmoking environment.)
5. Write in a log: feelings, food, activity and goal progress are all appropriate.
6. Develop a weekly plan for the activity that supports your goals.
7. Tell your friends and family about your goals and ask for their support.
8. Reward yourself when any goals are met (rewards should be non-food items, and should not be a day "off" from behaviors that promote your goals).
9. When goals are not met, check your log. What can you change to more effectively support your goals?
10. Periodically re-evaluate goals.

It has been firmly established that physical activity should be a part of our daily lives. Exercise enhances weight management and overall wellness by burning calories, speeding up metabolism, building muscle tissue, and balancing appetite with energy expenditure. More importantly, an active life decreases health risk and typically makes you feel good, and feel good about yourself. Look for opportunities to be active and have fun at the same time.

REFERENCES

Alters, S. and Schiff, W. *Essential Concepts for Healthy Living* (5th ed). Sudbury, MA., Jones and Bartlett. 2009.

American College of Sports Medicine (ACSM). *Exercise and Hypertension.*

American Heart Association (AHA). *Poor Teen Sleep Habits May Raise Blood Pressure, Lead to CVD.* News release December 10, 2008.

American Heart Association (AHA). *Heart Disease and Stroke Statistics—2009 Update.* 2009. www.aha.com

Canoy, M. P. et al. Abdominal Fat Distribution Predicts Heart Disease, *Circulation*, 2007.

Castelli, W. P., Chair, Women, smoking and oral contraceptives; Highlights of a consensus conference, Montreal, November 1997.

Center for Health and Health Care in Schools, School of Public Health and Health Services, George Washington University Medical Center. *Childhood Overweight: What the Research Tells Us.* September 2007 Update. www.healthinschools.org

Corbin, C. and Welk G. *Concepts of Physical Fitness* (15th ed). New York: McGraw-Hill. 2009.

Donatelle, R. J. and Davis, L. G. *Access to Health* (10th ed). Boston: Benjamin Cummings. 2007.

Flegal, K. M., Carrol, M. D., Kuczmarski, R. J., and Johnson, C. L. Overweight and Obesity in the United States: Prevalence and Trends, 1960–1994. *International Journal of Obesity and Related Metabolic Disorders,* 22: 39–47. 1998.

Frye, D. W. Contracting Officer. NHANES IV, Central Lipid Laboratory for National Health and Nutrition Survey. October 1999.

Gaesser, G. Obesity, Health, and Metabolic Fitness, *www.thinkmuscle.com/articles*

Gibbs, W. W. Obesity: An Overblown Epidemic? *Scientific American*, May 23, 2005.

Greenberg, J. et al. *Physical Fitness and Wellness* (2nd ed). Boston: Allyn and Bacon. 1998.

Hafen, B. Q., Karren, K. J., and Frandsen, K. J. *First Aid for Colleges and Universities* (7th ed). Boston: Allyn and Bacon. 1999.

The Heart Truth for Women: Women and Heart Disease, *www.hearttruth.gov*

Hoeger, W. W. K., Turner, L. W., and Hafen, B. Q. *Wellness Guidelines for a Healthy Lifestyle* (4th ed). Belmont, CA: Thomson Wadsworth. 2009.

Koop, C. E. Shape Up America! http://www.shapeupamericastore.org, 1994.

National Center for Health Statistics, U.S. Department of Health and Human Services, Centers for Disease Control and Prevention. Hyattsville, MD.

National Institutes on Aging, NIH, www.nia.nih.gov 2008.

National Institutes of Health, http://www.nhlbi.nih.gov/actintime/rhar/md.htm

National Institutes of Health. *Sixth Report on the Joint National Committee on Prevention, Detection, Evaluation and Treatment of High Blood Pressure.* 1997.

National Institutes of Health. Osteoporosis and Related Bone Disease, http://www.osteo.org

Ochoa, L. W., editor. *Women's Health and Wellness, an Illustrated Guide* (26th ed). Skokie, IL: Lippincott Williams & Wilkins. 2002.

Otis, C. L. and Goldingay, R. *The Athletic Woman's Survival Guide.* Champaign, IL: Human Kinetics Publishers. 2000.

Paffenbarger, R. et al. Physical Activity and Physical Fitness as Determinants of Health and Longevity. In C. Bouchard et al. *Exercise Fitness and Health.* Champaign, IL: Human Kinetics Publishers. 1990.

Payne, W. A. and Hahn, D. B. *Understanding Your Health* (6th ed). St. Louis, MO: Mosby. 2000.

Powers, S. K. and Dodd, S. L. *Total Fitness and Wellness.* San Francisco: Pearson Benjamin Cummings. 2009.

Rosato, F. *Fitness to Wellness: The Physical Connection* (3rd ed). Minneapolis: West. 1994.

Satcher, D. *Surgeon General's Report on Physical Activity and Health.* Atlanta, GA: CDC. 1996.

Sesso, H. D. and Paffenbarger, R. S. The Harvard Alumni Health Study, Harvard School of Public Health. Boston: 1956.

Seventh Report of the Joint National Committee on Prevention, Detection, Evaluation, and Treatment of High Blood Pressure (JNC VII). *Hypertension*, December 2003.

Springen, K. and Seibert, S. Artful Aging, *Newsweek*, January 17, p. 57. 2005.

Sullivan, P. W. et. al. Obesity, Inactivity, and the Prevalence of Diabetes and Diabetes-related Cardiovascular Comorbidities in the U.S., 2000–2002, *Diabetes Care,* 28: 1599–1603, 2009.

Surgeon General's Call to Action to Prevent and Decrease Overweight and Obesity, www.surgeongeneral.gov

Surgeon General's Report on Bone Health and Osteoporosis: What It Means to You. Washington, DC: U.S. DHHS. October, 2004.

Texas A&M University Human Nutrition Conference. College Station, TX. 1998.

Weinttraub, A. Yoga: It's Not Just An Exercise. *Psychology Today.* November, 2000.

Wilmore, J. H. Exercise, Obesity, and Weight Control, *Physical Activity and Research Digest.* Washington D.C.: President's Council on Physical Fitness & Sports. 1994.

World Health Organization (WHO). *Controlling the Obesity Epidemic.* Geneva: Author December 2008.

www.osteo.org

CONTACTS

American College of Sports Medicine (ACSM) http://www.acsm.org

American Heart Association
http://www.americanheart.org

American Medical Association
http://www.ama-assn.org

Franklin Institute of Science: interactive multimedia tour of the heart
http://www.fi.edu/biosci/heart.html

Dr. Koop's Community: health improvement info
http://www.drkoop.com

Stayhealthy.com: comprehensive Internet resources continuously updated
http://www.stayhealthy.com/

Go Ask Alice: sponsored by Columbia University Health Service; question & answer format
http://www.alice.columbia.edu/index.html

Centers for Disease Control and Prevention: Information and national health statistics plus more
http://www.cdc/gov

National Health Information Center: 100 organizations listed here to provide answers to health-related questions
http://nhic-nt.health.org/

Weight-control Information Network
www.win.niddk.nih.gov
1 WIN Way
Bethesda, MD 20892-3665
(toll-free number) 877-946-4627

RECOMMENDED READING

Working Out, Working Within by Jerry Lynch (Archer/Putnam, 1998)

The Athletic Woman's Survival Guide by Carol Otis & Roger Goldingay (Human Kinetics Publishers, 2000)

Strong Women Stay Young by Miriam E. Nelson (Bantam, 1997)

Habits Not Diets by James M. Ferguson (Bell, 1988)

ACTIVITIES

Notebook Activities

Self-Assessment of Cardiovascular Fitness

Healthy Back Test

Is Your Blood in Tune?

Is Osteoporosis in Your Future?

Name: _____ Section: _____ Date: _____

NOTEBOOK ACTIVITY

Self-Assessment of Cardiovascular Fitness

Once you've been exercising regularly for several weeks, you might want to assess your cardiovascular fitness level. Find a local track, typically one-quarter mile per lap, to perform your test. You may either run/walk for one and a half miles and measure how long it takes to reach that distance, or run/walk for twelve minutes and determine the distance you covered in that time. Use the chart below to estimate your cardiovascular fitness level based upon your age and gender. Note that females have lower standards for each fitness category because of their higher levels of essential fat.

	1.5-Mile Run (min:sec)		12-Minute Run (miles)	
Age*	Female (min:sec)	Male (min:sec)	Female (miles)	Male (miles)
	Good			
15–30	<12:00	<10:00	>1.5	>1.7
31–50	<13:30	<11:30	>1.4	>1.5
51–70	<16:00	<14:00	>1.2	>1.3
	Adequate for most activities			
15–30	<13:30	<11:50	>1.4	>1.5
31–50	<15:00	<13:00	>1.3	>1.4
51–70	<17:30	<15:30	>1.1	>1.3
	Borderline			
15–30	<15:00	<13:00	>1.3	>1.4
31–50	<16:30	<14:30	>1.2	>1.3
51–70	<19:00	<17:00	>1.0	>1.2
	Need extra work on cardiovascular fitness			
15–30	>17:00	>15:00	<1.2	<1.3
31–50	>18:30	>16:30	<1.1	<1.2
51–70	>21:00	>19:00	<0.9	<1.0

Please list the date, location, and amount of time it took you to complete 1.5 miles. _____
_____

or

Please list the date, location, and distance you traveled in twelve minutes. _____
_____

*Cardiovascular fitness declines with age.

If you are now at the Good level, your emphasis should be on maintaining this level for the rest of your life. If you are now at lower levels, you should set realistic goals for improvement.

Source: From *Health/Fitness Instructor's Handbook* by Edward Howley and B. Don Franks. Copyright © 1986. Reprinted by permission of Human Kinetics, Inc.

Name: _____ Section: _____ Date: _____

NOTEBOOK ACTIVITY

Healthy Back Test

These tests are among the ones used by physicians and therapists to make differential diagnoses of back problems. You and your partner can use them to determine if you have muscle tightness that may make you "at risk" for back problems. Discontinue any of these tests if they produce pain or numbness, or tingling sensations in the back, hips, or legs. Experiencing any of these sensations may be an indication that you have a low back problem that requires diagnosis by your physician. Partners should use great caution in applying force. Be gentle and listen to your partner's feedback.

Test 1—Back to Wall

Stand with your back against a wall, with head, heels, shoulders, and calves of legs touching the wall as shown in the diagram. Try to flatten your neck and the hollow of your back by pressing your buttocks down against the wall. Your partner should just be able to place a hand in the space between the wall and the small of your back.
- If this space is greater than the thickness of his/her hand, you probably have lordosis with shortened lumbar and hip flexor muscles.
  ❑ **Pass**   ❑ **Fail**

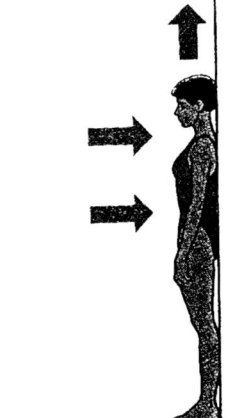

Test 2—Straight Leg Lift

Lie on your back with hands behind your neck. The partner on your left should stabilize your right leg by placing his/her right hand on the knee. With the left hand, your partner should grasp the left ankle and raise your left leg as near to a right angle as possible. In this position (as shown in the diagram), your lower back should be in contact with the floor. Your right leg should remain straight and on the floor throughout the test.
- If your left leg bends at the knee, short hamstring muscles are indicated. If your back arches and/or your right leg does not remain flat on the floor, short lumbar muscles or hip flexor muscles (or both) are indicated. Repeat the test on the opposite side. (Both sides must pass in order to pass the test.)
  ❑ **Pass**   ❑ **Fail**

Test 3—Thomas Test

Lie on your back on a table or bench with your right leg extended beyond the edge of the table (approximately one-third of the thigh off the table). Bring your left knee to your chest and pull the thigh down tightly with your hands. Your lower back should remain flat against the table as shown in the diagram. Your right thigh should remain on the table.
- If your right thigh lifts off the table while the left knee is hugged to the chest, a tight hip flexor (iliopsoas) on that side is indicated. Repeat on the opposite side. (Both sides must pass in order to pass the test.)
  ❑ **Pass**   ❑ **Fail**

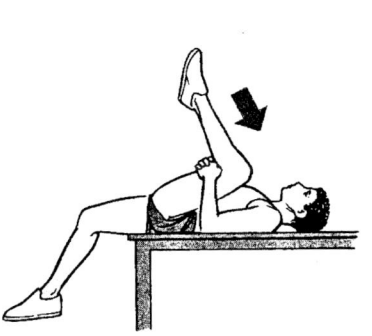

Test 4—Ely's Test

Lie prone; flex right knee. Partner gently pushes right heel toward the buttocks. Stop when resistance is felt or when partner expresses discomfort.
- If pelvis leaves the floor or hip flexes or knee fails to bend freely (135 degrees) or heel fails to touch buttocks, there is tightness in the quadriceps muscles. Repeat with left leg. (Both sides must pass to pass the test.)
  - ❏ Pass   ❏ Fail

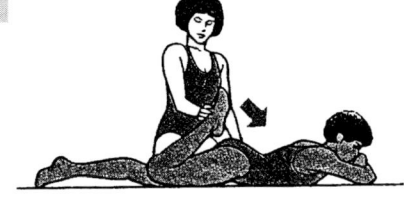

Test 5—Ober's Test

Lie on left side with left leg flexed ninety degrees at the hip and ninety degrees at the knee. Partner places right hip in neutral position (no flexion) and right knee in ninety-degree flexion; partner then allows the weight of the leg to lower it toward the floor.
- If there is no tightness in the iliotibial band (fascia and muscles on lateral side of leg), the knee touches the floor without pain and the test is passed. Repeat on the other side. (Both sides must pass in order to pass the test.)
  - ❏ Pass   ❏ Fail

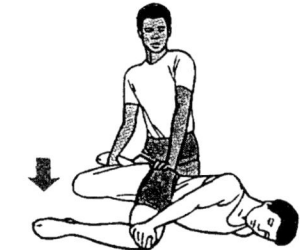

Test 6—Press-Up (Straight Arm)

Perform the press-up.
- If you can press to a straight-arm position, keeping your pubis in contact with the floor, and if your partner determines that the arch in your back is a continuous curve (not just a sharp angle at the lumbosacral joint), then there is adequate flexibility in spinal extension.
  - ❏ Pass   ❏ Fail

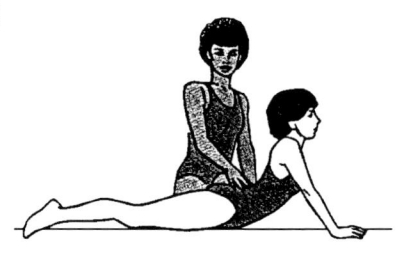

Test 7—Knee Roll

Lie supine with both knees and hips flexed ninety degrees, arms extended to the sides at shoulder level. Keep the knees and hips in that position and lower them to the floor on the right and then on the left.
- If you can accomplish this and still keep your shoulders in contact with the floor, then you have adequate rotation in the spine, especially at the lumbar and thoracic junction. (You must pass both sides in order to pass the test.)
  - ❏ Pass   ❏ Fail

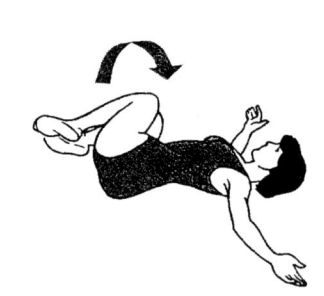

Healthy Back Ratings

Classification	Number of Tests Passed
Excellent	7
Very good	6
Good	5
Fair	4
Poor	1–3

Name: _____ Section: _____ Date: _____

NOTEBOOK ACTIVITY

Is Your Blood in Tune?

Instructions: The composition of your blood is very important when it comes to preventing CHD. You can easily have your physician check your blood-fat levels. Sometimes, this is done with a simple finger prick, but to be as accurate as possible, it should be done by having blood drawn from a vein after you have fasted for about twelve hours. Record the results of that assessment below by checking the appropriate rating.

_____ Total cholesterol is below 200: No further evaluation necessary, recheck in five years.

_____ Total cholesterol is 200–239 (borderline high cholesterol): Evaluate risk factors to see what lifestyle changes you can make (diet, exercise, and so forth). If your physician says you are not in high-risk category for CHD, active treatment is not necessary, but recheck in one to eight weeks.

_____ Total cholesterol is above 240 (high cholesterol): Analyze and measure HDL, LDL, and triglycerides.

Once the above is completed, answer the following questions:

Yes	No	
____	____	1. Is your total cholesterol no more than 4.5 × HDL cholesterol?
____	____	2. Is your cholesterol-to-HDL ration at least five to one?
____	____	3. Is your HDL reading above 35?
____	____	4. Is your LDL cholesterol less than 160?

If the answers to these questions are yes, your lipid profile is good. Regardless of how your lipid profile turned out, list the important changes you can make to lower your total cholesterol and increase your HDL cholesterol over the next twelve months.

1. _____

2. _____

3. _____

4. _____

5. _____

Source: From *Physical Fitness & Wellness, 2nd Edition,* by Greenberg, Dintiman & Oakes, Allyn and Bacon Publishers.

Name: _____ Section: _____ Date: _____

NOTEBOOK ACTIVITY

Is Osteoporosis in Your Future?

Risk Factors You CANNOT Control:

1. Are you female?
2. Do you have a family history of osteoporosis?
3. Are your ancestors from the British Isles, northern Europe, China, or Japan?
4. Are you very fair-skinned?
5. Are you small-boned?
6. Are you over age 35?
7. Have you had your ovaries removed, or did you have an early menopause?
8. Are you allergic to milk and milk products?
9. Have you never been pregnant?
10. Do you have cancer or kidney disease?
11. Do you have to take chemotherapy, steroids, anticonvulsants, or anticoagulants?

Risk Factors You CAN Control:

12. Do you smoke?
13. Do you drink alcohol?
14. Do you avoid milk and cheese in your diet?
15. Do you get very little exercise?
16. Do you drink a lot of soft drinks?
17. Is your diet high in protein?
18. Do you consume a lot of caffeine (five or more cups of coffee per day or equivalent)?
19. Are you amenorrheic (without a monthly period)?
20. Do you get less than 1,000 mg of calcium a day?
21. Is your body weight very low?
22. Do you go on extreme or crash diets?
23. Do you have a high sodium (salt) intake?

If you answered "yes" to three (3) of the above questions, you are at risk for osteoporosis and may want to ask your doctor to give you a bone density screening test. The more questions you answered "yes" to, the higher your risk of developing osteoporosis in the future.

Many clinical studies suggest that osteoporosis is a preventable disease. As you can see from the quiz, you can do several things right now to help prevent osteoporosis in your future.

Source: Adapted from *Marion Laboratories, Inc.*

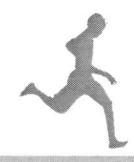

CHAPTER 5

Nutrition

"A man's health can be judged by which he takes two at a time—pills or stairs."

—Joan Welsh

OBJECTIVES

Students will be able to:
- Define the essential nutrients (carbohydrates, fats, proteins, vitamins, and minerals) and describe their roles in daily nutrition.
- Introduce and explain the USDA Food Guide Pyramid.
- Introduce guidelines for food labeling and explain how food labels describe the nutritional values of food.
- Define the four styles of vegetarianism.
- Discuss the roles of organic and functional foods.

Good, sound nutritional choices are necessary for maintaining a healthy lifestyle. Making the effort to obtain the essential nutrients through daily dietary intake is not something in which most Americans are proficient. In general, Americans eat too much salt, sugar, and fat and do not consume the recommended daily allowance (RDA) of vitamins and minerals.

Poor dietary habits, along with being physically inactive, is one of the major factors that results in Americans becoming increasingly overweight and obese. As noted in Chapter 4, being overweight or obese is a major risk factor for chronic health problems such as hypertension, cardiovascular disease, diabetes, and certain types of cancers. With this in mind, the importance of building a knowledge base that will allow an individual to develop sound, life-long nutritional habits and practices becomes clear.

Once an individual has made the effort to gather information that will allow him or her to make good nutritional choices, he or she must then make a concentrated effort to obtain the essential **macronutrients and micronutrients** through their daily food selections. **Macronutrients** provide energy in the form of calories. Carbohydrates, fats, and proteins make up the sources of macronutrients. **Micronutrients**, which include vitamins and minerals, regulate bodily functions such as metabolism, growth, and cellular development. Together, macronutrients and micronutrients are responsible for the following three tasks that are necessary for the continuance of life:

1. growth, repair, and maintenance of all tissues,
2. regulation of body processes, and
3. providing energy.

Because nutrition information is often filled with scientific terminology and unfamiliar jargon, it is many times misleading or appears to be overly complicated. Several government agencies, such as the U.S. Department of Agriculture (USDA) and the U.S. Department of Health and Human Services (DHHS), have teamed up in an effort to simplify and streamline nutritional information widely available to the general public in an effort to decrease the amount of misinformation on nutrition and increase the prevalence of practical, easy-to-apply, user-friendly information.

Dietary Guidelines for Americans

In 1980 the *Dietary Guidelines for Americans* was first published as a scientifically-based health promotion that attempted to reduce an individual's risk for chronic diseases through diet and increased levels of physical activity. The USDA and the DHHS have updated and republished these *Dietary Guidelines* every five years since their inception in 1980.

The most current version of the *Dietary Guidelines* was published in early 2005 (www.health.gov/dietaryguidelines/dga2005/html/executivesummary.htm). Despite the 2005 report containing more scientific and technical information than it has in the past, it continues to be an excellent source to aid in the building of a nutritious and healthy diet for the general population.

The recommendations stated by the *Dietary Guidelines* are interrelated and depend on each other. Therefore, it is the intent of the *Guidelines* to be used together in planning a healthy diet. However, it is still possible to achieve health benefits if just some of the recommendations are followed.

The following is a list of the key recommendations of the *Dietary Guidelines*.

Dietary Guidelines for Americans (pp. 120–124) from www.health.gov

Adequate Nutrients within Calorie Needs

Key Recommendations

- Consume a variety of nutrient-dense foods and beverages within and among the basic food groups while choosing foods that limit the intake of saturated and trans fats, cholesterol, added sugars, salt, and alcohol.
- Meet recommended intakes within energy needs by adopting a balanced eating pattern, such as the USDA Food Guide or the DASH Eating Plan.

Key Recommendations for Specific Population Groups

- *People over age 50.* Consume vitamin B12 in its crystalline form (i.e., fortified foods or supplements).
- *Women of childbearing age who may become pregnant.* Eat foods high in heme-iron and/or consume iron-rich plant foods or iron-fortified foods with an enhancer of iron absorption, such as vitamin C-rich foods.
- *Women of childbearing age who may become pregnant and those in the first trimester of pregnancy.* Consume adequate synthetic folic acid daily (from fortified foods or supplements) in addition to food forms of folate from a varied diet.
- *Older adults, people with dark skin, and people exposed to insufficient ultraviolet band radiation (i.e., sunlight).* Consume extra vitamin D from vitamin D-fortified foods and/or supplements.

Weight Management

Key Recommendations

- To maintain body weight in a healthy range, balance calories from foods and beverages with calories expended.
- To prevent gradual weight gain over time, make small decreases in food and beverage calories and increase physical activity.

Key Recommendations for Specific Population Groups

- *Those who need to lose weight.* Aim for a slow, steady weight loss by decreasing calorie intake while maintaining an adequate nutrient intake and increasing physical activity.
- *Overweight children.* Reduce the rate of body weight gain while allowing growth and development. Consult a healthcare provider before placing a child on a weight-reduction diet.
- *Pregnant women.* Ensure appropriate weight gain as specified by a healthcare provider.
- *Breast-feeding women.* Moderate weight reduction is safe and does not compromise weight gain of the nursing infant.
- *Overweight adults and overweight children with chronic diseases and/or on medication.* Consult a healthcare provider about weight loss strategies prior to starting a weight-reduction program to ensure appropriate management of other health conditions.

Physical Activity

Key Recommendations

- Engage in regular physical activity and reduce sedentary activities to promote health, psychological well-being, and a healthy body weight.
  - To reduce the risk of chronic disease in adulthood: Engage in at least thirty minutes of moderate-intensity physical activity, above usual activity, at work or home on most days of the week.
  - For most people, greater health benefits can be obtained by engaging in physical activity of more vigorous intensity or longer duration.
  - To help manage body weight and prevent gradual, unhealthy body weight gain in adulthood: Engage in approximately sixty minutes of moderate- to vigorous-intensity activity on most days of the week while not exceeding caloric intake requirements.
  - To sustain weight loss in adulthood: Participate in at least sixty to ninety minutes of daily moderate-intensity physical activity while not exceeding caloric intake requirements. Some people may need to consult with a healthcare provider before participating in this level of activity.
- Achieve physical fitness by including cardiovascular conditioning, stretching exercises for flexibility, and resistance exercises or calisthenics for muscle strength and endurance.

Key Recommendations for Specific Population Groups

- *Children and adolescents*. Engage in at least sixty minutes of physical activity on most, preferably all, days of the week.
- *Pregnant women*. In the absence of medical or obstetric complications, incorporate thirty minutes or more of moderate-intensity physical activity on most, if not all, days of the week. Avoid activities with a high risk of falling or abdominal trauma.
- *Breast-feeding women*. Be aware that neither acute nor regular exercise adversely affects the mother's ability to successfully breast-feed.
- *Older adults*. Participate in regular physical activity to reduce functional declines associated with aging and to achieve the other benefits of physical activity identified for all adults.

Food Groups to Encourage

Key Recommendations

- Consume a sufficient amount of fruits and vegetables while staying within energy needs. Two cups of fruit and two and one-half cups of vegetables per day are recommended for a reference 2,000-calorie intake, with higher or lower amounts depending on the calorie level.
- Choose a variety of fruits and vegetables each day. In particular, select from all five vegetable subgroups (dark green, orange, legumes, starchy vegetables, and other vegetables) several times a week.
- Consume three or more ounce-equivalents of whole-grain products per day, with the rest of the recommended grains coming from enriched or whole-grain products. In general, at least half the grains should come from whole grains.
- Consume three cups per day of fat-free or low-fat milk or equivalent milk products.

Key Recommendations for Specific Population Groups

- *Children and adolescents.* Consume whole-grain products often; at least half the grains should be whole grains. Children 2 to 8 years should consume two cups per day of fat-free or low-fat milk or equivalent milk products. Children 9 years of age and older should consume three cups per day of fat-free or low-fat milk or equivalent milk products.

Fats

Key Recommendations

- Consume less than 10 percent of calories from saturated fatty acids and less than 300 mg/day of cholesterol, and keep *trans* fatty acid consumption as low as possible.

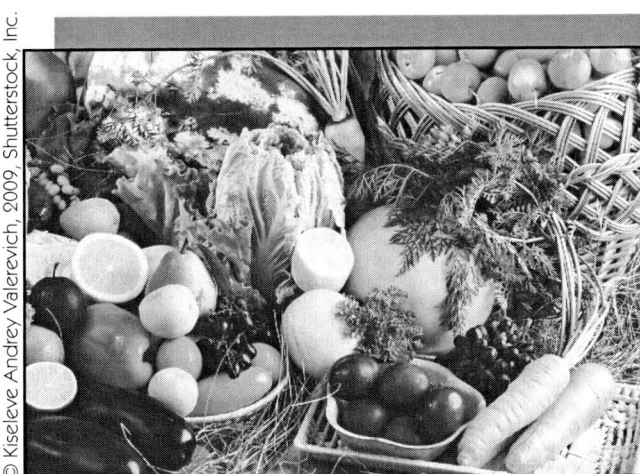

A variety of vegetables and fruits are important to a healthy diet.

- Keep total fat intake between 20 to 35 percent of calories, with most fats coming from sources of polyunsaturated and monounsaturated fatty acids, such as fish, nuts, and vegetable oils.
- When selecting and preparing meat, poultry, dry beans, and milk or milk products, make choices that are lean, low-fat, or fat-free.
- Limit intake of fats and oils high in saturated and/or *trans* fatty acids, and choose products low in such fats and oils.

Key Recommendations for Specific Population Groups

- *Children and adolescents.* Keep total fat intake between 30 to 35 percent of calories for children 2 to 3 years of age and between 25 to 35 percent of calories for children and adolescents 4 to 18 years of age, with most fats coming from sources of polyunsaturated and monounsaturated fatty acids, such as fish, nuts, and vegetable oils.

Carbohydrates

Key Recommendations

- Choose fiber-rich fruits, vegetables, and whole grains often.
- Choose and prepare foods and beverages with little added sugars or caloric sweeteners, such as amounts suggested by the USDA Food Guide and the DASH Eating Plan.
- Reduce the incidence of dental caries by practicing good oral hygiene and consuming sugar- and starch-containing foods and beverages less frequently.

Sodium and Potassium

Key Recommendations

- Consume less than 2,300 mg (approximately one teaspoon of salt) of sodium per day.
- Choose and prepare foods with little salt. At the same time, consume potassium-rich foods, such as fruits and vegetables.

Key Recommendations for Specific Population Groups

- *Individuals with hypertension, blacks, and middle-aged and older adults.* Aim to consume no more than 1,500 mg of sodium per day, and meet the potassium recommendation (4,700 mg/day) with food.

Alcoholic Beverages

Key Recommendations

- Those who choose to drink alcoholic beverages should do so sensibly and in moderation—defined as the consumption of up to one drink per day for women and up to two drinks per day for men.
- Alcoholic beverages should not be consumed by some individuals, including those who cannot restrict their alcohol intake, women of childbearing age who may become pregnant, pregnant and lactating women, children and adolescents, individuals taking medications that cannot interact with alcohol, and those with specific medical conditions.
- Alcoholic beverages should be avoided by individuals engaging in activities that require attention, skill, or coordination, such as driving or operating machinery.

Food Safety

Key Recommendations

- To avoid microbial foodborne illness:
  - Clean hands, food contact surfaces, and fruits and vegetables. Meat and poultry should not be washed or rinsed.
  - Separate raw, cooked, and ready-to-eat foods while shopping, preparing, or storing foods.
  - Cook foods to a safe temperature to kill microorganisms.
  - Chill (refrigerate) perishable food promptly and defrost foods properly.
  - Avoid raw (unpasteurized) milk or any products made from unpasteurized milk, raw or partially cooked eggs, or foods containing raw eggs, raw or undercooked meat and poultry, unpasteurized juices, and raw sprouts.

Key Recommendations for Specific Population Groups

- *Infants and young children, pregnant women, older adults, and those who are immunocompromised.* Do not eat or drink raw (unpasteurized) milk or any products made from unpasteurized milk, raw or partially cooked eggs, or foods containing raw eggs, raw or undercooked meat and poultry, raw or undercooked fish or shellfish, unpasteurized juices, and raw sprouts.
- *Pregnant women, older adults, and those who are immunocompromised.* Only eat certain deli meats and frankfurters that have been reheated to steaming hot.

Following the guidelines provided by the USDA and DHHS will not only improve an individual's overall health, it will also decrease their risk for chronic diseases such as heart disease, stroke, diabetes, obesity, and certain types of cancers.

Essential Nutrients

It is necessary for an individual to ingest more than forty different nutrients in order to maintain good health. Because no single food source contains all of these nutrients, variety in one's diet is essential. Eating a wide variety of foods will help ensure adequate intake of carbohydrates, fats, proteins, vitamins, and minerals.

Carbohydrates

Carbohydrates should be the body's main source of fuel. Between 55 and 60 percent of an individual's diet should be composed of carbohydrates. Of this 55 to 60 percent, 45 to 50 percent of total daily caloric intake should be from complex carbohydrates, leaving simple carbohydrates to account for less than 10 percent of the daily carbohydrate intake.

Complex carbohydrates are relatively low in calories (4 calories per gram), nutritionally dense, and are a rich source of vitamins, minerals, and water. Complex carbohydrates provide the body with a steady source of energy for hours. The best sources of complex carbohydrates are breads, cereals, pastas, and grains.

Dietary fiber, also known as roughage or bulk, is a type of complex carbohydrate that is present mainly in leaves, roots, skins, and seeds and is the part of a plant that is not digested in the small intestine. Dietary fiber helps decrease the risk of cardiovascular disease and cancer, and may lower an individual's risk of coronary heart disease. Table 5.1 lists good sources of dietary fiber.

Dietary fiber is either soluble or insoluble. Soluble fiber dissolves in water. It helps the body excrete fats and has been shown to reduce levels of blood cholesterol and blood sugar, as well as helping to control diabetes. Water-soluble fiber travels through the digestive tract in gel-like form, pacing the absorption of cholesterol, which helps prevent dramatic shifts in blood sugar levels. Soluble fiber is found primarily in oats, fruits, barley, and legumes.

Insoluble fiber does not dissolve easily in water; therefore, it cannot be digested by the body. Insoluble fiber causes softer, bulkier stool that increases peristalsis. This, in turn, reduces the risk of colon cancer by allowing food residues to pass through the intestinal tract more quickly, limiting the exposure and absorption time of toxic substances within the waste materials. Primary sources of insoluble fiber include wheat, cereals, vegetables, and the skins of fruits.

The recommended daily intake of fiber is 25–30 g per day. Health disorders associated with low fiber intake include constipation, diverticulitis, hemorrhoids, gall bladder disease, and obesity. Problems associated with ingesting too much fiber include losses of calcium, phosphorous, iron, and disturbances of the gastrointestinal system.

Simple carbohydrates are sugars that have little nutritive value beyond their energy content. Sugars that are found naturally in milk, fruit, honey, and some vegetables are examples of simple carbohydrates. Foods high in simple sugars are sometimes dismissed as "empty calories." Examples of these foods include candy, cakes, jellies, and sodas.

Fats

Fats are the body's primary source of energy, and supply the body with 9 calories of energy per gram ingested. While many Americans consume too many of their daily calories from fats (37 to 40 percent), dietary fat is not necessarily a "bad" component

Table 5.1
Good Sources of Dietary Fiber

Fruits	Grams
1 medium apple	4–5
1 banana	3
1 cup blueberries	5
10 dates	7
1 orange	3
1 pear	5
1 cup strawberries	3
1 watermelon slice	2–3

Vegetables	Grams
1 artichoke	4
1 raw carrot	2
1/2 cup cream style corn	6
1 cup chopped lettuce	1
1/2 cup green peas	6
1 cup cooked spinach	6
1 cup cooked squash	5–6
1 tomato	2

Legumes	Grams
1 cup cooked black beans	15
1 cup cooked green beans	3
1 cup pork and beans	18
1 cup cooked blackeyed peas	11
1 cup kidney beans	20
1 cup cooked navy beans	16
1 cup cooked pinto beans	19

Grains	Grams
1 bagel	1
1 whole-grain slice of bread	1–3
4 graham crackers	3
1 bran muffin	2
hot dog/hamburger bun	1
1 cup cooked oatmeal	7–9
1/2 cup Grape Nuts cereal	3.5
1 cup Nature Valley granola	7.5
3/4 cup Shredded Wheat cereal	4
1 cup cooked macaroni	1
1 cup cooked rice	2.5–4
1 cup cooked spaghetti	1–2

Other	Grams
1 cup almonds	15
1 cup cashews	8
1 cup shredded coconut	11
1 tbsp peanut butter	1
1/4 cup sunflower seeds	2

of an individual's diet at moderate levels of consumption. At moderate amounts, between 25 and 30 percent of daily calories, fat is crucial to good nutrition.

Fat has many essential functions: providing the body with stored energy, insulating the body to preserve body heat, contributing to cellular structure, and protecting vital organs by absorbing shock. Fat not only adds flavor and texture to foods and helps satisfy an individual's appetite because it is digested more slowly, it also supplies the body with essential fatty acids and transports fat-soluble vitamins A, E, D, and K. Fat is also necessary for normal growth and healthy skin, and is essential in the synthesis of certain hormones.

There are different types of dietary fat. Saturated fats are found primarily in animal products such as meats, lard, cream, butter, cheese, and whole milk. However, coconut and palm oils are two plant sources of saturated fat. A defining characteristic of saturated fats is that they typically do not melt at room temperature (an exception being the above mentioned oils that are "almost solid" at room temperature). Saturated fats increase low-density lipoproteins (LDL) or "bad cholesterol" levels and in turn increase an individuals risk for heart disease and colorectal cancer.

Table 5.2
What Is Your Upper Limit on Fat for the Calories You Consume?

Total Calories per Day	Saturated Fat in Grams	Total Fat in Grams
1,600	18 or less	53
2,000*	20 or less	65
2,200	24 or less	73
2,500*	25 or less	80
2,800	31 or less	93

*Percent Daily Values on Nutrition Facts Labels are based on a 2,000 calorie diet. Values for 2,000 and 2,500 calories are rounded to the nearest 5 grams to be consistent with the Nutrition Facts Label.

Trans fat is different from other types of fat in that it typically does not occur naturally in plant or animal products. While a small amount of trans fat is found naturally, the majority of trans fat is formed when liquid oils are made into solid fats (i.e., shortening and some margarines). Trans fat is made during hydrogenation—when hydrogen is added to vegetable oil. This process is used to increase the shelf life of foods and to help foods maintain their original flavor. Many fried foods and "store bought" sweets and treats have high amounts of this type of fat. While most individuals consume four to five times more saturated fat than trans fat, it is important to be aware of the amount of trans fat in one's diet because it raises LDL, "bad," cholesterol and increases the risk of coronary heart disease. Starting January 1, 2006, the Food and Drug Administration (FDA) requires all foods to list the amount of trans fat contained in the product on the Nutrition Facts panel. The exception to this new requirement is that if the total fat in a food is less than 0.5 g per serving and no claims are made about fat, fatty acid, or cholesterol content, trans fat does not have to be listed.

Unsaturated fats are derived primarily from plant products such as vegetable oils, avocados, and most nuts, and do not raise the body's blood cholesterol. Unsaturated fats include both monounsaturated and polyunsaturated fats. **Monounsaturated fats** are found in foods such as olives, peanuts, canola oil, peanut oil, and olive oil. **Polyunsaturated fats** are found in margarine, pecans, corn oil, cottonseed oil, sunflower oil, and soybean oil (see Table 5.3).

Table 5.3
Composition of Oils (%)

Type	Sat	Poly	Mono
safflower	9	75	16
sunflower	10	66	24
corn	13	59	28
soybean	14	58	28
sesame	14	42	44
peanut	17	32	51
palm	49	9	42
olive	14	8	78
canola	7	35	58

Table 5.4
Percentage of Fat Calories in Foods

Type of Food	Less than 15% of Calories from Fat	15%–30% of Calories from Fat	30%–50% of Calories from Fat	More than 50% of Calories from Fat
Fruits and Vegetables	Fruits, plain vegetables, juices, pickles, sauerkraut		French fries, hash browns	Avocados, coconuts, olives
Bread and Cereals	Grains and flours, most breads, most cereals, corn tortillas, pitas, matzoh, bagels, noodles, and pasta	Corn bread, flour tortillas, oatmeal, soft rolls and buns, wheat germ	Breakfast bars, biscuits and muffins, granola, pancakes and waffles, donuts, taco shells, pastries, croissants	
Dairy Products	Nonfat milk, dry curd cottage cheese, nonfat cottage cheese, nonfat yogurt	Buttermilk, low-fat yogurt, 1% milk, low-fat cottage cheese	Whole milk, 2% milk, creamed cottage cheese	Butter, cream, sour cream, half & half, most cheese, (including part-skim and lite cheeses)
Meats		Beef round; veal loin, round, and shoulder; pork tenderloin	Beef and veal, lamb, fresh and picnic hams	All ground beef, spareribs, cold cuts, beef, hot dogs, pastrami
Poultry	Egg whites	Chicken and turkey (light meat without skin)	Chicken and turkey (light meat with skin, dark meat without skin), duck and goose (without skin)	Chicken/turkey (dark meat with skin), chicken/turkey bologna and hot dogs, egg yolks, whole eggs
Seafood	Clams, cod, crab, crawfish, flounder, haddock, lobster, perch, sole, scallops, shrimp, tuna (in water)	Bass and sea bass, halibut, mussels, oyster, tuna (fresh)	Anchovies, catfish, salmon, sturgeon, trout, tuna (in oil, drained)	Herring, mackerel, sardines
Beans and Nuts	Dried beans and peas, chestnuts, water chestnuts		Soybeans	Tofu, most nuts and seeds, peanut butter
Fats and Oils	Oil-free and some lite salad dressings			Butter, margarine, all mayonnaise (including reduced-calorie), most salad dressings, all oils
Soups	Bouillons, broths, consomme	Most soups	Cream soups, bean soups, "just add water" noodle soups	Cheddar cheese soups, New England clam chowder
Desserts	Angel food cake, gelatin, some new fat-free cakes	Pudding, tapioca	Most cakes, most pies	
Frozen Desserts	Sherbert, low-fat frozen yogurt, sorbet, fruit ices	Ice milk	Frozen yogurt	All ice cream
Snack foods	Popcorn (air popped), pretzels, rye crackers, rice cakes, fig bars, raisin biscuit cookies, marshmallows, most hard candy, fruit rolls	Lite microwave popcorn, Scandinavian "crisps," plain crackers, caramels, fudge, gingersnaps, graham crackers	Snack crackers, popcorn (popped in oil), cookies, candy bars, granola bars	Most microwave popcorn, corn and potato chips, chocolate, buttery crackers

Source: American Heart Association/USDA.

Choose Sensibly for Good Health

- Choose a diet that is low in saturated fat and cholesterol and moderate in total fat.
- Choose beverages and foods to moderate your intake of sugars.
- Choose and prepare foods with less salt.
- If you drink alcoholic beverages, do so in moderation.

Fats and Oils

- Choose vegetable oils rather than solid fats (meat and dairy fats, shortening).
- If you need fewer calories, decrease the amount of fat you use in cooking and at the table.

Meat, Poultry, Fish, Shellfish, Eggs, Beans, and Nuts

- Choose two to three servings of fish, shellfish, lean poultry, other lean meats, beans, or nuts daily. Trim fat from meat and take skin off poultry. Choose dry beans, peas, or lentils often.
- Limit your intake of high-fat processed meats such as bacon, sausages, salami, bologna, and other cold cuts. Try the lower fat varieties (check the Nutrition Facts Label).
- Limit your intake of liver and other organ meats. Use egg yolks and whole eggs in moderation. Use egg whites and egg substitutes freely when cooking since they contain no cholesterol and little or no fat.

Dairy Products

- Choose fat-free or low-fat milk, fat-free or low-fat yogurt, and low-fat cheese most often. Try switching from whole to fat-free or low-fat milk. This decreases the saturated fat and calories but keeps all other nutrients the same.

Prepared Foods

- Check the Nutrition Facts Label to see how much saturated fat and cholesterol are in a serving of prepared food. Choose foods lower in saturated fat and cholesterol.

Foods at Restaurants or Other Eating Establishments

- Choose fish or lean meats as suggested. Limit ground meat and fatty processed meats, marbled steaks, and cheese.
- Limit your intake of foods with creamy sauces, and add little or no butter to your food.
- Choose fruits as desserts most often.

Following the tips here will help you keep your intake of saturated fat at less than 10 percent of calories. They will also help you keep your cholesterol intake less than the Daily Value of 300 mg/day listed on the Nutrition Facts Label.

FIGURE 5.1

Daily Diet Recommendations based on a 2,000-calorie pattern of a 19-Year-Old Female Who Does Less Than Thirty Minutes of Physical Activity a Day.

Go to MyPyramid.gov to get your personalized diet recommendation.

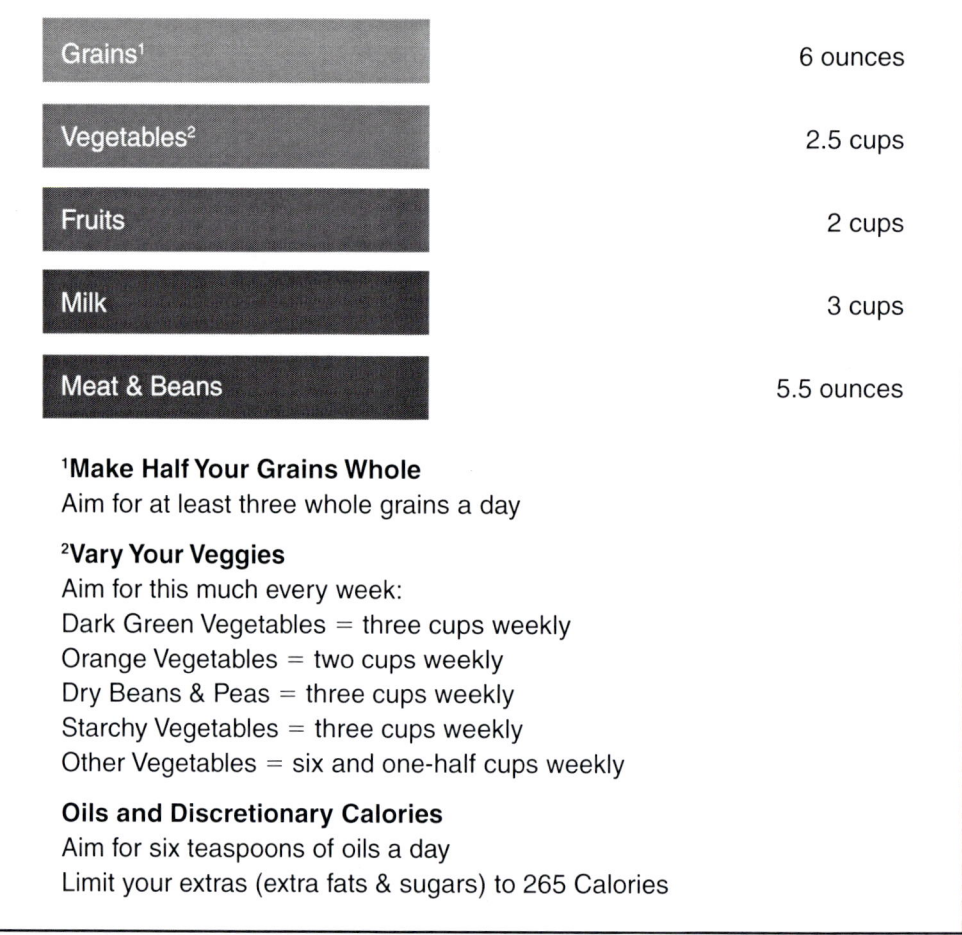

Grains[1]	6 ounces
Vegetables[2]	2.5 cups
Fruits	2 cups
Milk	3 cups
Meat & Beans	5.5 ounces

[1]**Make Half Your Grains Whole**
Aim for at least three whole grains a day

[2]**Vary Your Veggies**
Aim for this much every week:
Dark Green Vegetables = three cups weekly
Orange Vegetables = two cups weekly
Dry Beans & Peas = three cups weekly
Starchy Vegetables = three cups weekly
Other Vegetables = six and one-half cups weekly

Oils and Discretionary Calories
Aim for six teaspoons of oils a day
Limit your extras (extra fats & sugars) to 265 Calories

Source: From www.mypyramid.gov

Fats become counterproductive to good health when they are consumed in excess. Too much fat in many Americans' diets is the reason Americans lead the world in heart disease. Excess fat intake elevates blood cholesterol levels and leads to atherosclerosis, or a hardening of the arteries. Diets with excess fat have attributed to 30 to 40 percent of all cancers in men and 60 percent of all cancers in women, and have also been linked to cancer of the breast, colon, and prostate more frequently than any other dietary factor.

By following the guidelines listed in Table 5.2 on page 153 of this chapter, the level of saturated fat and trans fat consumed each day can be limited to 10 percent of that day's total calories.

Protein

Even though **proteins** should make up only 12–15 percent of total calories ingested, they are the essential "building blocks" of the body. Proteins are needed for the growth, maintenance, and repair of all body tissues, that is, muscles, blood, bones, internal organs, skin, hair, and nails. Proteins also help maintain the normal balance of body fluids and are needed to make enzymes, hormones, and antibodies that fight infection.

Proteins are made up of approximately twenty amino acids. An individual's body uses all twenty of these amino acids in the formation of different proteins. Eleven of the twenty are **non-essential amino acids**—they are manufactured in the body

Table 5.5
USDA Food Guide

The suggested amounts of food to consume from the basic food groups, subgroups, and oils to meet recommended nutrient intakes at twelve different calorie levels. Nutrient and energy contributions from each group are calculated according to the nutrient-dense forms of foods in each group (for instances, lean meats and fat-free milk). The table also shows the discretionary calorie allowance that can be accommodated within each calorie level, in addition to the suggested amounts of nutrient-dense forms of foods in each group.

Daily Amount of Food from Each Group (Vegetable Subgroup Amounts Are per Week)

Calorie Level	1,000	1,200	1,400	1,600	1,800	2,000	2,200	2,400	2,600	2,800	3,000	3,200
Food Group	Food group amounts shown in cup (c) or ounce-equivalents (oz-eq), with number of servings (srv) in parentheses when it differs from the other units. See note for quantity equivalents for foods in each group. Oils are shown in grams (g).											
Fruits	1 c (2 srv)	1 c (2 srv)	1.5 c (3 srv)	1.5 c (3 srv)	1.5 c (3 srv)	2 c (4 srv)	2 c (4 srv)	2 c (4 srv)	2 c (4 srv)	2.5 c (5 srv)	2.5 c (5 srv)	2.5 c (5 srv)
Vegetables	1 c (2 srv)	1.5 c (3 srv)	1.5 c (3 srv)	2 c (4 srv)	2.5 c (5 srv)	2.5 c (5 srv)	3 c (6 srv)	3 c (6 srv)	3.5 c (7 srv)	3.5 c (7 srv)	4 c (8 srv)	4 c (8 srv)
Dark green veg.	1 c/wk	1.5 c/wk	1.5 c/wk	2 c/wk	3 c/wk	3 c/wk	3 c/wk	3 c/wk	3 c/wk	3 c/wk	3 c/wk	3 c/wk
Orange veg.	.5 c/wk	1 c/wk	1 c/wk	1.5 c/wk	2 c/wk	2 c/wk	2 c/wk	2 c/wk	2.5 c/wk	2.5 c/wk	2.5 c/wk	2.5 c/wk
Legumes	.5 c/wk	1 c/wk	1 c/wk	2.5 c/wk	3 c/wk	3 c/wk	3 c/wk	3 c/wk	3.5 c/wk	3.5 c/wk	3.5 c/wk	3.5 c/wk
Starchy veg.	1.5 c/wk	2.5 c/wk	2.5 c/wk	2.5 c/wk	3 c/wk	3 c/wk	6 c/wk	6 c/wk	7 c/wk	7 c/wk	9 c/wk	9 c/wk
Other veg.	4 c/wk	4.5 c/wk	4.5 c/wk	5.5 c/wk	6.5 c/wk	6.5 c/wk	7 c/wk	7 c/wk	8.5 c/wk	8.5 c/wk	10 c/wk	10 c/wk
Grains	3 oz-eq	4 oz-eq	5 oz-eq	5 oz-eq	6 oz-eq	6 oz-eq	7 oz-eq	8 oz-eq	9 oz-eq	10 oz-eq	10 oz-eq	10 oz-eq
Whole grains	1.5	2	2.5	3	3	3	3.5	4	4.5	5	5	5
Other grains	1.5	2	2.5	2	3	3	3.5	4	4.5	5	5	5
Lean meat and beans	2 oz-eq	3 oz-eq	4 oz-eq	5 oz-eq	5 oz-eq	5.5 oz-eq	6 oz-eq	6.5 oz-eq	6.5 oz-eq	7 oz-eq	7 oz-eq	7 oz-eq
Milk	2 c	2 c	2 c	3 c	3 c	3 c	3 c	3 c	3 c	3 c	3 c	3 c
Oils	15 g	17 g	17 g	22 g	24 g	27 g	29 g	31 g	34 g	36 g	44 g	51 g
Discretionary calorie allowance	165	171	171	132	195	267	290	362	410	426	512	648

Source: USDA Food Guide.

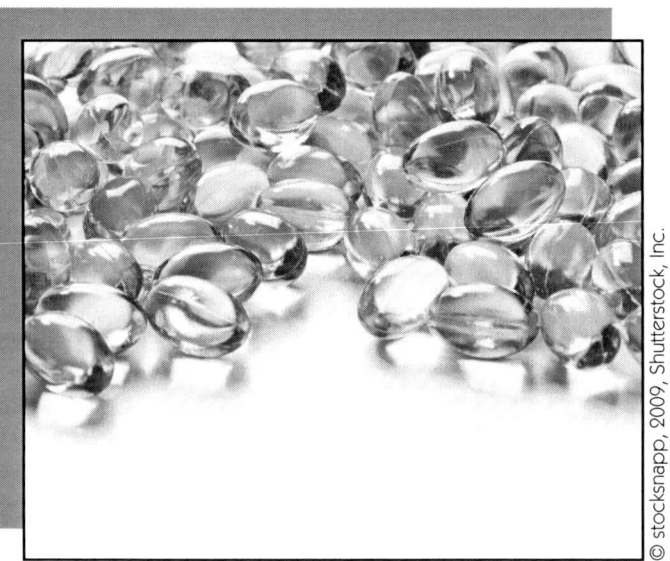

Fat-soluble vitamins, such as A, E, D and K, are stored in the body for relatively long periods of time.

if food proteins in a person's diet provide enough nitrogen. Nine of the twenty are **essential amino acids**—the body cannot produce these, and thus must be supplied through an individual's diet. All amino acids must be present at the same time for particular protein synthesis to occur.

The suggested RDA of protein for adults is 45 through 65 g per day (intake should not exceed 1.6 g/kg of body weight (1kg. = 2.2 lbs). A few exceptions to this rule should be noted: Overweight individuals need slightly less than the calculated "norm," and women who are pregnant or lactating need slightly more protein per pound of body weight than the calculation indicates.

It is inadvisable to consume more protein than the daily recommended dosage (45–65 g/day), particularly in the form of protein supplements. Excessive protein supplementation can damage the kidneys, increase calcium excretion, negatively affect bone health, inhibit muscle growth, and can be detrimental to endurance performance.

Individuals who are trying to maximize muscular strength, endurance, and growth should take in the recommended 1.5 g of protein per kilogram of body weight, as well as an additional 500 calories of complex carbohydrates. The recommended protein and additional complex carbohydrates will work together to provide the extra nutrients and glucose needed for the increased muscular work load.

Vitamins

Vitamins are necessary for normal body metabolism, growth, and development. They do not provide the body with energy, but they do allow the energy from consumed carbohydrates, fats, and proteins to be released. Although vitamins are vital to life, they are required in minute amounts. Due primarily to adequate food supply, vitamin deficiencies in Americans are rare. However, there are some situations that may alter an individual's requirements, including pregnancy and smoking. Non-smokers need to consume 60 mg of vitamin C each day; a smoker must ingest 100 mg of vitamin C each day in order to gain the same nutritional benefits. A man or a non-pregnant woman should consume 180–200 mcg of folic acid, while a pregnant woman should consume approximately 400 mcg of folic acid per day.

Vitamins are grouped as either fat soluble or water soluble. **Fat-soluble vitamins** are transported by the body's fat cells and by the liver. They include vitamins A, E, D, and K. Fat-soluble vitamins are not excreted in urine; therefore, they are stored in the body for relatively long periods of time (many months), and can build up to potentially toxic levels if excessive doses are consumed over time.

Water-soluble vitamins include the B vitamins and vitamin C. These vitamins are not stored in the body for a significant amount of time, and the amounts that are consumed and not used relatively quickly by the body are excreted through urine and sweat. For this reason, water-soluble vitamins must be replaced daily. Table 5.6 summarizes the functions of vitamins, lists the best sources for each vitamin, and outlines associated deficiency symptoms.

TABLE 5.6
Facts about Vitamins

Vitamin	Functions	Deficiency Problems	Effect of Excess Amounts	Dietary Sources
Fat Soluble				
Vitamin A	Allows normal vision in the dark; promotes health and growth of cells and tissues; protects health of skin and tissues in the mouth, stomach, intestines, and respiratory and uro-genital tract	Night blindness and other eye problems; dry, scaly skin; reproduction problems; poor growth	Birth defects, headaches; vomiting, double vision; hair loss; bone abnormalities; liver damage	Liver; fish oil; eggs; milk fortified with vitamin A; red, yellow, and orange fruits and vegetables; many dark green leafy vegetables
Vitamin D	Promotes absorption of calcium and phosphorus to develop and maintain bones and teeth	Osteoporosis and softening of the bones, rickets, defective bone growth	Kidney stones or damage, weak muscles and bones, excessive bleeding	Sunlight on the skin, cheese, eggs, some fish, fortified milk, breakfast cereals, and margarine
Vitamin E	Antioxidant and may protect against heart disease and some types of cancer	Nervous system problems	May interfere with vitamin K action and enhance the effect of some anticoagulant drugs	Vegetable oils and margarine, salad dressing and other foods made from vegetable oils, nuts, seeds, wheat germ, leafy green vegetables
Vitamin K	Helps blood clotting	Thin blood that does not clot	None observed	Green leafy vegetables, smaller amounts widespread in other foods
Water Soluble				
Vitamin C	Helps produce collagen; maintenance and repair of red blood cells, bones, and other tissues; promotes healing; keeps immune system healthy	Scurvy, excessive bleeding, swollen gums, improper wound healing	Diarrhea, gastrointestinal discomfort	Citrus fruits, berries, melons, peppers, dark leafy green vegetables, tomatoes, potatoes
Thiamin	Conversion of carbohydrates into energy	Fatigue, weak muscles, and nerve damage	None reported	Whole-grain, enriched grain products, pork, liver, and other organ meats
Riboflavin	Energy metabolism, changes tryptophan into niacin	Eye disorders, dry and flaky skin, red tongue	None reported	Milk and other dairy products; enriched bread, cereal, and other grain products; eggs; meat; green leafy vegetables; nuts; liver; kidney; and heart
Niacin	Helps the body use sugars and fatty acids, produce energy, enzyme function	Diarrhea, mental disorientation, skin problems	Flushed skin, liver damage, stomach ulcers and high blood sugar	Poultry, fish, beef, peanut butter, and legumes

(continued)

TABLE 5.6

Facts about Vitamins (continued)

Vitamin	Functions	Deficiency Problems	Effect of Excess Amounts	Dietary Sources
Vitamin B6	Converts tryptophan into niacin and serotonin, helps produce other body chemicals such as insulin, hemoglobin, and antibodies	Depression, nausea, mental convulsions in infants; greasy, flaky skin	Nerve damage	Chicken, fish, pork, liver, kidney, whole grains, nuts, and legumes
Folate	Produces DNA and RNA to make new body cells, works with vitamin B12 to form hemoglobin in red blood cells	Impaired cell division and growth, anemia	Medication interference, masking of vitamin B12 deficiencies	Leafy vegetables, orange juice and some fruits, legumes, liver, yeast breads, wheat germ, and some fortified cereals
Vitamin B12	Works with folate to make red blood cells, vital part of body chemicals	Anemia, fatigue, nerve damage, smooth tongue, very sensitive skin	None reported	Animal products and some fortified foods
Biotin	Metabolize fats, protein, and carbohydrates	Heart abnormalities, appetite loss, fatigue, depressions, and dry skin	None reported	Eggs, liver, yeast breads, and cereal
Pantothenic Acid	Metabolize protein, fat, and carbohydrates	Rare	Diarrhea and water retention	Meat, poultry, fish, whole-grain cereals, and legumes; smaller amounts in milk, vegetables, and fruits

Minerals

Minerals are inorganic substances that are critical to many enzyme functions in the body. Approximately twenty-five minerals have important roles in bodily functions. Minerals are contained in all cells and are concentrated in hard parts of the body—nails, teeth, and bones—and are crucial to maintaining water balance and the acid-base balance. Minerals are essential components of respiratory pigments, enzymes, and enzyme systems, while also regulating muscular and nervous tissue excitability, blood clotting, and normal heart rhythm. Table 5.7 outlines the major sources and functions of specific minerals, as well as lists deficiency symptoms for those minerals.

Two groups of minerals are necessary in an individual's diet: macrominerals and microminerals. **Macrominerals** are the seven minerals the body needs in relatively large quantities (100 mg or more each day). These seven minerals are: calcium, chloride, magnesium, phosphorus, potassium, sodium, and sulfur. In most cases, these minerals can be acquired by eating a variety of foods each day.

TABLE 5.7
Facts about Selected Minerals

Mineral	Functions	Deficiency Problems	Effect of Excess Amounts	Dietary Sources
Calcium	Helps build strong bones and teeth, control of muscle contractions and nerve function, supports blood clotting	Stunted growth in children, bone mineral loss in adults	Muscle and abdominal pain, calcium kidney stones	Milk and milk products, tofu, green leafy vegetables, fortified orange juice, and bread
Fluoride	Formation and maintenance of bones and teeth	Higher occurrence of tooth decay	Increased bone density, mottling of teeth, impaired kidney function	Fluoridated drinking water, tea, seafood
Iron	Helps carry oxygen to body tissues	Anemia, weakness, impaired immune function, cold hands and feet, gastrointestinal distress	Liver disease, arrhythmias, joint pain	Red meat, seafood, dried fruit, legumes, fortified cereals, green vegetables
Iodine	Component of thyroid hormones that help regulate growth, development, and metabolic rate	Enlarged thyroid, birth defect	Depression of thyroid activity, sometimes hyperthyroidism	Salt, seafood, bread, milk, cheese
Magnesium	Facilitates many cell processes	Neurological disorders, impaired immune function, kidney disorders, nausea, weight loss	Nausea, vomiting, nervous system depression, coma, death in people with impaired kidney function	Widespread in foods
Phosphorus	Works with calcium to build and maintain bones and teeth, helps convert food to energy	Bone loss, kidney disorders	Lowers blood calcium	Dairy products, egg yolks, meat, poultry, fish, legumes, soft drinks
Potassium	Vital for muscle contractions and nerve transmission, important for heart and kidney function, helps regulate fluid balance and blood pressure	Muscular weakness, nausea, drowsiness, paralysis, confusion, disruption of cardiac rhythm	Slower heart beat, kidney failure	Milk and yogurt, many fruits and vegetables (especially oranges, bananas, and potatoes)
Sodium	Maintains fluid and electrolyte balance, supports muscle contraction and nerve impulse transmissions	Muscle weakness, loss of appetite, nausea, vomiting	Edema, hypertension	Salt, soy sauce, bread, milk, meats
Zinc	Involved in production of genetic material and proteins, ability to taste, wound healing, sperm production, normal fetus development	Night blindness, loss of appetite, skin rash, impaired immune function, impaired taste, poor wound healing	Nausea and vomiting, abdominal pain	Seafood, meats, eggs, whole grains

Table 5.8
Antioxidants and Their Primary Food Sources

Vitamin A	Fortified milk; egg yolk; cheese; liver; butter; fish oil; dark green, yellow, and orange vegetables and fruits
Vitamin C	Papaya, cantaloupe, melons, citrus fruits, grapefruit, strawberries, raspberries, kiwi, cauliflower, tomatoes, dark green vegetables, green and red peppers, asparagus, broccoli, cabbage, collard greens, orange juice, and tomato juice
Vitamin E	Vegetable oils, nuts and seeds, dried beans, egg yolk, green leafy vegetables, sweet potatoes, wheat germ, 100 percent whole wheat bread, 100 percent whole grain cereal, oatmeal, mayonnaise
Carotenoids	Sweet potatoes, carrots, squash, tomatoes, asparagus, broccoli, spinach, romaine lettuce, mango, cantaloupe, pumpkin, apricots, peaches, papaya
Flavenoids	Purple grapes, wine, apples, berries, peas, beets, onions, garlic, green tea
Selenium	Lean meat, seafood, kidney, liver, dairy products, 100 percent whole grain cereal, 100 percent whole wheat bread

While **microminerals** are essential to healthy living, they are needed in smaller quantities (less than 100 mg per day) than macrominerals. Examples of these minerals include chromium, cobalt, copper, fluoride, iodine, iron, manganese, molybdenum, selenium, and zinc.

Antioxidants

Antioxidants are compounds that aid each cell in the body facing an ongoing barrage of damage resulting from daily oxygen exposure, environmental pollution, chemicals and pesticides, additives in processed foods, stress hormones, and sun radiation. Studies continue to show the ability of antioxidants to suppress cell deterioration and to "slow" the aging process. Realizing the potential power of these substances should encourage Americans to take action by eating at least five servings of a wide variety of fruits and vegetables each day (see Table 5.8).

There are many proven health benefits of antioxidants. Vitamin C speeds the healing process, helps prevent infection, and prevents scurvy. Vitamin E helps prevent heart disease by stopping the oxidation of low-density lipoprotein (the harmful form of cholesterol); strengthens the immune system; and may play a role in the prevention of Alzheimer's disease, cataracts, and some forms of cancer, providing further proof of the benefits of antioxidants.

Adequate amounts of vitamins, minerals, and antioxidants are crucial to good overall health. Table 5.9 lists the Recommended Daily Allowances and Adequate Intakes for selected nutrients.

Table 5.9
Dietary Reference Intakes (DRIs): Recommended Dietary Allowances (RDA) and Adequate Intakes (AI) for Selected Nutrients

	Recommended Dietary Allowances (RDA)													Adequate Intakes (AI)					
	Thiamin (mg)	Riboflavin (mg)	Niacin (mg NE)	Vitamin B_6 (mg)	Folate (mcg DFE)	Vitamin B_{12} (mcg)	Phosphorus (mg)	Magnesium (mg)	Vitamin A (mcg)	Vitamin C (mg)	Vitamin E (mg)	Selenium (mcg)	Iron (mcg)	Calcium (mg)	Vitamin D (mcg)	Fluoride (mg)	Pantothenic acid (mg)	Biotin (mg)	Choline (mg)
Males																			
14–18	1.2	1.3	16	1.3	400	2.4	1,250	410	900	75	15	55	11	1,300	5	3	5.0	25	550
19–30	1.2	1.3	16	1.3	400	2.4	700	400	900	90	15	55	8	1,000	5	4	5.0	30	550
31–50	1.2	1.3	16	1.3	400	2.4	700	420	900	90	15	55	8	1,000	5	4	5.0	30	550
51–70	1.2	1.3	16	1.7	400	2.4	700	420	900	90	15	55	8	1,200	10	4	5.0	30	550
>70	1.2	1.3	16	1.7	400	2.4	700	420	900	90	15	55	8	1,200	15	4	5.0	30	550
Females																			
14–18	1.0	1.0	14	1.2	400	2.4	1,250	360	700	65	15	55	15	1,300	5	3	5.0	25	400
19–30	1.1	1.1	14	1.3	400	2.4	700	310	700	75	15	55	18	1,000	5	3	5.0	30	425
31–50	1.1	1.1	14	1.3	400	2.4	700	320	700	75	15	55	18	1,000	5	3	5.0	30	425
51–70	1.1	1.1	14	1.5	400	2.4	700	320	700	75	15	55	8	1,200	10	3	5.0	30	425
>70	1.1	1.1	14	1.5	400	2.4	700	320	700	75	15	55	8	1,200	15	3	5.0	30	425
Pregnant	1.4	1.4	18	1.9	600	2.6	*	+40	750	85	15	60	27	*	*	3	6.0	30	450
Lactating	1.5	1.6	17	2.0	500	2.8	*	*	1,300	120	19	70	10	*	*	3	7.0	35	550

*Values for these nutrients do not change with pregnancy or lactation. Use the value listed for women of comparable age.

Source: Reprinted with permission from *Recommended Dietary Allowances,* 10th Edition by the National Academy of Sciences, courtesy of the National Academies Press, Washington, DC.

Progressive Effects of Dehydration

Percent loss of body water	Some progressive effects of dehydration
0–1 percent	Thirst
2–5 percent	Dry mouth, flushed skin, fatigue, headache, impaired physical performance
6 percent	Increased body temperature, breathing rate, and pulse rate; dizziness, increased weakness
8 percent	Dizziness, increased weakness, labored breathing with exercise
10 percent	Muscle spasms, swollen tongue, delirium
11 percent	Poor blood circulation, failing kidney function

Source: Adapted from "The American Dietetic Association's Complete Food and Nutrition Guide" (Minneapolis: Chronimed Publishing, 1996), p. 168.

Water

In many cases, **water** is the "forgotten nutrient." Although water does not provide energy to the body in the form of calories, it is a substance that is essential to life. Among other things, water lubricates joints, absorbs shock, regulates body temperature, maintains blood volume, and transports fluids throughout the body, while comprising 60 percent of an individual's body.

While it is clear that adequate hydration is crucial to proper physiological functioning, many people are in a semi-hydrated state most of the time. Whether exercising or not, hydration should be a continuous process. Prolonged periods of dehydration can result in as much as a 10 percent loss of intracellular water concentration and can result in death. Individuals more susceptible to dehydration include: persons who are overweight; deconditioned or unacclimitized to heat; very old and very young; and individuals who do not eat breakfast or drink water.

To ensure proper water balance and prevent dehydration, approximately six to eight eight-ounce glasses of water should be consumed each day an individual is not exercising. When working out, current recommendations for water intake are two to three eight-ounce cups of water before exercising, four to six ounces of cool water every fifteen minutes during the workout, and rehydrating thoroughly after the activity.

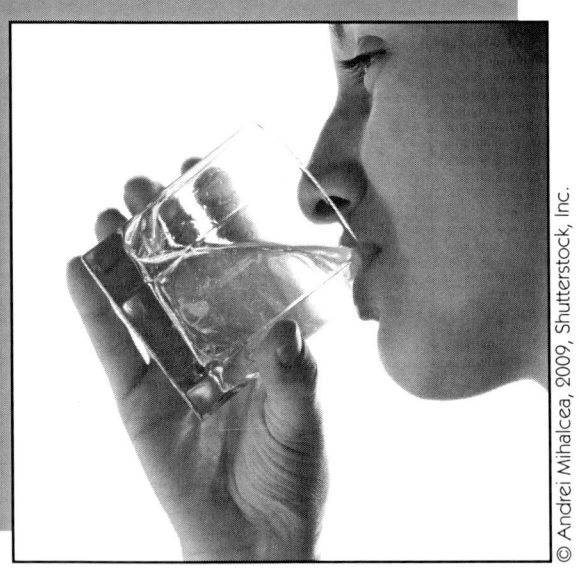

Water lubricates joints, absorbs shock, regulates body temperature, maintains blood volume, transports fluids throughout the body, and comprises 60 percent of your body.

The Food Guide Pyramid

The Food Guide Pyramid was originally created in 1992 by the federal government in an attempt to arm more Americans with the knowledge that would allow them to create a healthy, balanced, and tasty diet. Twelve years later, in 2004, the U.S. Department of Agriculture produced an expanded and updated version of that original Food Guide Pyramid (see Figure 5.2). Key to the new pyramid is the acknowledged necessity of balancing what an individual eats with the amount of physical activity in which he or she engages.

To make the pyramid portray the changes deemed necessary by the USDA, to promote optimal health, the pyramid was "flipped" onto its side so that all the food group bands run from the top of the pyramid to its base. The different size of each of the bands indicates how much food should be consumed from each food group. The bands are all wider at the base of the pyramid. This symbolizes the importance of eating, when possible, foods without solid fats and added sugar in each of the six bands or groups within the pyramid.

Grains

The color orange represents grains within the pyramid. When examining options of food choices within this group it is important to not only choose a majority on one's daily calories from grains, but also to remember that it is nutritionally prudent to make half of the grains chosen whole grains. Whole grains are defined by the American Association of Cereal Chemists as "food made from the entire grain seed, usually called the kernel, which consists of the bran, germ, and endosperm (AACC International Board of Directors, 1999) (see Figure 5.3 on page 167). If the kernel has been cracked, crushed, or flaked, it must retain nearly the same relative proportions of bran, germ, and endosperm as the original grain." Examples of easy-to-find whole grains include brown rice, bulgur (cracked wheat), popcorn, whole rye, wild rice, whole oats/oatmeal, whole-grain barley, and whole wheat. Selections of whole-grain products from this group will help an individual maximize their intake of dietary fiber as well as other nutrients. One serving from the grain group equals one slice of bread, half a bagel or one sixteen-inch tortilla.

What Counts as a Whole Grain Serving

- Cheerios – 2/3 cup
- Wheat Chex – 2/3 cup
- Oatmeal (hot, cooked) – 1/2 cup
- Quaker Oatmeal Squares or Toasted Oatmeal Cereal – 1/2 cup
- Grape Nuts – 1/5 cup
- Frosted Mini-Wheats (bite-sized) – 9 biscuits
- 100% whole-grain bread – 1 slice
- 100% whole-grain English muffin – 1 half
- Popcorn (popped) – 2 cups
- Sun Chips or baked tortilla chips – 1 oz. (about 15 chips)
- 100% whole-grain crackers (like Triscuits) – 4 crackers
- Whole-wheat pasta – 1/3 cup cooked
- Brown rice, bulgur, sorghum, or barley – 1/3 cup cooked

FIGURE 5.2

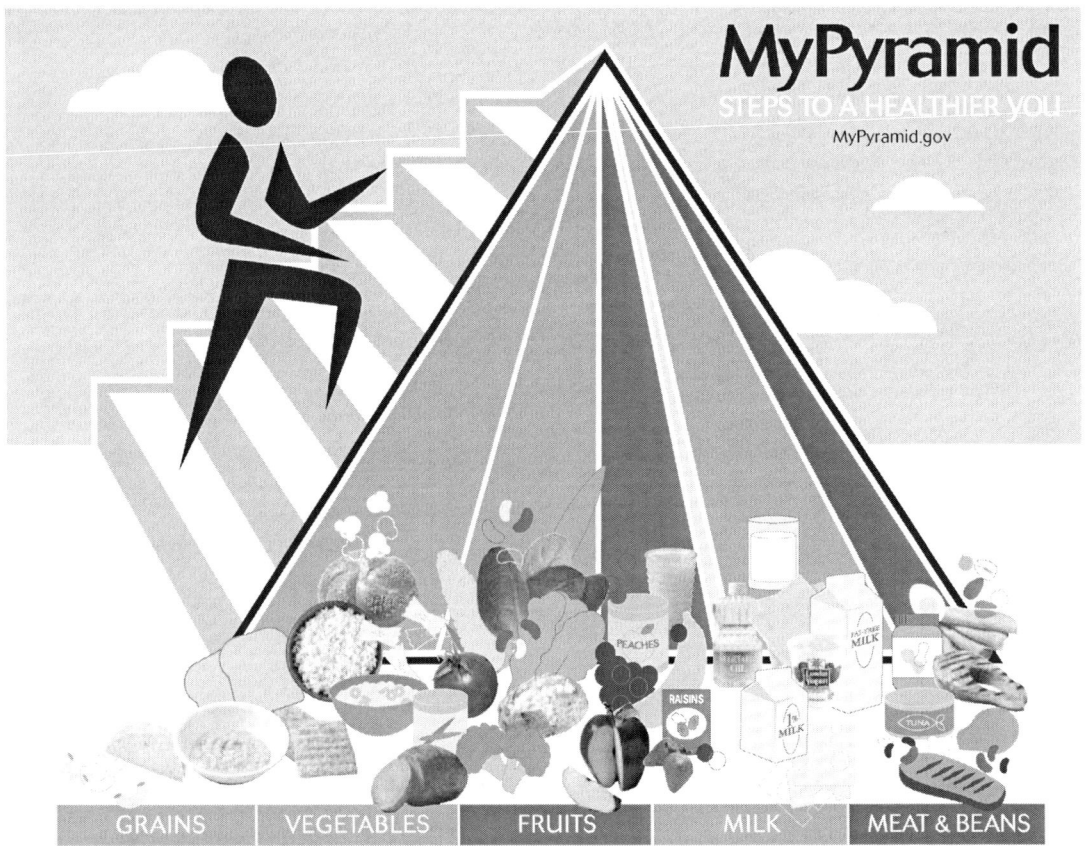

Source: From www.mypyramid.gov

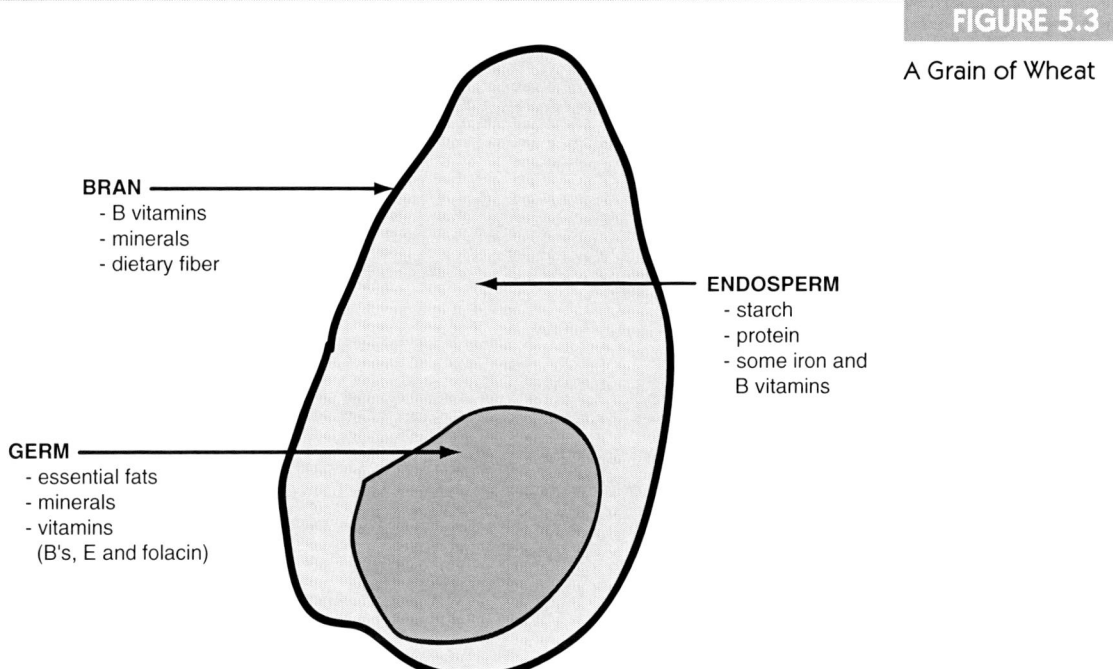

FIGURE 5.3

A Grain of Wheat

Vegetables

Green is the color within the pyramid that stands for vegetables. Vegetables are an excellent source of natural fiber, they are low in fat, and provide the body with vitamins, especially vitamins A and C. While all vegetables are good nutritional choices, to maximize the benefits of eating vegetables, one should vary the type of vegetables eaten. It is also important when choosing vegetables to ingest not only a variety of the brightly colored vegetables such as corn, squash, and peas, but also the green and orange vegetables such as carrots, yams, and broccoli. One serving from the vegetable group equals one cup of raw, lefty greens; half cup of other chopped vegetables; or three-quarter cup of vegetable juice.

Fruits

Fruits are represented in the pyramid by the color red. Fresh, canned, frozen, or dried fruits are all excellent sources of vitamins and minerals, most notably vitamin C. It is, however, important to watch for heavy, sugary syrups when selecting canned fruits. Fruits canned in lite syrups or the fruit's own natural juice allow an individual to take in the same amount of vitamins and minerals as their heavily syruped counterparts without adding unnecessary and/or unwanted sugar, fat, and calories to their diet. Fruit juices are another important part of many people's diet that should be monitored for "hidden" sugars and calories. When possible, freshly squeezed juices are an ideal alternative. Serving equivalents for the fruit group are: one serving equals one medium apple, banana, or orange; one melon wedge; half cup of chopped berries, or three-quarter cup of fruit juice.

Milk

Milk and other calcium-rich foods such as yogurt and cheese now make up the blue portion of the Food Guide Pyramid. Milk products are not only the body's best source of calcium, they are also an excellent source of protein and vitamin B12. To maximize the benefits of calcium-rich foods and minimize the calories, cholesterol, fat, and saturated fat per selection, low-fat and skim alternatives should be chosen. One serving from the milk group equals one cup of milk or yogurt, or one and a half ounces of cheese.

Meats and Beans

Purple is the designated color for meats and beans within the pyramid. Meats and beans are excellent sources of protein, iron, zinc, and B vitamins. It is important to be aware of the fact that many food selections within this food group can be relatively high in fat content, especially saturated fats. Lower fat alternatives within this group that remain a rich source of vitamins and minerals include beans, fish, poultry, and lean cuts of beef. Serving equivalents for the meat and beans group are as follows: one serving equals two to three ounces of cooked lean beef, poultry, or fish; one egg; half cup of cooked beans; or two tablespoons of seeds or nuts.

Oils

Oils are depicted by the yellow band within the Food Guide Pyramid. As in all other areas of the pyramid, it is important to choose your source(s) of oils carefully. As a general rule, oils such as olive oil, peanut oil, and canola oil contain unsaturated fats. These oils do not raise an individual's blood cholesterol and are therefore a healthier option.

Daily Activity

The steps along the side of the pyramid symbolize the importance of including exercise into each and every day of a person's life. When daily exercise does not occur, the benefits of even the wisest food or nutrition choices are minimized.

What Happened to the "Fat" Group?

When looking at the new Food Guide Pyramid, it appears that foods like cookies, candies, and sodas found in the former pyramid's "Fat Group" no longer are a part of the pyramid. These foods are typically high in fat, sugars, and "empty" calories, and though they are not mentioned or specifically depicted in the new pyramid, they should only be enjoyed sparingly or in moderation. These foods often taste great but, in general, they provide the body with very little nutritionally.

Due to the fact that one pyramid could not possibly match or meet the needs of all Americans, twelve different pyramids have been created. To determine which Food Guide Pyramid is the best match, you can go to the USDA's Web site at MyPyramid.gov and enter your age, gender, and activity level. This process takes only a few seconds and can personalize the amounts and types of grains, vegetables, fruits, milk products, meats, and beans you should consume each day to maximize your health benefits.

Because an individual's nutritional requirements vary based on their life circumstances, there is a range in the number of servings within each food group. Examples of factors that might influence the number of servings viewed as healthy for an individual could be age, activity level, gender—if the person is a woman, is she pregnant or lactating? The guidelines in Table 5.10 are from the USDA's Center for Nutrition Policy and Promotion, and they can help an individual determine the

Table 5.10

How Many Servings Do You Need Each Day?

Food group servings: Perceived, average daily consumed, and recommended* by gender/age group						
	Grains	Fruits	Vegetables	Milk	Meat, etc.	Other (fats, oils, and sweets)
Females 19–24						
Perceived	3.2	2.6	2.6	3.2	3.5	2.2
Consumed	4.2	0.8	1.7	1.2	1.6	3.0
Recommended	9	3	4	2	2.4	Use sparingly
Females 25–50						
Perceived	2.9	2.2	2.5	2.3	3.0	2.1
Consumed	4.6	0.8	2.0	1.0	1.7	3.2
Recommended	9	3	4	2	2.4	Use sparingly
Females 51+						
Perceived	2.5	2.4	2.6	2.1	2.7	1.6
Consumed	4.7	1.5	2.2	1.0	1.7	3.1
Recommended	7.4	2.5	3.5	3	2.2	Use sparingly
Males 19–24						
Perceived	2.9	2.1	2.2	3.1	3.7	2.1
Consumed	5.5	0.6	2.3	1.6	2.3	4.1
Recommended	11	4	5	2	2.8	Use sparingly
Males 25–50						
Perceived	2.9	2.2	2.4	2.2	3.4	2.1
Consumed	5.9	0.9	2.5	1.2	2.5	4.0
Recommended	11	4	5	2	2.8	Use sparingly
Males 51+						
Perceived	2.7	2.2	2.5	2.1	3.1	1.7
Consumed	6.2	1.3	2.7	1.1	2.4	4.5
Recommended	9.1	3.2	4.2	3	2.5	Use sparingly

*Recommended servings based on energy RDA for gender/age groups.
Source: Publication of the USDA Center for Nutrition Policy and Promotion, October 2000.

appropriate number of servings from each of the groups within the Food Guide Pyramid based on their current life circumstances.

Determining the appropriate number of servings from each of the food groups is extremely important when planning a healthy diet. However, this information is of little practical value unless a person also knows what constitutes an accurate serving size (see Figure 5.3). Table 5.12 on page 175 lists serving size equivalents for several common foods.

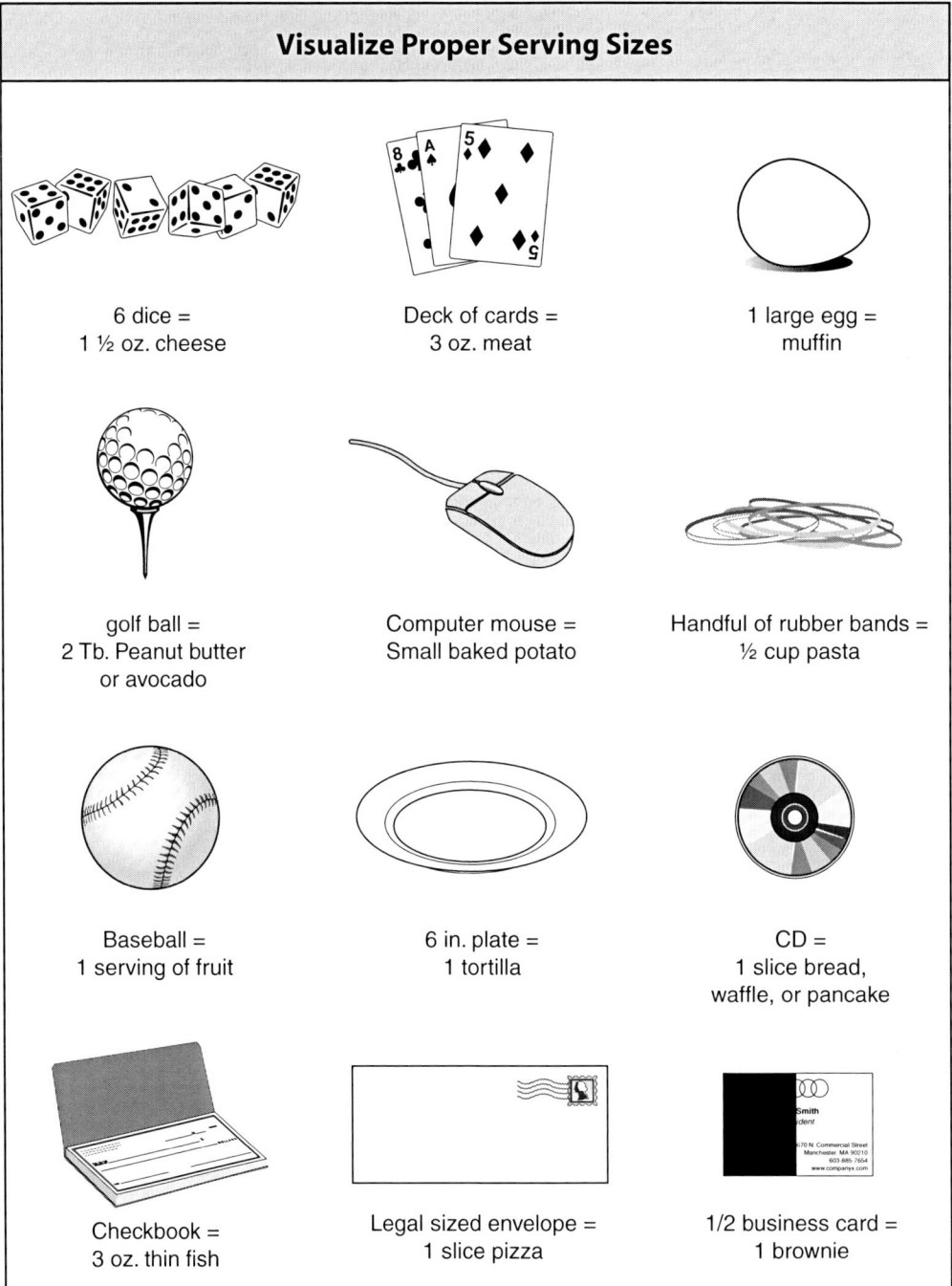

Other Issues in Nutrition

Organic Foods

Organic foods are foods that are grown without the use of pesticides. These chemical-free foods are much more difficult to grow because they are more vulnerable to disease and pests. Thus, they are not "high yield" crops. Due to the fact that they are less common, and harder to grow successfully, they are more expensive. Whether the expense is justified by the improved nutritional quality and overall health benefits is yet to be determined.

Functional Foods

Functional foods are foods that have benefits that go above and beyond basic nutrition. A person's overall health can be greatly affected by the food choices they make. Functional benefits of foods that have been consumed for decades are being discovered and new foods are being developed for their helpful dietary components. Table 5.11 lists examples of functional food components, their sources, and their potential benefits.

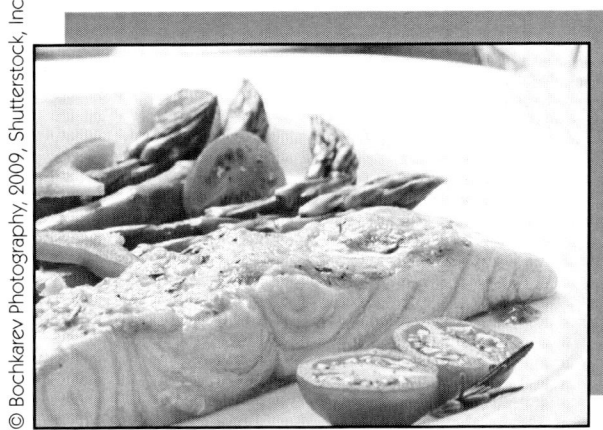

Salmon is a good source of Omega-3 fatty acids.

Vegetarianism

There have always been people who, for one reason or another (religious, ethical, or philosophical), have chosen to follow a vegetarian diet. However, in recent years, a vegetarian diet has become increasingly popular.

There are four different types of vegetarian diets. **Vegans** are considered true vegetarians. Their diets are completely void of meat, chicken, fish, eggs, or milk products. A vegan's primary sources of protein are vegetables, fruits, and grains. Because vitamin B12 is normally found only in meat products, many vegans choose to supplement their diet with this vitamin.

Lactovegetarians eat dairy products, fruits, and vegetables but do not consume any other animal products (meat, poultry, fish, or eggs).

Ovolactovegetarians are another type of vegetarians. They eat eggs as well as dairy products, fruits, and vegetables, but still do not consume meat, poultry, or fish.

A person who eats fruits, vegetables, dairy products, eggs, and a small selection of poultry, fish, and other seafood is a partial or **semivegetarian**. These individuals do not consume any beef or pork.

Vegetarians of all four types can meet all their daily dietary needs through the food selections available to them. However, because certain foods or groups of foods that are high in specific nutrients are forbidden, it is critical that a vegetarian is diligent in selecting his or her food combinations so that the nutritional benefits of the foods allowed are maximized. If food combinations from a wide variety of sources are not selected, nutritional deficiencies of proteins, vitamins, and minerals can rapidly occur and proper growth, development, and function may not occur. While a vegetarian diet can certainly be a healthy, low-fat alternative to the typical American diet, without diligent monitoring, it is not a guarantee of good health.

For many individuals who choose a vegetarian diet, it is more than simply omitting certain foods or groups of food, it is a way of living that they have embraced.

Table 5.11
Examples of Functional Components*

Class/Components	Source*	Potential Benefit
Carotenoids		
Beta-carotene	Carrots, pumpkin, sweet potato, cantaloupe	Neutralizes free radicals, which may damage cells; bolsters cellular antioxidant defenses; can be made into vitamin A in the body
Lutein, zeaxanthin	Kale, collards, spinach, corn, eggs, citrus	May contribute to maintenance of healthy vision
Lycopene	Tomatoes and processed tomato products, watermelon, red/pink grapefruit	May contribute to maintenance of prostate health
Dietary (functional and total) Fiber		
Insoluble fiber	Wheat bran, corn bran, fruit skins	May contribute to maintenance of a healthy digestive tract; may reduce the risk of some types of cancer
Beta glucan**	Oat bran, oatmeal, oat flour, barley, rye	May reduce risk of coronary heart disease (CHD)
Soluble fiber**	Psyllium seed husk, peas, beans, apples, citrus fruit	May reduce risk of CHD and some types of cancer
Whole grains**	Cereal grains, whole wheat bread, oatmeal, brown rice	May reduce risk of CHD and some types of cancer; may contribute to maintenance of healthy blood glucose levels
Fatty Acids		
Monounsaturated fatty acids (MUFAs)**	Tree nuts, olive oil, canola oil	May reduce risk of CHD
Polyunsaturated fatty acids (PUFAs)—omega-3 fatty acids—ALA	Walnuts, flax	May contribute to maintenance of heart health; may contribute to maintenance of mental and visual function
PUFAs—omega-3 fatty acids—DHA/EPA**	Salmon, tuna, marine, and other fish oils	May reduce risk of CHD; may contribute to maintenance of mental and visual function
Conjugated linoleic acid (CLA)	Beef and lamb; some cheese	May contribute to maintenance of desirable body composition and healthy immune function
Flavonoids		
Anthocyanins—cyanidin, delphinidin, malvidin	Berries, cherries, red grapes	Bolsters, cellular antioxidant defenses; may contribute to maintenance of brain function
Flavanols—catechins, epicatechins, epigallocatechin, procyanidins	Tea, cocoa, chocolate, apples, grapes	May contribute to maintenance of heart health
Flavanones—hesperetin, naringenin	Citrus foods	Neutralize free radicals, which may damage cells; bolster cellular antioxidant defenses
Flavonols—quercetin, kaempferol, isorhamnetin, myricetin	Onions, apples, tea, broccoli	Neutralize free radicals, which may damage cells; bolster cellular antioxidant defenses
Proanthocyanidins	Cranberries, cocoa, apples, strawberries, grapes, wine, peanuts, cinnamon	May contribute to maintenance of urinary tract health and heart health

Table 5.11
Examples of Functional Components*

Class/Components	Source*	Potential Benefit
Isothiocyanates		
Sulforaphane	Cauliflower, broccoli, broccoli sprouts, cabbage, kale, horseradish	May enhance detoxification of undesirable compounds; bolsters cellular antioxidant defenses
Minerals		
Calcium**	Sardines, spinach, yogurt, low-fat dairy products, fortified foods and beverages	May reduce the risk of osteoporosis
Magnesium	Spinach, pumpkin seeds, whole-grain breads and cereals, halibut, brazil nuts	May contribute to maintenance of normal muscle and nerve function, healthy immune function, and bone health
Potassium**	Potatoes, low-fat dairy products, whole-grain breads and cereals, citrus juices, beans, bananas	May reduce the risk of high blood pressure and stroke, in combination with a low-sodium diet
Selenium	Fish, red meat, grains, garlic, liver, eggs	Neutralizes free radicals, which may damage cells; may contribute to healthy immune function
Phenolic Acids		
Caffeic acid, ferulic acid	Apples, pears, citrus fruits, some vegetables, coffee	May bolster cellular antioxidant defenses; may contribute to maintenance of healthy vision and heart health
Plant Stanols/Sterols		
Free stanols/sterols**	Corn, soy, wheat, wood oils, fortified foods and beverages	May reduce risk of CHD
Stanol/sterol esters**	Fortified table spreads, stanol ester dietary supplements	May reduce risk of CHD
Polyols		
Sugar alcohols**—xylitol, sorbitol, mannitol, lactitol	Some chewing gums and other food	Applications may reduce risk of dental caries
Prebiotics		
Inulin, fructo-oligosaccharides (FOS), polydextrose	Whole grains, onions, some fruits, garlic, honey, leeks, fortified foods and beverages	May improve gastrointestinal health; may improve calcium absorption
Probiotics		
Yeast, *Lactobacilli*, *Bifidobacteria*, and other specific strains of beneficial bacteria	Certain yogurts and other cultured dairy and non-dairy applications	May improve gastrointestinal health and systemic immunity; benefits are strain-specific
Phytoestrogens		
Isoflavones—daidzein, genistein	Soybeans and soy-based foods	May contribute to maintenance of bone health, healthy brain and immune function; for women, may contribute to maintenance of menopausal health
Lignans	Flax, rye, some vegetables	May contribute to maintenance of heart health and healthy immune function

(continued)

Table 5.11

Examples of Functional Components* (continued)

Class/Components	Source*	Potential Benefit
Soy Protein		
Soy protein**	Soybeans and soy-based foods	May reduce risk of CHD
Sulfides/Thiols		
Diallyl sulfide, allyl methyl trisulfide	Garlic, onions, leeks, scallions	May enhance detoxification of undesirable compounds; may contribute to maintenance of heart health and healthy immune function
Dithiolthiones	Cruciferous vegetables	May enhance detoxification of undesirable compounds; may contribute to maintenance of healthy immune function
Vitamins		
A***	Organ meats, milk, eggs, carrots, sweet potato, spinach	May contribute to maintenance of healthy vision, immune function, and bone health; may contribute to cell integrity
B1 (Thiamin)	Lentils, peas, long-grain brown rice, brazil nuts	May contribute to maintenance of mental function; helps regulate metabolism
B2 (Riboflavin)	Lean meats, eggs, green leafy vegetables	Helps support cell growth; helps regulate metabolism
B3 (Niacin)	Dairy products, poultry, fish, nuts, eggs	Helps support cell growth; helps regulate metabolism
B5 (Pantothenic acid)	Organ meats, lobster, soybeans, lentils	Helps regulate metabolism and hormone synthesis
B6 (Pyridoxine)	Beans, nuts, legumes, fish, meat, whole grains	May contribute to maintenance of healthy immune function; helps regulate metabolism
B9 (Folate)**	Beans, legumes, citrus foods, green leafy vegetables, fortified breads and cereals	May reduce a woman's risk of having a child with a brain or spinal cord defect
B12 (Cobalamin)	Eggs, meat, poultry, milk	May contribute to maintenance of mental function; helps regulate metabolism and supports blood cell formation
Biotin	Liver, salmon, dairy, eggs, oysters	Helps regulate metabolism and hormone synthesis
C	Guava, sweet red/green pepper, kiwi, citrus fruit, strawberries	Neutralizes free radicals, which may damage cells; may contribute to maintenance of bone health and immune function
D	Sunlight, fish, fortified milk and cereals	Helps regulate calcium and phosphorus; helps contribute to bone health; may contribute to healthy immune function; helps support cell growth
E	Sunflower seeds, almonds, hazelnuts, turnip greens	Neutralizes free radicals, which may damage cells; may contribute to healthy immune function and maintenance of heart health

*Examples are not an all-inclusive list.
**FDA approved health claim established for component.
***Preformed vitamin A is found in foods that come from animals. Provitamin A carotenoids are found in many darkly colored fruits and vegetables and are a major source of vitamin A for vegetarians.

Source: Reprinted from International Food Information Council Foundation, 2007–2009. Originally printed in the 2007–2009 Foundation Media Guide on Food Safety and Nutrition.

Table 5.12
Food Guide Pyramid Serving Sizes

The USDA Food Guide Pyramid provides serving size recommendations to guide people in selecting their daily intake.

What counts as a serving?	How Many Servings Do You Need Each Day?		
	Children ages 2 to 6, women, some older adults (1,600 calories)	Older children, teen girls, active women, most men (2,200 calories)	Teen boys and active men (2,800 calories)
Grains Group (Bread, Cereal, Rice, and Pasta)—especially whole grain • 1 slice of bread • about 1 cup of ready-to-eat cereal • 1/2 cup of cooked cereal, rice or pasta	6	9	11
Vegetable Group • 1 cup of raw leafy vegetables • 1/2 cup of other vegetables—cooked or raw • 3/4 cup of vegetable juice	3	4	5
Fruit Group • 1 medium apple, banana, orange, pear • 1/2 cup of chopped, cooked, or canned fruit • 3/4 cup of fruit juice	2	3	4
Milk, Yogurt, and Cheese Group—preferably fat free or low fat • 1 cup of milk** or yogurt • 1 1/2 ounces of natural cheese (such as Cheddar) • 2 ounces of processed cheese (such as American)	2 or 3*	2 or 3*	2 or 3*
Meat and Beans (Meat, Poultry, Fish, Dry Beans, and Nuts)—preferably lean or low fat • 2–3 ounces of cooked lean meat, poultry, or fish These count as 1 ounce of meat: • 1/2 cup of cooked dry beans or tofu • 2 1/2 ounce soyburger • 1 egg • 2 tablespoons of peanut butter • 1/3 cup of nuts	2, for a total of 5 ounces	2, for a total of 6 ounces	3, for a total of 7 ounces

*Older children and teens ages 9 to 18 years and adults over age 50 need three servings daily. Others need two servings daily.
**This includes lactose-free and lactose-reduced milk products. Soy-based beverages with added calcium are an option for those who prefer a non-dairy source of calcium.

FIGURE 5.4

My Pyramid

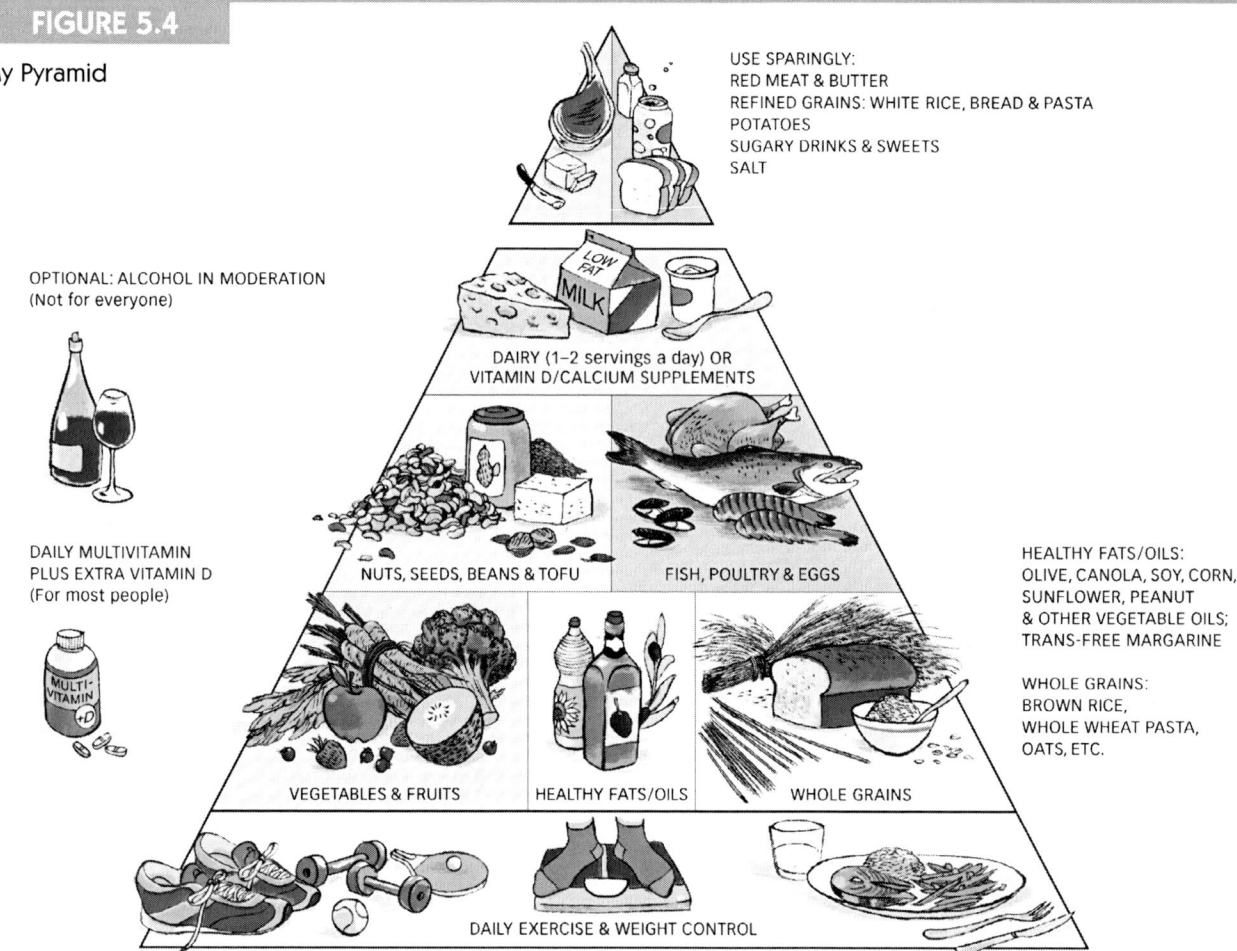

Source: Copyright © 2008 Harvard University. For more information about The Healthy Eating Pyramid, please see The Nutrition Source, Department of Nutrition, Harvard School of Public Health, http://www.thenutritionsource.org, and Eat, Drink, and Be Healthy, by Walter C. Willett, M. D. and Patrick J. Skerrett (2005), Free Press/Simon & Schuster Inc. Used with permission.

Reading and Understanding the Nutrition Facts Label

Beginning in May 1993, the federal government has required food manufacturers to provide accurate nutritional information about their products on their product labels. Because food labels are standardized, relatively straightforward, and easy to read, much of the guesswork has been taken out of good nutrition.

Ingredients are listed on food labels by percentage of total weight, in order from heaviest or highest to lowest. By reading the listing of ingredients, an individual can determine whether a food is relatively high in fat, sugar, salt, and so on.

Food labels are legally required to include the number of servings per container, serving size, and the number of calories per serving. They must also list the percentage of the daily value of total fat, saturated fat, and, beginning in January 2006, trans fat. Nutrition Facts Labels must also list the percentage of the daily value of cholesterol, sodium, total carbohydrates (including dietary fiber and sugars), proteins, vitamins, and minerals. Figure 5.5 provides an example of the required nutrition information found on packaged foods.

Food Label: Nutrition Facts FIGURE 5.5

Serving Size
Is your serving the same size as the one on the label? If you eat double the serving size listed, you need to double the nutrient and calorie values. If you eat one-half the serving size shown here, cut the nutrient and calorie values in half.

Calories
Are you overweight? Cut back a little on calories! Look here to see how a serving of the food adds to your daily total. A 5'4", 138-lb. active woman needs about 2,200 calories each day. A 5'10", 174-lb. active man needs about 2,900. How about you?

Total Carbohydrate
When you cut down on fat, you can eat more carbohydrates. Carbohydrates are in foods like bread, potatoes, fruits, and vegetables. Choose these often! They give you more nutrients than sugars like soda pop and candy.

Dietary Fiber
Grandmother called it "roughage," but her advice to eat more is still up-to-date! That goes for both soluble and insoluble kinds of dietary fiber. Fruits, vegetables, whole-grain foods, beans, and peas are all good sources and can help reduce the risk of heart disease and cancer.

Protein
Most Americans get more protein than they need. Where there is animal protein, there is also fat and cholesterol. Eat small servings of lean meat, fish, and poultry. Use skim or low-fat milk, yogurt, and cheese. Try vegetable proteins like beans, grains, and cereals.

Vitamins and Minerals
Your goal here is 100 percent of each for the day. Don't count on one food to do it all. Let a combination of foods add up to a winning score.

Nutrition Facts

Serving Size 1 cup (228g)
Servings Per Container 2

Amount Per Serving

Calories 250   Calories from Fat 110

	% Daily Value*
Total Fat 12g	18%
Saturated Fat 3g	15%
Trans Fat 3g	
Cholesterol 30mg	10%
Sodium 470mg	20%
Total Carbohydrate 31g	10%
Dietary Fiber 0g	0%
Sugars 5g	
Protein 5g	
Vitamin A	4%
Vitamin C	2%
Calcium	20%
Iron	4%

*Percent Daily Values are based on a 2,000 calorie diet. Your Daily Values may be higher or lower depending on your calorie needs:

	Calories	2,000	2,500
Total Fat	Less than	65g	80g
Sat Fat	Less than	20g	25g
Cholesterol	Less than	300mg	300mg
Sodium	Less than	2,400mg	2,400mg
Total Carbohydrate		300g	375g
Fiber		25g	30g

Calories per gram:
Fat 9 • Carbohydrates 4 • Protein 4

More nutrients may be listed on some labels.

Total Fat
Aim low. Most people need to cut back on fat! Too much fat may contribute to heart disease and cancer. Try to limit your calories from fat. For a healthy heart, choose foods with a big difference between the total number of calories and the number of calories from fat.

Saturated Fat
A new kind of fat? No—saturated fat is part of the total fat in food. It is listed separately because it's the key player in raising blood cholesterol and your risk of heart disease. Eat less!

Cholesterol
Too much cholesterol—a second cousin to fat—can lead to heart disease. Challenge yourself to eat less than 300 mg each day.

Sodium
You call it "salt," the label calls it "sodium." Either way, it may add up to high blood pressure in some people. So, keep your sodium intake low—2,400 to 3,000 mg or less each day.*

*The AHA recommends no more than 3,000 mg sodium per day for healthy adults.

Daily Value
Feel like you're drowning in numbers? Let the Daily Value be your guide. Daily Values are listed for people who eat 2,000 or 2,500 calories each day. If you eat more, your personal daily value may be higher than what's listed on the label. If you eat less, your personal daily value may be lower.

For fat, saturated fat, cholesterol, and sodium, choose foods with a low percent Daily Value. For total carbohydrate, dietary fiber, vitamins, and minerals, your daily value goal is to reach 100 percent of each.

g = grams (About 28 g = 1 ounce)
mg = milligrams (1,000 mg = 1 g)

You Can Rely on the New Label

Rest assured, when you see key words and health claims on product labels, they mean what they say as defined by the government. For example:

Key Words	*What They Mean*	*To Make* Health Claims About...	*The Food* Must Be...
Fat Free	Less than 0.5 g of fat per serving	Heart Disease and Fats	Low in fat, saturated fat, and cholesterol
Low Fat	3 g of fat (or less) per serving		
Lean	Less than 10 g of fat, 4 g of saturated fat, and 95 mg of cholesterol per serving	Blood Pressure and Sodium	Low in sodium
Light (Lite)	one-third less calories or no more than one-half the fat of the higher-calorie, higher-fat version; or no more than one-half the sodium of the higher-sodium version	Heart Disease and Fruits, Vegetables, and Grain Products	A fruit, vegetable, or grain product low in fat, saturated fat, and cholesterol, that contains at least 0.6 g soluble fiber, without fortification, per serving
Cholesterol Free	Less than 2 mg of cholesterol and 2 g (or less) of saturated fat per serving		

Other claims may appear on some labels.

> ### Why Is There No Percentage of Daily Value for Trans Fats?
>
> There have been scientific findings and reports that confirm a link between trans fats and an increased risk of coronary heart disease. However, none of the reports have recommended an amount of trans fat that the Food and Drug Administration could use to establish a daily value, and without a daily value, a percentage of that daily value cannot be calculated.

The bottom part of Nutrition Facts Labels on larger packages (typically any item that is not packaged for individual sale) contains a footnote with Daily Values (DVs) for 2,000- and 2,500-calorie-a-day diets. Because this information is not about a specific food product, it does not change from product to product. It shows recommended advice for all Americans. In the footnote section of the Nutrition Facts Label, the nutrients that have an upper limit or a set amount one wants to stay below are listed first. These nutrients include total fat, saturated fat, trans fat, sodium, and cholesterol. The amount of dietary fiber listed in this section is a minimum amount that should be consumed each day. The daily value for carbohydrates listed is a recommendation based on a 2,000-calorie-a-day diet, but it can vary slightly depending on the amount of fat and protein consumed.

When an individual takes the time to use the main body of the Nutrition Facts Label in conjunction with the footnote section of the label, he or she can get a very accurate picture of not only what source (carbohydrate, fat, or protein) their calories are coming from, but also how close they are coming to meeting the daily requirements necessary to maintain a high level of health.

Although product labels do have accuracy requirements, mistakes can be made and sometimes do occur. For this reason, it is wise to check the accuracy of food labels. One quick and easy way to do this is to divide the number of servings within the container—does it equal the serving size? For example, you have a product that the Nutrition Facts Label shows having a serving size of one-half cup and the number of servings per container is four. If you open the product and check it, does it contain two cups of that food? If so, the label is correct. Another way to check the accuracy of a nutrition label is to calculate the calories (grams of fat times nine, grams of protein and carbohydrates times four). Does the number calculated match the reported calories within 10 to 20 calories? If the numbers are way "off" one should be aware that the label is incorrect. See Figure 5.5 (Nutrition Facts Label) for an example of how to check for label accuracy based on reported calories.

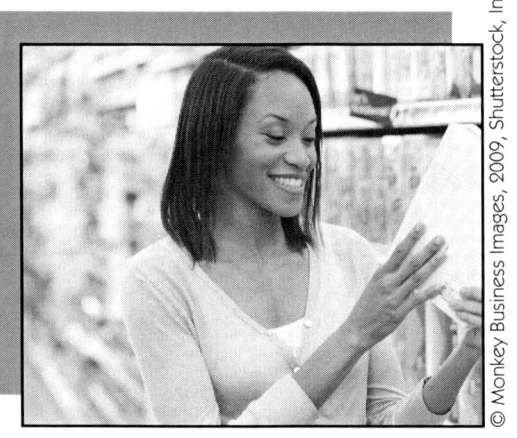
Reading labels while grocery shopping is important in preparing healthy meals.

Reported Total Calories per Serving = 250
Reported Calories from Fat = 110

The product contains a total of 12 g of fat. Fat contains 9 calories per gram of fat, so to check for accuracy of reported fat calories, multiply 12 × 9. This equals 108.

To check for accuracy of total number of calories, multiply the total grams of carbohydrates . . . 31 in this product, by 4 (the amount of calories per gram of carbohydrate). This equals 124 calories.

The total grams of protein . . . 5 in this product, by 4 (the amount of calories per gram of protein). This equals 20 calories.

To check for accuracy of the total number of calories per serving, add calories from fat, protein, and carbohydrates. If they are close to the number of calories per serving listed on the Nutrition Fact Label, the label is accurate.

108 + 124 + 20 = 252 actual vs. 250 reported

Both the total calories and fat calories listed on the Nutrition Facts Label were slightly low. Knowing this, an individual can more accurately determine when he or she has reached their nutritional limit.

REFERENCES

Donatelle, R. J. & Davis, L. G. *Access* to *Health* (9th ed). Boston: Allyn & Bacon. 2006.

Floyd, P. A., Mimms, S. E., and Yelding-Howard, C. *Personal Health: Perspectives & Lifestyles.*, Englewood, CO: Morton Publishing Company. 2007.

Hales, D. *An Invitation to Health* (8th ed). New York: Brooks/Cole Publishing Company. 1999.

Hoeger, W. and Hoeger, S. A. *Principles and Labs for Fitness and Wellness* (9th ed). Belmont, CA: Thomson Wadsworth. 2008.

Hoeger, W. W. K. and Hoeger, S. A. *Lifetime Physical Fitness and Wellness: A Personalized Program* (8th ed). Belmont, CA: Thomson Wadsworth. 2005.

Hyman, B., Oden, G., Bacharach, D., and Collins, R. *Fitness for Living.* Dubuque, Iowa: Kendall/Hunt. 2006.

http://www.ific.org/nutrition/functional/index.cfm?rederforprint = 1

Powers, S. K., Todd, S. L. and Noland, J. J. *Total Fitness and Wellness* (2nd ed). Boston: Allyn & Bacon. 2005.

Prentice, W. E. *Fitness and Wellness for Life* (6th ed). New York: WCB McGraw-Hill. 1999.

Pruitt, B. E. & Stein, J. *HealthStyles* (2nd ed). Boston: Allyn & Bacon. 1999.

Robbins, G., Powers, D., and Burgess, S. *A Wellness Way of Life* (4th ed). New York: WCB McGraw-Hill. 1999.

Rosato, F. *Fitness for Wellness* (3rd ed). Minneapolis: West. 1994.

Webmaster@noah.cuny.edu

http://www.cfsan.fda.gov/~dms/transfat.html

http://www.ganesa.com/food/foodpyramid.gif

http://www.healthdepot.com

http://www.health.gov/dietaryguidelines/dga2000.htm

http://www.health.gov/dietaryguidelines/dga2000/document/aim.htm

http://www.health.gov/dietaryguidelines/dga2000/document/choose.htm

http://www.health.gov/dietaryguidelines/dga2005/document/html/executivesummary.htm

http://www.health.gov/dietaryguidelines/dga2005/document/html/chapter1.htm

http://vm.cfsan.fda.gov/~dms/foodlab.html

http://www.ers.usda.gov/AmberWaves/June05/Features?Will2005WholeGrain.htm

http://www.aaccnet.org/definitions/wholegrain.asp

CONTACTS

American Dietetic Association
Get Nutrition Fact Sheets at
American Dietetic Association
Consumer Education Team
216 West Jackson Boulevard
Chicago, IL 60606
(send a self-addressed, stamped envelope), call 800–877–1600, ext. 5000 for other publications or 800–366–1655 for recorded food/nutrition messages

American Obesity Association
1250 24th Street, NW, Suite 300
Washington, DC 20037
800–98–OBESE

Department of Nutrition Sciences
University of Alabama at Birmingham
Birmingham, AL 35294

Calorieking.com

Fitday.com

http://www.caloriesperhour.com/index_food.html

ACTIVITIES

Notebook Activities

- Food Processor
- Dietary Analysis Project
- Cholesterol Levels Measured
- Create a Personalized Nutrition Plan

Name: _____ Section: _____ Date: _____

NOTEBOOK ACTIVITY

Food Processor

Record all that you eat and drink for three days. Include at least one weekend day and one weekday for a total of three days. Use as much detail as possible, including amount and type of food. The more accurate your record, the more accurate your analysis will be. Be honest and specific!

EXAMPLES:
1 cup of fruity pebbles
1 cup of 1% milk
1 small package of peanut M&Ms (6 oz.)
1 large coffee, black (8 oz.)

Take your food list, and go to room 150 in the Read building (the computer lab.) **Bring your student ID and get a lab log-on ID and password if you don't already have one. This will take an extra ten to fifteen minutes.** Secure a food processor instruction sheet from the shelves and follow the directions. Input all your food for the three days together. There is no need to separate the days. You may need to make some substitutions; however, the food inventory list has much to choose from. If you have problems, ask the personnel behind the help desk for assistance.

Print out everything—that should be **4 printouts**:

1. Profile
2. Comparison
3. Single Nutrient
4. Bar Graphs

Please staple everything together in the order you ran them off. Good Luck!

Note: Most people overestimate their activity level and underestimate their food intake. Be as accurate as possible! Most individuals fall into a moderate activity level.

If you have problems finding a food item, backspace several times and then double click to see that you are spelling the item correctly. Sometimes you will find *carrots* where you could not find *carrot*—change plurals to singular and vice versa. Finally, think of other names for food items—such as toaster pastry instead of pop tart.

*Remember, eat as normally as possible.

For additional information and benefits, complete the following Dietary Analysis Project.

Name: _____ Section: _____ Date: _____

NOTEBOOK ACTIVITY

Dietary Analysis Project

I. Carbohydrates

1. Look at your analysis sheet and list below each day's intake, then find the average calories that you consumed for the time period you entered.

   Day 1 _____, 2 _____ 3, _____ (ex. credit 4, _____ 5, _____ 6, _____ 7, _____)

   Total calories divided by 3(7) days = _____ Average intake

2. Look at your analysis sheet and list below each day's carbohydrate intake, then find the average grams of carbs that you consumed for the time period you entered

   Day 1 _____, 2 _____ 3, _____ (ex. credit 4, _____ 5, _____ 6, _____ 7, _____ g)

   Total carbs divided by 3(7) days = _____ Average intake

3. Now calculate the percentage of energy in your diet from carbohydrate. Use the formula below and use your **average** carb grams and your average calorie intake.

   Average grams of CHO ( ) × 4 × 100 = _____ % of energy from carbohydrates average calories consumed (_____)

4. Did your carb intake meet the RDA's recommendations that 55–65 percent of your total calories come from carbohydrate? _____ yes _____ no

5. If not, what carbohydrate-rich foods do you need to eat more or less of to meet these requirements?

   _____

   _____

6. List below each day's fiber intake and then determine the average grams of fiber you consumed

   Day 1 _____, Day 2 _____, Day 3 _____, Day 4 _____, Day 5 _____, Day 6 _____, Day 7 _____

   Total grams of fiber/days (i.e., 30 g/3 days = 10 grams per day average intake)

   _____/_____ = _____ g fiber

7. Did this amount meet the recommendations to consume 20–35 g of fiber a day? _____
   If not, what foods do you need to eat more of to increase your fiber intake?

   _____

   _____

II. Fats

8. Look at your analysis and list your daily intakes of the following types of fat, and then determine the average intakes for the period recorded.

	Total Fat	Saturated Fat	Cholesterol	MUS	PUS
Day 1	_____	_____	_____	____	____
Day 2	_____	_____	_____	____	____
Day 3	_____	_____	_____	____	____
Day 4	_____	_____	_____	____	____
Day 5	_____	_____	_____	____	____
Day 6	_____	_____	_____	____	____
Day 7	_____	_____	_____	____	____
Average	_____	_____	_____	____	____

9. Now calculate the percentage of energy in your diet from fat. Use the formula below and use your **average** total fat grams (as listed in #7 and your average calorie intake).

$$\frac{\text{Average of fat (\_\_\_\_)} \times 9}{\text{Average calories consumed (\_\_\_\_)}} \times 100 = \underline{\hspace{1cm}} \text{ \% of energy from fat}$$

10. Did your fat intake meet the RDA's recommendations that 20–30 percent of your total calories come from fat? ____yes ____ no

11. If not, what foods do you need to eat less of to meet these requirements?

_____

_____

12. What was your average intake of cholesterol? _____ Does your cholesterol intake fall within the recommendations of consuming no more than 300 mg of cholesterol each day? _____ yes _____ no

13. If your intake was above 300 mg per day, what foods do you need to eat less of to reduce your cholesterol intake?

_____

_____

Name: _____ Section: _____ Date: _____

III. Protein

14. List each day's protein intake below.

    Day 1 ____, Day 2 ____, Day 3 ____, Day 4 ____, Day 5 ____, Day 6 ____, Day 7 ____

    According to your Dietary Analysis, how many grams of protein did you consume per day (average) during this time? ____ (i.e., total protein intake = 300 g/3 days = 100 g per day average)

15. Now calculate the percentage of energy in you diet from protein. Use the formula below and use your **average** protein grams (as listed in #1 and your average calorie intake).

    $$\frac{\text{Average g of protein (\_\_\_\_)}}{\text{Average calories consumed (\_\_\_\_)}} \times 4 \times 100 = \underline{\qquad} \% \text{ of energy from protein}$$

    Does this amount follow the dietary recommendations for protein intake (12–15 percent of your total calorie intake)? ____

16. The minimum recommendations for protein intake are as follows:

    .8 g – .9 g of protein per kg of body weight

    Determine your protein needs according to these recommendations (kg = #/2.2)

    Body weight in #/2.2 = ____ × (.8 or .9) = ____ g needed minimum

    My minimum protein needs are _____. I consumed _____ g of protein for a difference of +, − _____ g.

17. What foods do you need to consume more/less of to meet your protein requirements?

    _____

    _____

18. Did your protein come more from animal or plant sources? _____

19. If you would exercise regularly (3 × week for 30 minutes), you would need about 1.2–1.4 g of protein/kg of body weight. Calculate your protein requirements.

    Body weight (kg) × 1.2–1.4 g protein = _____ g needed.

20. Look at your food printout and calculate your average servings of fruits and veggies according to the food guide pyramid's serving sizes suggestions. Then compare your averages to the USDA's analysis of your fruits and veggies intake. Remember French fries and chips are not veggies. One-half cup cooked red, yellow, or green veggies or one cup leafy is a serving of veggies and one medium fruit or one-half or three-quarter cup juice is a serving of fruit.

    Average fruit intake _____ USDA intake _____

    Average veggie intake _____ USDA intake _____

21. Based on the total analysis of your diet, what health problems might you experience if you continue to eat in this manner?

22. What is the most important thing you learned about your diet after doing this analysis?

Name: _____ Section: _____ Date: _____

NOTEBOOK ACTIVITY

Cholesterol Levels Measured

Have a cholesterol test performed by a licensed individual, and turn in the actual results from the test.

Name: _____ Section: _____ Date: _____

NOTEBOOK ACTIVITY

Create a Personalized Nutrition Plan

1. Go to the U.S. Department of Agriculture's Web site at http://www.mypyramid.gov.

2. Enter the following information in the My Pyramid section:
   Age
   Gender
   Activity Level

3. Submit the information you have entered.

4. Print the information you are given and attach it to this sheet.

5. Use the MyPyramid Worksheet that is based on the number of calories you should be consuming (choose from 1,800 calories, 2,000 calories, or 2,400 calories) and complete this worksheet for three consecutive days. Attach completed worksheets to this sheet.

Name: _____ Section: _____ Date: _____

MyPyramid Worksheet

Check how you did today and set a goal to aim for tomorrow

Write in Your Choices for Today	Food Group	Tip	Goal Based on a 1800 calorie pattern.	List each food choice in its food group*	Estimate Your Total
_____ _____ _____ _____	**GRAINS**	Make at least half your grains whole grains	**6 ounce equivalents** (1 ounce equivalent is about 1 slice bread, 1 cup dry cereal, or ½ cup cooked rice, pasta, or cereal)	_____ _____ _____	_____ ounce equivalents
_____ _____ _____ _____	**VEGETABLES**	Try to have vegetables from several subgroups each day	**2 ½ cups** Subgroups: Dark Green, Orange, Starchy, Dry Beans and Peas, Other Veggies	_____ _____ _____	_____ cups
_____ _____ _____ _____	**FRUITS**	Make most choices fruit, not juice	**1 ½ cups**	_____ _____ _____	_____ cups
_____ _____ _____ _____	**MILK**	Choose fat-free or low fat most often	**3 cups** (1 ½ ounces cheese = 1 cup milk)	_____ _____ _____	_____ cups
_____ _____ _____ _____	**MEAT & BEANS**	Choose lean meat and poultry. Vary your choices—more fish, beans, peas, nuts, and seeds	**5 ounce equivalents** (1 ounce equivalent is 1 ounce meat, poultry, or fish, 1 egg, 1 T. peanut butter, ½ ounce nuts, or ¼ cup dry beans)	_____ _____ _____	_____ ounce equivalents
_____ _____ _____ _____	**PHYSICAL ACTIVITY**	Build more physical activity into your daily routine at home and work.	At least **30 minutes** of moderate to vigorous activity a day, 10 minutes or more at a time.	*Some foods don't fit into any group. These "extras" may be mainly fat or sugar—limit your intake of these.	_____ minutes

How did you do today? ☐ Great   ☐ So-So   ☐ Not so Great

My food goal for tomorrow is: _____

My activity goal for tomorrow is: _____

From www.mypyramid.gov

Name: _____ Section: _____ Date: _____

MyPyramid Worksheet

Check how you did today and set a goal to aim for tomorrow

Food Group	Tip	Goal Based on a 2000 calorie pattern.	List each food choice in its food group*	Estimate Your Total
GRAINS	Make at least half your grains whole grains	**6 ounce equivalents** (1 ounce equivalent is about 1 slice bread, 1 cup dry cereal, or ½ cup cooked rice, pasta, or cereal)		_____ ounce equivalents
VEGETABLES	Try to have vegetables from several subgroups each day	**2 ½ cups** Subgroups: Dark Green, Orange, Starchy, Dry Beans and Peas, Other Veggies		_____ cups
FRUITS	Make most choices fruit, not juice	**2 cups**		_____ cups
MILK	Choose fat free or low fat most often	**3 cups** (1 ½ ounces cheese = 1 cup milk)		_____ cups
MEAT & BEANS	Choose lean meat and poultry. Vary your choices—more fish, beans, peas, nuts, and seeds	**5 ½ ounce equivalents** (1 ounce equivalent is 1 ounce meat, poultry, or fish, 1 egg, 1 T. peanut butter, ½ ounce nuts, or ¼ cup dry beans)	*Some foods don't fit into any group. These "extras" may be mainly fat or sugar—limit your intake of these.	_____ ounce equivalents
PHYSICAL ACTIVITY	Build more physical activity into your daily routine at home and work.	At least **30 minutes** of moderate to vigorous activity a day. 10 minutes or more at a time.		_____ minutes

Write in Your Choices for Today

How did you do today? ☐ Great   ☐ So-So   ☐ Not so Great

My food goal for tomorrow is: _____

My activity goal for tomorrow is: _____

From www.mypyramid.gov

Name: _____ Section: _____ Date: _____

MyPyramid Worksheet

Check how you did today and set a goal to aim for tomorrow

Food Group	Tip	Goal Based on a 2400 calorie pattern.	Write in Your Choices for Today	List each food choice in its food group*	Estimate Your Total
GRAINS	Make at least half your grains whole grains	**8 ounce equivalents** (1 ounce equivalent is about 1 slice bread, 1 cup dry cereal, or ½ cup cooked rice, pasta, or cereal)	_____	_____	_____ ounce equivalents
VEGETABLES	Try to have vegetables from several subgroups each day	**3 cups** Subgroups: Dark Green, Orange, Starchy, Dry Beans and Peas, Other Veggies	_____	_____	_____ cups
FRUITS	Make most choices fruit, not juice	**2 cups**	_____	_____	_____ cups
MILK	Choose fat-free or low fat most often	**3 cups** (1 ½ ounces cheese = 1 cup milk)	_____	_____	_____ cups
MEAT & BEANS	Choose lean meat and poultry. Vary your choices—more fish, beans, peas, nuts, and seeds	**6 ½ ounce equivalents** (1 ounce equivalent is 1 ounce meat, poultry, or fish, 1 egg, 1 T. peanut butter, ½ ounce nuts, or ¼ cup dry beans)	_____	_____	_____ ounce equivalents
PHYSICAL ACTIVITY	Build more physical activity into your daily routine at home and work.	At least **30 minutes** of moderate to vigorous activity a day, 10 minutes or more at a time.	_____	_____	_____ minutes

*Some foods don't fit into any group. These "extras" may be mainly fat or sugar—limit your intake of these.

How did you do today? ☐ Great ☐ So-So ☐ Not so Great

My food goal for tomorrow is: _____

My activity goal for tomorrow is: _____

From www.mypyramid.gov

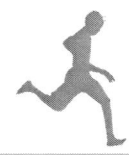

CHAPTER 6

Lifetime Weight Management

"Thou shouldst eat to live; not live to eat."

—Socrates, 469 BC–399 BC

OBJECTIVES

Students will be able to:
- Identify problems associated with fast food dining.
- Discuss diet supplements.
- Present guidelines for a successful weight-loss program.
- Identify a healthy Body Mass Index.
- Identify causes of obesity and complications associated with obesity.
- Discuss the importance of activity for weight management.
- Recognize the pitfalls of Fad Dieting.

Why have Americans gained so much weight over the last fifty years (see Figure 6.1)? Approximately two-thirds of adult Americans are overweight, and typically so are their children. The causes are numerous and complex. The bottom line is nutritional balance (see Figure 6.2): calories eaten versus calories expended. However, even if some folks exercise and attempt to eat healthy, it is more complicated than that. Because our society has become increasingly automated, Americans are saving lots of energy in the form of stored fat. "Easier," "automated," "instant," and "remote control" are all terms which describe using less energy. Saving energy relates to moving less, which means saving calories. A person who moves less typically stores more fat. Chapter 3 discusses lifestyle activity, which means looking for opportunities to expend more energy—like taking the stairs instead of the elevator. Every time you drive through for fast food, think of all of the energy you are saving. Another culprit in contributing to larger Americans is the Internet, games, texting, and so on. Balancing sedentary activities with playing baseball, tag, and climbing trees is important.

Causes of Obesity and Being Overweight

Patrick O'Neil, director of the Weight Management Center at the Medical University of South Carolina in Charleston, determined that 40 percent of people's weight problems are due to whom they choose for their parents. Gene pool plays a big role in body size. Through evolution we are programmed to hunt and gather, then

FIGURE 6.1

Percentage of Adults Who Are Obese,* by State

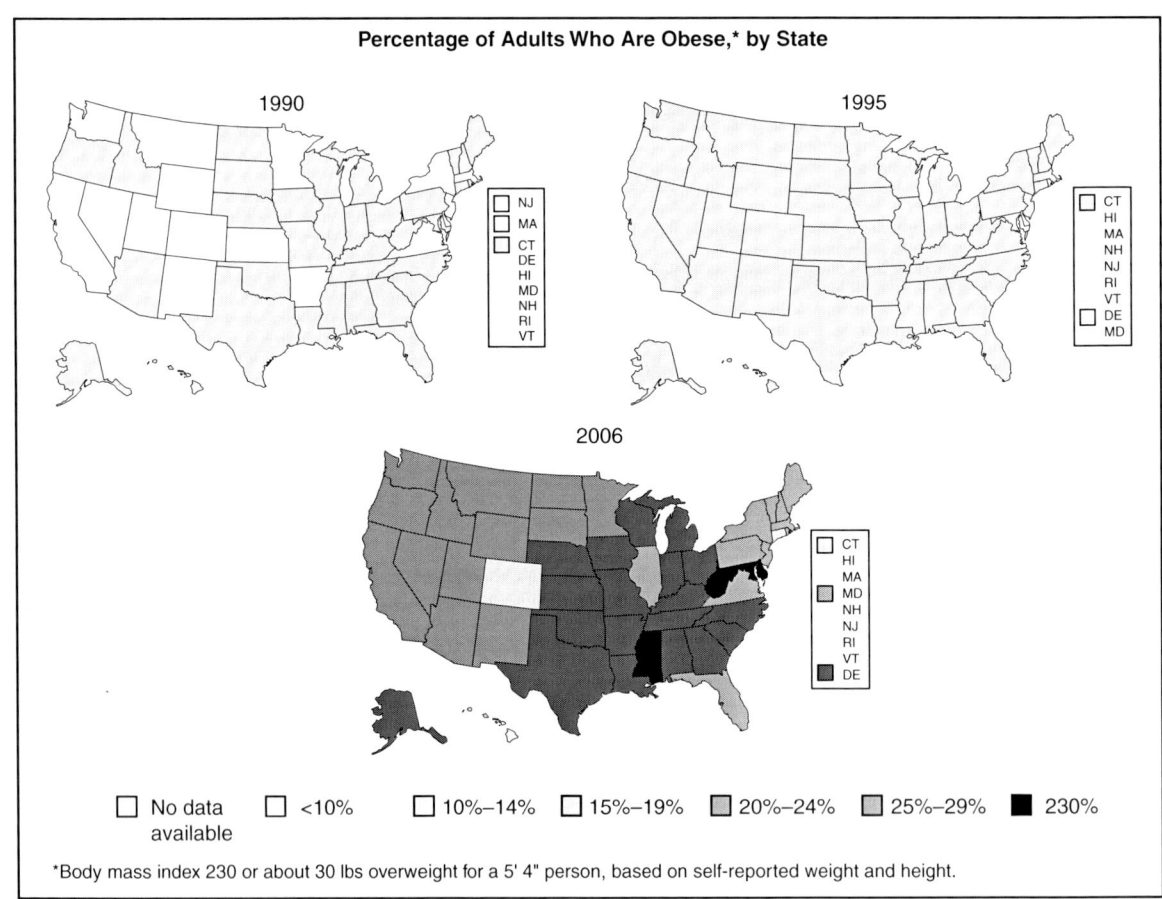

*Body mass index 230 or about 30 lbs overweight for a 5' 4" person, based on self-reported weight and height.

Source: Behavioral Risk Factors Surveillance System, CDC.

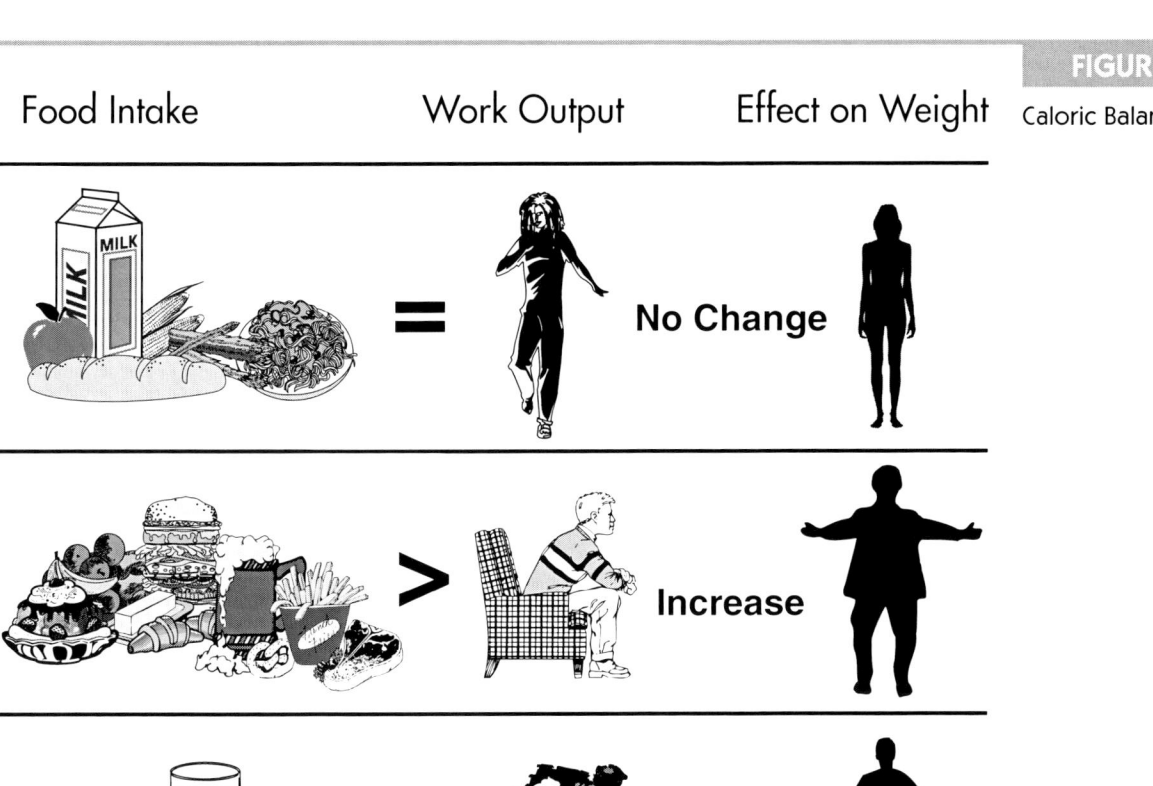

FIGURE 6.2 Caloric Balance

eat plenty as the food is available to store energy. Dr. O'Neil quotes the old adage, "Genes load the gun, but environment pulls the trigger." We typically learn eating patterns and develop a familiarity with certain types of foods that we eat when we are younger. Starting with what we eat as infants through adulthood, we learn particular eating styles.

Foods have changed. Fifty years ago foods were less processed. There was less convenience food. Foods were eaten more in their wholesome state. Portion sizes were smaller than they are today. Today's small McDonald's Happy Meal French fries were the "regular" size when McDonald's opened. A McDonald's Super Size serving of French fries contains 540 calories with 230 calories coming from fat. It is only in the last 20 years that convenience stores and fast-food eateries have offered the 42-ounce size of sweetened soft drinks. A 42-ounce Dr. Pepper has 525 calories. Many in the health industry think that the increase in corn syrup sweetened soft drink consumption has contributed to America's obesity problem, especially childhood obesity. Portion control is a critical component in weight management. Check product labels to determine how much food is considered a serving, as well as how many calories, grams of fat, and so on, are in a serving. Many prepackaged foods contain two or more servings—always read the label! See What Counts as a Serving on page 175. Trans-fatty acids have entered the diet via hydrogenation, a process by which liquid oils (which are unsaturated and healthy) are reconstituted to a solid convenient form. As you recall from the nutrition chapter, the problem with ingesting trans-fatty acid is that it raises LDL (the bad cholesterol) and lowers HDL (the good cholesterol). Results from Nurses' Health Study determined that a diet high in trans-fatty acids is highly associated with an increase in cardiovascular risk. A diet high in trans fats also may be linked to an increased abdominal fat measurement, as well as to an increase in the risk of Type 2 diabetes (IUFOST, 2006). What you eat, when you eat, and how much you eat make a difference. How you choose to eat makes a difference as well. Do you sit down and enjoy your food, or do you eat on the run?

Although the causes of overweight and obesity are complex and numerous, the risks of being overweight or obese are very real and tangible. An individual who is overweight is at increased risk for conditions such as high blood pressure, high cholesterol, stroke, heart disease, obesity, diabetes, and certain types of cancers. For most Americans, food is plentiful. Americans are typically not malnourished due to a lack of food, but the World Health Organization (WHO) predicts that there will soon be a world epidemic of overweight and malnourished people resulting from the unhealthy types of foods that are being eaten. A person living on only fast food that is high in sodium, fat, and cholesterol and low in vitamins and fiber can experience a lack of some essential nutrients. Eating a variety of foods such as vegetables, fruits, whole grains, low-fat dairy, fish, lean cuts of meat (or other quality protein), and beans are the building blocks of a solid nutritional practice.

Chapters 3 and 4 emphasized the importance of regular activity for overall health. Exercise can help you get fit and stay fit and is a critical aid in efforts to lose weight. The three largest contributors to overweight are lack of exercise, eating choices and behaviors, and genetics. Exercise may be the most significant. Sobering studies show that most people who successfully lose weight will have gained it back within two years time. The 5 percent that successfully maintain weight loss have exercise in their life—it is part of their lifestyle (see Figure 6.3). It isn't important to take up running or any activity you are uncomfortable doing. The important thing is to just move!

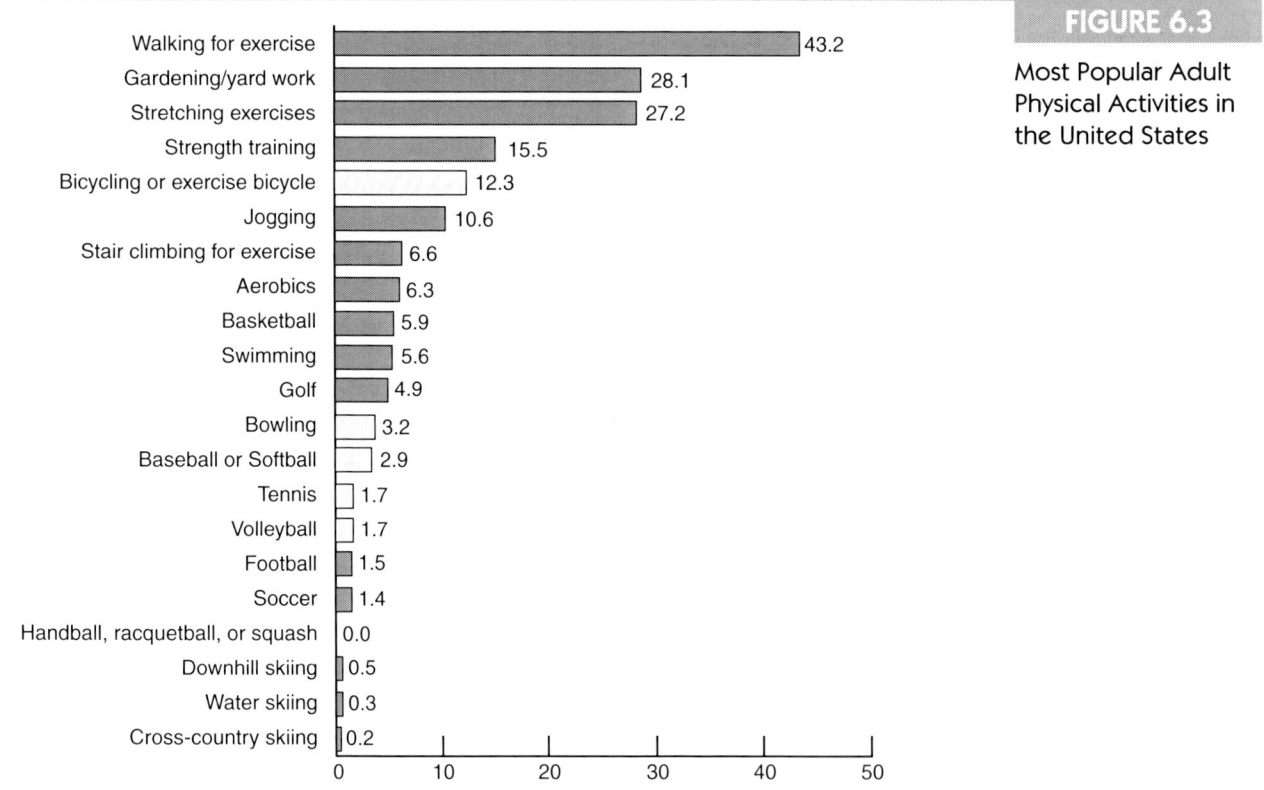

FIGURE 6.3

Most Popular Adult Physical Activities in the United States

Note: Data are weighted to the U.S. population and age-adjusted to the year 2000 population standard. "Participation" in activity reported as being done at least once during the past two weeks.

Source: Centers for Disease Control and Prevention, National Health Interview Survey (NHIS), 1998, Atlanta.

Body Image

The media, advertising, and the fashion industry portray women, as well as men, as thin (or fit), beautiful, and youthful. This is an ideal that is difficult to attain and nearly impossible to maintain. It is important to note that glamorous magazine cover models' pictures are airbrushed with imperfections deleted, so that the final product is an almost perfect unachievable image. It wasn't too long ago that the ideal for a woman's body was "fat is where it's at" instead of the current preoccupation with "thin is in." Many of the great masters' paintings portray the female image as having desirable traits such as soft, round, and fleshy bodies. The 50's had curvy movie stars such as Marilyn Monroe. In the 60's, the Twiggy look was in. In the 70's, it was Farrah Fawcett Fit. In the 80's, it was the fit look with Cindy Crawford. In the 90's, Kate Moss exemplified the gaunt heroin look. As Americans grow in size, the current unobtainable look is very thin. The Body Mass Index of Playboy models and Miss America contestants lowered significantly from the 1970's to the 1990's. Even wealthy celebrities who can afford personal chefs, trainers, registered dieticians, and top consultants sometimes battle with their weight.

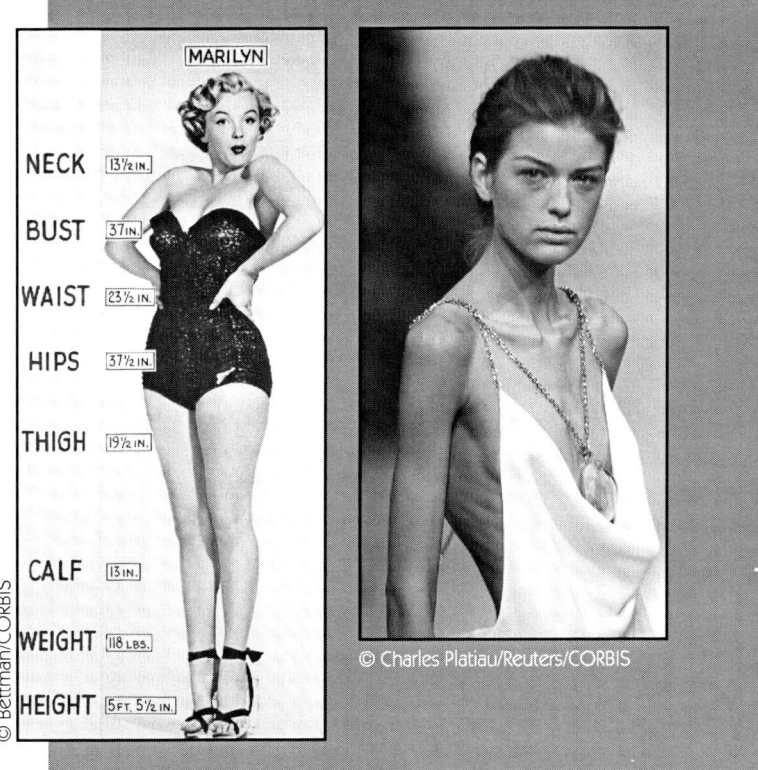

Body image is affected by a person's attitudes and beliefs, as well as outside influences such as family, social pressures, and the media.

A person's body image is how a person sees him or herself in his or her mind. Body image is affected by a person's attitudes and beliefs, as well as by outside influences such as family, social pressures, and the media. It is important to have good perspective. If you are a pear, you may gain weight and become a bigger pear, or you may lose weight and become a smaller pear. You cannot become a different shape, nor can you diet down to a thin waif. Accept yourself for who you are; then work on behavior changes to become healthier. The fringe benefit to becoming healthier is that you will most likely fit better in your jeans. You will also feel better while you reduce your risk of heart disease and diabetes.

It's All about Balance and Portion Size!

- One small chocolate chip cookie is equivalent to walking briskly for ten minutes.
- The difference between a large gourmet chocolate chip cookie and a small chocolate chip cookie could be about forty minutes of raking leaves (200 calories).
- One hour of walking at a moderate pace (twenty min/mile) uses about the same amount of energy that is in one jelly-filled doughnut (300 calories).
- A fast-food "meal" containing a double-patty cheeseburger, extra-large fries, and a twenty-four-ounce soft drink is equal to running two and one-half hours at a ten min/mile pace (1,500 calories).

(Surgeon General, 2005)

What Is a Healthy Body Weight?

There is no single ideal body weight; rather there is a range of healthy body weights that are acceptable for a certain height. Activity level, age, eating patterns, body composition, pregnancy or lactation, and gender, as well as genetic predisposition, can determine weight. You may find that your body seems to change, but it hovers around the same weight. The **set-point theory** postulates that the body regulates metabolism in order to maintain a certain weight, much the same as a thermostat regulates temperature. If fat stores fall below the "set" point, then the body responds by increasing appetite. If we overeat, then appetite may be reduced or all of the calories available may not be stored. Set-point gradually creeps up with poor health habits. Lowering your set-point takes patience and regular physical activity.

Body Mass Index or **BMI** is a simple way to determine if your body weight falls within a healthy range. Because BMI is a ratio between weight and height, there are certain populations that cannot use this parameter as a gauge of body composition. Persons with a large amount of muscle mass will have a higher BMI. Athletes, body builders, pregnant or lactating women, young children, or sedentary older populations should not use BMI as a reliable measure for health risk. Even so, BMI is considered superior to traditional height-weight charts. See Table 6.1 to determine your BMI.

Table 6.1
Body Mass Index Table

To use the table, find the appropriate height in the left-hand column labeled Height. Move across to a given weight (in pounds). The number at the top of the column is the BMI at that height and weight. Pounds have been rounded off.

BMI	19	20	21	22	23	24	25	26	27	28	29	30	31	32	33	34	35
Height (inches)								Body Weight (pounds)									
58	91	96	100	105	110	115	119	124	129	134	138	143	148	153	158	162	167
59	94	99	104	109	114	119	124	128	133	138	143	148	153	158	163	168	173
60	97	102	107	112	118	123	128	133	138	143	148	153	158	163	168	174	179
61	100	106	111	116	122	127	132	137	143	148	153	158	164	169	174	180	185
62	104	109	115	120	126	131	136	142	147	153	158	164	169	175	180	186	191
63	107	113	118	124	130	135	141	146	152	158	163	169	175	180	186	191	197
64	110	116	122	128	134	140	145	151	157	163	169	174	180	186	192	197	204
65	114	120	126	132	138	144	150	156	162	168	174	180	186	192	198	204	210
66	118	124	130	136	142	148	155	161	167	173	179	186	192	198	204	210	216
67	121	127	134	140	146	153	159	166	172	178	185	191	198	204	211	217	223
68	125	131	138	144	151	158	164	171	177	184	190	197	203	210	216	223	230
69	128	135	142	149	155	162	169	176	182	189	196	203	209	216	223	230	236
70	132	139	146	153	160	167	174	181	188	195	202	209	216	222	229	236	243
71	136	143	150	157	165	172	179	186	193	200	208	215	222	229	236	243	250
72	140	147	154	162	169	177	184	191	199	206	213	221	228	235	242	250	258
73	144	151	159	166	174	182	189	197	204	212	219	227	235	242	250	257	265
74	148	155	163	171	179	186	194	202	210	218	225	233	241	249	256	264	272
75	152	160	168	176	184	192	200	208	216	224	232	240	248	256	264	272	279
76	156	164	172	180	189	197	205	213	221	230	238	246	254	263	271	279	287

Source: www.nhlbi.gov

A BMI over 25 is considered overweight and a BMI over 30 is considered obese. A higher BMI may indicate you are at an elevated risk for heart disease, Type 2 diabetes, and most of the conditions related to obesity. Underweight is a BMI of 18.5 or below. It is interesting to note that on the catwalks of New York and Paris, models now have to weigh in and are unable to participate if they are below a BMI of 18. It is encouraging that the fashion world is participating in increasing awareness regarding the dangers of being too thin.

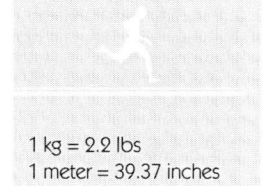

1 kg = 2.2 lbs
1 meter = 39.37 inches

$$BMI = \frac{\text{weight in kilograms}}{\text{height in meters squared}}$$

Body composition is one of the five health-related fitness components discussed in Chapter 3. A person's body composition is a measure of health, estimating the amount of fat mass relative to the lean body mass. Lean body mass is comprised of muscle, bone, and internal organs. Body composition is a more accurate indicator of overall fitness than using a person's body weight.

The ideal range for college-aged females is 18–23 percent body fat and 12–18 percent body fat for college-aged men. Essential fat is that fat which is necessary for normal physiological functioning. If a female gets below 11–13 percent of essential body fat, she typically experiences hormonal disturbances and may have menstruation cessation. Essential fat for men is around 3 percent body fat.

There are numerous different methods to determine an estimate of percent body fat. Skinfold calipers are commonly used in schools. At health fairs, bioelectrical impedence is a simple and inexpensive test to administer. The accuracy of this method is highly questionable due to variations in hydration levels in people throughout the day. The air displacement method uses pressure sensors inside an airtight chamber to measure the amount of air displaced by the person inside the chamber. This is a bulky and expensive container. Hydrostatic weighing is popular with laboratories and athletic centers. The clinicians determine how much a person weighs under water. Dual energy X-ray absorptiometry (DEXA) is the preferred method in research facilities. Each method has pros and cons. If measuring a percentage of body fat in a pre- and post-comparison, it is important to replicate the same environment and to use the same technique in the post-test that was used for the pre-test.

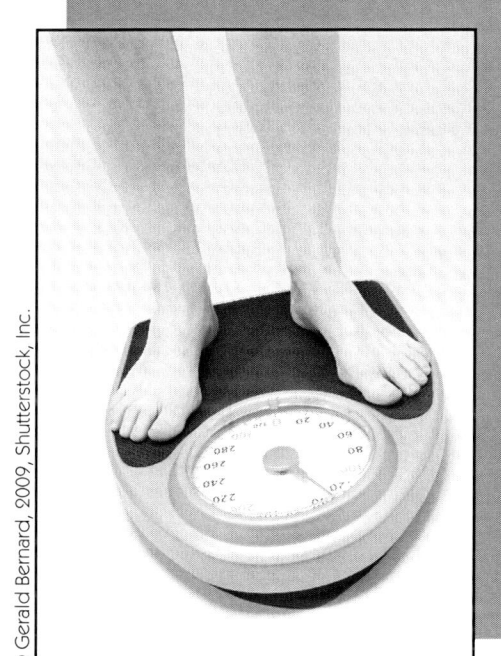

Body composition is a more accurate indicator of overall fitness than is a person's body weight.

Determining Caloric Needs

Caloric needs are different for every individual. To a large degree, each person's need is determined by their current body weight and by the level of physical activity they choose to engage in. See Table 6.2 to determine your own daily caloric needs. Notice the different caloric requirement for active individuals compared to sedentary individuals.

Table 6.2

Estimated Calorie Requirements (in Kilocalories) for Each Gender and Age Group at Three Levels of Physical Activity[a]

Estimated amounts of calories needed to maintain energy balance for various gender and age groups at three different levels of physical activity. The estimates are rounded up to the nearest 200 calories and were determined using the Institute of Medicine equation.

Gender	Age (years)	Activity Level[b,c,d]		
		Sedentary[b]	Moderately Active[c]	Active[d]
Child	2–3	1,000	1,000–1,400[e]	1,000–1,400[e]
Female	4–8	1,200	1,400–1,600	1,400–1,800
	9–13	1,600	1,600–2,000	1,800–2,200
	14–18	1,800	2,000	2,400
	19–30	2,000	2,000–2,200	2,400
	31–50	1,800	2,000	2,200
	51+	1,600	1,800	2,000–2,200
Male	4–8	1,400	1,400–1,600	1,600–2,000
	9–13	1,800	1,800–2,200	2,000–2,600
	14–18	2,200	2,400–2,800	2,800–3,200
	19–30	2,400	2,600–2,800	3,000
	31–50	2,200	2,400–2,600	2,800–3,000
	51+	2,000	2,200–2,400	2,400–2,800

[a]These levels are based on Estimated Energy Requirements (EER) from the Institute of Medicine Dietary References Intakes macronutrients report, 2002, calculated by gender, age, and activity level for reference-sized individuals. "Reference-size," as determined by IOM, is based on median height and weight for ages up to age 18 years of age and median height and weight for that height to give a BMI of 21.5 for adult females and 22.5 for adult males.

[b]Sedentary means a lifestyle that includes only the light physical activity associated with typical day-to-day life.

[c]Moderately active means a lifestyle that includes physical activity equivalent to walking about 1.5 to 3 miles per day at 3 to 4 miles per hour, in addition to the light physical activity associated with typical day-to-day life.

[d]Active means a lifestyle that includes physical activity equivalent to walking more than 3 miles per day at 3 to 4 miles per hour, in addition to the light physical activity associated with typical day-to-day life.

[e]The calorie ranges shown are to accommodate needs of different ages within the group. For children and adolescents, more calories are needed at older ages. For adults, fewer calories are needed at older ages.

Source: USDA.

Obesity

Overweight is defined as an excess of body weight to some height standard, or a BMI between 25 and 30. **Obesity** is a term that refers to excess fat with an accompanying loss of function and an increase in health problems (see Figure 6.4), or a BMI of 30 or more. **Creeping obesity** is a gradual increase of percent body fat as activity decreases with age. This typically results in a one-half to one pound fat gain per year, with an approximate simultaneous loss of one-half pound of fat-free mass or muscle. Consider that if you overeat just 100 calories per day, you will gain one pound in a month. An extra ten pounds can sneak up on you in one year.

Obesity Prevention

Activity is the optimal way to manage current weight or successfully lose weight. The key is to exercise, maintain a healthy diet throughout your life, and avoid gaining excess weight. Participate in planned exercise as well as increased lifestyle activity.

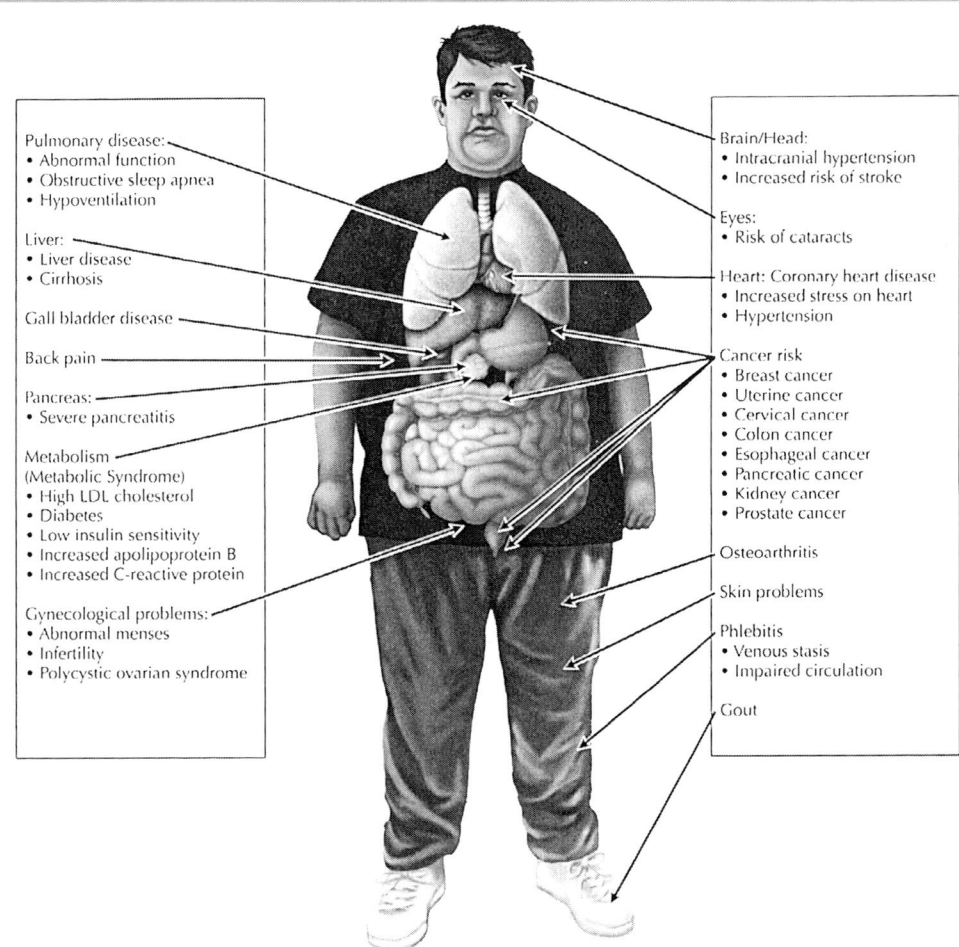

FIGURE 6.4

Medical Cost Associated with Obesity $100 Billion

Source: From *Concepts of Physical Fitness* 15th edition, by Charles Corbin et al. Copyright © 2009 by McGraw-Hill Companies. Reprinted by permission of The McGraw-Hill Companies, Inc.

Establish support systems to help you with exercise adherence and healthy lifestyle habits.

How Does Activity Help Obesity?

There is only a 2 to 3 percent success rate for people who lose weight to actually maintain weight loss (Texas A&M University Human Nutrition Conference, 1998). Those who are successful are usually committed to a regular exercise routine. Exercise greatly increases the likelihood of success with a maintenance program after weight loss. Weight gain occurs with inactivity; activity is the best way to reduce the size of fat stores. Even a small weight loss, 10 percent of your weight, helps boost the basal metabolic rate, which is often suppressed when a person diets without exercise. Activity, specifically weight training, has been shown to increase a person's confidence and self-esteem, regardless of actual weight loss.

How Do I Lose Weight?

The bottom line is that in order to lose weight, the calories you take in must be less than the calories that you expend. Once you have determined what your daily caloric needs are, then estimate how many calories you are actually eating on a regular basis. The recommended weight loss is one-half to one pound per week. Losing weight faster often signifies a short-term fix, indicating that the weight loss

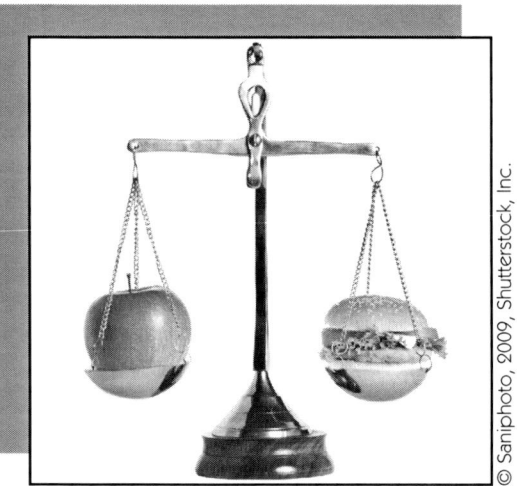

The bottom line is that in order to lose weight, the calories you take in must be less than the calories you expend.

will be difficult to maintain. Fast weight loss is often followed by fast weight gain. This is called yo-yo dieting, and often the weight gain is a bit more than what was initially lost. Repeated bouts of weight loss/gain like this can gradually add unwanted excess weight. Studies have shown that yo-yo dieting through the years can make it more difficult to lose weight in the future. This also adds stress to your cardiovascular system because the workload on your heart constantly fluctuates.

In order to change your lifestyle habits to lose weight, you must change your behaviors. Determine what behaviors and everyday patterns seem to sabotage your efforts. Is it the donut cart mid-morning at the office? Is it going through the drive-through at 2 a.m. after going out with friends? Anticipate these challenges and plan ahead. Use the behavior change activity at the end of Chapter 1 in order to focus on your goal. Most likely your goal will include examining your current diet. Use your results from the diet analysis activity at the end of Chapter 5 (Nutrition). In order to lose a pound, there needs to be an approximate 3,500 caloric deficit. Eating 500 calories less per day over the week may cause that to occur, or expending an extra 500 calories per day may cause that to occur. The best option is to include both. Exercise is the key to losing weight, and is also the key to maintaining weight loss. The importance of movement illustrates how critical it is to find an activity that you enjoy so that you can embrace it for the rest of your life. Walking is the most popular activity in the United States (refer back to Figure 6.3). See Table 6.3 to determine a reasonable schedule for you to lose weight with a walking and caloric restriction program.

If you eat less food than you regularly eat as you might on a calorie restricted diet, the body's natural tendency is to slow the basal metabolic rate up to 30 percent. Exercise does the opposite—it will increase your metabolism. Staying active when trying to lose weight is critical because it burns calories, increases metabolism, and preserves muscle (see Table 6.4). Fad diets accompanied by no exercise often result in weight lost with an actual increase in percent body fat due to the loss of lean body mass. See the example below of Sally and the school dance to see the effects of fad diets versus a change in lifestyle.

Sally was invited to the annual spring dance with her sweetheart. She wanted desperately to lose the "freshman 15"—the extra pounds she had put on in the previous year in order to fit into her favorite little black dress.

Table 6.3

Countdown to Weight Loss

The combination of walking and cutting calories results in greater weight loss than either alone.

If you walk (minutes)	&	If you cut daily calories by	Days to Lose Weight				
			5 lb.	10 lb.	15 lb.	20 lb.	25 lb.
30		400	27	54	81	108	135
30		800	16	32	48	64	80
45		400	23	46	69	92	115
45		800	14	28	42	56	70
60		400	21	42	63	84	105
60		800	13	26	39	54	65

Source: cdc.gov

Table 6.4

How Much Physical Activity Do I Need?

It really depends on what your health goals are. Here are some guidelines to follow:

Goal	Physical Activity Level for Adults
Reduce the risk of chronic disease	At least 30 minutes of a moderate intensity physical activity, **above usual activity**, most days of the week.
Manage body weight and prevent gradual unhealthy body weight gain	Approximately 60 minutes of moderate intensity physical activity most days of the week while not exceeding calorie needs.
Maintain weight loss	At least 60 to 90 minutes of moderate intensity physical activity most days of the week while not exceeding calorie needs. Some people may need to talk to their healthcare provider before participating in this level of physical activity.

Source: cdc.gov

Option 1: Sally has two weeks before the event. She decides to crash diet. Sally drinks water and two ounces of fruit juice a day. She succeeds in losing thirteen pounds of water, fat, and muscle weight. Along the way, Sally is hungry, which leads to headaches and severe moodiness. She has little energy and sleeps through class. At the dance, Sally fits into her dress, but she is extremely fatigued. Because severe dieting can also cause an individual's blood pressure to plummet, resulting in dizziness, light-headedness, and fatigue, Sally has no energy. After the dance, Sally engages in some binge-eating behaviors. In several days' time, she gains back all the weight she lost. Unfortunately she does not gain back the muscle she lost, so her body fat increases.

Option 2: Sally can think now of next year's dance. She begins a program of walk-jogging for thirty minutes five days a week. With each workout, she burns approximately 150–200 calories. Those 150 calories burned five days a week equals 750 calories each week. It will take Sally about a month to lose one pound if she does not limit her eating. If she sticks to this rather conservative program, Sally will have lost about twelve pounds in a year's time. Not only will Sally fit into her dress, but she will have established a habit and she has positively changed her lifestyle, her attitude, her body composition, her measurements, her lean body mass, and she has:

- increased her muscular endurance
- increased her cardiovascular endurance
- reduced her risk of mental anxiety and depression
- improved her sleep patterns
- dealt with her stress in a positive manner
- increased her cognitive abilities
- reduced her risk of dying prematurely
- reduced her risk of heart disease, diabetes, high blood pressure
- reduced the risk of some cancers
- helped reduce risk of osteoporosis
- most likely decreased her mile time

Top Ten Reasons to Give Up Dieting

10. DIETS DON'T WORK. Even if you lose weight, you will probably gain it all back, and you might gain back more than you lost.

9. DIETS ARE EXPENSIVE. If you didn't buy special diet products, you could save enough to get new clothes, which would improve your outlook right now.

8. DIETS ARE BORING. People on diets talk and think about food and practically nothing else. There's a lot more to life.

7. DIETS DON'T NECESSARILY IMPROVE YOUR HEALTH. Like the weight loss, health improvement is temporary. Dieting can actually cause health problems.

6. DIETS DON'T MAKE YOU BEAUTIFUL. Very few people will ever look like models. Glamour is a look, not a size. You don't have to be thin to be attractive.

5. DIETS ARE NOT SEXY. If you want to be more attractive, take care of your body and your appearance. Feeling healthy makes you look your best.

4. DIETS CAN TURN INTO EATING DISORDERS. The obsession to be thin can lead to anorexia, bulimia, bingeing, and compulsive exercising.

3. DIETS CAN MAKE YOU AFRAID OF FOOD. Food nourishes and comforts us, and gives us pleasure. Dieting can make food seem like your enemy, and can deprive you of all the positive things about food.

2. DIETS CAN ROB YOU OF ENERGY. If you want to lead a full and active life, you need good nutrition, and enough food to meet your body's needs.

And the number one reason to give up dieting:

1. Learning to love and accept yourself just as you are will give you self-confidence, better health, and a sense of well-being that will last a lifetime.

Source: From Council on Size & Weight Discrimination with permission. www.cswd.org

Dieting or cutting back on calories is considered "severe" when an individual ingests fewer than 800 calories in a day. It is impossible to get all the nutrients you need with less than 1,000–1,200 calories daily. Physiological and psychological problems can result from chronic caloric restriction. Much of the weight lost with severe caloric restriction is in the form of muscle. Cardiac muscle can be weakened to the point that it is no longer able to pump blood through the body—resulting in death. See complications of eating disorders in Chapter 2.

Weight Loss Guidelines

If you would like to lose weight in a positive manner as Sally did in option #2, follow the guidelines set by the American College of Sports Medicine (see the box on page 205).

Dietary Supplements

Eating a healthy diet with fruits, vegetables, whole grains, quality proteins, and unsaturated fats, as well as restricting refined white flour and sugar, is the best method for obtaining an adequate supply of nutrients in your diet. Dietary supplements are popular and provide a means for delivering these nutrients in a more

Guidelines for a Successful Weight Loss Program

The American College of Sports Medicine has put together the following eleven guidelines in an effort to help individuals recognize potentially successful weight loss programs and avoid unsound or dangerous weight loss programs.

1. Prolonged fasting and diet programs that severely restrict caloric intake are scientifically unsound and can be medically dangerous.
2. Fasting and diet programs that severely restrict caloric intake result in the loss of large amounts of water, electrolytes, minerals, glycogen stores, and other fat-free tissues, but with minimal amounts of fat loss.
3. Mild caloric restriction (500–1,000 calories less than usual per day) results in smaller loss of water, electrolytes, minerals, and other fat-free tissues and is less likely to result in malnutrition.
4. Dynamic exercise of large muscle groups helps to maintain fat-free tissue, including lean muscle mass and bone density, and can result in a loss of body weight (primarily body fat).
5. A nutritionally sound diet resulting in mild caloric intake restrictions, coupled with an endurance exercise program, along with behavior modification of existing eating habits, is recommended for weight reduction. The rate of weight loss should never exceed two pounds per week.
6. To maintain proper weight control and optimal body fat levels, a lifetime commitment to proper eating habits and regular physical activity is required.
7. A successful weight loss plan can be followed anywhere—at home, work, restaurants, parties, and so on.
8. For a plan to be successful, the emphasis must be on portion size.
9. Successful weight loss plans incorporate a wide variety of nutritious foods that are easily accessible in the supermarket.
10. A weight loss plan must not be too costly if it is to be successful.
11. The most essential aspect of a weight loss program is that it can be followed for the rest of an individual's life.

convenient, but often less effective, form. It is a good idea to check with a health professional before beginning supplementtion. Taken in concentrations higher than the recommended daily allowance, some nutrients have undesirable side effects, and some are even toxic.

Unfortunately some individuals think that if one pill is good, two or more must be better. In most cases this is simply not true. Sometimes, an excess of nutrients can be detrimental as is the case with fat-soluble vitamins A, D, E and K. Megadoses of many vitamins, minerals, and other supplements can cause kidney and liver damage and interact adversely with other supplements, herbs, and drugs. It is possible to interfere with absorption of other nutrients when ingesting megadoses of some supplements. In general, consuming more than the RDA of vitamins and minerals is discouraged. A registered dietician or physician may prescribe supplements for some populations or certain medical conditions (for instance, people who are pregnant, have anemia, are elderly, or are certain types of vegetarians).

Weight Loss Products

Appetite suppressants claim to help diminish a person's appetite, cut cravings, and increase overall energy and possibly increase metabolism. Over time this may result in weight loss, but consider the negative side effects. Appetite suppressants often contain

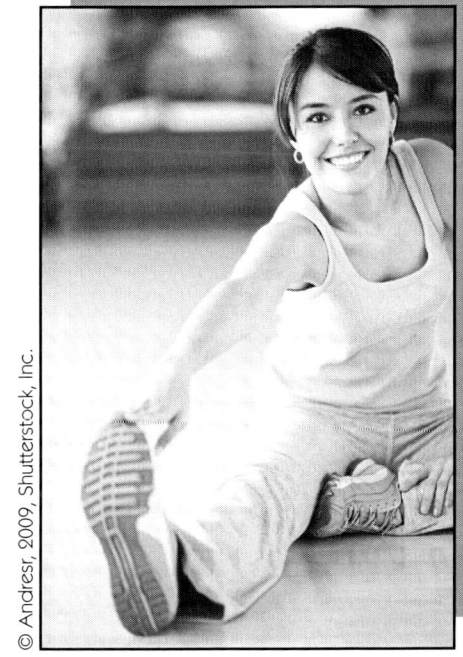

The most essential aspect of a weight loss program is that it can be followed for the rest of an individual's life.

high levels of caffeine, guarana, or Ma Huang (an herbal form of ephedra) that can cause hypertension, cardiac arrhythmia, myocardial infarction, and/or stroke that can and has led to premature death of the person consuming this type of dietary supplement. Examples of commonly used supplements include Hydroxycut, Xenadrine-EFX, and Trim Spa.

In 1997, fenfluramine and dexfenfluramine (fen/phen) were withdrawn from the market due to a link to the development of a heart valve problem. Serious illness and, in some cases, death occurred. Even FDA-approved drugs need to be used cautiously. In the 1960's and the 1970's amphetamines were often prescribed for weight loss, and in the 1920's weight loss pills were found to contain tapeworm eggs (Hales, 2007). Diet aids and supplements that have gone through rigorous testing and been approved by the FDA still need to be approached with common sense and caution.

Metabolism boosters are various supplements that speed up or boost an individual's basal metabolism. Most of these types of products claim to act in a way that increases the building of lean muscle mass. Examples of such supplements are creatine phosphate, chromium picolinate, and HMB. Megathin, Microlean, and Metabolife (now banned by the FDA) have appetite suppressants as well as metabolism boosters. Long-term effectiveness and safety of these types of supplements are unknown.

There are two types of weight loss programs, clinical and nonclinical. A clinical program is typically offered in a healthcare facility with a team of licensed health professionals. The following are examples of nonclinical programs: Jenny Craig, Nutrasystem, Weight Watchers, and Slimfast. Jenny Craig and Nutrasystem sell prepackaged foods which are convenient, but typically are higher in cost. Weight Watchers teaches participants the value of foods on a point system. The positive aspect of Weight Watchers is that participants are taught how to choose, shop, and prepare foods. Group support is essential and highly recommended after the goal weight is attained. Weight loss maintenance is one of the most difficult aspects of dieting, so support from others is often a significant help. Two other programs that offer group support are TOPS (Take Off Pounds Sensibly) and Overeaters Anonymous (OA). Programs such as Slimfast replace one or two meals with shakes or bars. Unless a person learns to make wise choices on their own, it is doubtful that weight loss will be maintained.

Low-carbohydrate high-protein diets are popular. The Zone, Atkins, Sugar-Busters, Protein Power, and the South Beach Diet are all examples of this type of diet. Although there are some variation in the diets, all advocate severely limiting carbohydrate foods such as pasta, potatoes, bread, cereals, juices, sweets, and even fruits and vegetables. Protein-rich foods are plentiful. Steak, ham, bacon, eggs, fish, chicken, and cheese are allowed to be eaten in unlimited quantities for some diets.

The basis for the low-carbohydrate diet is that during digestion, carbohydrates are converted into glucose, which serves as fuel for every cell in a person's body. When blood glucose levels begin to rise, insulin, the hormone that allows the entry of glucose into the cells, is released. This process lowers the level of glucose in the bloodstream. If the available glucose is not rapidly used for normal cellular functions or physical activity, the glucose is converted to and stored as body fat. Individuals who support this type of diet believe that if a person eats fewer carbohydrates and more protein, they will produce less insulin, and as insulin levels drop, the body will look to its own fat stores to meet energy needs.

While research has shown that people participating in low-carbohydrate high-protein diets do initially loose weight more rapidly than an individual who maintains a more nutritionally balanced diet but decreases calorie intake and increases physical activity, these same studies show that at the one-year mark weight loss for many of the dieters in both groups was not significantly different. Low carbohydrate diets also have the potential to result in the loss of B vitamins, calcium, and potassium. This can lead to osteoporosis, constipation, bad breath, and fatigue. Before starting on this type of diet, consider that because the diet is high in protein, and therefore high in fat, it may carry an increased risk for heart disease.

Fad diets

Fad diets are risky because they...

- tend to be very low in calories
- are limited to a few foods, limiting key nutrients and minerals
- produce only short-term, rapid weight loss—not long-term weight management
- ignore the importance of physical activity in healthy weight loss
- increase risks for certain diseases or health complications
- take the pleasure and fun out of eating
- alter metabolism, making it easier to regain the weight after the diet has ceased

Diets That Don't Work

1. **"Magical"/Same Foods Diets** (i.e., grapefruit, cabbage soup, Subway diet)
   - *Pros*—usually the single food is a nutritious food
   - *Cons*—too few calories, risk of overeating, lacking of specific nutrients, lack variety, do not teach healthy eating habits, do not encourage exercise

2. **High-Protein Diets** (i.e., Atkins)
   - *Pros*—weight loss does occur
   - *Cons*—high in saturated fat and cholesterol increasing risk for heart disease; high protein puts strain on liver and kidneys; lacks vitamins, minerals, complex carbohydrates, and fiber; weight loss is water weight, not fat; lack of carbs causes a condition called ketosis with symptoms of nausea, weakness, and dehydration

3. **Liquid Diets** (i.e., Slimfast)
   - *Pros*—drinks have vitamins, minerals, and high-quality protein
   - *Cons*—do not teach new ways of eating, no long-term weight loss, very low in calories

4. **Gimmicks, Gadgets, and Other "Miracles"**
   - *Pros*—none
   - *Cons*—may be harmful, expensive, do not teach healthy eating, do not encourage exercise

Effective Weight Loss Questionnaire

1. *Could you follow the diet for the rest of your life?* Good health and permanent weight loss require a lifestyle change, not just a temporary modification.

2. *Does the diet promise quick results?* If so, you're probably losing water and lean muscle tissue. Weight loss of one-half to two pounds a week is safe and will more likely be kept off.

3. *Does the diet accommodate your lifestyle?* Any diet that does not allow much freedom or flexibility is less likely to be followed permanently.

4. *Is the diet very low in calories?* Any diet that is below 1,200 calories per day could be dangerous. You may not be getting enough energy and nutrients. You may feel deprived and frustrated, both physically and mentally. In the long run, metabolism slows in order to conserve energy with very low calorie diets.

5. *Does the diet eliminate or restrict certain food groups?* Many diets leave out one or more food groups. Restricting a type of food may result in elimination of essential nutrients in the diet causing health risks. A balanced diet modeled after the Food Guide Pyramid and including a variety of foods should be followed.

6. *Does the diet call for unusual items or require you to go to a specialty store?* Unusual foods or supplements may be very costly and hard to obtain. They may also contain dangerous ingredients that are not regulated by the Food and Drug Administration.

7. *Will someone make money on the diet?* If yes, BEWARE! The diet could be a quick way for someone to make a lot of money.

8. *Is the author or supplier reputable?* To check for validity and credibility of a book, diet, or supplement, view the list of references provided and check the credentials of the author.

Fad Diets

Each year billions of dollars are spent in the weight loss industry. Unfortunately, many of these dollars are spent on diet plans that are unhealthy, cannot be maintained long term, or simply do not work. The lure of a quick and easy way to "melt away" the pounds is too tempting for many individuals, and although the diets are more times than not ineffective in the long term, weight loss hopefuls are willing to give almost anything a chance. To avoid the pitfalls of an unsuccessful, unreliable, or even dangerous weight loss plan, one should always take the time to check out as much factual information as possible from a variety of sources (see Figures 6.5a and 6.5b). The boxed information on page 207 is a list of some fad diets that are currently popular and the theories and possible shortcomings within these diets.

FIGURE 6.5a

Guide to the Ratings

Overall score is based on adherence to nutritional guideline and the results of expert evaluations of each diet book. Expert evaluation ratings are derived from results of panel survey on the books' nutritional and scientific information, exercise recommendations, ease of use, menus, and meal plans. **Nutrition analysis** was based on a week of menus from each book, using The Food Processor software

RATINGS

Diet books
what the experts say

These seven diet books have never been put to the acid test of a large clinical trial (unlike the diets that we rate on page 16). We rated them based on an expert-panel questionnaire and our own analysis of nutritional quality.

Books are listed in rank order of overall score. Scores of "Eat, Drink, & Weigh Less," "You on a Diet," and "The Abs Diet" were very close to one another.

All the books offered fairly healthful menus. But when our panelists evaluated the nutrition advice, they found noticeable differences in the restrictiveness of various books. They also found variations in the quality of exercise information and the explanations of the science and nutrition behind the plans.

Our nutritional analysis is based on the 2005 U.S. Dietary Guidelines for Americans. The guidelines are updated every five years and represent a broad scientific consensus.

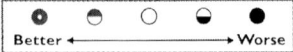
Better ← → Worse

THE BEST LIFE DIET
Bob Greene (Simon & Schuster), $26
What it is The diet's first phase involves exercise and a recommended eating schedule. Calorie reduction starts in phase two. You eat enough healthful foods to satisfy hunger but no more. Includes tools to customize diet and exercise plans.
Pros and cons Reviewers liked personalized advice and section on exercise. Extensive discussion of "emotional eating" might help some. Dieters might be discouraged when they don't lose weight in phase one. Straightforward recipes use common ingredients.

Rating
Overall score .... ◐
Expert evaluation .... ◐
  Science .... ◐
  Nutrition .... ◐
  Exercise .... ◐
  Ease of use .... ◐
  Meal plans .... ◐
Nutrition analysis .... ●
Percent of calories
  Fat 30
  Saturated fat 6
  Carbohydrates 47
  Protein 23
Fiber, g/1,000 cal. 22
Fruits & veg., daily serv. 8
Average daily calories 1,520

EAT, DRINK, & WEIGH LESS
Mollie Katzen and Walter Willett, M.D. (Hyperion), $14.95
What it is Harvard nutrition researcher Walter Willett teamed up with cookbook author Mollie Katzen for this book based on the Mediterranean diet. Premise is that by "mindfully" following this diet, you can lose weight while enjoying eating. Little full-fat dairy or red meat. Up to one egg and one glass of wine a day.
Pros and cons Sample diet had 1,910 calories per day—too many to allow most people to lose weight. Reviewers liked book's scientific accuracy but thought the exercise chapter too brief.

Rating
Overall score .... ◐
Expert evaluation .... ◐
  Science .... ◐
  Nutrition .... ◐
  Exercise .... ○
  Ease of use .... ◐
  Meal plans .... ◐
Nutrition analysis .... ●
Percent of calories
  Fat 39
  Saturated fat 8
  Carbohydrates 45
  Protein 17
Fiber, g/1,000 cal. 19
Fruits & veg., daily serv. 16
Average daily calories 1,910

YOU ON A DIET
Michael F. Roizen, M.D., and Mehmet C. Oz, M.D. (Simon & Schuster), $25
What it is The physician-authors devote more than half the book to background on appetite, metabolism, and behavior. Diet starts with a two-week "rebooting program." Monotonous breakfasts and lunches cut down cravings. Sugar, saturated fat, and refined flour products are banned.
Pros and cons Most reviewers thought the diet lacked detail and was too restrictive, and some were skeptical that habits can change for good in two weeks. Most recipes were very simple.

Rating
Overall score .... ◐
Expert evaluation .... ○
  Science .... ◐
  Nutrition .... ◐
  Exercise .... ◐
  Ease of use .... ○
  Meal plans .... ○
Nutrition analysis .... ●
Percent of calories
  Fat 33
  Saturated fat 6
  Carbohydrates 48
  Protein 19
Fiber, g/1,000 cal. 18
Fruits & veg., daily serv. 13
Average daily calories 1,520

Source: Copyright © 2007 by Consumer Union of U.S., Inc. Yonkers, NY 10703-1057, a nonprofit organization. Reprinted with permission from the June 2007 issue of *Consumer Reports®* for educational purposes only. No commercial use or reproduction permitted. www.ConsumerReports.org

Healthy Habits

Healthy Weight Gain

Although they are in the minority, many people struggle to gain weight. It is important for individuals who feel that they are "too thin" to recognize that there are healthy and unhealthy ways of accomplishing their goal of weight gain. Overeating all types of foods will simply result in an increase in body fat.

Adding lean body mass through strength training and a slight caloric increase is a much healthier alternative. Chapter 3 outlines the benefits of muscular fitness, as well as presents helpful guidelines for beginning a strength training regimen. Nutrition information on page 177 of Chapter 5 identifies ways to add calories in an appropriate portion and manner to maximize their benefits.

from ESHA Research. For diets that had a short introductory phase and a longer weight-loss phase, we evaluated the latter. Higher scores went to menus that conformed most closely to the recommendations of the 2005 U.S. Dietary Guidelines for Americans: 20 to 35 percent of calories from fat, with less than 10 percent from saturated fat; 45 to 65 percent from carbohydrates; 10 to 35 percent from protein; more than 14 grams of fiber per 1,000 calories. **Average daily calories** and servings of fruits and vegetables are listed in the Ratings for information only and are not part of the overall nutrition score. Guidelines call for 6 to 9 servings in a 1,400 to 1,900 calorie diet.

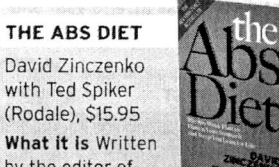

THE ABS DIET
David Zinczenko with Ted Spiker (Rodale), $15.95
What it is Written by the editor of Men's Health magazine, the diet promises "a six-pack in 6 weeks" by eating six meals a day featuring "power 12" foods. Includes about 100 pages of illustrated exercises.
Pros and cons Reviewers were skeptical of the promise of rapid weight loss and disliked emphasis on whey supplements. Fitness program deemed easy to follow but possibly too strenuous for beginners and more appealing to men.

Rating
Overall score ....◐
Expert evaluation ....○
  Science..................................○
  Nutrition...............................○
  Exercise................................◐
  Ease of use...........................○
  Meal plans............................○
Nutrition analysis ....●
Percent of calories
  Fat..27
  Saturated fat 7
  Carbohydrates 49
  Protein..................................24
Fiber, g/1,000 cal. 20
Fruits & veg., daily serv. 7
Average daily calories.......1,890

THE SOUTH BEACH DIET
Arthur Agatston, M.D. (Rodale), $24.95
What it is Slightly more permissive version of the Atkins diet is based on the premise that eating low-glycemic foods decreases cravings for sugar and refined carbs. In the first phase, fruits, sugar, and grains are banned. Phase two allows some fruit, high-fiber grains, and dark chocolate.
Pros and cons Reviewers thought the simplicity of diet would appeal to some but criticized overuse of the glycemic index and the too-short exercise section. Recipes seemed easy to prepare, but some called for unusual ingredients.

Rating
Overall score ....◐
Expert evaluation ....○
  Science..................................○
  Nutrition...............................○
  Exercise................................◐
  Ease of use...........................◐
  Meal plans............................◐
Nutrition analysis ....◐
Percent of calories
  Fat..39
  Saturated fat 9
  Carbohydrates 38
  Protein..................................22
Fiber, g/1,000 cal. 19
Fruits & veg., daily serv. 13
Average daily calories.......1,340

THE SONOMA DIET
Connie Guttersen, R.D., Ph.D. (Meredith), $24.95
What it is An updated lower-carb diet with a Mediterranean theme, its 10-day "wave 1" bans most sweet or refined foods. The longer wave 2, where most weight loss takes place, permits fruits and wine. You calculate portions by filling sectors of small plates with specified food categories.
Pros and cons Reviewers found the overall diet healthful but complex and needlessly restrictive. They felt the book stinted on exercise. Recipes were rather elaborate to prepare.

Rating
Overall score ....◐
Expert evaluation ....○
  Science..................................○
  Nutrition...............................◐
  Exercise................................◐
  Ease of use...........................○
  Meal plans............................○
Nutrition analysis ....◐
Percent of calories
  Fat..36
  Saturated fat 8
  Carbohydrates 39
  Protein..................................24
Fiber, g/1,000 cal. 20
Fruits & veg., daily serv. 10
Average daily calories.......1,390

ULTRA-METABOLISM
Mark Hyman, M.D. (Scribner), $25
What it is The author designed the diet around his theory that people get fat because their systems become toxic, inflamed, stressed, and imbalanced. Initial "detox" phase and longer "rebalancing" phase. Eliminate: white rice, refined grains, grain-fed or processed red meats, caffeinated beverages.
Pros and cons Reviewers felt book's theory goes beyond scientific evidence and was overly restrictive and complicated. Exercise section judged somewhat brief but practical.

Rating
Overall score ....○
Expert evaluation ....◐
  Science..................................◐
  Nutrition...............................○
  Exercise................................◐
  Ease of use...........................◐
  Meal plans............................◐
Nutrition analysis ....◐
Percent of calories
  Fat..41
  Saturated fat 8
  Carbohydrates 41
  Protein..................................18
Fiber, g/1,000 cal. 22
Fruits & veg., daily serv. 12
Average daily calories.......1,660

FIGURE 6.5b

Guide to the Ratings
Overall score is based on adherence to nutritional guideline and the results of published randomised clinical studies (exception noted in footnote) that reported three- to six-month short-term and one-year long-term results and together studied at least 40 subjects per diet. **Study results**, including short- and long-term weight-loss and

RATINGS
Diet plans What the studies say

Better ◐ ◔ ○ ◕ ● Worse

No need to wonder about losing weight on these diets; they've all been tested in clinical trials published in scientific journals. Plans are listed in rank order of overall score. Even the highest-rated diets generally produced less than a 10 percent weight loss after a year and had dropout rates of more than one in five participants. Weight Watchers, Jenny Craig, and Slim-Fast scores were very close together.

VOLUMETRICS
What it is Based on research at Penn State, diet aims to maximize the amount of food available per calorie, mainly by use of reduced-fat products, liberal addition of vegetables, and low-fat cooking techniques. Encourages first course of broth-based soup or low-calorie salad to take the edge off appetite.

Pros and cons Recent clinical trials show best overall weight loss of any diet evaluated. We judged the recipes appetizing but somewhat time-consuming to prepare.

Rating
Overall score ....◔
Study results
  Short-term
    Weight loss ....◔
    Dropout rate ....◔
  1 year
    Weight loss ....◔
    Dropout rate ....○
Nutrition analysis ....◐
Percent of calories
  Fat 23
  Saturated fat 7
  Carbohydrates 55
  Protein 22
Fiber, g/1,000 cal. 20
Fruits & veg., daily serv. 14
Average daily calories 1,500

WEIGHT WATCHERS
What it is Venerable program uses weekly meetings and weigh-ins for motivation and behavioral support for diet and exercise changes, or you can sign up for similar support online. Dieters either earn or spend "points" with food and exercise or consume specified foods with "Core" plan. Vegetarian menu available.

Pros and cons Behavioral support is proven to increase adherence to any diet. Scored average on weight loss in this group but first in long-term adherence. We judged recipes to be appetizing and fairly easy to prepare.

Rating
Overall score ....◔
Study results
  Short-term
    Weight loss ....○
    Dropout rate ....○
  1 year
    Weight loss ....○
    Dropout rate ....○
Nutrition analysis ....◐
Percent of calories
  Fat 24
  Saturated fat 7
  Carbohydrates 56
  Protein 20
Fiber, g/1,000 cal. 20
Fruits & veg., daily serv. 11
Average daily calories 1,450

JENNY CRAIG
What it is Dieters sign up for individual counseling and meal plans at company outlets, by phone, or online. Centerpiece of diet is eating Jenny Craig-prepared foods of single-serving entrées and snacks, supplemented by dairy, salads, and other vegetables you prepare yourself. Vegetarian menu available.

Pros and cons Diet requires minimal food preparation and meets dietary guidelines. Published study of actual client histories revealed high dropout rate, though those who stuck with plan lost considerable weight. Clinical trial had better adherence.

Rating
Overall score ....◔
Study results [1]
  Short-term
    Weight loss ....◔
    Dropout rate ....○
  1 year
    Weight loss ....◔
    Dropout rate ....○
Nutrition analysis ....◐
Percent of calories
  Fat 18
  Saturated fat 7
  Carbohydrates 62
  Protein 20
Fiber, g/1,000 cal. 16
Fruits & veg., daily serv. 6
Average daily calories 1,520

SLIM-FAST
What it is Brand line of controlled-calorie shakes and bars, widely available in drugstores and supermarkets. Company Web site provides weekly menus. On standard meal plan, a bar or shake for breakfast and lunch, with additional food. For dinner, a low-calorie meal you fix yourself.

Pros and cons Menu we analyzed meets dietary guidelines. Convenient for people with little time or inclination to cook. Clinical studies show above-average long-term weight loss but high long-term dropout rate.

Rating
Overall score ....◔
Study results
  Short-term
    Weight loss ....◔
    Dropout rate ....◔
  1 year
    Weight loss ....◔
    Dropout rate ....●
Nutrition analysis ....◐
Percent of calories
  Fat 22
  Saturated fat 6
  Carbohydrates 57
  Protein 21
Fiber, g/1,000 cal. 21
Fruits & veg., daily serv. 12
Average daily calories 1,540

1 One study used was a longitudinal study of all enrollees in Jenny Craig's premium plan for a one-year period, published in the February 2007 International Journal of Obesity.

Healthy Food Shopping

The National Heart, Lung, and Blood Institute Obesity Guidelines (www.nhlbi.nih.gov/health/public/heart/obesity/lose_wt/shop.htm) list the following suggestions to help individuals prepare healthier home cooked meals in shorter periods of time. They recommend reading labels while shopping—paying particular attention to serving sizes and the number of servings in the container. Comparing the total number of calories in similar products and choosing the product containing the lower number of total calories will result in a healthier meal. Finally, make cooking at home easier and healthier by shopping for quick, low-fat food items and filling kitchen cabinets with a supply of lower calorie staples such as:

- fat-free or low-fat milk, yogurt, cheese, and cottage cheese
- light or diet margarine

dropout rates, were derived from published studies of each diet. **Nutrition analysis**, done in 2005, was based on a week of menus from each book or program, using The Food Processor software from ESHA Research. For diets that had a short introductory phase and a longer weight-loss phase, we evaluated the latter. Higher scores went to menus that conformed most closely to the recommendations of the 2005 U.S. Dietary Guidelines for Americans: 20 to 35 percent of calories from fat, with less than 10 percent from saturated fat; 45 to 65 percent from carbohydrates; 10 to 35 percent from protein; more than 14 grams of fiber per 1,000 calories. **Average daily calories** and servings of fruits and vegetables are listed in the Ratings for information only and are not part of the overall nutrition score. Guidelines call for 6 to 9 servings in a 1,400 to 1,900 calorie diet.

eDIETS

What it is Well-established online subscription diet site offers 24 meal plans customized for various eating preferences and desired weight loss. Membership includes access to support groups, experts, menu plans, recipes. The standard eDiets.com weekly menu we analyzed met dietary guidelines and delivered the number of calories promised.

Pros and cons Customizable plans are appealing, especially for those with wheat or lactose intolerances, but clinical studies find average adherence and below-average weight loss.

Rating
Overall score ....◐
Study results
  Short-term
    Weight loss ....◐
    Dropout rate ....○
  1 year
    Weight loss ....◐
    Dropout rate ....○
Nutrition analysis ....●
Percent of calories
  Fat 23
  Saturated fat 5
  Carbohydrates 53
  Protein 24
Fiber, g/1,000 cal. 19
Fruits & veg., daily serv. 12
Average daily calories 1,450

THE ZONE DIET (men's menu)

What it is The "Zone," as conceived by Barry Sears, is a the ideal balance of foods to keep your blood sugar and hormones ready to fight obesity and diseases. To stay in the Zone, every meal must consist of 30% fat calories, 30% protein, and 40% carbs. Diet allows many fruits, practically no grains except oatmeal.

Pros and cons We judged the recipes simple to prepare and the meal plan to have a good nutritional profile, but figuring out the diet without a meal plan involves a lot of math. Weight loss below average.

Rating
Overall score ....◐
Study results
  Short-term
    Weight loss ....○
    Dropout rate ....○
  1 year
    Weight loss ....◐
    Dropout rate ....○
Nutrition analysis ....●
Percent of calories
  Fat 27
  Saturated fat 7
  Carbohydrates 42
  Protein 30
Fiber, g/1,000 cal. 21
Fruits & veg., daily serv. 17
Average daily calories 1,660

ORNISH DIET

What it is Ultra-low-fat vegetarian regimen bans all meat, fish, oils, alcohol, sugar, and white flour. Ornish's clinical studies have shown that strictly following the diet can prevent or reverse disease. He believes it's easier to make drastic changes in diet than small ones.

Pros and cons Provides the most food per calorie of any diet evaluated. Lower in fat than guidelines recommend. Studies show average long-term weight loss and below-average long-term adherence.

Rating
Overall score ....○
Study results
  Short-term
    Weight loss ....○
    Dropout rate ....○
  1 year
    Weight loss ....○
    Dropout rate ....◐
Nutrition analysis ....○
Percent of calories
  Fat 6
  Saturated fat 1
  Carbohydrates 77
  Protein 16
Fiber, g/1,000 cal. 31
Fruits & veg., daily serv. 17
Average daily calories 1,520

ATKINS DIET

What it is This grand-daddy of low-carb diets starts with a two-week induction period that bans practically all carbs. The longer "ongoing weight loss" phase is only slightly less restrictive, gradually adding more vegetables, fruit, and wine.

Pros and cons There's growing evidence that dieters aren't as hungry on Atkins as on some other diets. But many find it too restrictive, so long-term adherence is below average; long-term weight loss is average. Its nutritional profile is far outside dietary guidelines.

Rating
Overall score ....◐
Study results
  Short-term
    Weight loss ....◐
    Dropout rate ....○
  1 year
    Weight loss ....○
    Dropout rate ....◐
Nutrition analysis ....●
Percent of calories
  Fat 60
  Saturated fat 20
  Carbohydrates 11
  Protein 29
Fiber, g/1,000 cal. 12
Fruits & veg., daily serv. 6
Average daily calories 1,520

- sandwich breads, bagels, pita bread, English muffins, low-fat tortillas
- plain cereal, dry or cooked
- rice and pastas, dry beans, and peas
- fresh, frozen, canned fruits in light syrup or juice
- fresh, frozen, or no-salt-added canned vegetables
- low-fat or no-fat salad dressings and sandwich spreads
- mustard and ketchup
- jam, jelly, or honey
- salsa, herbs, and spices

Bar exam

Energy Bars Flunk

By Bonnie Liebman and David Schardt

"For $50,000 or $100,000 you can be in the bar business," Brian Maxwell, president and CEO of PowerBar Inc, told Food Processing magazine last year.

That's one reason that supermarket, health food store, and drug store shelves carry a burgeoning selection of bars. (You can often find them at the front counter, with the other "impulse" items.) Sales of energy bars rose more than 50 percent last year, to $114 million, according to the trade publication Supermarket News. And energy is just the beginning.

To create a niche for a new bar in a dog-eat-dog marketplace, each manufacturer needs a new twist. Names like Ironman and Steel sell, but they're no longer enough. Viactiv and Luna bars are targeted at women. Protein Revolution, Pure Protein, and Perfect Solid Protein push the nutrient that muscles are made of. GeniSoy and Soy Sensations stake a claim on soy. Clif and Boulder go the natural route. And Think! promises to boost your brain power with herbs and vitamins.

This is one hot market. Why else would Nestlé have bought PowerBar, Kraft have bought Balance Bar, and Rexall Sundown have bought Met-Rx? So when it comes to advertising, chances are we ain't seen nothin' yet.

Do you need any of this stuff? This month we take a look at some of the biggest and boldest bars around. But first, a short course on the "energy" scam.

Energy for Sale

Luckily for food companies out to make a buck, "energy" has a double meaning. To most people, a food that supplies "energy" makes you feel energetic. But to scientists and the literal-minded regulators at the Food and Drug Administration, "energy" means calories.

That's right. To the folks who are in charge of keeping food labels honest, any food with calories is an "energy" food.

Never mind that no more than one in a million consumers would ever guess that, especially when ads for energy bars show people running, leaping, and otherwise looking energetic. Never mind that a simple disclosure on labels could explain to consumers that an "energy food" means simply that it "contains calories." Years after the Center for Science in the Public Interest (publisher of *Nutrition Action*) petitioned the FDA to require that kind of disclosure, the agency still hasn't lifted a finger to let consumers in on the energy secret.

Taking advantage of this irresistible loophole, companies have hit on a clever marketing scheme. While few people compete in long-distance athletic events, millions slog through a demanding day with no time for lunch. Marketing "energy" to the average office worker, stay-at-home mom, or just about anyone was a stroke of genius that's paying off big-time...but not necessarily for you.

"I caution people not to replace wholesome food with energy bars," says Elizabeth Applegate, a nutritionist and exercise expert at the University of California at Davis. "Manufacturers don't put everything you need from food into them. We don't even know everything in food that *should* be put in them."

Applegate, who consults for the food industry, does advise some people to eat energy bars, but not because they make the eater more energetic. "If you're going to grab a candy bar or a box of cookies or two bags of M&Ms from a vending machine for lunch, it's better to have an energy bar," she says.

Why? "Most bars are low in saturated and hydrogenated [*trans*] fat. And they can have as much as five grams of fiber and a handful of vitamins and minerals, just like a bowl of breakfast cereal.

"But if the wrappers are starting to accumulate on the floor of your car, back off," she adds. "You're better off with real food, like a sandwich on whole-grain bread, fresh fruit, and some baby carrots."

High-Carb Bars

"Don't bonk," say ads for PowerBars. The original PowerBar, launched in 1987 was designed to keep athletes from bonking—that is, running out of gas in the middle of a marathon or other long-distance event. The high-carbohydrate, low-fat bars consist largely of high-fructose corn syrup and grape and pear juice concentrate, with added vitamins and

(continued)

Source: Nutrition Action Health Letter, December 2000 by Bonnie Liebman & David Schardt. Copyright 2000 by Center for Science in the Public Interest. Reproduced by permission of Center for Science in the Public Interest via Copyright Clearance Center.

minerals. They have a taffy-like texture that seems more functional than flavorful.

It didn't take long for competitors (and PowerBar itself) to come up with energy bars that taste more like food than fuel. Clif, Boulder, PowerBar Harvest, and others started adding real food—like oats, nuts, and fruit—to their recipes. The final products taste like something between cookies and granola bars. But judging by the little research that's been done, there's nothing special—other than convenience—about getting your carbs in a compact wrapper.

David Pearson and colleagues at Ball State University in Muncie, Indiana, conducted one of the few studies on high-carb bars, though so far only a summary has been published.[1] First, nine trained cyclists rode for an hour to lower the levels of stored carbohydrate (glycogen) in their muscles. The next day, they rode for another half-hour and then sprinted.

After a one-hour rest, the cyclists were randomly assigned to eat 1,000 calories' worth of Power-Bars, Tiger's Milk bars, or cinnamon-raisin bagels over a four-hour period. An hour later, they rode for another hour while the researchers measured their energy output and blood sugar levels.

"The bagels resulted in the same aerobic performance as the energy bars," says Pearson, whose study was funded by Nabisco. "There's no magic to the bars. As long as you're getting the same number of calories and carbs in each food, there's no advantage to eating energy bars, and they're much more expensive."

Of course, most people don't even need carbs when they exercise. "High-calorie, carbohydrate-dense bars are really only for athletes doing long-term exercise," Pearson explains. "People think, 'if top-grade athletes eat these bars, I need them for *my* workout.' That's a misconception."

Pearson's hard-pedaling cyclists performed better with bars (or food) than with just water because they needed carbs. But unless you're running, cycling, cross-country skiing, or doing some other aerobic activity continuously for more than an hour at a stretch, you don't need a quick carb fix.

"The bar wouldn't empty out of your stomach before the event is over," says Pearson. What's more, he adds, "most people burn off fewer calories in the workout than they get from the bar."

So the next time you run a marathon, you may find it easier to pack some high-carb bars instead of bagels. (Some experts recommend taking one bite every ten minutes until the bar is gone.) But if you're just looking for a snack or pick-me-up after a game of tennis, save your money.

40-30-30 Bars

With the high-carb field sewn up, competitors like Balance, Ironman, and ProZone entered the market with bars that have a 40-30-30 ratio of carbohydrates to protein to fat, as touted by the best-selling diet book *The Zone*.

"The companies that market these bars have done a fabulous job of getting people to think that one bar makes their whole diet 40-30-30," notes Applegate.

Reaching 40-30-30 in a bar isn't difficult. It simply means replacing some of the high-fructose corn syrup with protein (from whey or soy protein isolate or casein) and with fat (often palm kernel oil).

Palm kernel oil is popular because it's saturated enough to stay solid at room temperature, so the coating doesn't smear all over your hands. Whether it smears all over the walls of your arteries is another question. Palm kemel oil is twice as saturated as lard.

It's not clear who is supposed to be eating 40-30-30 bars. And that's one secret to their success.

A bar that isn't for anyone in particular is for everyone. They're for athletes (real or would-be) who want to stay "in the zone." (Long before—and one reason why—Barry Sears' diet book became a best seller, that term applied to athletes at the top of their game.) They're for people who want to lose weight. And they're for people who want the "sustained energy" that the bars promise in order to get them through the day.

Of course, no published studies show how 40-30-30 bars like Balance or Ironman affect performance or weight loss for any of those groups. One small study concluded that an Ironman bar didn't raise blood sugar levels as rapidly or as much as a (high-carbohydrate) PowerBar.[2] Of course, a quick rise in blood sugar is precisely what an athlete wants.

"A 40-30-30 bar doesn't have enough carbohydrate for an athlete," says Ball State's Pearson. "But if you're sitting behind a desk and you want a bar instead of a Big Mac for lunch, you're better off with a 40-30-30 bar than a high-carbohydrate

(continued)

bar, because it's closer to what you'd get in a typical American diet."

That's not to say that the highly processed milk and soy protein, high-fructose corn syrup, oils, vitamins, and minerals are anything approaching an ideal food. Missing are the vegetables, beans, low-fat diary, and other real foods that can cut the risk of cancer, heart disease, and stroke (see cover story).

"If you're using bars in place of a meal, look for at least 10 to 15 grams of protein," says Applegate. "I also recommend eating at least one real food—like a piece of fresh fruit or some carrots or low-fat cheese sticks—with the bar."

Ads boast that the new Balance Gold bars "taste like a candy bar!" That's because they are candy bars…with some extra soy or milk protein and vitamins. Balance Outdoor bars use more natural ingredients, like soy pieces, fruit, and nuts. But watch out.

"You can still get a lot of calories from these bars," says Pearson. The 200-odd calories may not seem like much, but 200 calories in roughly two ounces of food means that bars are calorie-dense.

For a quick snack, you're better off with an apple, a handful of grape tomatoes, or some other fruit or vegetable that fills you up with fewer calories.

High-Protein Bars

They've got names like Ultimate Lo Carb, Met-Rx Protein Plus, Promax, Protein Fuel, Protein Revolution, Pure Protein, Solid Protein, and Steel. They're often bigger in calories (250 or so) and size (as much as three ounces), for people who want bigger muscles. Body builders—not dieters, soccer moms, or busy Yuppies—are the typical target audience.

Do They Work?

"Protein needs increase with exercise, whether it's strength training or endurance," says Applegate. But that doesn't mean that people need protein bars.

"You can easily get the protein from food," she explains. "The bars are more expensive and it's just food protein they put in there. People are surprised to hear that. They think, 'it's exactly what my muscles need.'"

Few companies have studies to show that their "proprietary blends" of milk or soy protein and other ingredients like "growth factors" and glutamine trump the competition.

Take Met-Rx's blend, which is called metamyosyn. Two published studies have tested its impact in healthy people in exercise programs. One found that overweight policemen gained more muscle mass and strength on metamyosyn than they did on another protein supplement, but the measurements were outdated and inexact.[3]

"The results of this study are interesting, but it needs to be repeated using more sophisticated methods of body composition assessment before definitive conclusions can be made," says Rick Kreider of the University of Memphis.

The other study, using more exact measures, found that Met-Rx was no better than a high-carbohydrate supplement at increasing muscle mass and strength in college football players.[4]

Supplement Bars

"Just taste these delicious, satisfying *new* energy sources for women," say ads for Viactiv. "Boost bars are the ideal snack and help give you the energy to do the things you want to do," says the company's Web site.

Yes, you do get calories from these bars. You also get the same vitamins and minerals that you'd find in a vitamin pill. The main difference is that someone might take a pill along with a bowl of lentil soup, a plate of stir-fried vegetables and chicken, or a fruit salad. But Mead Johnson's clever marketing for its Boost bars persuades people—especially women—to eat a fortified candy bar *instead* of real food…and to think they're healthier and more energetic as a result.

Soy protein bars like GeniSoy and Soy Sensations may help lower your cholesterol. But it's too early to say if their phytoestrogens can cut the risk of breast and prostate cancers. In fact, some preliminary studies suggest that consuming more soy may raise the risk of breast cancer in some people (see *Nutrition Action*, Sept. 1999 and Jan./Feb. 2000).

And soy isn't the only new twist. Think! bars sell nothing less than brain power. As if the name weren't enough, the labels and the company Web site (www.thinkproducts.com) note that the bars have "ginkgo biloba to stay sharp" and other "mind enhancing" ingredients, which have an "impact on

(continued)

brain and nerve cell function." But don't expect the company to supply evidence to back up its claims.

"We're not claiming it helps you think," insists Garrett Jennings, the inventor of Think!, the "Food for Thought" bar. Think! bars contain Jennings's secret blend of amino acids, fatty acids, and herbs.

Good published studies show no significant impact on thought or memory in people given the amounts of ginkgo or ginseng (60 mg each) or the other ingredients in Think! Bars. (A recent study found that 160 mg of a proprietary blend of ginseng and ginkgo modestly improved the "quality" of memory in middle-aged men and women, but until it's published, we can't draw any conclusions.)

"But if somebody feels great after a Think! bar," asks Jennings, "who cares if that's just a placebo effect?"

The information for this article was compiled by Jackie Adriano.

[1]*J. Strength Cond. 10:* 1996.
[2]*J. Amer. Diet. Assoc. 100:* 97, 2000.
[3]*Ann. Nutr. Metab. 44:* 21, 2000.
[4]*J. Exercise Physiol.* (online) 2: 24, 1999.

Fast Foods/Eating Out

People eat more meals outside the home than ever before. Due to their quick service and relatively low food prices, fast-food chains are the most frequent source for meals eaten away from home. Each day 50 million people line up inside or drive through outside service lanes of one of the over 160,000 fast-food establishments in this country.

When meals are prepared with speed and convenience as the primary focus, good nutrition will, in most cases, suffer. A great majority of fast foods are high in fat, calories, and salt, and low in many of the essential nutrients and dietary fiber.

However, fast food does not have to mean "junk food." While it may take a little more thought and discretion, quick and healthy alternatives do exist. Depending on what ingredients are used and how the food is prepared, fast foods served in restaurants can be healthy. Most restaurants have nutritional information about the foods they serve posted in the dining area or on their menus. By taking a couple of extra minutes to think about their best and most nutritious options, an individual can make dining out more nutritious, filling, and healthy.

Another pitfall of eating meals prepared away from home is the quality of food an individual is served. In an effort to be competitive, many restaurants serve well beyond an adequate portion size. To control portion sizes when eating out, order from the senior citizens or kids menus, share the entrée with a friend, or take part of the food home for a later meal.

Another way to eat healthy when dining out is to select foods that are steamed, broiled, baked, roasted, or poached rather than foods that are fried or grilled. Asking if the restaurant will trim visible fat off the meat or serve butter, sauces, or dressings "on the side" is another way to ensure a healthy and tasty meal.

Fitness or Fatness

Our food choices and habits, our exercise habits, and our genetic make-up all play a role in our ability to maintain a healthy weight. Managing weight is brought about most successfully by a lifestyle choice, not a short-term diet. Even if both of your parents are overweight and you didn't have good nutrition emphasized when you were young, you can make wise choices for yourself today.

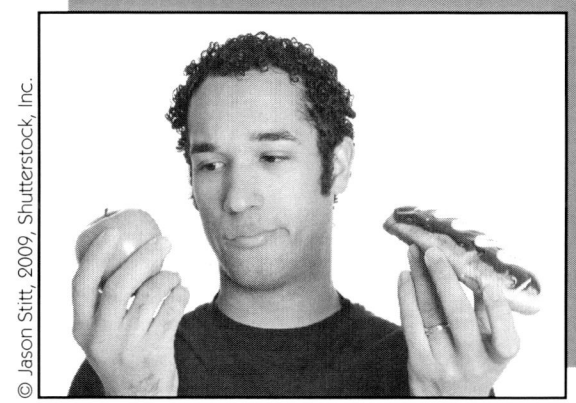

Our food choices and habits, our exercise habits, and our genetic make-up all play a role in our ability to maintain a healthy weight.

Tips for Healthy Dining at Home and Away

When restaurant eating, ask for a to-go box right away and put half of your order in it as soon as it comes.

Order a dinner salad, but share the entree with a friend when eating out.

Order water with your meal rather than a soda—save money and calories.

Opt for your traditional foods made in a "light" version.

Use a smaller plate to encourage smaller portions.

Drink a glass of water before your meal.

Eat your salad first.

Eat slowly. Put your eating utensil down and enjoy your meal or converse between bites. Eat breakfast regularly.

Have healthy snacks in your backpack or briefcase or car always.

Try eating fruits for dessert.

Trim visible fat off meat and take skin off poultry before cooking.

Try to use less refined sugar and processed flour in food preparation. Try whole wheat flour or unbleached white flour.

Wean yourself off sodas—or try to cut way down on your intake.

Read labels: minimize corn syrup, trans fat, coconut oil, palm kernel oil, and cocoa butter.

Use added fats like salad dressings minimally—try dipping your fork into the dressing before skewering the lettuce.

Avoid supersizing your meal.

Make small positive changes to encourage healthful behaviors. If you are overweight or obese, even a small 5 percent to 10 percent weight loss can have a favorable effect on your overall health risk.

REFERENCES

American Heart Association. Heart Disease and Stroke Statistics. 2009 Update.

Bishop, A. *Step Up to Wellness: A Stage Based Approach* (1st ed). Needham Heights, MA: Allyn & Bacon. 1999.

The Center for Health and Healthcare in Schools, School of Public Health and Health Services, George Washington University Medical Center. *Childhood Overweight: What the Research Tells Us*. March 2005 Update. www.healthinschools.org

Corbin, C. and Welk, G. *Concepts of Physical Fitness* (15th ed). Dubuque, IA: McGraw-Hill. 2009.

Donatelle, R. J. *Access to Health* (9th ed). Boston: Allyn & Bacon. 2006.

Flegal, K. M., Carrol, M. D., Kuczmarski, R. J., and Johnson, C. L. Overweight and Obesity in the United States: Prevalence and Trends, 1960–1994. *International Journal of Obesity and Related Metabolic Disorders* 22:39–47. 1998.

Floyd, P., Mims, S., and Yelding-Howard, C. *Personal Health: Perspectives and Lifestyles*. Morton Publishing Co. 2007.

Gibbs, W. W. Obesity: An Overblown Epidemic? *Scientific American*, May 23, 2005.

Hahn, D. B. and Payne, W. A. *Understanding Your Health*. McGraw-Hill. 2008.

Hales, D. *An Invitation to Wellness* (Instructor Ed.). Thomson-Wadsworth, 2007.

Hoeger, W. W. K. and Hoeger, S. A. *Lifetime Physical Fitness and Wellness: A Personalized Program* (10th ed). Belmont, CA: Wadsworth. 2009.

http://ahha.org

http://www.cdc.gov/nccdphp/dnpa/healthyweight/physical_activity/index.htm

http://www.nhlbi.nih.gov/health/public/heart/obesity/lose_wt/shop.htm

http://www.reachout.com.au/default.asp?ti=2249

http://www.cfsan.fda.gov/~dms/foodlab.html

http://www.win.niddk.nih.gov/publications/tools.htm

http://www.womhealth.org.au/studentfactsheets/bodyimage.htm

Hyman, B., Oden, G., Bacharach, D., and Collins, R. *Fitness for Living.* Dubuque, IA: Kendall-Hunt Publishing Co. 2006.

IUFOST, International Union of Food Science and Technology Bulletin. Trans-fatty Acids, May 2006.

O'Neil, Patrick. Weight Management Center, Medical University of South Carolina. 2009. www.muschealth.com

Powers, S. K., Todd, S. L., and Noland, U. J. *Total Fitness and Wellness* (2nd ed). Boston: Allyn & Bacon. 2005.

Prentice, W. E. *Fitness and Wellness for Life* (6th ed). New York: WCB McGraw-Hill. 1999.

Pruitt, B. E. and Stein, J. *Health Styles.* Boston: Allyn & Bacon. 1999.

Rosato, F. *Fitness for Wellness* (3rd ed). Minneapolis: West. 1994.

Satcher, D. Surgeon General's Report on Physical Activity and Health. Atlanta: U.S. Department of Health and Human Services, CDC. 1996.

Texas A&M University, Student Health Services. Fad Diets: Promise or Profit, 77, 2002.

Texas A&M University Human Nutrition Conference. College Station, TX. 1998.

Wilmore, J. H. Exercise, Obesity, and Weight Control, *Physical Activity and Research Digest.* Washington, DC: President's Council on Physical Fitness and Sports. 1994.

World Health Organization (WHO). Management of Severe Malnutrition: A Manual for Physicians and other Senior Health Workers. Geneva: Author. 1999.

World Health Organization (WHO). Obesity: Preventing and Managing the Global Epidemic — Report of WHO Consultation on Obesity. Geneva, June 1997.

Surgeon General's Call to Action to Prevent and Decrease Overweight and Obesity. 2005. www.surgeongeneral.gov

Diet Books: What the Experts Say, *Consumer Reports,* June 2007, 14–15.

Diet Plans: What the Studies Say, *Consumer Reports,* June 2007, 16–17.

RECOMMENDED READING

Eat, Drink and Be Healthy: The Harvard Medical School Guide to Healthy Eating by Walter C. Willett, M.D. Simon and Schuster Source, 2001.

The Spectrum: A Scientifically Proven Program to Feel Better, Live Longer, Lose Weight, and Gain Health. Ballantine Books, 2007.

ACTIVITIES

Notebook Activities

Body Mass Index Calculator

Facts about My Favorite Fast-Food Meal

Name: _____ Section: _____ Date: _____

NOTEBOOK ACTIVITY

Body Mass Index Calculator

In order to complete this Body Mass Index assignment, go to http://www.cdc.gov/nccdphp/dnpa/bmi/calc-bmi.htm

Body Mass Index is a mathematical formula that correlates highly with body fat. This weight calculation helps determine whether you are at a healthy weight or have too much fat.

$$\text{The formula for BMI} = \frac{\text{Weight (kg)}}{\text{Height (m)}^2}$$

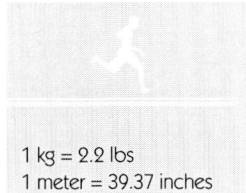

1 kg = 2.2 lbs
1 meter = 39.37 inches

Note:

If you are under the age of 20 years, you have the option of using the BMI-by-age calculator.

1. Enter your weight and height using English or metric measurements. What is your BMI? _____

2. What is your weight status according to your BMI calculation? _____

3. Click on "What does this all mean?"
   How can two individuals, one fit and one unfit, who weigh the same and are the same height have the same BMI?

4. What does your BMI tell you about your health risk?

       <18   Underweight
     19–26   Healthy Weight (low risk)
     27–29   Overweight (medium risk)
     30–40   Obese (high risk)
       >40   Morbidly obese (very high risk)

A BMI of 25 or higher is associated with an increased health risk of conditions that include coronary heart disease, certain forms of cancer, stroke, high blood pressure, and non insulin-dependent diabetes.

Source: www.cdc.gov

Name: _____ Section: _____ Date: _____

NOTEBOOK ACTIVITY

Facts about My Favorite Fast-Food Meal

1. List your favorite fast-food meal in the space provided below—be specific and detailed. Include anything you consume with the meal and the quantity (i.e., large beverage, four ketchup or salsa packets, etc.).

2. Go to the restaurant and obtain a nutritional analysis of their foods. This information is generally available as a pamphlet. You might also be able to obtain this information from the restaurant's Web site.

3. Determine and list the following for your meal:

    A. total number of calories

    B. grams of total fat

    C. grams of saturated fat

    D. grams of trans fat

4. Use Table 6.2 on page 200 to determine your daily calorie allowance based on your age, gender, and activity level. List that information in the space provided below.

    Age:

    Gender:

    Activity Level:

    Estimated Daily Caloric Allowance:

5. Using Table 5.2 on page 153 of Chapter 5 (What Is Your Upper Limit on Fat for the Calories You Consume) and your estimated daily caloric allowance, judge how "healthy" your food choice was in relation to the total number of calories it contains and the number of grams of total fat, saturated fat, and trans fat it contains. When you are looking at these numbers, remember that the calorie allowance and the limit on fat is for all food consumed within a twenty-four-hour period, and the meal listed is probably only about one-third of the calories and fat you will consume during this time period. In the space below, use the numbers you compared and briefly describe how "healthy" your choice was.

6. Other than never eating this meal, what modifications could reasonably be made to keep this meal in your diet but make it a more nutritionally sound choice?

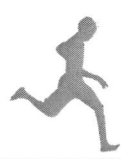

CHAPTER 7

Relationships

"It's not about getting what you want, it's about wanting what you've got."

— Sheryl Crow

OBJECTIVES

Students will be able to:
- List and describe the three elements of a healthy relationship.
- List five ways to reduce the risk of date rape.
- Identify the differences between males and females and how these differences relate to communication.
- List warning signs of an unhealthy relationship.
- Identify types of abuse and describe the cycle of abuse and why it's difficult for the victim to end the relationship.

Healthy Relationships

There are numerous types of relationships that exist. They range from casual acquaintances to life-long partners. It is important to realize the different types and stages that relationships grow into, as well as what represents a healthy relationship.

Positive Self-Worth

The first step to having a healthy relationship is developing a positive self-worth. This self-worth comes from many different sources. These may include family members, close friends, co-workers, occupation, achievements, and so on. A couple of questions to answer might include: (1) Whom do you see in the mirror? (2) Would you want a relationship with you? A positive self-worth is represented in confidence, a healthy body, and a positive attitude about yourself and others. This is not to say that one has to be completely healthy in order to have a healthy relationship, but the closer to this goal the better relationships typically will be.

Healthy relationships include open communication, compromise, trust, respect, caring, selflessness, as well as many other attributes. Researchers have found that 70 to 93 percent of messages sent come from nonverbal communication. Nonverbal communication includes unwritten and unspoken information; these can be both intentional and unintentional. Some examples include smiling, eye contact, nodding, leaning closer, crossed arms, looking off in another direction, and even rolling eyes. Mismatch of verbal and nonverbal communication can cause confusion. When this happens, people tend to believe the nonverbal communication more readily, which comes from the old saying, "Actions speak louder than words." With this in mind, pay attention to the messages you are sending nonverbally. As mentioned earlier, some individuals will lean closer to let a person know they are interested in them or in what is being said. There are different spatial zones that exist. There is an acceptable amount of space or a "zone" that individuals claim as their personal space. Depending upon the circumstance, geographic location (such as a crowded city), or culture one grew up in, this zone changes. For example, this zone is larger when an individual is in a public or social environment, but typically becomes smaller when they are in a more personal or intimate setting. If your personal zone becomes too small for your comfort level, take two steps backward to increase the size of the space.

Open Communication

Open communication involves actively listening, talking effectively, and body language. Minimize or alleviate other distractions in order to maximize open communication with your partner or friend. This may include turning off the radio, the television, or maybe getting away from other friends and/or roommates. During a discussion truly listen to the other person. Do not interrupt or simply wait until they are finished speaking to interject your thought or advice. So much of the time people only hear the first part of a sentence or a concept because they are busy forming their thoughts and ideas of how they are going to reply. Periodically confirm the main points that you are hearing. Do this before proceeding with the conversation. Do this several times during the discussion, as well as at the end, to make certain that you agree on the conclusion and the important points discussed. Be open to questions. Do not continuously lead the conversation. Let the other person talk and listen to what they have to say.

As for talking effectively, be straightforward and say what you mean. Do not beat around the bush and hope that your partner can read your mind. If you say you do not care about a certain situation, then mean that you do not care. If you

> ## Spelling a Healthy Relationship
>
> (adapted from Kuriansky, 2002)
>
> **H**onesty—always tell the truth even if it will initially hurt.
> Harmony—enrich one another's differences.
> Heart—give your whole heart.
> Honor—hold others in high regard.
> Happy—be happy with each other.
>
> **E**mpathy—be able to understand what each other feel.
> Equality—treat the other as your equal.
> Energetic—be spontaneous, relationships take energy.
> Enthusiasm—be excited about being together.
> Empowerment—support each other.
>
> **A**cceptance—know that you approve of each other just the way they are.
> Accommodation—make adjustments for each other's needs.
> Appreciation—be grateful for each other.
> Adaptability—be able to make changes when necessary.
> Agreements—make an agreement and hold to it.
>
> **L**ove—should be unconditional.
> Loyalty—be devoted, never betray each other.
> Listening—actively listen, it makes the other person feel important.
> Laughter—have fun together.
> Lust—sparks the union.
>
> **T**rust—being able to relax around the other person.
> Talking—communication is the key.
> Time—spend time together. Nothing is more important than time.
> Tenderness—treat each other with kindness.
> Thoughtfulness—show consideration in thoughts and actions.
>
> **H**ome—create a safe haven.
> Healing—work together to heal new and old wounds.
> Humility—admit when you are wrong.
> Hope—for a better tomorrow when things are not at their best.
> Homework—relationships are not easy, they do require constant work.
>
> **Y**ES! Say yes as often as you can.

have an opinion, let your partner know what it is. Friends and partners will not always agree on every decision; therefore, compromise is important in a healthy relationship.

Compromise

In order to come to an appropriate compromise, discuss the pros and cons about a certain situation and then come to a mutual agreement. An individual will not always get what they want, but sometimes an idea synthesizes from the two and is much better. Sometimes it is important to concede and let the other individual get what they desire, and other times this gesture must be returned. Problems typically occur when one person is always conceding.

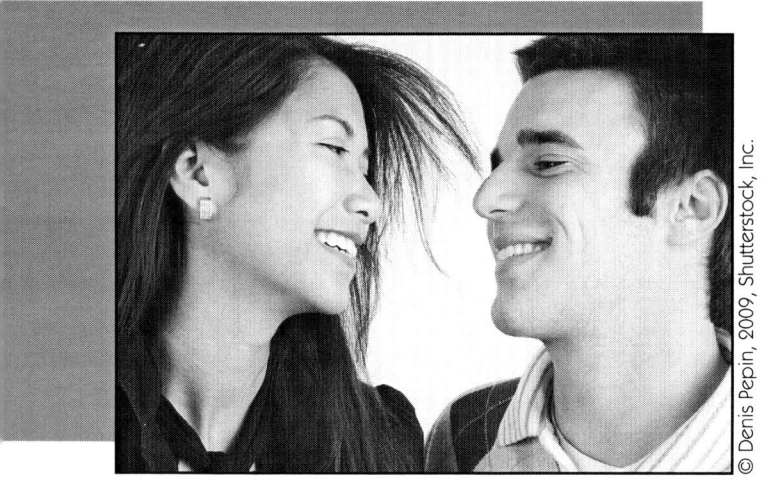

Healthy relationships include open communication, compromise, trust, respect, and caring.

Trust

Trust is an integral element in a healthy relationship. From friendship to life-long partner, individuals must be able to trust the people they spend time with. Trust takes time to develop. Be cautious and do not expose deep feelings and internal ideas too early, but at the same time give others a chance to build trust little by little. In a relationship built upon trust one can discuss issues with confidence and know that these ideas will be kept private if necessary. Another element associated with trust is that in this person's absence one can trust the friend's ideas and actions. A relationship built upon trust can have incredible rewards. With this added element each person is comfortable being himself or herself and the relationship can develop to a completely different level. When complete trust exists many problems such as jealousy are non-existent in the relationship.

Types of Relationships

There are many types of relationships, which fulfill many different needs. We begin with our family relationships, parents, siblings, aunts, uncles, and so on. This is the core of our foundation. In today's society we have many different structures that represent "family." Some individuals are raised by both of their biological parents, or maybe just one parent, others by grandparents, and others are adopted, to name a few. These initial relationships have a huge impact upon how we relate with others. What type of relationship do you have with your parents? Is it close? What changes would you make in your relationships with family members if you had the chance? Who has impacted you the most in your family? Was this a positive or negative impact? When there is a good foundation of healthy relationships with family members this typically carries over to friendships and intimate relationships.

There are different levels of friendship: casual, close, and intimate. Each of these friendships can be very beneficial. The key ingredients to a successful friendship include steadfastness, honesty, reliability, and trust. Casual friendships are good for camaraderie, someone to see a movie with, or eat lunch. In close friendships, there is typically a greater investment of time and emotional energy. Benefits typically seen with close friendships are those that can stand the test of time. There is a connection beyond the surface and a history with this person. Typically close friends know more about you than a casual acquaintance and can be called upon more easily in a time of need.

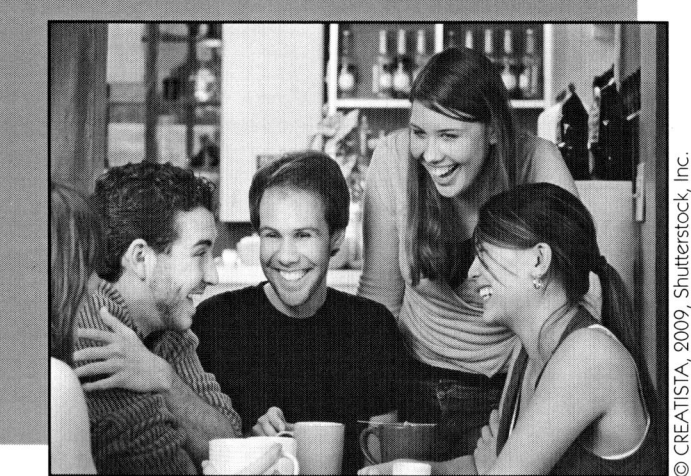

There are many types of relationships, which fulfill many needs.

The Ten Commandments of a Healthy Relationship

(Kuriansky, 2002)

1. I will do my best to be the happiest person I can be.
2. I will be honest in my dealings with my partner.
3. I will keep my agreements.
4. I will have integrity about my actions.
5. I will honor all others I am in a relationship with.
6. I will practice forgiveness for others and myself.
7. I will nurture my spiritual soul and that of others.
8. I will accept others for who they are without judging them or insisting they change to suit me.
9. I will be open to suggestions and change when it's in the best interest for both of us.
10. I will trust in the powers that be what happens is for the best.

This chapter would not be complete without the mention of cyber-relationships. More often people are meeting others and developing relationships over the Internet. This can be very beneficial in that you can express your opinions and thoughts anonymously and receive feedback. It can also help fill a void on a lonely Friday night. Use this method of meeting people with extreme caution and never give your full name, address, or other personal information for the entire world to see. As detailed in this chapter, a student was murdered by an individual he had met over the Internet. Remember, you never know exactly to whom you are talking through the Internet. Be cautious when using MySpace or posting personal information on the Internet. It is relatively easy for criminals to piece together random information and figure out where you live or what your usual routine is.

True-Life Stories

Man Indicted in Death of A&M Student
31-year-old could get life in Internet-luring incident.

A San Antonio man accused of posing as a woman on the Internet and luring a Texas A&M University junior to an out-of-town rendezvous was indicted Wednesday on charges of murdering the student.

A San Marcos grand jury handed up the first-degree felony indictment, saying there was enough evidence for Kenny Wayne Lockwood, 31, to be charged with the early-April shooting death of Kerry Jason Kujawa, 20, of Richmond, Texas.

If convicted, Lockwood faces five to 99 years or life in prison for the crime.

Hays County Sheriff's Department authorities said evidence shows Lockwood probably shot and killed Kujawa between April 7 and 9 in San Antonio, put the body in the trunk of a car and then dumped it west of Dripping Springs.

Kujawa's body was recovered April 19, almost two weeks after he left College Station for San Antonio.

Concerns about Kujawa's disappearance were not reported to police for almost two weeks, a delay perpetuated by Lockwood, according to police who said friends and family received e-mail messages from a person they presumed to be Kujawa.

Authorities said Lockwood was logging on to the computer as Kujawa.

A&M police and the Texas Rangers knew Kujawa had excitedly told friends and family that he was meeting face-to-face for the first time with a female friend he met in January over the Internet.

That person was Kelley Lynn McCauley, a 21-year-old female pre-law student at A&M who had several online suitors during the past year, but existed only in Lockwood's mind, according to the investigation. Lockwood pretended to be "Kelley."

The inquiry led to Lockwood's doorstep in San Antonio where he lived with his parents. Computer records showed Lockwood would regularly log on the Internet as Kelley, often spending hours in chat rooms talking to strangers.

The break in the case came when A&M students came forward with a telephone number and details of the Kelley they thought Kujawa met while online.

Lockwood's carefully crafted online identity was flirtatious and imaginative. Authorities said Lockwood continued to lie after killing Kujawa, telling others online that "she" and Kujawa were engaged and "she" would soon meet his parents.

Authorities said Lockwood confessed to the crime a week after Kujawa's body was discovered.

Texas Ranger Frank Malinak, who is based in Bryan and assisted in the case, said it's unfortunate it took Kujawa's death for people to learn about the dangers of meeting others over the Internet.

"I just hope people are more wary of these chat rooms, because you never know who you are communicating with," Malinak said. "You may be talking to a truthful and forthright individual or you may be talking to murder.com."

Lockwood has been in the Hays County Jail on $500,000 bail since April 27, when he was arrested for Kujawa's murder.

Source: From *Bryan-College Station Eagle,* July 6, 2000 by Kelly Brown. Copyright © 2000 by Bryan-College Station Eagle. Reprinted by permission.

Don't Be Fooled! There Are Risks!

The following are things to be aware of:

DON'T disclose:
- phone number
- address
- actual email address (use Hotmail or other free email service)

Also, watch out that your personal signature lines on those services do not include the personal information you are trying to guard.

How Do I Know They're Legit?
- WhoIsHe.com/WhoIsShe.com and CheckMate.com. On-line services to do background checks.
- Ask the person if they'd be will for you to contact some personal references.
- Make sure that you have numerous contacts with the individual prior to agreeing to meet in person. This should include several contacts of different sorts, including phone or snail mail.

The Big Meeting

So, you think you've met your match. You've checked him out and allowed him to check you out. You have sent pictures and email and talked on the phone.

Just as with a blind date, let someone know where you are and whom you are with. Better yet, bring them along and have them be in the same restaurant to keep their eyes peeled.

Meet in a public place.

Carry your cell or pager and have someone page you at a certain time. Tell your friend if you don't answer, they should worry.

Take your own car or cab.

If things get uncomfortable, leave (even if it's through the back door).

Meet on your home turf if you can. This, of course, follows the above guidelines of a public place and such.

If you meet them at their place away from your city, don't stay with them. Get a hotel and arrange your own transportation. The expense of that is worth the safety. Don't tell them where you are staying.

Source: www.selfcounseling.com with permission.

Stages of Relationships

These are some of the most common stages of a relationship. Not all relationships will have all of these stages, nor will they all proceed in this exact order.

- The first look
- Getting to know one another
- Finding out you like this person
- Establishing boundaries—who needs more or less space?
- Sexual attraction
- Falling in love

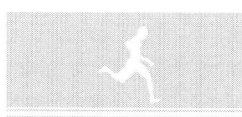

Rules about Sexual Health

Smart sex in the new millennium requires that you:

- Protect yourself (through abstinence or condoms).
- Never make a mistake or allow an exception to safe sex practices.
- Ease up on using protection only if both partners were virgins when they met, or if both have tested negative for AIDS and other STIs, and then had sex with each other exclusively.
- Talk about your sexual history. Say something like, "Before we have sex, we need to talk about diseases, safe sex, and our sexual pasts."
- Discuss what method you are going to use for safe sex.
- Find ways to enjoy intimacy other than through sex.

- Looking beyond the surface
- Commitment
- Playing house
- Living together
- Valleys and mountains—the ups and downs of a long-term relationship

Dating

Dating is the process of getting to know other people as well as yourself while growing with and from each relationship. Typically a date is stimulated by physical attraction, which can lead to emotional and physical intimacy. One of the outcomes of this process can be finding someone with whom we can happily spend the rest of our life. This process can be incredibly exciting and frustrating all at the same time. There are so many people with whom to meet and enjoy their company. Each new relationship exposes one to new and exciting experiences. While dating, your abilities, strengths, and interests can be maximized. As you are learning who you are and what you like, you should prioritize which characteristics are important and which are not. There is so much to be learned during the dating process. How do you relate to your partner in an intimate setting? What expectations do you have for the person with whom you want to live the rest of your life? As mentioned earlier, after the initial physical attraction, individuals may choose to become emotionally and/or physically intimate. There are many responsibilities that follow when taking this next step. There is more at risk—mentally, physically, and financially. A scenario to contemplate is: How long does it take the average person to decide to buy a car? Or maybe a house? How long will these items be an influence on an individual's life? How long does the average person contemplate sexual intercourse? What are some of the repercussions associated with intercourse and how long will this affect an individual's life? It is best to fully consider the consequences before proceeding. Make sure that you and your partner are ready to deal with the consequences. For more information on protection against sexually transmitted infections and pregnancy, see Chapter 8.

Some of the best places to meet people: doing something you enjoy—for example, music store, coffee shop, workout facility, sporting events, bookstore, museum, lake, church, club, concert, class, or convention.

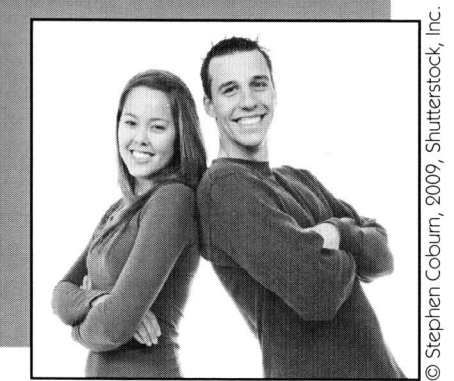

Levels of passion, intimacy, and commitment change over time as a relationship matures.

When and What Type of Love Is It?

There are probably as many different definitions of love as there are people in this world. For this reason, it makes answering "When is it love?" very difficult. One definition of love is a strong affection or liking for someone or something. Some signs it might be love include: verbally expressing affection, such as saying "I love you"; feeling happier or more secure when this person is present; putting the other person's interests before yours (in a healthy give-and-take relationship); respecting the other person for who they are; and not minding the other person's idiosyncrasies (adapted from Strong et al., 2006).

Historically, there are several different models of love. Two common ones are described below. The first is Sternberg's (1988) love triangle which includes three components: passion, intimacy, and commitment. Passion tends to occur at the beginning of relationships, peaks relatively quickly, and then reduces to a stable level. Passion generates romance, physical attraction, and sometimes intercourse. Intimacy is the feeling of closeness that exists between two people. Intimacy tends to peak slower than passion and then gradually reduces to a lower level. This level typically changes throughout a relationship. Commitment is the decision to further a loving relationship with another individual. The level of commitment typically rises slowly in the beginning, speeds up, and then gradually levels off. Sternberg describes the various types of love as a composition of different combinations of these three components. These various kinds of love change over time as the relationship matures.

John Lee (1973) describes six styles of loving:

EROS – passionate love
    Becomes sexually involved quickly
    Intense focus on partner and shares all of him/herself
    Quick to develop, quick to end

LUDUS – game-playing love
    Love and sex are seen only as fun, an activity, a diversion
    Move from partner to partner and often have several at a time
    Passion for the game, not the partner

STORGE – friendship love
    Long-term commitment
    Strong and secure, places less emphasis on passion

MANIA – obsessive love
    Turbulent and ambivalent
    Intense mental preoccupation, but little satisfaction
    Likely to be possessive and jealous

PRAGMA – realistic love
    Rational and practical
    Often for evolutionary and economic purposes
    Intense feelings may develop once a partner is chosen

AGAPE – altruistic love
    Generous, unselfish giving of oneself
    Less emphasis on passion and sexuality

Some Things to Do on a Date

1. Sit outside and visit.
2. Feed the ducks at the park.
3. Make a meal together.
4. Go for a bike ride.
5. Go to a baseball game.
6. Draw a picture together.
7. Enjoy a romantic moonlit picnic.
8. Play a game of pool.
9. Sightsee in a nearby town.
10. Grill some steaks outside for dinner together.
11. Go see a comedian.
12. Make s'mores (over a campfire or stove).
13. Have dinner at a very quaint restaurant.
14. Go to the zoo.
15. Go to an amusement park.
16. Take a recreational class together.
17. Go hiking.
18. Stop and read all of the historic landmarks.
19. Lie in a hammock.
20. Tie-dye two T-shirts.
21. Play I Spy.
22. Go to the ballet.
23. Play chess.
24. Host a dinner buffet for your closest friends.
25. Make a cake together.
26. Go white-water rafting.
27. Play games at the local arcade.
28. Share a five-course meal.
29. Wait in line all night together for tickets.
30. Rent a jeep and go to the lake.
31. Discuss the three most memorable events in your life.
32. Finger-paint a picture.
33. Go to a yoga class.
34. Gather food for a good cause.
35. Dress up for Halloween and hand out candy.
36. Read a book together.
37. Teach a Sunday school class together.
38. Go scuba diving.
39. Have your cholesterol levels checked.
40. Volunteer for a fund-raiser.
41. Go roller blading.
42. Rent his and her movies and watch them together.
43. Play a board game.
44. Go ice-skating.
45. Play tennis.
46. Go canoeing.
47. Spend an evening counting your blessings.
48. Visit your state capitol.
49. Run a 5K.
50. Go to the circus.
51. Visit a national park.
52. Study religious texts together.
53. Donate blood.
54. Go to a water park.
55. Take a class in self-defense.
56. Pick fruit from an orchard.
57. Adopt your own clean-up spot.
58. Baby-sit together.
59. Go to a county fair.
60. Spend an evening massaging each other.
61. Play hide-and-seek.
62. Make homemade ice cream.
63. Go to church/temple/mosque together.
64. Ride a tandem bike.
65. Dress up as clowns and visit the children's ward at a hospital.
66. Go Hawaiian by hosting a luau.
67. Play Frisbee.
68. Go to a basketball game.
69. See a talent show.
70. Go fishing.
71. Take a hot-air balloon ride.
72. Visit a haunted house.
73. Go play in the rain (and get drenched)!
74. Dress up for a special night out on the town.
75. Write a poem.
76. Go on a hayride.
77. Pick out and cut a Christmas tree.
78. Do laundry together.
79. Go for a walk on campus on a foggy night.
80. Go for a moonlight swim.
81. Lend support during a tough time.
82. Go to a bed and breakfast.
83. Share what you wish to have accomplished by the time you are 30, 40, and so on.
84. Pray together.

Rating Safe Sex Activities

Safer sex activities include:
- Dry kissing
- Hugging
- Frottage (rubbing against each other)
- Massage
- Telephone sex
- Tantric sex (extended love-making techniques from the Orient that don't involve penetration)

Riskier activities include:
- Open mouth or deep tongue kissing
- Oral sex (with condoms or dental dams)
- Vaginal intercourse with a condom

Unsafe sex activities include:
- Vaginal intercourse without a condom (even if pulling out before ejaculation)
- Oral sex without a condom (even if pulling out before ejaculation)
- Oral sex or vaginal penetration without a condom during a woman's period
- Anal sex without a condom

Date Rape

How to decrease the odds for date rape (Floyd et al., 2007):
- Develop clear lines of communication with the person you are dating.
- Communicate and clearly understand what each of you want and expect from the date.
- Do not use psychoactive substances, including alcohol, in dating situations.
- Do not give clues or display body language that is flirtatious or indicates you are interested in having sex when you are not. For example, allowing a date to visit your bedroom may send a message that you are interested in becoming intimate.
- Do not be coerced into unwanted sexual activities.

If you are the victim of date rape, remember it is not your fault. Seek medical treatment and counseling immediately. There are hotlines and other contact information listed at the end of this chapter.

Taming the Green-Eyed Monster

Jealousy typically comes from a lack of self-esteem and/or lack of confidence. Jealousy will undermine an otherwise healthy relationship and drive potential partners away. Realizing you are the jealous type is the first step in solving the problem. Then you can begin work on your self-confidence. Realize what your strong points are and focus on them. Exercise on a regular basis. Studies show that individuals who exercise on a regular basis feel better about themselves. Walk with confidence and feel good about who you are. Look in your past, is there anything that has happened to make you insecure? Evaluate what happened and what could be different in the future so those past "ghosts" do not haunt you.

What to Do for a Jealous Partner

Reassure their importance to you on a regular basis and let them know there is no need for their jealous tendencies. Let your partner know in a constructive manner that you do not care for their jealous tendencies. Take your partner to meet your friends and co-workers and include them in social gatherings.

Differences between Males and Females

(Adapted from Godek, 1997)

The following are generalizations, trends, and some personal observations.

- **Men** hear "sex" when you say "romance."
- **Women** hear "love" when you say "romance."

- **Men** can easily separate their sexuality from their feelings.
- **Women** connect many emotional issues with their sexuality.

- **Men** communicate to gather information.
- **Women** communicate to create relationships.

- **Men** view relationships in a hierarchical manner.
- **Women** view relationships as a vast interlocking network.

- **Men** are aroused visually and quickly.
- **Women** are aroused through sensation and slowly.

- **Men** have been taught to hide their tender feelings.
- **Women** have been taught to hide their angry feelings.

- **Men** have been taught to suppress their gentle side.
- **Women** have been taught to suppress their aggressive side.

Left-brain vs. Right-brain. Men typically are associated with left-brained dominance (see Table 7.1), with their cognitive style being more logical (focusing more on problems and solutions). Whereas, women typically are associated with right-brained dominance, with emphasis on communication and emotions (Kuriansky, 2003).

So, what does this mean? Men and women approach simple as well as complex relationships very differently. The first step to a healthy relationship is to realize these differences exist. Secondly, respect these differences. Then you can begin to understand the differences, where they come from, and make your relationship

Table 7.1

How Differences in Brain Dominance Affect Behavior

Left Brain (Male)	Right Brain (Female)
Values power or being in control	Values love and communication
Needs approval and acceptance	Needs appreciation and attention
Fulfilled by achieving goals	Fulfilled by expression and relating
More interested in news and sports	More interested in romance novels and self-help
Comfortable with gadgets and hi-tech	Comfortable with gab groups

Source: Adapted from Kuriansky, 2003.

a healthier one. Always work toward compromise and find the best solution to fulfill your relationship. As stated earlier, the above characteristics are simply generalizations, not the rule. In the recent past there have been trends to meet more in the middle with some of these characteristics. Inevitably when you have two different sets of ideas and philosophies arguments will occur. Realize that long-term stress can have a detrimental effect on your relationship. Try to engage in stress-relieving techniques discussed in Chapter 2. A typical response to increased stress is arguing. Always try to argue fairly, which sometimes is hard to do when individuals are tired and stressed.

Rules for Arguing Fairly

(Adapted from Godek, 1997)

1. Stay with the initial issue, do not bring up everything that is bothering you.
2. Stay in the present, do not bring up past problems and issues.
3. Say what you feel.
4. Do not generalize. ("You always…" "You are just like your mother…")
5. Do not threaten (verbally or physically).
6. Absolutely, no violence. (Men: Not even the slightest touch. Women: This includes slapping his face.)
7. State your needs as specific requests for different behavior.
8. Work toward a solution. Do not add fuel to the fire.

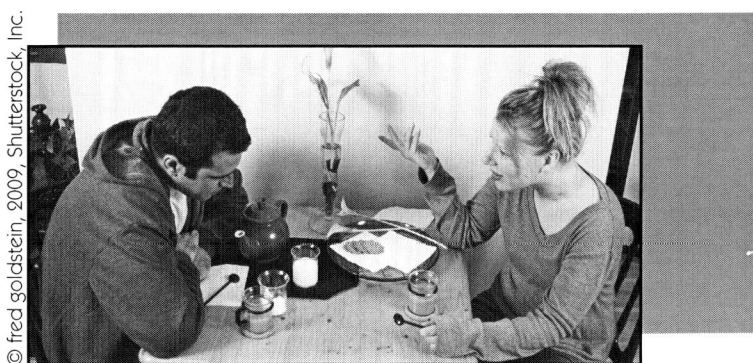
Always try to be fair when arguing.

The most common topics couples argue about include:

- When to see each other
- How often to see each other
- Flirting with other people
- Being late
- Forgetting important dates (birthdays and anniversaries)
- Being faithful
- Who spends how much money and on what
- How you spend time (watching too much TV and going out with friends)
- The amount or type of sex you have
- Family (when and whom to visit)

(Kuriansky, 2003)

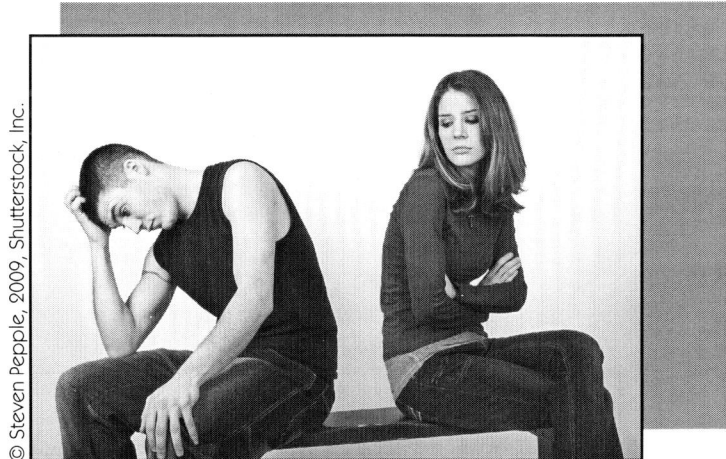
Disagreements happen in every relationship.

Ending a Relationship

In most cases the first individual you date will not be the person you marry. There are many reasons that exist to end a relationship. Some of these include initial misperceptions, changes in life routes, surfacing unattractive behaviors, infidelity, or even boredom. Typically only one individual sees a need for the change in the relationship, which makes ending a relationship a difficult situation.

On the Sending End

Always try to be as tactful as possible. Remember that at one point you were interested enough in this person to pursue a relationship. Be open and honest about the reason(s) you wish to end the relationship. The worst way to end a relationship is to ignore the other person. This leads your partner on and fosters confusion.

On the Receiving End

Listen carefully to what the person is saying and do not respond desperately or defensively. If your partner has brought up some characteristics that *you* would like to change, slowly work toward this change for yourself. If this truly is the end of this relationship, realize and accept that there will be a better match for you at some point in the future.

One definition of **love** is a passionate affection of one person for another. Another definition is "The emotion evoked when two souls resonate or 'fit together' naturally. It is close, but still not perfect" (Godek, 1997). There is no one exact definition that sums up all of the meanings of the word *love*. It is very different and personal to each individual.

Different types of love exist with regard to partners, parents, children, and friends. Within a loving relationship there are five important elements:

1. honesty,
2. loyalty,
3. thoughtfulness,
4. sharing,
5. sacrifice.

Honesty is the foundation that relationships are formed upon. Without this one cannot deepen or enrich a relationship further. Loyalty is also incredibly important. Your partner must always realize where your loyalty lies regardless if they are present. This loyalty also builds the foundation to further enhance your relationship. Thoughtfulness is an expression of how you feel about the other person. These actions should indicate to your partner how important they are to you. Another fulfilling element of a loving relationship includes sharing. This includes sharing possessions as well as experiences. Most experiences are enhanced if accompanied by someone you love. This could include a trip, dinner, sporting activity, and the menial tasks that go along with life. Finally sacrifice, loving someone enough to do without so they may have what they desire. This is sacrificing without being a martyr, because it is freely given without strings attached.

I Do or I Do Not

In today's society, it is unfortunate that many individuals treat marriage as a dating game. If the relationship gets too rough, they will just get a divorce. This casual attitude toward marriage diminishes the meaning of the vows that are taken when a couple marries.

There are many things to consider when contemplating marriage. Is this the person with whom you truly want to spend the rest of your life? Are we compatible? Do we have similar values? These are just a few of the questions that should be asked.

The question of compatibility is one that takes time to answer. Some characteristics that comprise compatibility include similar interests, ways of doing things, as well as the ability to compromise when you do not see "eye to eye." Do you both like to participate in outdoor or indoor activities? Are your activity levels similar? Do you need structure to your life or is spontaneity more your style? Are you both outgoing or do you complement each other with some differences? What are your long-term goals and are they similar to your partner's? Do you have similar views on finances? Are you thrifty or extravagant? Do both of you want children? This is not to say that you and your ideal partner have to be identical. In fact, it is helpful to have some differences (within reason) to help complement the other's weaknesses. For example, if one of you is somewhat overreactive and the other one is more grounded, then you will probably balance one another out. Problems arise when there are so many differences that you cannot relate or the differences simply irritate one another. With this said, it is very helpful to have similar interests and ways of doing things that can carry past the initial infatuation stage.

Values are defined as beliefs or standards. Are your values similar? For example, how you treat other people, volunteer work, religion, and child rearing. What do you hold very dear to your heart? Are there any specific lines that you would never cross and expect the same out of a life-long partner? Some examples include drug use, infidelity, or lying. What are your views of marriage? What does this word mean to you, and is it similar to the meaning your partner places on it?

Tips for a Successful Marriage

- Always respect your spouse.
- Not only love your spouse, but like him or her too.
- Remember that a relationship is not 50/50, it is 100/100 (Godek, 1997). If you only try to give 50 percent (or your fair share) you will definitely fall short of the combined 100 percent that is needed.
- Don't expect perfection from yourself or your partner.

Ten Characteristics of a Happy Marriage

(Floyd et al., 2007)

1. They are giving people, meeting their emotional needs by doing for others—and they do not keep score.
2. They have a strong sense of commitment, do not take their happiness for granted, and are determined to make their marriages work.
3. They do not lose themselves in the relationship. They value their independence—the right to form their own opinions, make their own decisions, pursue their own goals—marital harmony is a top priority.
4. They have vigorous sexual drives. Sex plays a central and profoundly important role in the marriage.
5. They like to talk, sharing their thoughts about all sorts of subjects. They are open and direct, not manipulative.
6. They have a positive outlook on life.
7. They express appreciation and are generous with praise.
8. They have strong spiritual or religious convictions and commit themselves to a spiritual lifestyle, though they may not be affiliated with an organized church.
9. They recognize the needs of others, respect their differences, consider their feelings, and put themselves in the other person's shoes.
10. They are willing to grow, change, and work hard at their marriages. They know that a good relationship requires flexibility and effort to keep it alive.

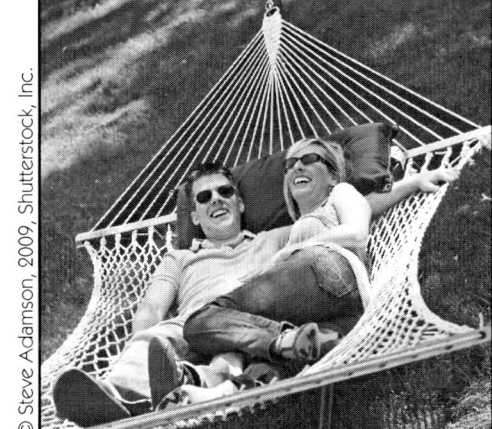

People in successful marriages are willing to grow, change, and work hard at their marriages. A good relationship requires flexibility and effort to keep it alive.

Unhealthy Relationships

As discussed earlier it takes a lot to have a healthy relationship. Many times there is a process of growing through unhealthy relationships in order to achieve your final goal. Some signs of an unhealthy relationship include (Kuriansky, 2002):

- You feel insecure and weak around each other.
- You suffer from low self-esteem as a result of what happens between you.
- You are dishonest with each other.
- You spend more time feeling hurt than feeling good about how you treat each other.
- You find yourself complaining to others about your relationship.
- You are unable to talk about your feelings or problems with your partner, much less solve them.
- You are unable to resolve your differences together.
- You become unenthusiastic about life because of what goes on between you.
- Your trust is irrevocably broken.
- Seemingly small things erode your relationship, like trickling water that wears away at a rock over time.
- Priorities other than each other constantly present themselves.
- What goes on between you interferes with other aspects of your life.

Abusive Relationships

Sometimes unhealthy relationships progress further into abusive relationships (see Table 7.2). This can be physical, emotional, or both in nature and typically cycles through repetitive phases. These phases include:

- **The honeymoon phase** may consist of flowers, apologies, and acting in a manner that originally attracted the abused to the abuser. This phase may last a day, a week, or sometimes longer.
- **The tension phase** typically builds slowly over time. This phase may consist of small insults that build into public humiliation and belittling.
- **The explosion phase** typically happens in the privacy of a home or away from witnesses. Behaviors during this phase can include but are not limited to hitting, throwing down stairs, rape, and in some cases death. This is a dangerous cycle with high stakes.

Table 7.2

Warning: This Relationship May Be Dangerous to Your Health

What you see:	What your partner says:
Blaming	"I love you, but you make me hit you."
Hypermasculine behavior	"I make all the decisions in this family."
Emotional abuse	"You are so stupid. I don't know why I married you."
Isolation	"I don't like your friend Linda, and I don't want you going to the store with her."
Intimidation	"Just like I kicked that dog, I can kick you."
Coercion and threats	"If you don't do what I say, I'll leave you. You can't make it without me."
Economic abuse	"You don't need to make any more money. I can give you what you need when you ask me for it."

Source: Floyd et al., 2007.

As mentioned earlier, this cycle typically continues to repeat itself many times with each cycle increasing in intensity.

When this happens, it is definitely time to get out of the relationship. Sometimes this is incredibly hard for the abused partner because their self-esteem is so low. They honestly feel the only person that would "put up" with them is their partner, so they feel very trapped. The abusing partner typically isolates their partner from friends and family over an extended period of time. This evolves into a very controlling and abusive relationship. Many times the abuser will threaten their partner's life if they try to leave. If this is the case, do not let your partner know you are thinking about leaving. Wait until you know your partner will be gone for an extended period of time and call someone whom your partner does not know for help. There are numerous help lines listed at the end of this chapter.

In some instances restraining orders are necessary to keep an individual from stalking or harassing. Be very careful in these situations because they can and have become life threatening. Remember that if you are in an abusive relationship more likely than not this individual will continue to abuse you until the relationship is over. Also, the abuse will typically escalate over time. The incidence of physical violence in college dating relationships is reported as 20 percent to 50 percent, varying from slapping and hitting to more life-threatening violence (Floyd et al., 2007).

ADDITIONAL READINGS

Berkowitz, B. and Gittines, R. *What Men Won't Tell You But Women Need to Know.* New York: Avon. 2008.

Botting, K. and Botting, D. *Sex Appeal—The Art and Science of Sexual Attraction.* New York: St. Martin's Press. 1995.

Carter, S. *Getting to Commitment.* New York: M. Evans and Co. 2000.

Glass, L. *Attracting Terrific People—How to Find and Keep the People Who Bring You Joy.* New York: St. Martin's Press. 1998.

Gray, J. *Men Are from Mars, Women Are from Venus.* New York: HarperCollins. 2004.

Tannen, D. *You Just Don't Understand: Women and Men in Conversation.* New York: William Morrow. 2001.

REFERENCES

Floyd, P. et al. *Personal Health: Perspectives & Lifestyles* (4th ed). Englewood, CO: Morton Publishing Co. 2007.

Godek, G. *Love: The Course They Forgot to Teach You in School.* Naperville, IL: Casablanca Press. 1997.

Kuriansky, J. *The Complete Idiot's Guide to a Healthy Relationship* (2nd ed). New York: Alpha Books. 2002.

Kuriansky, J. *The Complete Idiot's Guide to Dating* (3rd ed). New York: Alpha Books. 2003.

Lee, J. A. *Colours of love: an exploration of the ways of loving.* New York: New Press. 1973.

Sternberg, R. J. *The Triangle of Love: Intimacy, Passion, Commitment.* New York: Basic Books. 1988.

Strong, B. et al. *Human Sexuality: Diversity in Contemporary America* (6th ed). McGraw-Hill. 2006.

CONTACTS

American Association for Marriage and Family Therapy

202-452-0109

American Social Health Association
800-227-8922
www.ashastd.org

Christian Singles International
www.christiansinglesinternational.com

Family Violence Prevention Information
800-777-1960

Gay and Lesbian Medical Association
459 Fulton Street, Suite 107
San Francisco, CA 94102
415-255-4547
www.glma.org

National Domestic Violence Hotline
800-799-SAFE (7233)

National Victim Center
800-FYI-CALL

Parents, Families, and Friends of Lesbians and Gays (PFLAG)
1101 14th Street NW, Suite 1030
Washington, DC 20005
202-638-4200

TAMU Student Life Gender Issues Education Services (GIES)
979-845-1107
www.glbtpn.tamu.edu/resources.html

ACTIVITIES

In-Class Activities

Discussion questions:
- What do you value most in a friendship?
- What is the most mysterious thing about the opposite sex?
- What is the one thing that the opposite gender simply doesn't "get" about your gender?
- Describe your idea of a perfect date.
- Have you ever been infatuated? Describe the feeling. Describe the relationship.
- Have you ever been in love? Describe the feeling. Describe the relationship.

The "Perfect" Mate

Notebook Activities

Relationship Readiness Assessment for Singles
How Strong Is the Communication and Affection in Your Relationship?
Relationship Report Card
Interactive Relationship Assessment Scale
Are You in an Abusive Relationship?

Name: _____ Section: _____ Date: _____

IN-CLASS ACTIVITY

The "Perfect" Mate

Directions: In the space below, write down all the qualities of a "perfect" mate for you. Then go back over the list and write the codes that apply in the blank to the left.

Qualities of my "Perfect" Mate:

_____ 1.
_____ 2.
_____ 3.
_____ 4.
_____ 5.
_____ 6.
_____ 7.
_____ 8.
_____ 9.
_____ 10.
_____ 11.
_____ 12.
_____ 13.
_____ 14.
_____ 15.
_____ 16.
_____ 17.
_____ 18.
_____ 19.
_____ 20.

Codes:
D Your dad has this quality.
M Your mom has this quality.
+ You have this quality.
− You wish you had this quality.
B You think both partners need this quality to be happy.
* These are the three most important qualities.

Source: Copyright © 1993 by The Center for Applied Research in Education.

Name: _____ Section: _____ Date: _____

NOTEBOOK ACTIVITY

Relationship Readiness Assessment for Singles

www.relationshipcoachingnetwork.org

Many singles feel that they are ready for a committed relationship. Readiness is understanding the difference between recreational dating for fun and a committed long-term relationship. This assessment will help you begin to define what being "ready" means for you. Go to the www.relationshipcoaching-network.org website, and click on the statements which apply to you. At the end click on "Get Score."

- I have a vivid "vision" of what I want for my life and my relationship. ❏
- I am clear about my values and live by them. ❏
- I have clearly defined my life purpose and put it into action daily. ❏
- I know where and how I want to live. ❏
- I have written goals and an action plan to help me achieve my vision. ❏
- I am living my life fully and in alignment with my vision, values, and life purpose. ❏
- I know what I will not tolerate in a relationship and don't tolerate them. ❏
- I know what I can't live without in a relationship and don't settle for less. ❏
- I know what values I must share with a partner. ❏
- I have a written list of requirements and will not enter a relationship if even one is missing. ❏
- I know that only I can be responsible for my own life and success. ❏
- I am clear about what I need for a relationship to function for me on a daily basis. ❏
- I am clear about what I need emotionally to feel loved in a relationship. ❏
- I am clear about my boundaries and how to enforce them to get my needs met. ❏
- I ask for what I need and want, and take responsibility for the outcome. ❏
- I do not expect a relationship to meet all my needs and make me happy. ❏
- I have a support system to supplement meeting my social and emotional needs. ❏
- I have inner strength which helps me be self-reliant and proactive about my needs. ❏
- I understand what did and didn't work for me in previous relationships. ❏
- I understand which positive and negative relationship patterns I risk repeating. ❏
- I am aware of the traits that my parents exhibit that drive my partner choices. ❏
- I am aware of specific traits of my parents in myself. ❏
- I am aware of habits, patterns, and values I have inherited from my family. ❏
- I understand my past patterns of choosing partners. ❏
- I understand my past relationship attitudes, choices, and actions/behaviors. ❏
- I am clear about what personality traits and qualities I most value in a partner. ❏
- I am clear about what interests/activities I must share with a partner. ❏
- My past relationship experiences do not impact my present relationships. ❏
- I have forgiven my parents for my past and present unmet needs. ❏
- I have let go of relationships which are damaging to me. ❏
- I have forgiven people who have hurt me. ❏

Source: From Steele, David. *Conscious Dating: Finding the Love of Your Life in Today's World.* Campbell, CA: RCN Press, 2006. © 2006 by Relationship Coaching Institute, used with permission. www.relationshipcoachingnetwork.org

- I have sought forgiveness from people who I may have hurt. ❏
- I am able to forgive myself for my past mistakes. ❏
- I trust that everyone does the best they can at all times. ❏
- I am aware of, and own, my emotional issues when they arise in a relationship. ❏
- I do not gossip or talk about others. ❏
- I clearly communicate what I want and need; I don't make people guess. ❏
- I deal positively with misunderstandings and disagreements when they occur. ❏
- I own my judgments and accept differences with others. ❏
- I do not get defensive and "take personally" the things that people say about me. ❏
- I make requests rather than complain. ❏
- I regularly practice active listening, give validation, and express appreciation. ❏
- I am careful about what I promise and keep my word. ❏
- I am aware of how I come across and affect others. ❏
- I am surrounded by caring people. ❏
- I add value to everyone in my community. ❏
- I spend my social time with healthy, happy, able people. ❏
- I have positive relationships with my parents, siblings, children, and ex. ❏
- I have a close circle of friends and we gather regularly. ❏
- I take extraordinary care of the people I have chosen to love. ❏
- I am a member of two or more communities (hobbies, spiritual, professional, etc.) ❏
- I am satisfied with my work/career. ❏
- I support my present lifestyle and am preparing for my future security. ❏
- I have no financial or legal problems. ❏
- I am happy and successful being single. ❏
- I am living the life that I want as a single person. ❏
- I am ready and available for commitment. ❏
- I am healthy in mind, spirit, and body. ❏
- I take initiative and responsibility for choosing who I want in my life and don't wait to be chosen. ❏
- I have clearly defined guidelines for sexual involvement that I adhere to. ❏
- I am authentic and do not try to make myself more appealing to attract a partner. ❏
- I am able to communicate my issues and needs to dating partners. ❏
- I balance my heart with my head and make careful relationship choices. ❏
- I do not interpret infatuation, attraction, attachment, and/or good sex as "love". ❏
- I do not expect a relationship to "rescue" me from emotional or financial problems. ❏
- I understand and use the "Law of Attraction" (like attracts like). ❏
- I scout, sort, and screen potential partners effectively. ❏
- I am clear whether I am seeking a short-term recreational relationship or am ready to seek a long-term committed relationship. ❏
- I effectively disengage from prospective partners who are not a fit for me. ❏
- I use my community support system to scout for me. ❏
- I am actively involved in activities and groups of people highly aligned with me. ❏
- I am balancing my partner search with investing in myself and living my vision. ❏

Get Score

Name: _____ Section: _____ Date: _____

NOTEBOOK ACTIVITY

Relationship Report Card

Grade yourself and your partner in twenty-five key relationship skills.

- A = Passionate, exciting, fulfilling; not perfect—but clearly excellent
- B = Very good, solid, better-than-most, consistent, improving
- C = Average, adequate, acceptable, okay, ho-hum, static
- D = Below average, dismal, unhappy, bad—but not hopeless
- F = Hopeless, dangerous; tried everything, didn't work

Description

The Relationship Report Card allows you to grade yourself and your partner on *a number of very specific skills* that contribute to successful relationships. It measures *actions,* not *emotions.* It is an exercise that will give you a realistic picture of how you act in your relationship. And by *comparing* how both you and your partner act in your relationship, it will give you insights into the dynamics of yourselves as a unique couple.

The Relationship Report Card measures *behavior,* not *character.* It is a technique for allowing you to focus on specific aspects of behavior, one-at-a-time. It does *not* judge *personality*! You're not a *bad person* if you have a C+ sense of humor; and you're not a *superior person* if you have A+ communication skills.

The goals of this exercise are: 1) to raise your awareness by giving you an objective look at how the two of you act as a couple, 2) to identify strengths and help you appreciate them, 3) to identify areas that need improvement, 4) to help your partner see you as you perceive yourself, 5) to help your partner see himself or herself as you see him or her, 6) to help you see your partner as he or she perceives himself or herself, and 7) to help you see yourself through your partner's eyes.

Instructions

- Each of you grades yourself and your partner.
- While grading, ask yourself, "How well do I (or my partner) exemplify/act on this particular skill?"
- Regarding choosing grades: Your first inclination is probably the right one. Rely more on your intuitive side—your gut reaction—than on your analytical side.
- Use "pluses" and "minuses" to fine-tune your grading. (A "B" is clearly a "B"—but a "B+" is nearly an "A"!)
- During the grading process, don't talk about the grades you're giving. You may talk about the process, but don't share your grades until later.
- Customize the Relationship Report Card. There are blanks at the bottom of the form where you can add topics and skills that you consider to be important.
- Most people take six to ten minutes to complete the grading process. (Although some folks fly through it in sixty seconds, and others ponder it for half an hour!)

Source: Copyright © 1997 by Gregory J.P. Godek. Reprinted from the book *Love: The Course They Forgot to Teach You in School* with permission of its publisher, Sourcebooks, Inc. (800-432-7444). This is a tool for increasing awareness, not a validated psychological test.

- Note: The goal is not to get "straight A's." We all have a wide variety of characteristics, strengths, and weaknesses. The goal is to improve, not to be perfect!
- When you have both completed the grading process, compare your grades. Start at the top of the list, and share the grades you gave yourself and your partner.
- For each skill, discuss the discrepancies between how you graded yourself compared to how your partner graded you.
- Some questions to consider: What was your reasoning behind various grades? Are you satisfied, dissatisfied, happy, embarrassed, or proud of your grades? What might you do to get a better grade? What kind of help can you offer your partner?

Name: _____ Section: _____ Date: _____

NOTEBOOK ACTIVITY

Relationship Report Card

Grade yourself—and your partner—using the school-type evaluation of A+ through F.

Relationship skill	Grade yourself	Grade your partner
❑ Affection	_____	_____
❑ Arguing skills	_____	_____
❑ Attitude	_____	_____
❑ Commitment	_____	_____
❑ Communication	_____	_____
❑ Considerateness	_____	_____
❑ Couple thinking	_____	_____
❑ Creativity	_____	_____
❑ Financial responsibility	_____	_____
❑ Flexibility	_____	_____
❑ Generosity	_____	_____
❑ Gift-giving	_____	_____
❑ Honesty	_____	_____
❑ Household management	_____	_____
❑ Listening skills	_____	_____
❑ Lovemaking	_____	_____
❑ Patience	_____	_____
❑ Playfulness	_____	_____
❑ Romance	_____	_____
❑ Self-awareness	_____	_____
❑ Self-esteem	_____	_____
❑ Sense of humor	_____	_____
❑ Sensitivity	_____	_____
❑ Spontaneity	_____	_____
❑ _____		
❑ _____		
❑ _____		
❑ _____		
❑ _____		

Name: _____ Section: _____ Date: _____

NOTEBOOK ACTIVITY

Interactive Relationship Assessment Scale

www.selfcounseling.com

Answer all questions. Circle the number which best represents your situation or answer, and then click the score button to see your results.

1. How well does your partner meet your needs?

1	2	3	4	5
Poorly		Average		Very Good

2. In general, how satisfied are you with your relationship?

1	2	3	4	5
Unsatisfied		Average		Very Satisfied

3. How good is your relationship compared to most?

1	2	3	4	5
Poor		Average		Excellent

4. How often do you wish you hadn't gotten in this relationship?

1	2	3	4	5
Very often		Average		Never

5. To what extent has your relationship met your original expectations?

1	2	3	4	5
Hardly at all		Average		Completely

6. How much do you love your partner?

1	2	3	4	5
Not much		Average		Very much

7. How many problems are there in your relationship?

1	2	3	4	5
Very many		Average		Very few

Total Score _____

A total score of 7 indicates low satisfaction, and a score of 35 indicates high satisfaction. If you scored in the 7–14 range, you might want to consider consulting a counselor about your relationship.

Source: www.selfcounseling.com

Name: _____ Section: _____ Date: _____

NOTEBOOK ACTIVITY

Are You in an Abusive Relationship?

Check any of the questions below to which you can truthfully answer "yes."

_____ Are you afraid of your partner?

_____ Does your partner monitor your comings and goings?

_____ Does your partner control who you can and cannot talk to?

_____ Are you forced to have sex against your will?

_____ Are you told what you can and cannot wear?

_____ Are you verbally or physically abused for looking at another man (woman)?

_____ Has your partner threatened to harm your children?

A "yes" response to any of these questions signals trouble and the need to get help.

Source: Dr. Carolyn Ramsey, in an article by Laura B. Randolph, "Battered Women: How to Get and Give Help," *Ebony,* September, 1994.

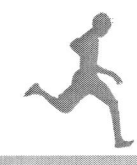

CHAPTER 8

Sexuality

"A healthy attitude is contagious but don't wait to catch it from others. Be a carrier."

—Source Unknown

OBJECTIVES

Students will be able to:
- Identify structures of the female and male sexual anatomy.
- Describe the stages of the menstrual cycle and pregnancy.
- Explain the benefits and drawbacks of each barrier method and hormonal method of pregnancy prevention.
- Identify the options in the case of an unplanned pregnancy.
- Identify and discuss the following issues concerning sexually transmitted infections: transmission, prevention, type, vaccines, asymptomatic infections, treatment, and consequences if left untreated.
- Discuss the influence the media have on attitudes and beliefs about relationships and sexuality.

The purpose of this chapter is to familiarize students with the female and male anatomy and gender-specific cycles. Information will be presented on parenthood and the options that exist when pregnancy prevention is not effective. Additional material will be presented detailing various sexually transmitted infections (STIs), the health risks associated with contraction of STIs, and various preventative measures and techniques in sexually transmitted infections and pregnancy.

Anatomy

Female Sexual Anatomy

The female anatomy consists of multiple integral parts both externally and internally (see Figure 8.1). The **vulva** includes visible external genitalia. The **mons pubis** is the soft fatty tissue covering the pubic symphysis (joint of the pubic bones). This area is covered with pubic hair that begins growing during puberty. The **labia majora** include two longitudinal folds of skin that extend on both sides of the vulva and serve as protection for the inner parts of the vulva. The **labia minora** are the delicate inner folds of skin that enclose the urethral opening and the vagina. These skin flaps, which contain sweat and oil glands, extensive blood vessels, and nerve endings, are hairless and sensitive to touch. When sexually stimulated, the labia minora swell and darken. The **clitoris** is usually the most sensitive part of the female genitalia. The clitoris consists of erectile tissue, which becomes engorged with blood, resulting in swelling during sexual arousal that enables it to double in size. The **clitoral hood** consists of inner lips, which join to form a soft fold of skin, or hood, covering and connecting to the clitoris. The **urethra** is approximately 2.5 cm below the clitoris and functions as the opening for urine to be excreted from the bladder. Because the urethra is located close to the vaginal opening, some irritation may result from vigorous or prolonged sexual activity. The most common problem

FIGURE 8.1

The Human Female Reproductive System

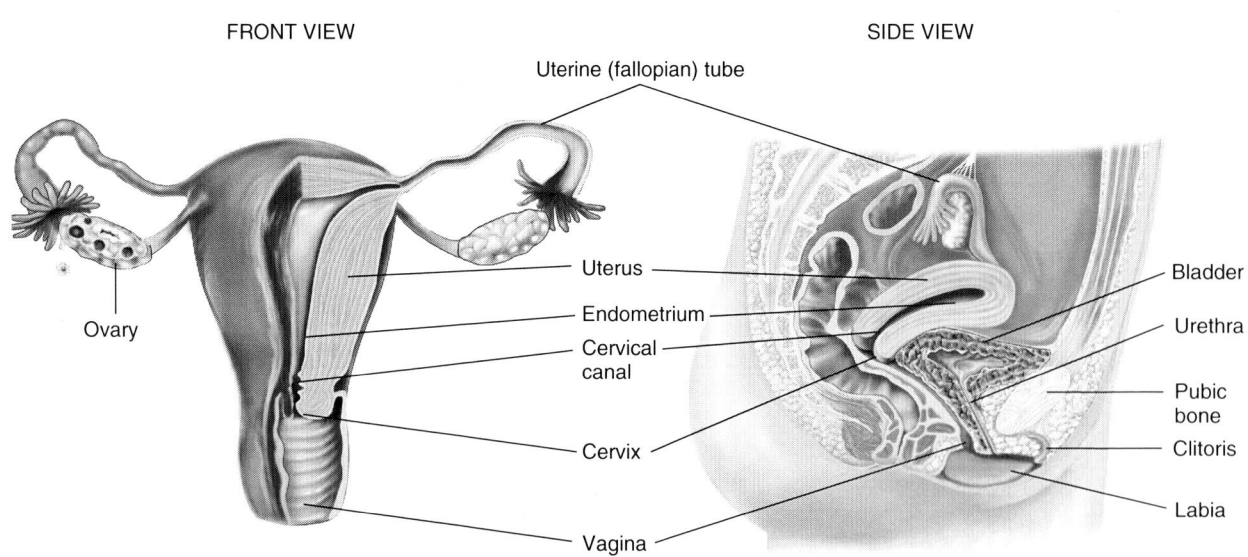

Source: From *Biology: Understanding Life* by Alters and Alters, © 2006 by Alters and Alters. Reproduced with permission of John Wiley & Sons, Inc.

associated with this is the development of urinary tract infections. The **vagina** is located between the urethral opening and the anus. The **hymen** is the small membrane around the vaginal opening that is believed to tear during initial intercourse, with tampon use, while riding a horse, or other various types of athletic activities. The only function of the hymen is to protect the vaginal tissues early in life. The **perineum** is the smooth skin located between the labia minora and the anus. During childbirth this area may tear or be cut (episiotomy) as the newborn passes out of the vagina. The **anal canal** is located just behind the perineum and allows for elimination of solid waste. The anal canal is approximately an inch long with two sphincter muscles, which open and close like valves.

Internally, just past the vagina, is the cervix, which connects the vagina and the uterus. The uterus is the hollow, pear-shaped muscular organ about the size of a fist when a female is not pregnant. This is the organ in which the fetus develops during pregnancy. The upper expanded portion is referred to as the fundus (see Figure 8.2), and the lower constricted part is the cervix. On each side of the uterus there is a **fallopian tube**, which is quite narrow and approximately four inches in length. Because of the narrow passageway within these tubes, infection and scarring may cause fertility problems. Most women have a right and a left fallopian tube. These tubes extend from the ovaries to the uterus and transport mature ovum. Fertilization usually takes place within the fallopian tubes. The opening between the fallopian tube and the uterus is only about as wide as a needle. On each end of the

FIGURE 8.2

An Anterior View of the Female Reproductive Organs Showing the Relationship of the Ovaries, Uterine Tubes, Uterus, Cervix, and Vagina

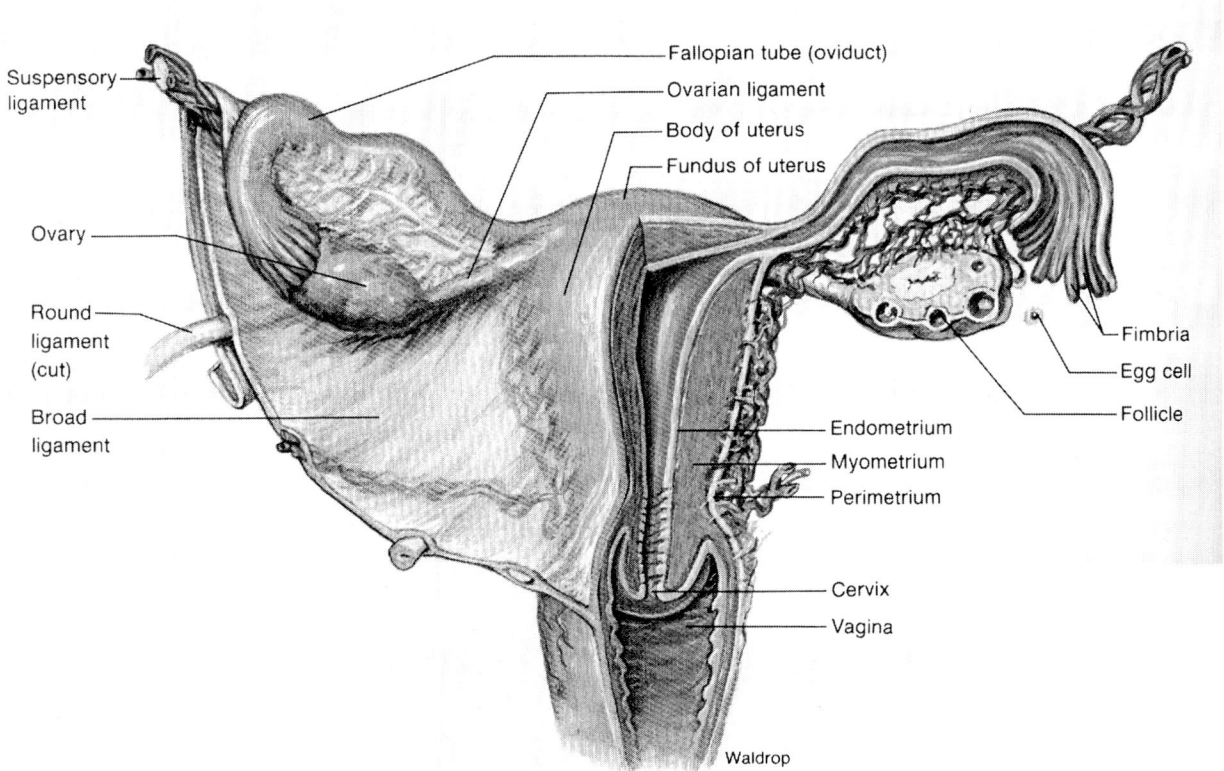

Source: From *Sexuality: Insights and Issues,* third edition. Copyright © 1993 by Jerrold Greenberg, Clint Buess, and Kathleen D. Mullen. Reprinted by permission of the authors.

fallopian tubes are the **ovaries**, where eggs are produced and released usually once a month. Each ovary is about the size of a large olive. At birth, a female's ovaries contain 40,000 to 400,000 immature ova, of which approximately 450 will mature and be released during the reproductive years. The ovaries also produce the hormones estrogen and progesterone, both of which help regulate the menstrual cycle (Crooks and Baur, 2007).

The female *sexual response* consists of four phases:

1. **Excitement:**
   Vaginal lubrication begins and the vagina, clitoris, labia majora and minora all fill with blood. The nipples swell, and there is increased tension in many voluntary muscles.

2. **Plateau:**
   The vaginal opening usually decreases in diameter due to swelling, the uterus usually increases in size, and the labia majora and minora become more swollen and engorged.

3. **Orgasm:** and
   The muscles of the vaginal wall undergo rhythmic contractions. The number of contractions may range from three to as many as twelve. Involuntary contraction of other muscles may take place as well.

4. **Resolution:**
   Blood rapidly returns to the rest of the body from the vagina, clitoris, labia majora, and minora, resulting in reduced swelling. At this time the breasts also return to their original size.

Male Sexual Anatomy

The external male sexual structures include the penis and scrotum. The **penis** is an organ through which semen and urine pass, and is structured into three main sections: the root, the shaft, and the glans penis (see Figure 8.3). The root attaches the penis within the pelvic cavity at the base, while the shaft, or the tube-shaped body of the penis, hangs freely. The **glans penis** is covered by a loose portion of tissue called the **foreskin**, which may be removed during a surgery known as circumcision. A penis without foreskin is circumcised, while one with the foreskin intact is uncircumcised. Uncircumcised men should gently pull the foreskin back when they bathe to wash the foreskin and tip of the penis. At the base of the glans is a rim known as the corona. On the underside is a triangular area of highly sensitive skin called the frenulum, which attaches the glans to the foreskin. The glans penis is the soft, fleshy, enlarged tissue at the end of the shaft, with the urethral opening at the tip. The **scrotum** is the pouch of skin, which hangs from the root of the penis and holds the two testicles. Covered sparsely with hair, the scrotum is divided in the middle by a ridge of skin, showing the separation of the testes. The surface changes of the scrotum help maintain a moderately constant temperature within the testes (~93 degrees F), which is important for maintaining good sperm production (Crooks and Baur, 2007).

The male internal sexual structures include the testes, epididymus, vas deferens, seminal vesicles, and prostate and Cowper's glands. The **testes** are the reproductive ball-shaped glands inside the scrotum, which are also referred to as testicles. Sperm and hormone production are the two main functions of the testes (Crooks and Baur, 2007). Sperm are formed constantly, beginning during puberty, inside the highly coiled thin tubes called seminiferous tubules within each testis. Between the seminiferous tubules are cells that produce sex hormones. One such important sex hormone is testosterone, which stimulates the production of sperm. On top of each testis is another tightly coiled tube, the **epididymis**, where nearly mature sperm complete

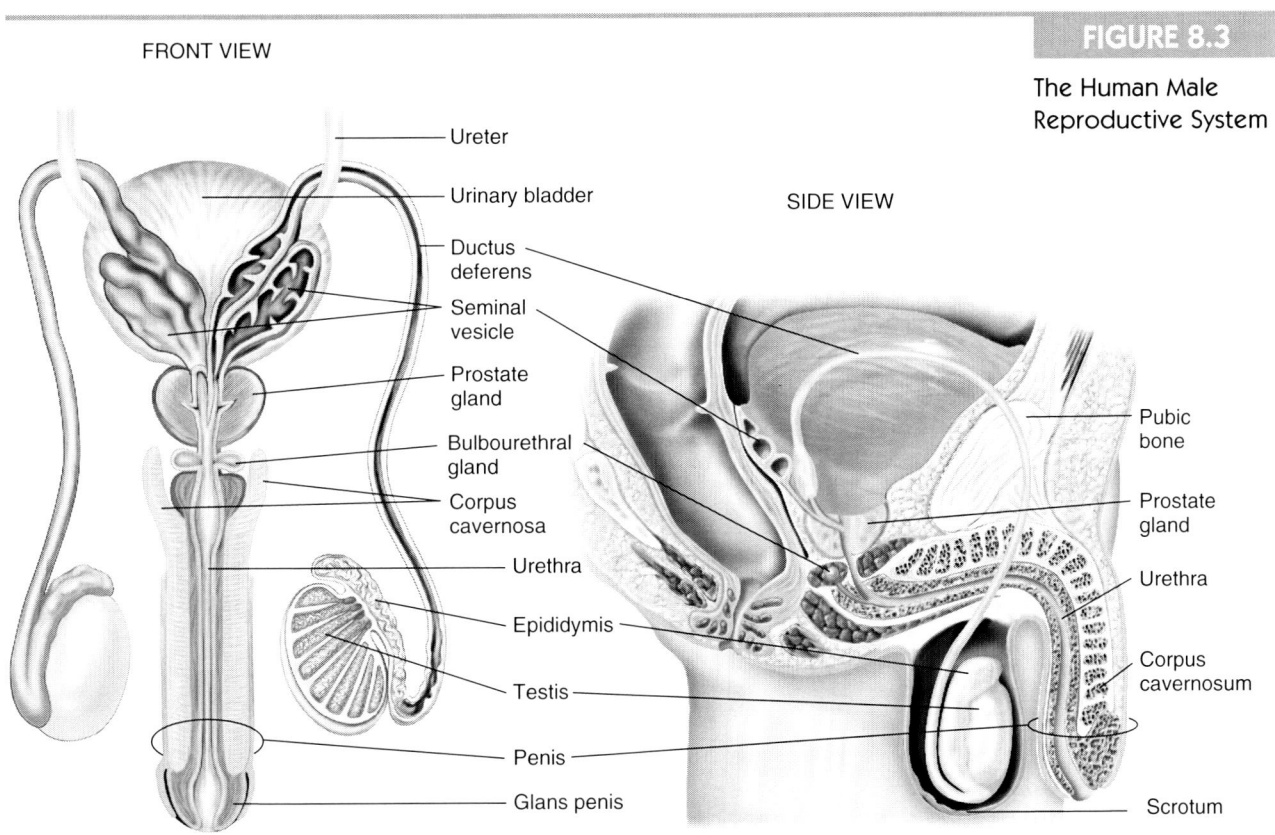

FIGURE 8.3

The Human Male Reproductive System

Source: From Biology: Understanding Life by Alters and Alters, © 2006 by Alters and Alters. Reproduced with permission of John Wiley & Sons, Inc.

the maturation process (Crooks and Baur, 2007). Mature sperm are stored in the epididymis until they are released during ejaculation. The **vas deferens** is a long tube through which sperm travel during ejaculation. The epididymis is connected to the **seminal vesicle** via the vas deferens, which is responsible for contracting and pushing the sperm to the seminal vesicle. Located beneath the bladder are the two small seminal vesicles, which secrete a fluid that provides nourishment as well as an environment conducive to sperm mobility. After the sperm have combined with the seminal fluid, they reach the prostate where another substance is added. A thin, milky fluid is produced by the prostate and secreted into the urethra during the time of emission of semen, which enhances the swimming environment for the sperm (Crooks and Baur, 2007). Below the prostate and attached to the urethra are the two pea-sized **Cowper's glands,** responsible for depositing a lubricating fluid for sperm and a coating for the urethra. If there are sperm in the urethra from a previous ejaculation, they will mix with the Cowper's fluid and become a pre-ejaculate lubricant fluid. Ejaculation occurs at peak sexual excitement when the prostate muscle opens and sends the seminal fluid to the urethra where it is then forced out through the urethral opening, forming semen.

Sperm facts:

- Sperm are produced at an average rate of 1,500 per second per testicle.
- It takes about one hundred days for sperm to mature.
- The average ejaculation contains about a teaspoon of semen and 200–500 million sperm.
- At least thirty-two different chemicals have been found in semen. They include more than twenty amino acids, glucose, citric acid, fructose, vitamin C, vitamin B12, zinc, potassium, calcium, and copper.

- The average time a sperm survives in the female reproductive tract is three to five days.
- Sperm can live in the man's body up to six weeks.
- Sperm that are not ejaculated get broken down and reabsorbed or are washed away in urine. (ETR Associates, 2007a)

The shaft of the penis can change dramatically during *sexual arousal*. During sexual excitement, tiny muscles inside the shaft tissue called corpus spongiosum and corpus cavernosa relax and open, allowing inflow of blood. As these tissues fill with blood, the penis becomes longer, thicker, and less flexible, resulting in an erection. Although sexual sensitivity is unique among individuals, the glans penis is particularly important in sexual arousal due to its high concentration of nerve endings. When a man is either sexually aroused or cold, the testes are pulled close to the body (Crooks and Baur, 2007).

Sexual Orientation

The components of sexuality are gender identity (biological gender, as determined by chromosomes and sexual organs), social sex role (adherence to cultural norms for feminine and masculine behavior), and sexual orientation. Sexual orientation is distinguished by emotional, romantic, sexual, or affectionate attraction to individuals of a particular gender. Sexual orientation often becomes apparent during puberty, when hormonal changes are taking place in the body. Three sexual orientations are commonly recognized:

1. "heterosexual," attraction to individuals of the opposite gender;
2. "homosexual," attraction to individuals of the same gender;
3. "bisexual," attraction to members of both genders.

Persons with a homosexual orientation are sometimes referred to as "gay" (both men and women) or "lesbian" (women only). Sexual orientation is different from sexual behavior because it refers to feelings and self-concept. Persons may or may not express their sexual orientation in their behaviors. Homosexual orientation is not limited to a particular type of person. Gay men and lesbians are of all ages, cultural backgrounds, races, religions, and nationalities.

Alfred Kinsey, a sex researcher in the mid-1900s, developed a 7-point continuum representing sexual orientation (see Figure 8.4). He used this scale to study the sexual behaviors and preferences of the American population. The scale ranges from 0 to 6, with 0 representing exclusive heterosexual behavior, 3 representing bisexual behavior, and 6 representing exclusive homosexual behavior. This scale recognizes that many individuals do not fit solely into one of the three previously described sexual orientations.

A term often witnessed in association with homosexuality is homophobia. In general, *phobia* means an irrational, excessive, or persistent fear of something or a particular situation. *Homophobia* is defined as irrational fear of homosexuals or homosexuality. An additional component of this definition, however, is hatred since many homophobic individuals express their emotions of fear in physically aggressive ways. Homophobic behaviors range from avoiding hugging same-gender friends to name-calling, as well as physical attacks. Homophobia can also be explained as a continuum,

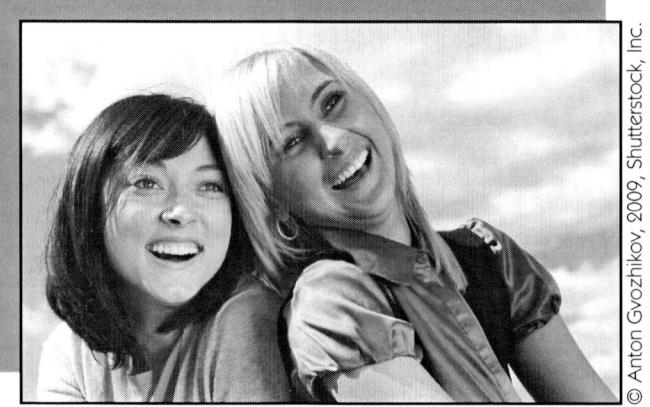

People may or may not express their sexual orientation in their behaviors.

FIGURE 8.4

Kinsey Scale of Sexual Behavior Kinsey believed that some people did not fit into strict same-gender or opposite-gender sexual behavior. His scale of sexual behavior reflects this belief.

0	1	2	3	4	5	6
Exclusive heterosexual experience	Heterosexual with incidental homosexual experience	Heterosexual with substantial homosexual experience	Equal heterosexual and homosexual experience	Homosexual with incidental heterosexual experience	Homosexual with substantial heterosexual experience	Exclusively homosexual experience

which at one end is described as feeling uncomfortable around a homosexual individual, the middle representing fear, and finally the other end of the continuum representing hatred. Homophobia has led to many discriminatory practices toward homosexuals in employment, housing, and insurance coverage, as well as in many other facets of life.

Readiness for Sexual Activity

Deciding whether you are ready for sexual activity is a very important and personal decision. It is a decision that has numerous physical, spiritual, and emotional implications and should not be taken lightly. Typically individuals have very different timelines at which they feel comfortable participating in different types of sexual activity. Different sexual activities include: vaginal/penal, anal/penal, oral/vaginal, or oral/penal intercourse. Some individuals consider themselves "virgins" if they have not had vaginal/penal intercourse, but have participated in other sexual activities. It is important to realize there are very real risks associated with all forms of sexual activity, which include and are not limited to sexually transmitted infections (STIs). It is also important that you decide what you would like out of a relationship and when you feel comfortable with beginning a specific sexual activity. Some individuals view sexual activity as a very casual event and others wait until they are married to participate in any sexual activity. When making this decision it is important that the individual has considered most if not all of the implications of their actions. Examples of these implications will be provided throughout this chapter.

One of the most important tools to use with your partner is communication. An individual must be able to talk openly and honestly to their prospective sexual partner about their wishes and beliefs on this subject. Talking can bring you closer because it develops a sense of trust. It can also help you learn more about your partner and remind both of you about the risks of sexual activity. The benefits of waiting include: more time to get to know your partner without the pressures sex can add to a relationship, freedom from worries about unplanned pregnancy and STIs, as well as building a stronger relationship based on friendship and trust, without the confusion sex can add (ETR Associates, 2007b). According to the 2007 Youth Risk Behavior Survey conducted by the CDC, the percentage of high school students who had ever had sexual intercourse decreased from 57.4 percent for males and 50.8 percent for females in 1991

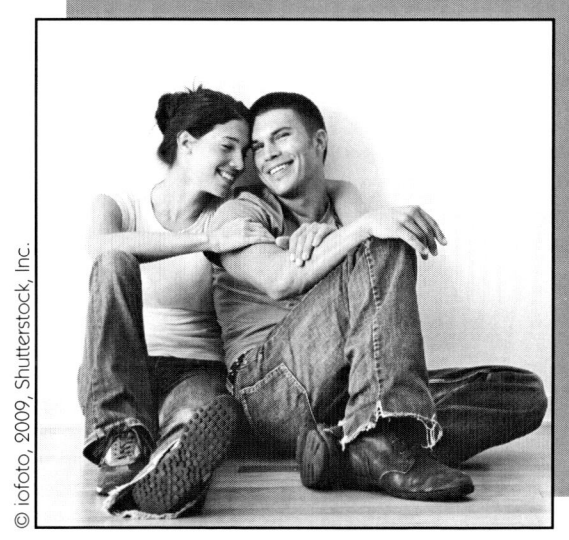

It is important to decide what you would like out of a relationship and if/when you feel comfortable beginning a specific sexual activity.

to 49.8 percent and 45.9 percent, respectively, in 2007. This decline has also decreased the number of teenage pregnancies, as well as the spread of STIs in this age group.

If you decide the time is right to become sexually active, you should stay informed about and decide which contraception method and STI protection makes sense for you and your partner. Think about how an unplanned pregnancy, STI, or a break-up would affect you and your long-term plans. Purchase some condoms. Learn the difference between "YES" and "NO". If you hear "no", "maybe", or if you hear nothing, STOP and talk to your partner. Always respect and adhere to what a person is saying. Make sure any "yes" is absolute and certain. Do not use mind-altering substances such as drugs and alcohol (including beer). These substances decrease your decision-making ability. This is problematic for using a condom consistently and correctly and for listening for the "yes" answer described above (ETR Associates, 2008).

Sex, Lies, and Condom Use

In a series of focus groups with 92 sexually active, young, ethnically and racially diverse individuals, aged 15 to 20, in five American cities, researchers focused on their views and motivations for sex and for condom use. Most found it difficult to believe that people their age used condoms every single time they had sex. Although they acknowledged that everyone is at risk for sexually transmitted diseases, the young people saw their own risk as minimal.

The genders had very different motives both for engaging in sex and for using condoms. In the interviews, young women said they engaged in sexual relations because of a desire for physical intimacy and a committed relationship. They generally reported having sex only with men they cared for and deeply trusted and expected that these men would be honest and forthright about their sexual history. This trust played a significant role in their decision whether to insist on condom use.

In contrast, few of the young men said "relationships" were an important dimension of their sexual involvements. Their primary motivation was a desire for physical and sexual satisfaction. Most said they were not interested in commitment and viewed emotional expectations as a complication of becoming sexually involved with a woman. The young men also admitted to making judgments about "types" of girls. To them, young women they didn't care about were "sluts" with whom they used a condom for their own protection.

Which partner determined whether a couple would use a condom? In these interviews, the answer was the women—if they chose to do so.

Regardless of race or ethnicity, many of the young women were adamant in demanding that their partners use condoms–and many young men said they would not challenge such a demand out of fear of losing the opportunity for sex. Men often expected potential partners to want to use condoms and described themselves as "suspicious" of women who did not.

Both sexes named two primary reasons for using condoms: preventing pregnancy and protecting against sexually transmitted diseases. Young women saw an unwanted pregnancy as an occurrence that would be disruptive, expensive, and could "ruin" their lives and their parents' lives. Young men saw condom use as a way of protecting themselves against emotional entanglements and paternity issues.

The young people were most strongly motivated to use condoms when they did not know a potential sexual partner well or were at the earliest states of sexual involvement with others. Nearly all said they solicited information about a potential partner's sexual history from this person or from friends. Rather than directly asking about the number of past partners, they more often relied on feelings and visual observations. Some admitted to lying when asked about their own sexual experience in order to avoid being seen as promiscuous. Once a couple had sex without a condom, both partners—but especially women—found it awkward to resume condom use because doing so would imply a lack of trust.

Source: "In the Heat of the Moment: A Qualitative Study on Motivating Condom Use Among Sexually Active Young People," prepared by Michaels Opinion Research for the Henry J. Kaiser Family Foundation, June 2001 with permission.

Reproduction

Menstrual Cycle

The menstrual cycle typically lasts twenty-eight days, with a range of twenty-five to forty days. Day one of the cycle is the first day of menstruation. The cycle ends with the next menstruation (see Figure 8.5). The follicular phase begins with menstruation and terminates when ovulation occurs. The follicular phase can be very unpredictable (typically fourteen days, but can be as little as ten or as long as twenty-five). Stress, illness, and many other factors can change when a female ovulates. This can cause problems when individuals are trying to control whether they become

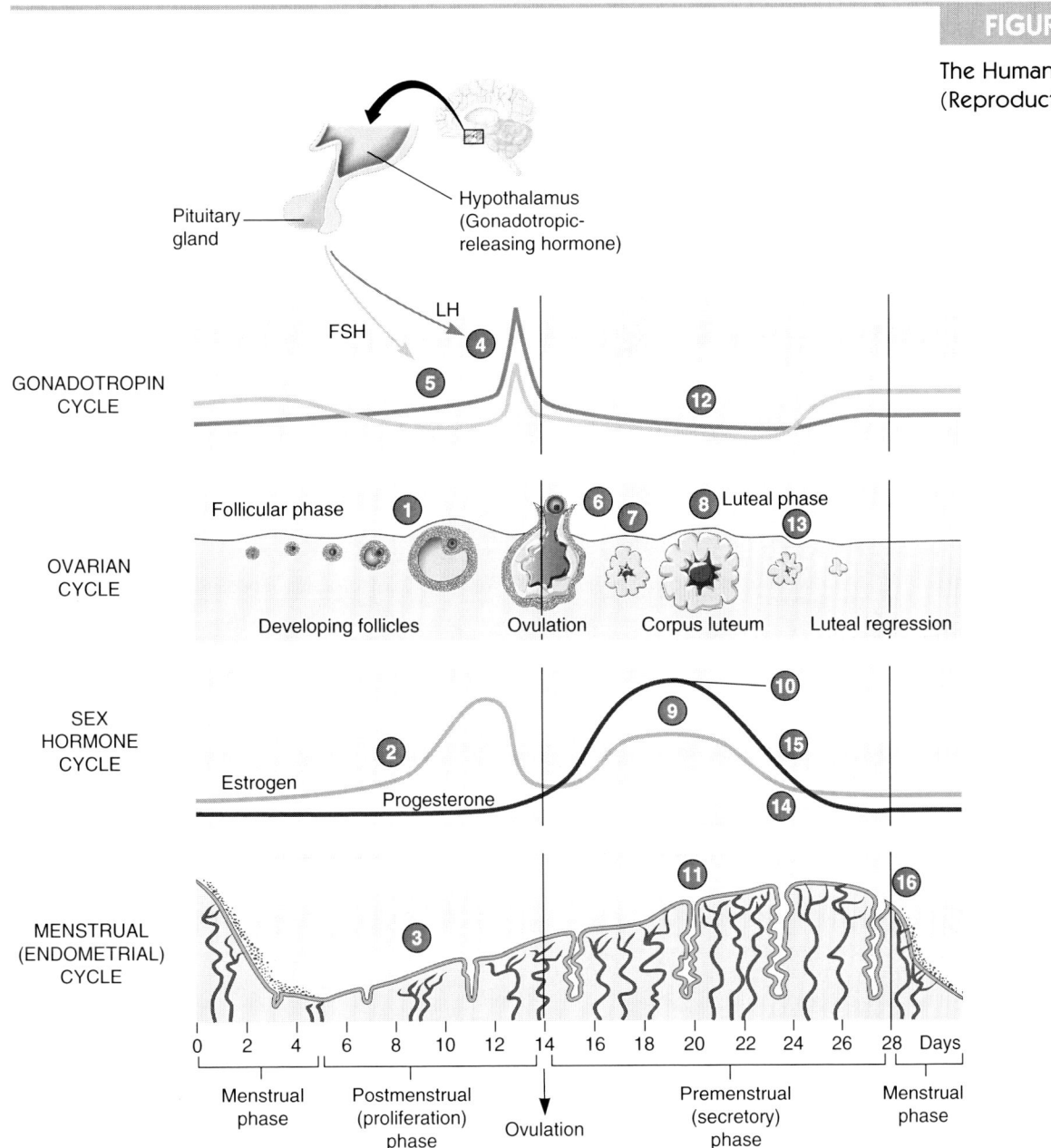

FIGURE 8.5

The Human Menstrual (Reproductive) Cycle

Source: From *Biology: Understanding Life* by Alters and Alters, © 2006 by Alters and Alters. Reproduced with permission of John Wiley & Sons, Inc.

pregnant or not. The length of the luteal phase is much more predictable (typically thirteen to fifteen days), beginning with ovulation and ending when the next menstrual cycle begins.

Premenstrual syndrome (PMS) can occur from one to ten days before a woman's period. This syndrome can consist of feeling bloated, diarrhea, nausea, backache, and/or cramping. Behaviors that can help ease PMS symptoms include:

- decrease salt and sugar intake,
- do not consume caffeine, and
- exercise regularly.

Ovarian Cycle

During the ovarian cycle immature eggs (follicles) are maturing and moving toward the surface of the ovary. The follicle and the ovarian surface open and allow the egg to float out. At the time of ovulation some women may feel a twinge or pain in the lower abdomen or back. After ovulation, the egg is swept into a fallopian tube (where fertilization typically occurs; see Figure 8.6) by fimbrae and the cilia (tiny hairs) and travels to the uterus. If the egg is not fertilized, it simply disintegrates or flows out with vaginal secretions, usually before menstruation. If the egg is fertilized, it will attach itself to the endometrium (internal lining of the uterus) in order to develop (see Figure 8.7).

Endometrial Cycle

The endometrial cycle consists of three phases:

1. the menstrual,
2. proliferative, and
3. progestational (secretory).

FIGURE 8.6

The Egg

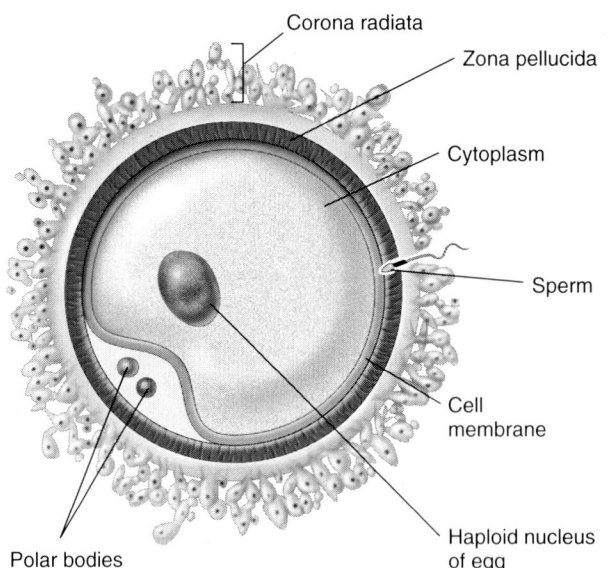

Source: Alters, Sandra, *Biology: Understanding Life*, 3rd Edition © 2000 Jones and Bartlett Publishers, Sudbury, MA. www.jbpup.com. Reprinted with permission.

FIGURE 8.7

From Fertilization to Implantation

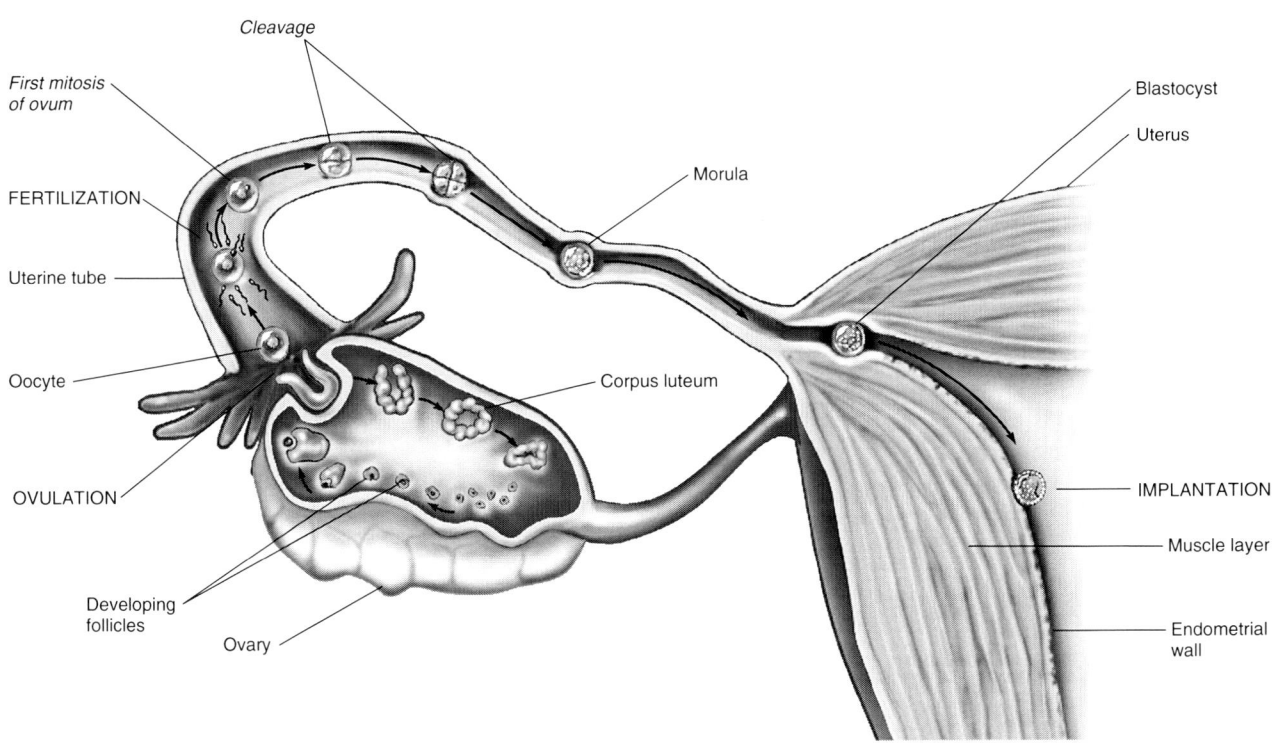

Source: From *Biology: Understanding Life* by Alters and Alters, © 2006 by Alters and Alters. Reproduced with permission of John Wiley & Sons, Inc.

The menstrual phase lasts approximately four to seven days, when the lining of the uterus is sloughed off and flows out of the uterus through the vagina, along with blood and other vaginal secretions. The proliferative phase lasts from the completion of the menstrual phase until a day or two after ovulation. During this time the endometrium is regenerating the layer that was sloughed off with new epithelial cells. During the progestational phase the endometrium becomes twice as thick as it did during the proliferative phase. It develops a cushion-like surface, thereby possessing the ability to nourish an implanted fertilized ovum. During the end of the progestational phase, if fertilization has not occurred, the endometrium begins to deteriorate. These phases repeat throughout the reproductive years until fertilization or menopause occurs.

Pregnancy

Pregnancy is usually divided into three trimesters, each of which last approximately three months or thirteen weeks (see Figure 8.8). Typically fertilization occurs twelve to eighteen days after the beginning of the menstrual cycle. There are many variables that can impact the timing of fertilization, including irregular periods, extreme exercise, illness, stress, a missed contraceptive pill, as well as many other factors. As soon as fertilization occurs the cells begin to divide and multiply. The fertilized egg implants in the uterus after approximately one week after fertilization. For most women the first sign(s) of pregnancy include a missed period, nausea, or excessive fatigue. Home pregnancy kits are 97–99 percent accurate if used

FIGURE 8.8

Prenatal Development of Fetus

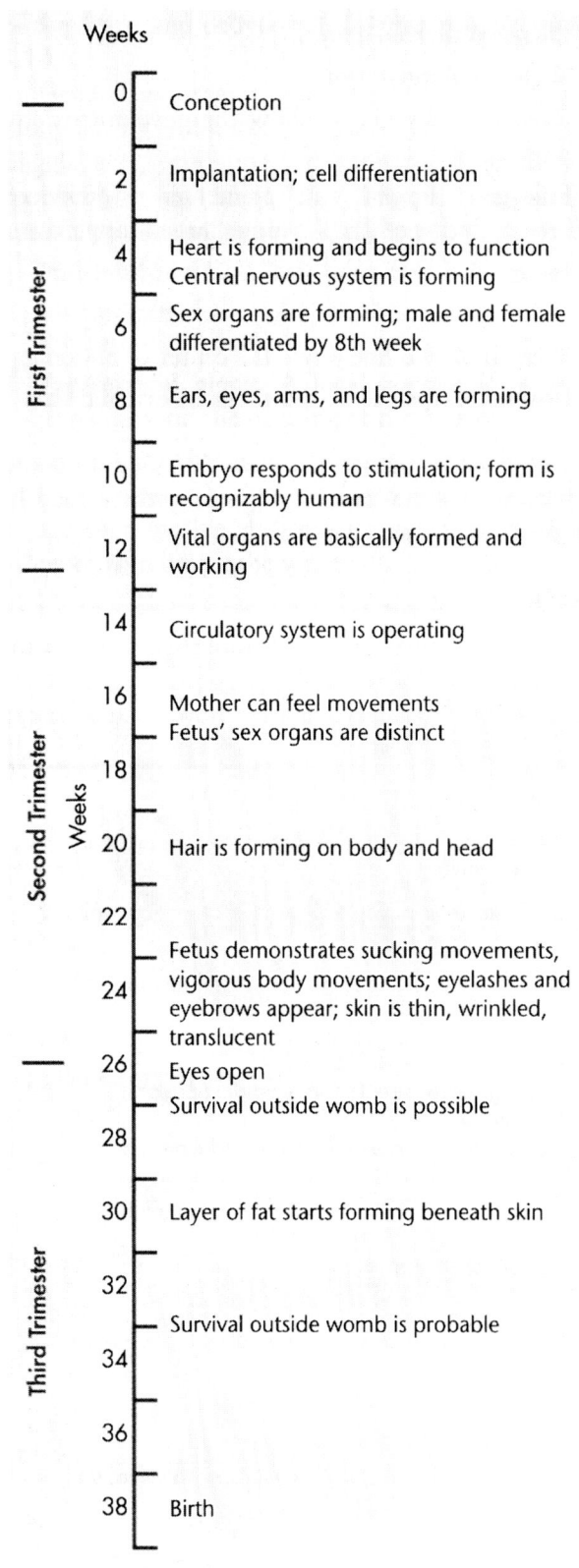

Source: From *Personal Health: Perspectives and Lifestyles* by Floyd et al. (2007).

correctly. These tests can detect human chorionic gonadotropin (HCG) within two to three weeks of fertilization. HCG is the hormone secreted by the placenta to help sustain the pregnancy for the first trimester. During the second and third trimesters the HCG levels decrease and the levels of estrogen and progesterone are sufficient to sustain the pregnancy to term. This is believed to be the reason morning sickness ends for most women after the first trimester. The embryo develops very rapidly during the first trimester. During these three months, all of the major organs are formed. Therefore, it is imperative to see a physician as soon as an individual thinks she may be pregnant to begin taking prenatal vitamins and change any habits that could be harmful to the developing embryo. The pregnancy is dated utilizing the first day of the last menstrual period (LMP). The heartbeat can be seen during a sonogram as early as the sixth or seventh week when the embryo is approximately 5 mm long. During the second and third trimesters the fetus is growing larger and stronger in preparation for delivery. Typically the mother will begin to feel the movements of the fetus between the sixteenth and twentieth weeks. This is referred to as "quickening." After an additional month or so, these movements can be felt externally by friends or family members. Thirty-six weeks is considered a full-term pregnancy, but typically delivery does not occur until around the fortieth week.

Sexually Transmitted Infections and Pregnancy

Sexually transmitted infections (STIs) can be passed from a pregnant woman to the baby before, during, or after the baby's birth. Syphilis can cross the placenta and infect the baby while it is in the uterus. Chlamydia, gonorrhea, genital herpes, and hepatitis B can be transmitted from the mother to the baby during delivery as the baby passes through the birth canal. HIV can cross the placenta during pregnancy, during the delivery, and can infect the baby through breast milk. If an STI is transmitted, it can result in stillbirth, low birth weight (less than five pounds), conjunctivitis, pneumonia, infection of the baby's blood stream, neurological damage, blindness, deafness, acute hepatitis, meningitis, chronic liver disease, and cirrhosis. Most of these can be prevented if the mother receives routine prenatal care, including screening tests for STIs. The CDC *Guidelines for Treatment of Sexually Transmitted Infections* (2006a) recommend that pregnant women be screened on their first prenatal visit for STIs, which may include: chlamydia, gonorrhea, syphilis, hepatitis B and C, and HIV. Chlamydia, gonorrhea, and syphilis can be treated and cured with antibiotics during pregnancy. There is no cure for most viral STIs, such as genital herpes and HIV. Below is a list of annual occurrences of specific STIs and the estimated number of pregnant women who are infected in the United States:

STIs	Estimated Number of Pregnant Women
Herpes	880,000
Chlamydia	100,000
Gonorrhea	13,200
Hepatitis B	16,000
HIV	6,400
Syphilis	<1,000

(CDC, 2008)

Pregnancy Prevention

Abstinence from Penile/Vaginal Intercourse

Effectiveness:
- in preventing pregnancy: 100 percent
- in preventing STIs—100 percent

Advantages:
- No worries
- No medical or hormonal side effects
- Protects against unwanted pregnancy

Disadvantages:
- Very few people choose lifetime celibacy or abstinence from sexual intercourse.
- People often forget to protect themselves against pregnancy or STIs when they stop abstaining.

Withdrawal Method

The man will pull his penis out of the vagina before he ejaculates to keep sperm from joining an egg.

Effectiveness:
- in preventing pregnancy: 73–96 percent
- in preventing STIs—NONE

Advantage:
- Can be used when no other method is available

Disadvantages:
- Requires great self-control, experience, and trust
- Not for men who ejaculate prematurely
- Not for men who do not know when to pull out
- Not recommended for teenagers

Fertility Awareness-based Methods (FAMs)
- A woman must chart her menstrual cycle and must be able to detect certain physical signs in order to predict "unsafe" days.
- She must abstain from intercourse or use barrier contraceptives during nine or more "unsafe" days each menstrual cycle.
- Check temperature daily. Before ovulation waking temperatures remain low, after ovulation temperatures rise until the next menstrual cycle begins.
- Check cervical mucus daily. Before ovulation the mucus is wet and similar to a raw egg white, after ovulation the cervical fluid dries up quickly.
- Record menstrual cycles on calendar to determine if she has regular or irregular cycles. This method is more effective for those with regular menstrual cycles.
- Remember that the sperm can live up to 120 hours after ejaculation. If a female ovulates within 120 hours after unprotected sexual intercourse the possibility of pregnancy exists.

*More specific information can be found at www.birth-control-comparison.info/fam.htm

Effectiveness:
- in preventing pregnancy: 75–99 percent
- in preventing STIs—NONE

Advantages:
- No medical or hormonal side effects
- Calendars, thermometers, and charts are easy to obtain

Disadvantages:
- Requires expert training before effective use
- Taking risks during "unsafe" days
- Poor record keeping
- Illness and lack of sleep affect body temperatures
- Vaginal infections and douches change mucus
- Cannot use with irregular periods or temperature patterns

Male Condom

The male condom is a latex sheath, placed over the penis prior to intercourse (see Figure 8.9).

Effectiveness:
- in preventing pregnancy: 83–98 percent
- in preventing STIs—85–98 percent

FIGURE 8.9
Using a Condom

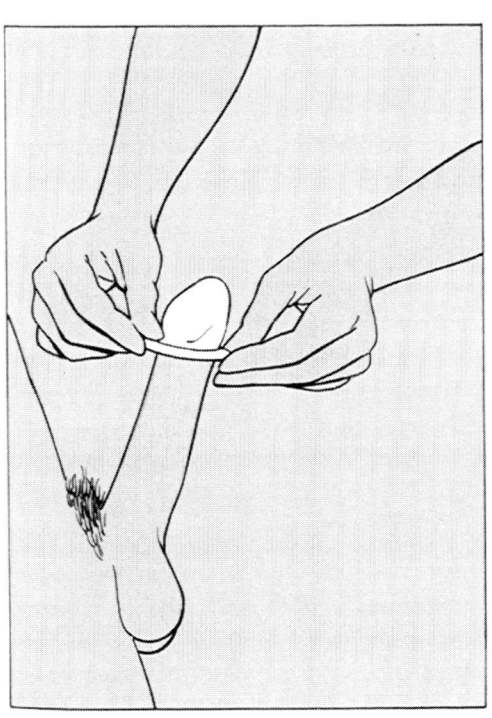

(a) The wrong way

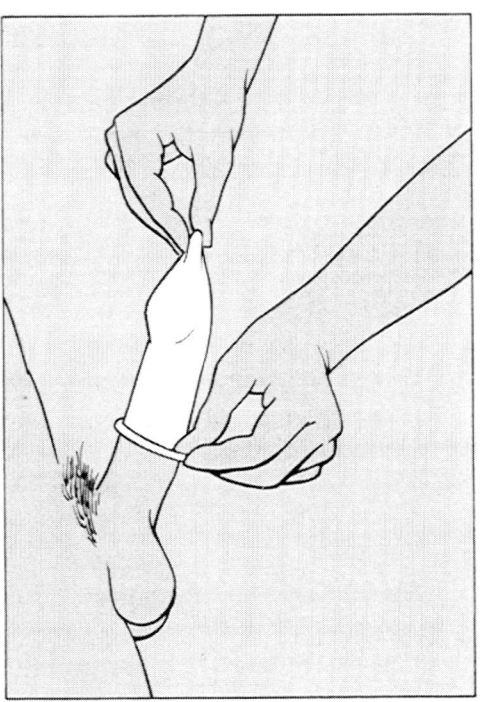

(b) The right way: Pinch the top of the condom, leaving 1/2 inch at the top to catch the semen; hold the tip of the condom and unroll the condom until it reaches the pubic hair.

Source: From *Sexuality: Insights and Issues,* third edition. Copyright © 1993 by Jerrold Greenberg, Clint Buess, and Kathleen D. Mullen. Reprinted by permission of the authors.

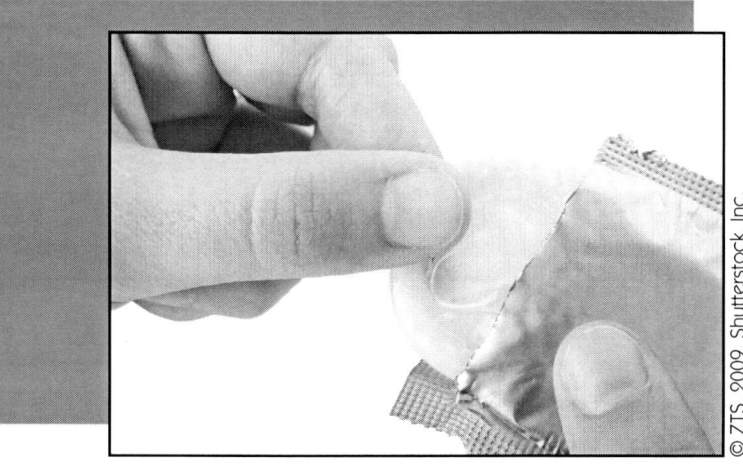
Other than abstinence, use of a condom is the most effective way to prevent STIs.

To increase pregnancy prevention effectiveness also use spermicide or have female utilize another form of contraception.

Do not use oil-based lubricants such as Vaseline or lotion, which will cause the condom to break. Use only water-based lubricants such as KY jelly once the condom is on the penis.

Advantages:

- Most effective way to prevent STIs besides abstinence
- Easy to buy (inexpensive)
- Easy to carry
- Only way for male to protect himself from unplanned pregnancy
- Can help relieve premature ejaculation

Problems:

- Possible allergies to latex
- Less sensation
- Condom breakage
- Sometimes interrupts "the mood"
- Human error: withdrawal without holding the condom in place; using after the expiration date; opening the package with teeth, fingernails, or sharp objects can damage the condom; storage of condoms in a warm place such as a wallet in a back pocket can decrease effectiveness.

The Pill

The pill (oral contraceptive pills) is a prescription medication containing the hormones estrogen and/or progesterone, which usually prevent the release of the egg, thickens the cervical mucus, and reduces the buildup of the endometrial lining within the uterus. The sperm is thus unable to penetrate the egg, and/or the fertilized egg is prevented from implanting in the uterus.

Effectiveness:

- in preventing pregnancy: 92–99.7 percent
- in preventing STIs—NONE

Advantages:

- Nothing to put into place before intercourse
- Regular and shorter periods
- Decreases chances of developing ovarian and endometrial cancers, non-cancerous breast tumors, ovarian cysts, pelvic inflammatory disease, and osteoporosis
- Decreased incidence of tubal pregnancies
- Ability to become pregnant returns quickly when use is stopped

Disadvantages:

- Less effective when taken with some drugs
- Must be taken daily (within the same two hour period)

- Rare but serious health risks, including: blood clots, heart attack, and stroke, which are more common for women over 35 and/or who smoke cigarettes (ARHP, 2008). This increased risk is found in most of the hormonal contraceptive methods. This is due to an increased correlation of cardiovascular disease most likely from the formation of atherosclerosis in women who smoke and use hormonal contraceptive methods. This risk also increases as women age, smoke, and use hormonal contraceptive methods.
- Side effects can include temporary irregular bleeding, weight gain, breast tenderness, and nausea.

Women who experience any of the following symptoms while taking the pill should call their physician immediately:

- Abdominal pains (severe)
- Chest pain or shortness of breath
- Headaches (severe)
- Eye problems, such as blurred vision
- Severe leg or arm pain or numbness
(http://www.fwhc.org/birth-control/thepill.htm)

Mini-pills

Mini-pills (oral contraceptive pills) are a prescription medication containing progesterone only, which usually prevents the release of the egg, thickens the cervical mucus, and reduces the buildup of the endometrial lining within the uterus. The sperm is thus unable to penetrate the egg, and/or the fertilized egg is prevented from implanting in the uterus.

Effectiveness:

- in preventing pregnancy: 87–99.7 percent (slightly less than regular birth control pills)
- in preventing STIs—NONE

Advantages:

- Nothing to put into place before intercourse
- Avoids typical side effects of regular birth control pills
- Has no estrogen
- Ability to become pregnant returns quickly when use is stopped

Disadvantages:

- Less effective when taken with some drugs
- MUST be taken at the same time every day
- Increased risk of ectopic pregnancy
- Increased risk of functional ovarian cysts

Vaginal Ring

The female will insert a small, flexible ring deep into the vagina for three weeks and take it out for the fourth week. It releases combined hormones that protect against pregnancy for one month. The ring uses hormones similar to the estrogen and progesterone made by a woman's ovaries to prevent the ovaries from releasing an egg, thickens the cervical mucus, and reduces the buildup of the endometrial lining within the uterus. The sperm is thus unable to penetrate the egg, and/or the fertilized egg is prevented from implanting in the uterus.

Effectiveness:
- in preventing pregnancy: 92–99.7 percent
- in preventing STIs—NONE

Advantages:
- Protects against pregnancy for one month
- No pill to take daily
- Does not require a "fitting" by a clinician
- Does not require the use of spermicide
- Ability to become pregnant returns quickly when use is stopped
- Nothing to put into place before intercourse
- More regular and shorter periods
- Reduces the risk of ovarian and endometrial cancers, pelvic inflammatory disease, non-cancerous growths of the breasts, ovarian cysts, and osteoporosis
- Fewer occurrences of ectopic pregnancy

Disadvantages:
- Increased vaginal discharge
- Vaginal irritation or infection
- Cannot use a diaphragm or cap for a backup method of birth control
- Rare but serious health risks, including blood clots, heart attack, and stroke—women who are 35 and older and/or smoke are at a greater risk. This increased risk is found in most of the hormonal contraceptive methods. This is due to an increased correlation of cardiovascular disease most likely from the formation of atherosclerosis in women who smoke and use hormonal contraceptive methods. This risk also increases as women age, smoke, and use hormonal contraceptive methods.
- Temporary irregular bleeding, weight gain, breast tenderness, and nausea

Women who experience any of the following symptoms while using the ring should call their physician immediately:
- Abdominal pains (severe)
- Chest pain or shortness of breath
- Headaches (severe)
- Eye problems, such as blurred vision
- Severe leg or arm pain or numbness
  (http://www.fwhc.org/birth-control/vaginal-ring.htm)

Contraceptive Patch
The female will place a thin plastic patch on the skin of the buttocks, stomach, upper outer arm, or upper torso once a week for three weeks in a row. Use a new patch each week. Do not use a patch for the fourth week. The patch releases combined hormones that protect against pregnancy for one month. The patch uses hormones similar to the estrogen and progesterone made by a woman's ovaries to prevent the ovaries from releasing an egg, thickens the cervical mucus, and reduces the buildup of the endometrial lining within the uterus. The sperm is thus unable to penetrate the egg, and/or the fertilized egg is prevented from implanting in the uterus.

Effectiveness:
- in preventing pregnancy: 99 percent (for women who weigh 197 pounds or less) 92 percent (for women who weigh 198 pounds or more)
- in preventing STIs—NONE

Advantages:
- Protects against pregnancy for one month
- No pill to take daily
- Nothing to put into place before intercourse
- Ability to become pregnant returns quickly when use is stopped
- More regular and shorter periods
- Reduce the risk of ovarian and endometrial cancers, pelvic inflammatory disease, non-cancerous growths of the breasts, ovarian cysts, and osteoporosis
- Fewer occurrences of ectopic pregnancy

Disadvantages:
- Skin reaction at the site of application
- Menstrual cramps
- May not be effective for women who weigh more than 198 pounds
- Rare but serious health risks, including blood clots, heart attack, and stroke—women who are 35 and older and/or smoke are at a greater risk. This increased risk is found in most of the hormonal contraceptive methods. This is due to an increased correlation of cardiovascular disease most likely from the formation of atherosclerosis in women who smoke and use hormonal contraceptive methods. This risk also increases as women age, smoke, and use hormonal contraceptive methods.
- Temporary irregular bleeding, weight gain, breast tenderness, and nausea

Some women may not be able to use contraceptive patches because of the risk of serious health problems. Women over 35 who smoke or have any of the following conditions should not use the patch:

- History of heart attack or stroke
- Chest pain
- Blood clots
- Unexplained vaginal bleeding
- Severe high blood pressure
- Diabetes with kidney, eye, nerve, or blood vessel complications
- Known or suspected cancer
- Known or suspected pregnancy
- Liver tumors or liver disease
- Headaches with neurological symptoms
- Hepatitis or jaundice
- Disease of the heart valves with complications
- Require long bed rest following surgery
- Allergic reaction to the patch

Women who have a family history of breast cancer, diabetes, high blood pressure, high cholesterol, headaches or epilepsy, depression, gallbladder disease, kidney disease, heart disease, irregular periods, or are breast-feeding may not be able to use the patch.

Women who experience any of the following symptoms while using the contraceptive patch should call their physician immediately:

- Abdominal pains (severe)
- Chest pain or shortness of breath
- Headaches (severe)
- Eye problems, such as blurred vision
- Severe leg or arm pain or numbness
  (http://www.fwhc.org/birth-control/patch.htm)

Depo-Provera
Depo-Provera is a hormone shot injected into the arm or buttocks every twelve weeks, which will prevent the release of the egg, less often thickens the cervical mucus and reduces the build up of the endometrial lining within the uterus thereby preventing conception, and/or the fertilized egg from implanting in the uterus.

Effectiveness:

- in preventing pregnancy: 97–99.7 percent
- in preventing STIs—NONE

Advantages:

- Protects against pregnancy for twelve weeks
- No daily pill
- Nothing to put into place before intercourse
- Can be used by some women who cannot take the pill (oral contraceptive)
- Decreases incidence of endometrial and ovarian cancer, as well as iron deficiency anemia (ARHP, 2008)
- Can be used while breast-feeding

Disadvantages:

- Studies released in 2004 show that Depo-Provera is associated with a loss of bone density resulting in an increased risk of osteoporosis. The bone loss appears not to be reversed when the woman stops the Depo-Provera injections (U.S. Department of Health and Human Services).
- Side effects include irregular bleeding, headaches, depression, nausea, loss of monthly period, weight gain, nervousness, and dizziness
- Side effects cannot be reversed until medication wears off (up to twelve weeks)
- May cause delay in getting pregnant after shots are stopped (up to twelve to eighteen months)
- Should not be used continuously for more than two years

Diaphragm and Femcap
Latex cup (diaphragm) or silicone cup (Femcap) requires fitting by a clinician. The diaphragm or cap is coated with spermicide before placement in the vagina. The diaphragm or cervical cap combined with spermicide act by destroying the sperm and preventing the sperm from reaching the egg. After intercourse, the Femcap should be left in place for eight hours.

Effectiveness:

in preventing pregnancy:

- Diaphragm with spermicide—86–94 percent

- Femcap with spermicide—84–91 percent for women who have never given birth; 68–74 percent for women who have given birth
- in preventing STIs—NONE

Advantages:
- Femcap can be inserted many hours before sexual intercourse
- Diaphragm can be inserted two hours before sexual intercourse
- Does not alter the menstrual cycle; easy to carry with you, comfortable
- No major health concerns
- Can last several years

Disadvantages:
- Can be messy
- Possibility of allergies to latex, silicone, or spermicide
- Cannot use with vaginal bleeding or an infection
- Diaphragm—can only be left in place for up to twenty-four hours
- Diaphragm—increased risk of bladder infection
- Femcap—difficult for some women to use
- Femcap—can only be left in place for up to forty-eight hours

Over-the-Counter Contraceptives for Women
- Female condom—insert vaginal pouch deep into vagina prior to intercourse
- Spermicide, foam, jelly, or cream—insert deep into vagina prior to intercourse

Effectiveness:

in preventing pregnancy:
- Female condom—79–95 percent
- Spermicide, foam, jelly, or cream—71–82 percent

in preventing STIs:
- Female condom—similar to the male condom, but not quite as effective, due to possible folding
- Spermicides, foam, jelly, and cream in preventing STIs—NONE

Advantages:
- Easy to purchase in drugstores, supermarkets, etc.
- Increased sensation compared to the male condom
- Erection not necessary to keep female condom in place

Disadvantages:
- Outer ring of female condom may slip into vagina during intercourse
- Possible difficulty inserting the pouch
- More difficult preparation
- Possible allergies to spermicide

IUD
The intrauterine device (IUD) requires a health care professional to insert a small plastic device through the cervix and into the uterus. The IUD contains copper or hormones that impede conception or rarely prevent implantation of a fertilized egg. IUDs can last one to ten years.

Effectiveness:
- in preventing pregnancy: 99.2–99.9 percent
- in preventing STIs—NONE

Advantages:
- Nothing to put into place before intercourse
- Para Gard (copper IUD) may be left in place for up to ten years; Mirena (hormone IUD) may be left in place for up to five years
- No daily pills
- Ability to become pregnant returns quickly when use is stopped

Disadvantages:
- May cause cramping (copper IUD)
- Spotting between periods
- Heavier and longer periods
- Increased risk of tubal infection, which may lead to infertility if inserted when a women has an STI
- Rarely, the wall of the uterus is punctured

Contraceptive Implant

Contraceptive implants are soft capsules, about 1.5 inch long, placed under the skin in a woman's upper inner arm. The capsules release progestin, which usually prevents the release of the egg, thickens the cervical mucus, and reduces the buildup of the endometrial lining within the uterus. The sperm is thus unable to penetrate the egg, and/or the fertilized egg is prevented from implanting in the uterus. Implanon is currently being used in the United States and is a single rod that releases a hormone called etonogestrel which lasts three years. Contraceptive implants can be removed at any time.

Effectiveness:
- in preventing pregnancy: 99 percent
- in preventing STIs—NONE

Advantages:
- Can be worn for three years
- Affects fertility one month at a time
- Has no estrogen

Disadvantages:
- Increased risk of heart attack
- Increased risk of stroke

Sterilization

Sterilization is an operation performed on the female (tubal ligation) or male (vasectomy). The tubal ligation is intended to permanently block a woman's fallopian tubes, where sperm typically unite with the eggs.

A vasectomy is performed to permanently block a man's vas deferens tubes, which transport sperm.

Effectiveness:
- in preventing pregnancy: 99.5–99.9 percent
- in preventing STIs—NONE

Table 8.1
Prevention of Sexually Transmitted Infections (STIs) and Pregnancy

Birth Control Method	Effectiveness in Preventing Pregnancy (Perfect Use)	Effectiveness in Preventing Pregnancy (Typical Use)	Effectiveness in Preventing Sexually Transmitted Infections (Typical Use)
Abstinence from Penile/Vaginal Intercourse		100%	100%
Fertility-based Methods (FAMs)	99%	75%	0%
Male Condom	98%	85%	less than 100%
Oral Contraceptive Pill	99%	92%–99%	0%
Mini-Pill		87–99%	0%
Depo-Provera Injection		97–99%	0%
Diaphragm w/ Spermicide	94%	84%	0%
Female Condom	95%	79%	less than 100%
Spermicides used alone	82%	71%	0%
Intrauterine Device		99%	0%
Contraceptive Implant		99%	0%
Sterilization		over 99%	0%
Vaginal Ring		92–99%	0%
Contraceptive Patch	99%	92–99%	0%
Withdrawal Method	96%	73%	0%
Femcap w/ Spermicide	91%	68%	0%

Source: (Planned Parenthood, 2005) (www.youngwomanshealth.org/sexuality_menu.html, 2003).

Advantages:
- Permanent protection against pregnancy
- No lasting side effects
- No effects on sexual pleasure
- Protects woman whose health would be seriously threatened by a pregnancy

Disadvantages:
- Mild bleeding or infection after the surgery
- Some people eventually regret being unable to have children later in life
- Reaction to anesthetic
- Not usually reversible if you change your mind
- Rarely, tubes reopen, allowing pregnancy to occur
- Rare complications with tubal ligation include bleeding and injury to the bowel
- Vasectomy—infection or blood clot can occur in or near the testicles; often there is temporary bruising, swelling, or tenderness of the scrotum

Go to www.arhp.org/crc and use this interactive program to help you choose the birth control method that is right for you.

Emergency Contraception "The Morning After Pill"

There is considerable public confusion about the difference between emergency contraception (EC) pills and medication abortion (RU-486). Pregnancy begins when a pre-embryo completes implantation into the lining of the uterus (ACOG, 1998). EC helps prevent pregnancy, whereas medication abortion terminates pregnancy. Hormonal methods of contraception, including EC, prevent pregnancy by inhibiting ovulation and fertilization (ACOG, 1998). More specifically, EC works by delaying or inhibiting ovulation, and/or altering tubal transport of sperm and/or ova (thereby inhibiting fertilization), and/or altering the endometrium (thereby inhibiting implantation) (Trussell and Jordan, 2006).

After unprotected intercourse, emergency contraception may be utilized. This treatment has been in place for several years in other countries, but only recently became available in the United States. The medication should be taken within 120 hours of unprotected sexual intercourse. The sooner the medication is begun, the higher the effectiveness for pregnancy prevention. There are two types of ECs. The first one contains both estrogen and progestin. When taken within seventy-two hours of unprotected intercourse, ECs that contain both estrogen and progestin reduce the risk of pregnancy by 75 percent. The combination pills are taken in two doses, twelve hours apart.

The other type of ECs only contains progestin. When taken within twenty-four hours of unprotected intercourse, progestin-only ECs were found to reduce the risk of pregnancy by 95 percent (Ellertson et al., 2003). The progestin-only ECs are taken in two doses, twelve hours apart or at the same time.

The emergency contraceptive method is typically used in cases of unanticipated sexual intercourse, contraceptive failure, or sexual assault.

Some common side effects include substantial nausea and vomiting. These side effects generally subside within forty-eight hours. This is not to be used as a regular method of birth control. As with many of the other pregnancy prevention methods, this one offers no protection against the contraction of STIs.

Unplanned Pregnancy

This can be a very exciting and/or frightening time in an individual's life. The thought of pregnancy conjures up many emotions, such as the realization of life changes, increased responsibility, happiness, and worry all at the same time. Pregnancy and the responsibilities of parenthood are tremendous. It is important to realize these potential consequences of unprotected intercourse or failed pregnancy prevention. It is a good idea to discuss how you might handle this situation with your potential sexual partner. In the event of an unplanned pregnancy, there are several options, none of which are easy and all can be life altering. These will be discussed in the following sections.

Parenthood

Parenthood has been described in many words. Many agree it is one of the best things that can happen, while for others parenthood is quite difficult and challenging. For most, this phase of life (given its rewards and demands) is a blend of these two perspectives. These differences of opinion are often influenced by the stage of life during which the individual becomes a parent, combined with factors such as other life circumstances (whether the parent will be a single parent or not), as well as the personality and financial situation of the new parent. Parenthood usually will dramatically alter the lifestyle to which an individual has become accustomed. Initially, it is an end to restful nights, spur-of-the-moment trips, and many social activities. New parents now have an individual who is solely dependent upon them twenty-four hours a day for attention, love, food, clothing, safety, and shelter. This can be overwhelming physically, mentally, and financially even for the most prepared parents. It is also a time of tremendous joy, as well as many special moments, such as your baby's first smile, giggle, word, or step. As the child grows they are less dependent upon you for the basic necessities, but those needs change into dance lessons, soccer practice, and slumber parties, to name a few. The commitment to becoming a parent is large and one that never ends and can be very difficult to face alone.

Adoption

For many, present life circumstances do not permit them to remain the caregiver in the best interest of their child. Many factors, such as the age of the parent and economic circumstance, come to bear upon this complex and often difficult decision. For the vast majority this is indeed a most difficult decision to reach. The bond that ties the newborn child and parent(s) is enormous. Usually this course is taken in an attempt to be unselfish and provide the child with improved opportunities in life which might otherwise be unavailable to them. Many adoption agencies exist to help make this option as painless as possible. There are many different types of adoptions. Some allow the biological parents to remain a part of the child's life; others do not, but provide a mechanism whereby the child can eventually obtain information regarding the biological parents. Often this information can be made available only after the adopted child enters adolescence or adulthood.

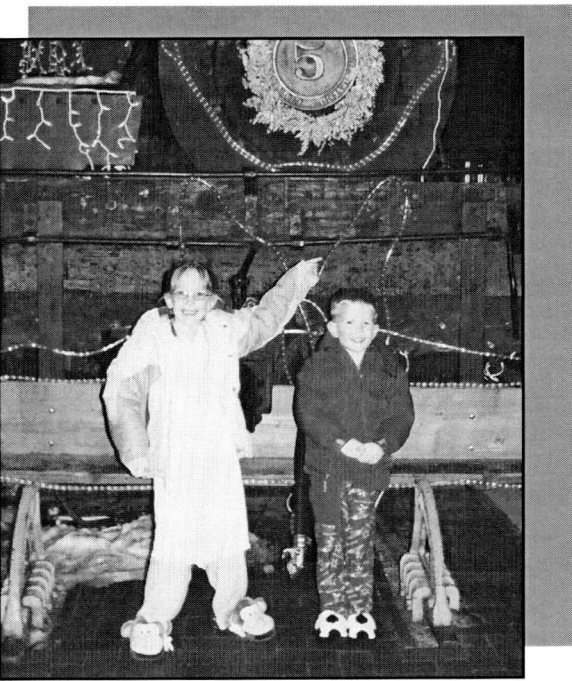

Parenthood can be both overwhelming and a time of tremendous joy.

Abortion

Some individuals cannot (due to medical reasons) or do not want to carry the embryo to term, and therefore choose abortion. This decision is reached for various reasons. Sometimes this is felt to be the best decision because of the circumstances of conception (such as a rape resulting in pregnancy). Some believe they cannot disclose a pregnancy to their parents or partner and see no other alternative. Others are not ready to become parents and do not want to complete the pregnancy.

Abortion was made legal throughout the United States in 1973. Since that time, abortion has become the most often performed outpatient surgery. Today, abortion is about ten times safer than giving birth. The cost of an abortion depends upon the stage of the pregnancy and which clinic is providing the service. During the first trimester (up to twelve weeks) the cost is usually between $450 and $1,275. During the second trimester (thirteen to twenty-four weeks) the cost increases to $600 to $6,000. Some insurance plans will cover abortion costs. There are some potential complications associated with abortion. The complications can include an incomplete abortion, which means the procedure would need to be repeated; an infection, which can usually be treated with antibiotics; or perforation of the uterine wall.

There are several types of abortion procedures available, depending on the stage of the pregnancy. Medical abortion (Mifepristone, RU-486, or nonsurgical abortion) is an option up to eight weeks since the last menstrual period (LMP). Surgical vacuum aspiration abortion is the procedure used to empty the uterus and can be performed between six and twelve weeks since the LMP. Last, the dilation and evacuation procedure can be performed between thirteen and twenty-four weeks since the LMP. After and during an abortion there is typically mild to very strong cramping for one to three hours, as well as bleeding and/or spotting for three to six weeks. A normal menstrual period should begin within four to eight weeks. Usually clinics will offer counseling before and after an abortion. Due to the emotional nature of any decision associated with pregnancy, counseling is highly recommended.

As mentioned earlier, pregnancy is accompanied by many emotions and lasting effects for both partners. There is no easy route once pregnancy has occurred. It is a good idea to discuss your values and ideas of what you would do in the event of an unplanned pregnancy with your prospective sexual partner. It is best to fully consider all of the options before making a decision.

Sexually Transmitted Infections (STIs)

There are more than thirty infections that are primarily spread through sexual activity (see Table 8.7 on pages 294–297, near the end of this chapter, for a partial listing). In the United States, there are more than 65 million people currently living with an incurable STI. An additional 19 million people become infected with one or more STIs each year (see Figure 8.14, on page 285), of which approximately half are not curable (SIECUS, 2008) or www.siecus.org. STIs are transmitted during vaginal, oral, anal sexual activity, or in some cases by simply touching an infected area. STIs can be transferred not only to the genitalia area, but also to the mouth, eyes, nose, and other orifices of the body. You can become infected if someone's blood, semen, vaginal secretions, or precum goes into your body during vaginal, anal, or oral sex (see Table 8.2). Many individuals who become infected with STIs are asymptomatic (without symptoms) and thus become silent carriers. This is one of the reasons STIs have reached epidemic proportions. There are many health problems that can result if an asymptomatic STI carrier is not treated. Some of these health problems include infertility, ectopic pregnancies, and genital cancers, particularly cervical cancer in women. Therefore, it is very important to know your sexual history and be tested for STIs regularly.

Table 8.2

Is It Safe?

Types of Sexual Contact	Can I Get Pregnant?	Can I Get an STI?	How Can I Protect Myself?
Vaginal Intercourse	Yes	Yes, any STI	Condom
Anal Intercourse	No	Yes, any STI	Condom
Oral Sex	No	Yes, any STI	Condom, plastic food wrap, latex dam
Genital Touching (skin-to-skin)	Rarely*	Yes, herpes, HPV, and syphillis	Condom, plastic food wrap, latex dam
Kissing	No	Yes**	Don't kiss when herpes sores are on mouth
Abstinence***	No	No	

*If precum enters the vagina.
**If herpes virus is present on or around the mouth.
***Abstinence means no sexual contact, including genital (skin-to-skin) touching.

Levels of Risk

Sexual behaviors have different levels of risk for different STIs (Figure 8.12 on page 283). Using condoms lowers the risk of transmitting STIs in association with anal, oral, or vaginal intercourse. The following list depicts risk, assuming no protection is used for the following behaviors.

High Risk
- Anal intercourse
- Vaginal intercourse
- Oral sex on a man with ejaculation
- Oral sex on a man without ejaculation
- Oral sex on a woman
- Oral-anal contact

Low Risk
- Intimate kissing
- Casual kissing
- Touching, massage

No Risk
- Masturbation
- Talking, fantasy (ACHA, 2004)

Bacterial STIs

Chlamydia

Chlamydia is caused by a bacteria-like intracellular parasite called *Chlamydia trachomati*. Chlamydia is typically spread during vaginal, oral, or anal sex and can infect other body parts such as the eyes, nose, or throat where chlamydia can also be contracted. Symptoms in males include a thin, clear-whitish urethral discharge, itching or burning during urination, pain, or swelling in the testes and a low-grade fever. In females, symptoms include moderate vaginal discharge, itching or burning during urination, abdominal pain, bleeding between periods, nausea, headaches, and a low-grade fever. If symptoms occur, they will typically begin one to three weeks after infection. Seventy-five percent of infected females and 51 percent of infected males are asymptomatic (without symptoms). The long-term effects of untreated chlamydia can include infertility in both males and females from scarring in the testicles and fallopian tubes. Chlamydia infections are the leading cause of preventable infertility and ectopic pregnancies. In up to 40 percent of women with untreated chlamydia, infection can spread into the uterus and fallopian tubes, causing pelvic inflammatory disease (PID). Most infections respond to tetracycline, doxycycline, or erythromycin, but not penicillin. It is very important that all partners be treated to decrease the spread of infection, as well as prevent reinfection. Chlamydia is estimated to be the most common bacterial STI in the United States (Figure 8.10), with approximately three to four million new cases occurring each year (ASHA, 2004). Adolescents and young adults have the highest infection rates (Figure 8.11). College students account for over 10 percent of the infected cases which are on the rise (Donatelle, 2006).

FIGURE 8.10

Chlamydia—Rates by Sex: United States, 1984–2004

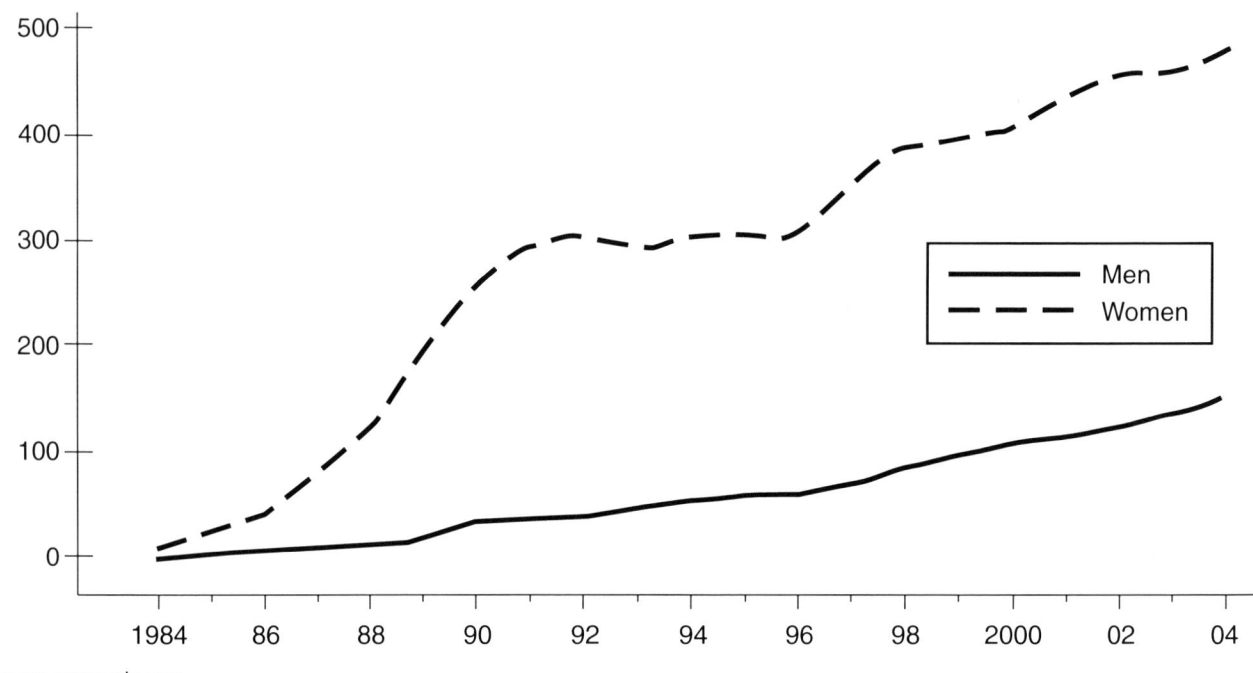

Source: www.cdc.gov

FIGURE 8.11

Chlamydia—Positivity among 15- to 24-Year-Old Women Tested in Family Planning Clinics by State: United States and Outlying Areas, 2004

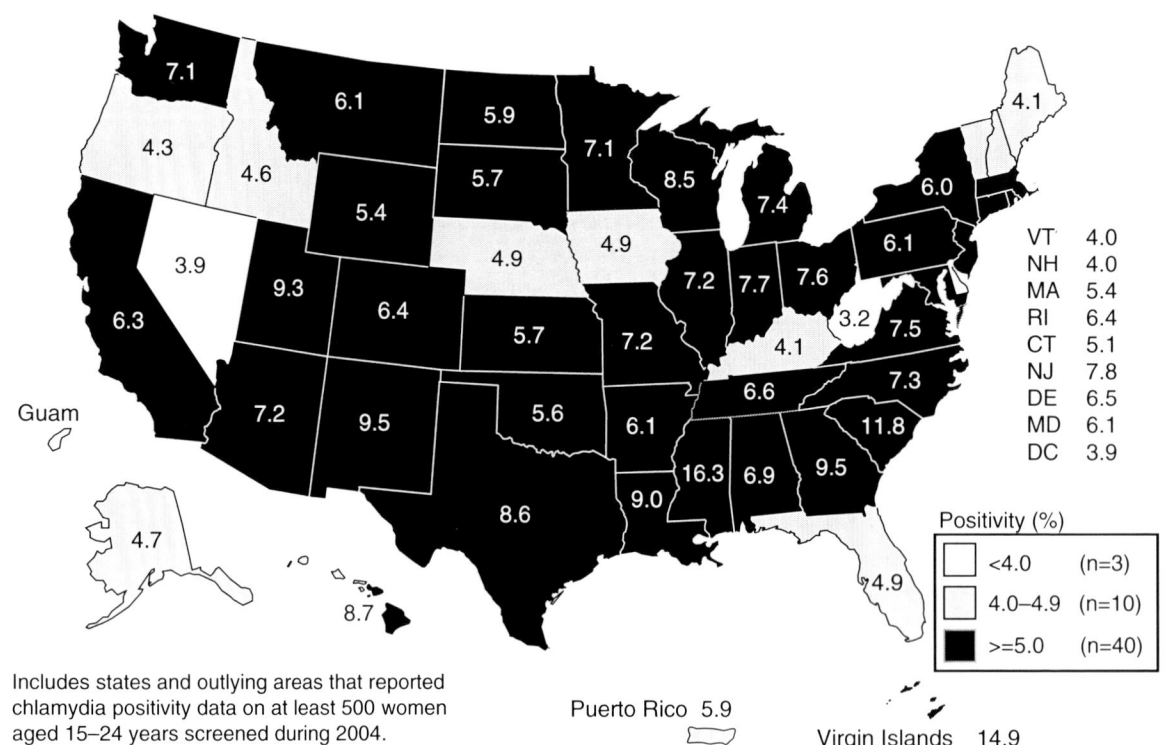

Includes states and outlying areas that reported chlamydia positivity data on at least 500 women aged 15–24 years screened during 2004.

Source: Regional Infertility Prevention Projects; Office of Population Affairs; Local and State STD Control Programs; Centers for Disease Control and Prevention 2004.

FIGURE 8.12

STI Risk Sheet

Unprotected vaginal or anal intercourse:
- Bacterial Vaginosis
- Chlamydia
- Cytomegalovirus (CMV)
- Gonorrhea
- Hepatitis B
- Herpes Simplex
- Human Immunodeficiency Virus (HIV)
- Human Papilloma Virus (HPV, Warts)
- Pelvic Inflammatory Disease (PID)
- Pubic Lice
- Scabies
- Syphilis
- Trichomoniasis

*Safer Sex Tip: Always use condoms.

Unprotected oral sex:
("blow job," "giving head," "going down," "rimming")
- Cytomegalovirus (CMV)
- Gonorrhea
- Hepatitis B
- Herpes (including cold sores)
- Human Immunodeficiency Virus (HIV)
- Human Papilloma Virus (HPV, Warts)
- Syphilis

*Safer Sex Tip: Use dental dams, non-lubricated or flavored condom, or female condoms.

Unprotected manual sex:
("hand job" or "fingering")
- Bacterial Vaginosis
- Cytomegalovirus (CMV)
- Herpes Simplex
- Human Papilloma Virus (HPV, Warts)
- Pubic Lice
- Scabies

*Safer Sex Tip: Use gloves or condoms.

Source: Adapted from www.scarleteen.com.

Gonorrhea

Gonorrhea is caused by the bacterium called *Neisseria gonorrhea*. Infection is found primarily in the linings of the urethra, vagina, mouth, and rectum (Crowley, 2006). Symptoms in males include a foul-smelling thick, creamy white, yellow, or yellow-green discharge from the penis, painful urination, blood or pus in the urine, and enlarged lymph nodes in the groin area. In females, the symptoms include similar discharge from the vagina, pain during urination, pelvic pain, or irregular and painful menstruation. If symptoms are present, they usually appear about one week after exposure. Many individuals are asymptomatic *(5 to 20 percent of infected males and 60 to 80 percent of females).* The long-term effects of untreated gonorrhea can cause infertility in both males and females, as a result of infection and scarring in both testicles and in the fallopian tubes. Gonorrhea remains one of the major

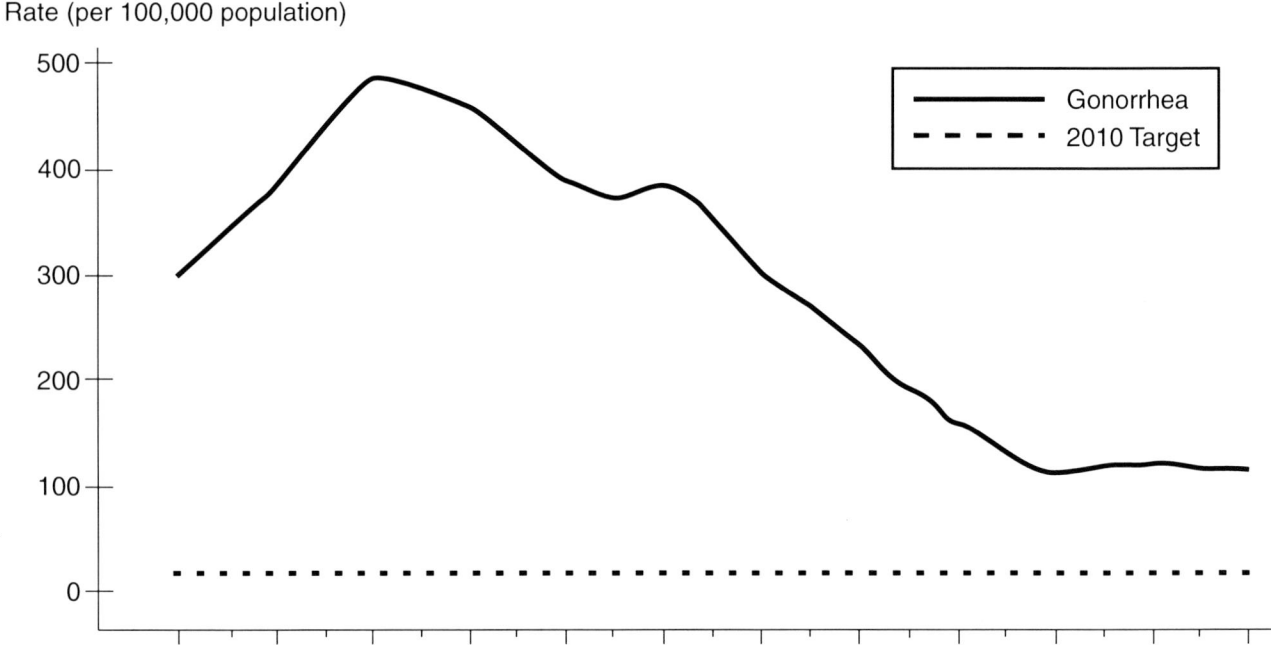

FIGURE 8.13

Gonorrhea—Rates: United States, 1970–2004 and the *Healthy People 2010* Target

Note: The *Healthy People 2010* target for gonorrhea is 19.0 cases per 100,000 population.
Source: www.cdc.gov.

causes of PID (Figure 8.13 and 8.15). Most infections respond to penicillin, tetracycline, spectinomycin, cefixime, or ceftriaxone. It is very important that all partners be treated to decrease the spread of the infection, as well as to prevent reinfection.

Pelvic Inflammatory Disease (PID)

PID is a general term that refers to an infection of the uterus, fallopian tubes, or other reproductive organ. Chlamydia and gonorrhea are the most common STIs (if left untreated) that lead to PID. Damage to the fallopian tubes and tissues in and near the uterus and ovaries can result from PID. This damage occurs from the inflammation and results in scarring of these tissues. This scarring can lead to serious consequences including infertility, ectopic pregnancy, abscess formation, and chronic pelvic pain. Each year, it is estimated that more than 1 million women will experience an episode of PID.

More than 100,000 women become infertile each year as a result of PID (CDC, 2008 or www.cdc.gov/std/PID/STDFact-PID.htm). Annually more than 150 women die from PID or complications associated with this infection.

The more sexual partners a woman has had, the higher her risk of developing PID. This is because of the potential for more exposure to STIs. Most of the time there are no symptoms associated with PID. Meanwhile, the infection is causing serious long-term damage to the woman's reproductive organs. If symptoms exist, they can include lower abdominal pain, fever, unusual vaginal discharge, painful intercourse or urination, irregular menstrual bleeding, or pain in the right upper abdomen. PID can be cured with Ofloxacin, Levofloxacin, or Metronidazole. Antibiotic treatment does not reverse any damage that has already occurred to the reproductive organs.

FIGURE 8.14

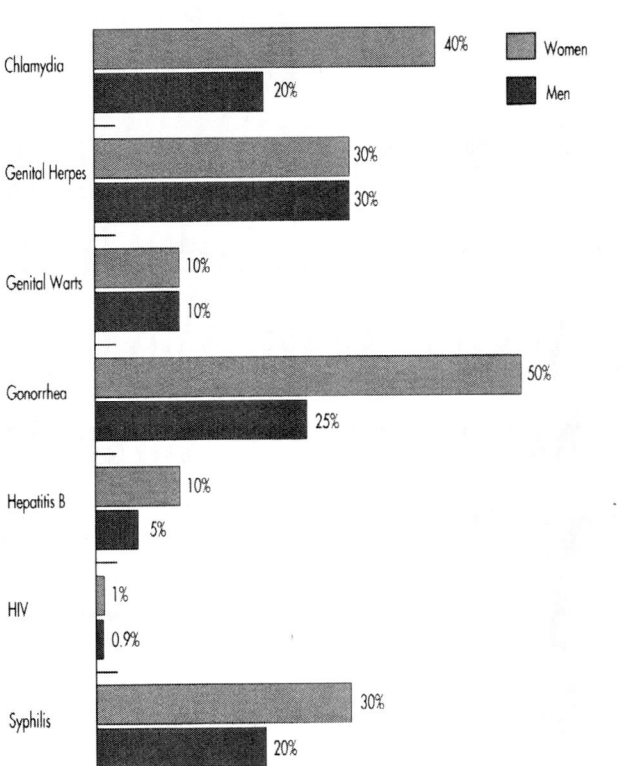

Rates for Contracting Various STIs after One Heterosexual Unprotected Intercourse with an Infected Partner

Source: Centers for Disease Control and Prevention.

FIGURE 8.15

Gonorrhea—Rates by State: United States and Outlying Areas, 2004

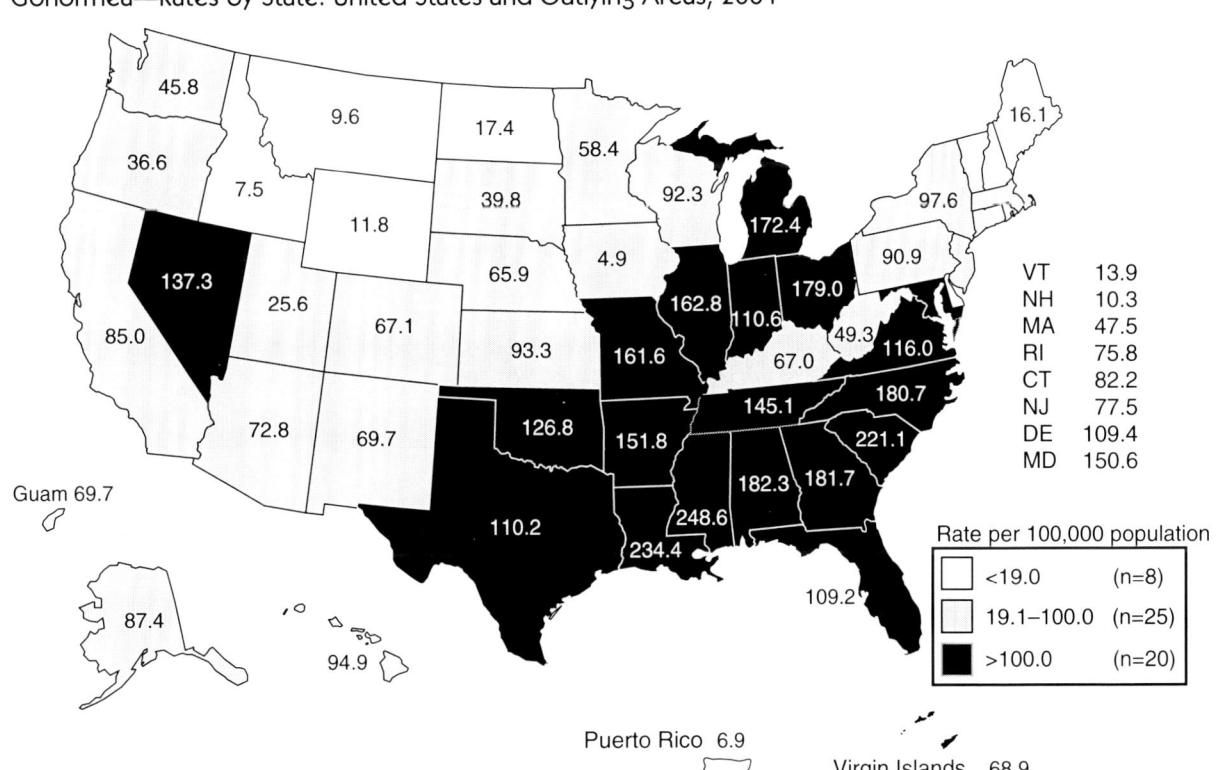

Note: The total rate of gonorrhea for the United States and outlying areas (Guam, Puerto Rico, and Virgin Islands) was 112.1 per 100,000 population. The *Healthy People 2010* target is 19.0 cases per 100,000.

Source: www.cdc.gov.

It is critical for any woman who has symptoms of PID to be evaluated by a physician immediately. The longer treatment is delayed for PID the more likely she is to become infertile due to the damage to the reproductive organs.

Syphilis

Syphilis is a serious bacterial infection caused by the spirochete *Treponema pallidum*. Syphilis can be contracted and spread through vaginal, oral, or anal sex, as well as through blood and blood products. This disease can be debilitating and even fatal if left untreated. A person may be unknowingly infected with syphilis and transmit it to others. In the United States, over 36,000 cases of syphilis were reported in 2006 (CDC, 2008) or www.cdc.gov/std/syphilis/STDFact-syphilis.htm. The actual incidence of syphilis is much higher than reported (see Figures 8.16 and 8.17). It is estimated that for every case of syphilis that is reported, three are not (Crooks and Baur, 2007).

This disease has three stages.

1. During the first stage, a painless sore (chancre) about the size of a dime may appear at the point where the bacteria first entered the body, usually three weeks after contact. This sore may appear around or in the vagina, on the penis, or inside the mouth or anus. Sores inside the vagina or anus are often unnoticed and may disappear on their own if not treated; however, the bacterial infection remains.
2. The second stage occurs two to eight weeks after the exposure and includes flu-like symptoms and possible hair loss, a rash on the palms of hands and soles of feet, as well as over the entire body.

FIGURE 8.16

Primary and Secondary Syphilis—Rates: United States, 1970–2004 and the *Healthy People 2010* Target

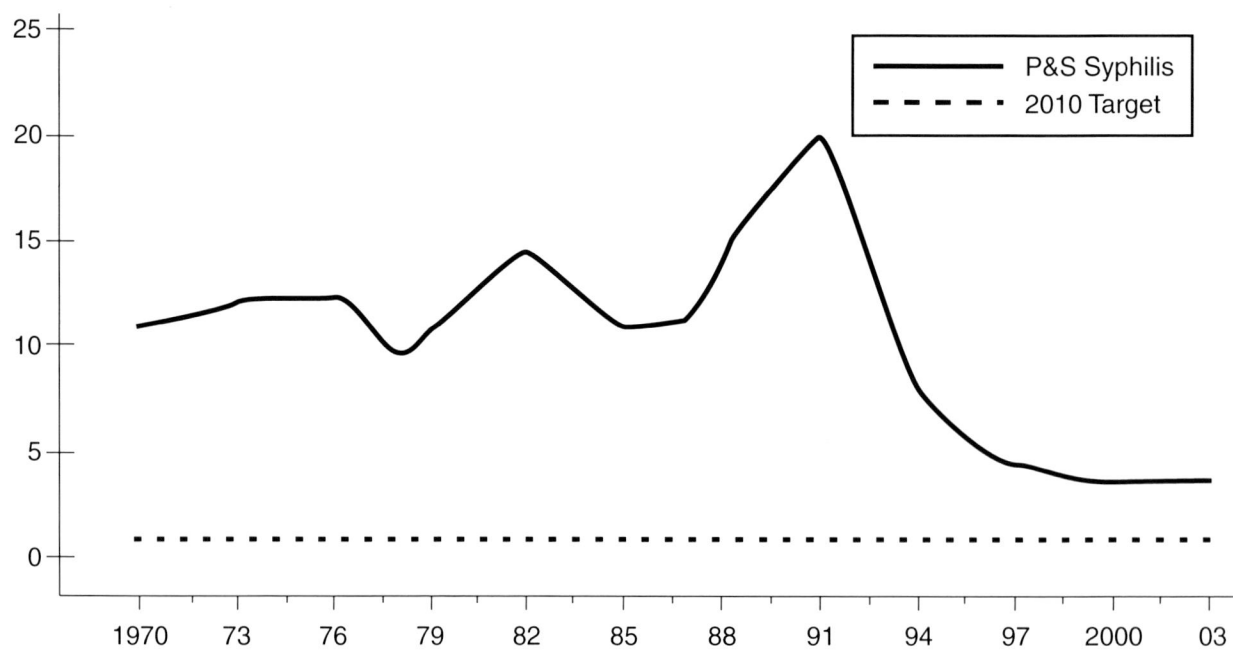

Note: The *Healthy People 2010* target for P&S syphilis is 0.2 cases per 100,000 population.
Source: www.cdc.gov.

FIGURE 8.17

Primary and Secondary Syphilis—Rates by State: United States and Outlying Areas, 2004

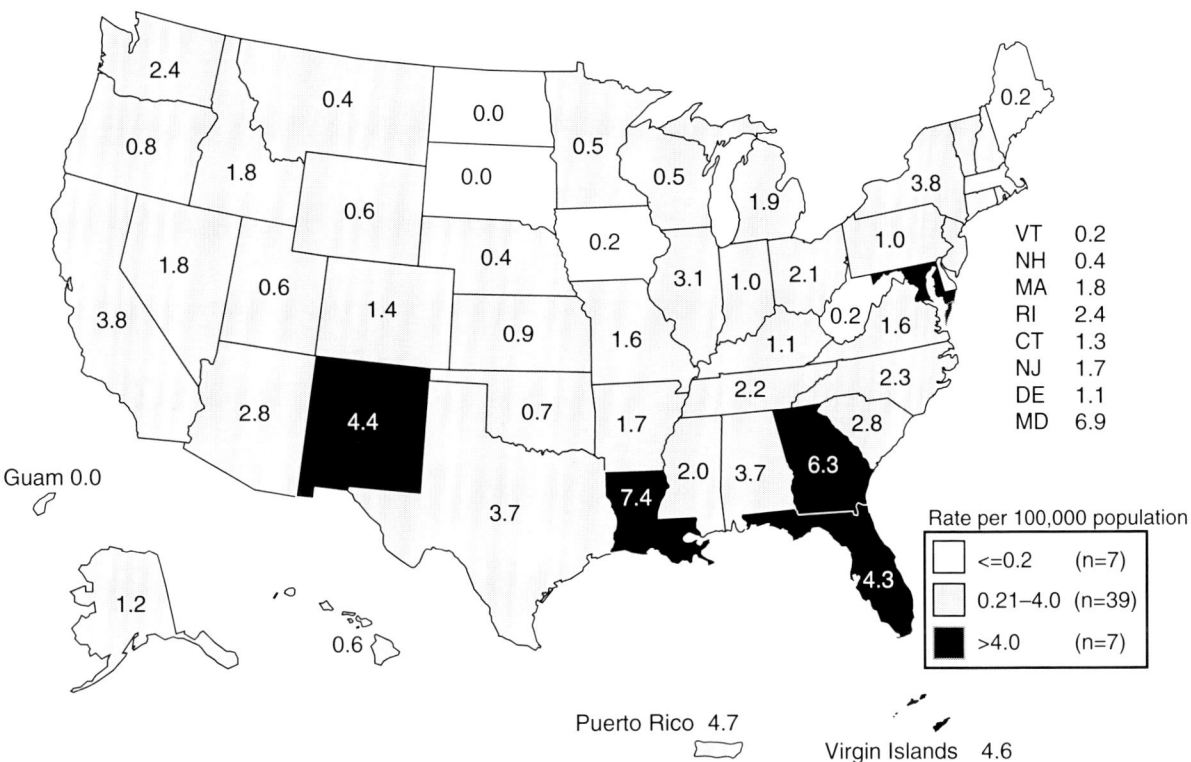

Note: The total rate of P&S syphilis for the United States and outlying areas (Guam, Puerto Rico, and Virgin Islands) was 2.8 per 100,000 population. The *Healthy People 2010* target is 0.2 cases per 100,000 population.
Source: www.cdc.gov.

3. The tertiary (third stage) syphilis can appear five to twenty-five years after the initial exposure. Symptoms of this stage may include skin lesions, mental deterioration, loss of balance and vision, loss of sensation, shooting pains in the legs, and heart disease (Crooks and Baur, 2007).

See a physician immediately if there is any chance you have been exposed to syphilis. A simple blood test can usually determine whether or not you have the disease. However, if you become infected two to three weeks prior to testing, the blood test may not be sensitive enough to detect the antibodies. Syphilis can be treated with the proper antibiotics, most commonly penicillin injections.

There have been several resistant strains that have developed when individuals did not take the full prescription dose. Always take all of the antibiotics that are prescribed to you; don't save them for later or stop them just because you feel better and NEVER take someone else's medication.

Go to www.thebody.com/surveys/sexsurvey.html to take this absolutely anonymous test and discover your risk for HIV or other STIs.

Viral STIs

Genital Herpes

Genital herpes is a chronic, life-long infection caused by the herpes simplex virus (HSV). There are two types of HSV (Type 1 and Type 2), both of which can infect any area of the body, producing lesions (sores) in and around the vaginal area, on the penis, around the anal opening, on the buttocks or thighs, in or around the mouth, and in the eyes possibly causing blindness (Donatelle, 2006). Herpes can be contracted and spread through vaginal, oral, or anal sex, as well as skin-to-skin contact.

A newborn may be infected with genital herpes while passing through the birth canal (Crooks and Baur, 2007). Infection in the newborn can cause mental retardation, blindness, or even death (Crooks and Baur, 2007). Therefore, it is important that an infected pregnant female inform her physician of the infection so that the physician can watch for an outbreak and perform a cesarean section (C-section) if necessary. Current estimates indicate that 45 million people (more than one in five Americans) have genital herpes (CDC, 2008) or www.cdc.gov/std/herpes/STDFactherpes.htm. Each year there are approximately one million new cases of genital herpes (ASHA, 2004). There are many more individuals who have genital herpes and are asymptomatic. The symptoms vary, and many people have no noticeable symptoms. Symptoms will most commonly occur within two to twenty days after infection. Early symptoms may include a tingling or burning sensation in the genitals, lower back pain, pain when urinating, and flu-like symptoms. A few days later, small red bump(s) may appear in the genital area. Later, these bumps can develop into painful blisters, which then crust over, form a scab, and heal. Sometimes the diagnosis can be made by physical examination alone. For testing, the physician collects a small amount of fluid from the sores to see if the herpes virus is present. It may take up to two weeks to receive the results. If no sores are present, testing may be difficult. However, a blood test does exist to determine if an individual does have the herpes virus. It is expensive and does not indicate the location of the infection. Although herpes is a chronic, life-long viral infection, the symptoms can be treated. Treatment of genital herpes outbreaks, especially when begun early, shortens the duration of the outbreak and reduces the symptoms (Marr, 2007). Medications used include acyclovir, famcyclovir, and valacyclovir. Individuals with more than six outbreaks per year may be treated with preventative (prophylactic) suppressive therapy.

HIV/AIDS

Human Immunodeficiency Virus (HIV)/Acquired Immune Deficiency Syndrome (AIDS) was first identified in the United States in June 1981 by the Centers for Disease Control and Prevention (CDC). HIV is the virus that causes AIDS and is transmitted in one of four ways:

1. vaginal, oral, or anal sex;
2. sharing a needle for piercing, tattoos, or drugs including steroids;
3. blood products infected with HIV;
4. from mother to child during pregnancy, delivery or breast milk.

The highest concentrations of HIV are found in bodily fluids such as blood, semen, vaginal secretions, and breast milk (Floyd et al., 2007). Infection can occur when any of these fluids from an infected person comes into direct contact with the bloodstream or mucous membranes of another person (see Table 8.4). Trace amounts are found in tears, saliva, and other body fluids but have not been found to transmit infection. HIV is *not* spread by casual contact. It is not known if all individuals infected with this virus will develop AIDS. Women are more likely to become infected

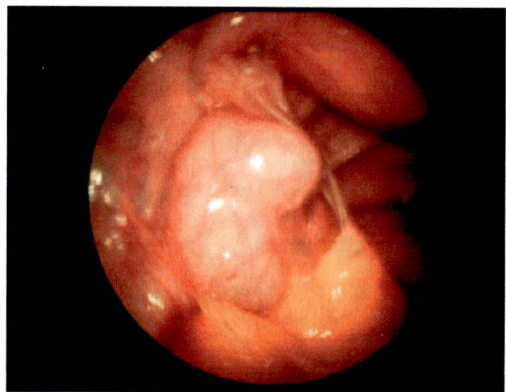

Hydrosalpinx—resulting from Chlamydia—closed, swollen and water-filled left fallopian tube in a young woman.

Excerpted from *The Secret Epidemic; STIs on Campus* © American College Health Association, PO Box 28927, Baltimore, MD 21240.

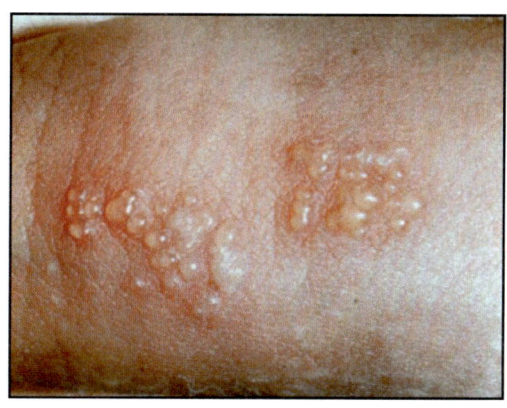

Penis with vesicles (blisters) from genital herpes.

Excerpted from *The Secret Epidemic; STIs on Campus* © American College Health Association, PO Box 28927, Baltimore, MD 21240.

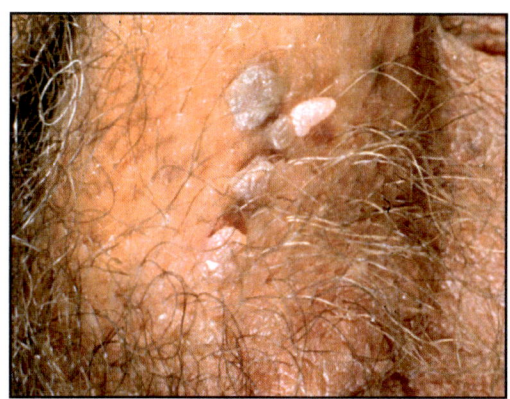

Genital warts on the penis.

From *Visuals Unlimited* © Science VU/Visuals Unlimited

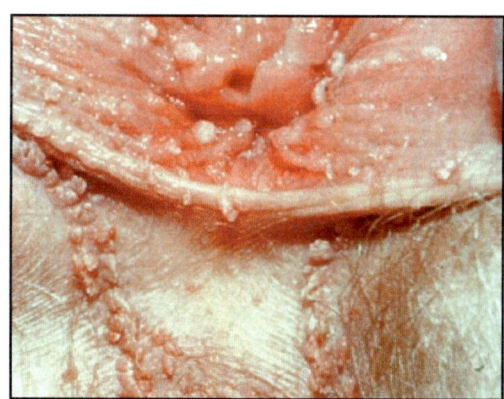

Papillary (HPV) genital warts of female.

Excerpted from *The Secret Epidemic; STIs on Campus* © American College Health Association, PO Box 28927, Baltimore, MD 21240.

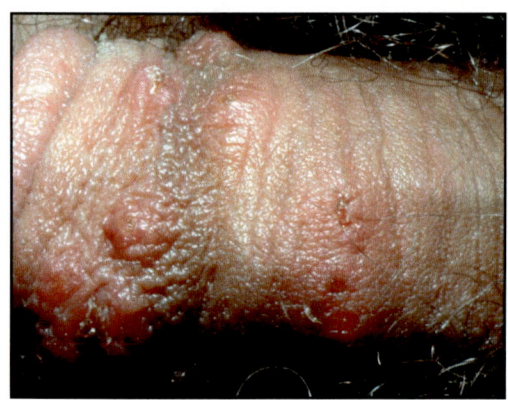

Genital herpes infection characterized by recurring cycles of painful blisters on the genitalia.

From Steven J. Nussenblatt/Custom Medical Stock Photo

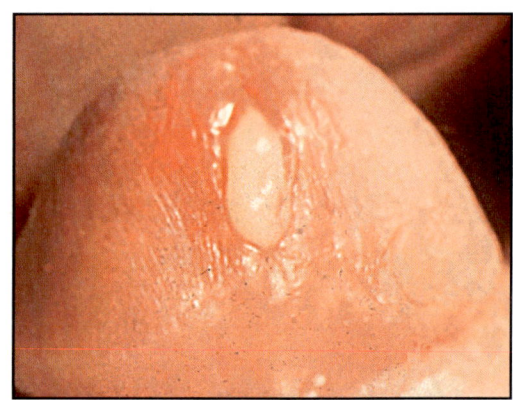

Gonorrheal discharge from the penis.

From *Visuals Unlimited* © Science VU/Visuals Unlimited

Table 8.4:

AIDS Cases by Transmission Category

Six common transmission categories are male-to-male sexual contact, injection drug use, male-to-male sexual contact and injection drug use, high-risk heterosexual (male-female) contact, mother-to-child (perinatal) transmission, and other (includes blood transfusions and unknown cause).

Following is the distribution of the estimated number of cases of AIDS among adults and adolescents by transmission category in the fifty states and the District of Columbia. A breakdown by sex is provided where appropriate.

Transmission Category	Estimated # of AIDS Cases, in 2006		
	Adult and Adolescent Male	Adult and Adolescent Female	Total
Male-to-male sexual contact	16,001	-	16,001
Injection drug use	4,410	2,385	6,795
Male-to-male sexual contact and injection drug use	1,803	-	1,803
High-risk heterosexual contact*	4,558	7,196	11,754
Other**	217	220	437

*Heterosexual contact with a person known to have, or to be at high risk for, HIV infection.
**Includes hemophilia, blood transfusion, perinatal exposure, and risk not reported or not identified.

Transmission Category	Estimated # of AIDS Cases, through 2006*		
	Adult and Adolescent Male	Adult and Adolescent Female	Total
Male-to-male sexual contact	465,965	-	465,965
Injection drug use	170,171	74,718	244,889
Male-to-male sexual contact and injection drug use	68,516	-	68,516
High-risk heterosexual contact**	65,241	108,252	173,493
Other***	13,893	6,596	20,489

*Includes persons with a diagnosis of AIDS from the beginning of the epidemic through 2006.
**Heterosexual contact with a person known to have, or to be at high risk for, HIV infection.
***Includes hemophilia, blood transfusion, perinatal exposure, and risk not reported or not identified.
Source: From the CDC HIV/AIDS Surveillance Report: Cases of HIV Infection and AIDS in the United States and Dependent Areas. 2006b.

with HIV during heterosexual sex than males, because the concentration of virus is higher in semen than it is in vaginal secretions (Floyd et al., 2007).

An individual may be asymptomatic or may have some of the symptoms, which include:

- fatigue,
- dry cough,
- fever,
- night sweats,

- diarrhea,
- skin rashes,
- swollen lymph nodes,
- recurrent vaginal yeast infections,
- unexplained weight loss.

Typically six weeks to six months is required after the initial infection to detect the HIV antibodies in a blood test (Floyd et al., 2007). The average time from infection until AIDS diagnosis is about ten years. There is no known cure at the present for HIV or AIDS. There are numerous drugs/cocktails (mixture of different types of drugs) that exist to boost the immune system and interfere with the replication of the virus, therefore delaying the onset of AIDS.

The best way to avoid contracting HIV is to abstain from vaginal, oral, or anal sex or have a mutually monogamous relationship with an uninfected partner. Other ways to protect yourself include HIV testing before becoming sexually active, consistent and correct use of latex condoms with all sexual acts (vaginal, oral, and anal), avoid sharing needles for anything, and do not have sex with anyone known or suspected of using injectable drugs including steroids.

More than 45 percent of those diagnosed with AIDS were infected with HIV in their teens and twenties (Floyd et al., 2007). (See Tables 8.5 and 8.6.) About 56,000 people became infected with HIV in the past year (CDC, 2008) or www.cdc.gov/nchhstp/newsroom/WADPressrelease-112408.htm.

HPV

The Human Papilloma Viruses (HPV) cause warts on various parts of the body. There are more than one hundred types of HPV, about half of which can cause genital infections (Crooks and Baur, 2007). These viruses can be transmitted by vaginal, oral, or anal sex, as well as skin-to-skin contact. Genital warts or condyloma may appear three weeks to eight months after infection, with an average of three months (Crooks and Baur, 2007). As with many of the other STIs, an individual may be infected and never show signs or symptoms of the virus. Genital warts may be brown, pink, red, yellow, or grayish in color. The warts are typically found on the vaginal opening, cervix, perineum, labia, inner walls of the vagina, or anal area in females and on the foreskin or shaft of the penis, anal area, or urethra in males. Genital warts can cause bleeding and obstruction in the urinary and/or anal openings. There is a strong association between HPV infection and cancers of the cervix, vagina, vulva, penis, and anus (Crooks and Baur, 2007). In 2006, the FDA approved Gardasil, the first vaccine developed to prevent certain types (16 and 18) of HPV, which cause 70 percent of cervical cancers and against types 6 and 11, which cause approximately 90 percent of genital warts. The vaccine is designed for females age 9–26. Ideally, the vaccine would be given before an individual becomes sexually active and is exposed to the viruses. In order for the vaccine to be effective, it must be given in three different doses over a six month period. Also, it is imperative that all sexually active females receive an annual Pap test with the first test occurring three years after the onset of sexual activity. Numerous studies show there are many false positive results from Pap tests detecting precancerous cells on the cervix if performed too close to the first vaginal intercourse experience. One such study in college students showed that in 91 percent of women with new HPV infections, HPV became undetectable within two years (Ho, 1998). Most HPV infections appear to be temporary and are most likely eradicated by the body's immune system. During this exam HPV is typically the only STI that can be detected visually, with the exception of genital herpes, if the female is having an outbreak. It is typically necessary to receive a blood or urine test to detect other types of STIs. It is not known

Table 8.5
AIDS Cases by Age
Of the **estimated number** of AIDS cases in the fifty states and the District of Columbia persons' ages at time of diagnosis were distributed as follows.

Age (Years)	Estimated # of AIDS Cases in 2006	Cumulative Estimated # of AIDS Cases, through 2006*
Under 13	38	9,156
Ages 13–14	73	1,078
Ages 15–19	401	5,626
Ages 20–24	1,669	36,225
Ages 25–29	3,423	117,099
Ages 30–34	4,349	197,530
Ages 35–39	6,402	213,573
Ages 40–44	7,298	170,531
Ages 45–49	5,628	107,207
Ages 50–54	3,687	59,907
Ages 55–59	2,071	32,190
Ages 60–64	955	17,303
Ages 65 or older	835	15,074

*Includes persons with a diagnosis of AIDS from the beginning of the epidemic through 2006.
Source: From the CDC HIV/AIDS Surveillance Report: Cases of HIV Infection and AIDS in the United States and Dependent Areas. 2006b.

Table 8.6
AIDS Cases by Top Ten States/Dependent Areas
The ten states or dependent areas **reporting** the highest number of AIDS cases were:

State/Dependent Area	# of AIDS Cases in 2006
New York	5,495
Florida	4,932
California	3,960
Texas	2,998
Pennsylvania	1,893
Maryland	1,626
Georgia	1,605
Illinois	1,382
North Carolina	1,229
New Jersey	1,065

State/Dependent Area	# of Cumulative AIDS Cases through 2006*		
	Adults or Adolescents	Children (<13)	Total
New York	174,908	2,354	177,262
California	142,254	664	142,918
Florida	104,084	1,530	105,614
Texas	69,735	392	70,127
New Jersey	48,750	778	49,528
Illinois	33,620	282	33,902
Pennsylvania	33,417	365	33,782
Georgia	31,734	231	31,965
Maryland	30,252	319	30,571
Puerto Rico	29,511	400	29,911

*Includes persons with a diagnosis of AIDS from the beginning of the epidemic through 2006.
Source: From the CDC HIV/AIDS Surveillance Report: Cases of HIV Infection and AIDS in the United States and Dependent Areas. 2006b.

if HPV directly causes cancer or if it combines with other cofactors such as infections or smoking to increase the risk of developing cancer. A few HPV types have been found to be at least partly responsible for more than 90 percent of cancers of the cervix. These HPV types seem to be the same ones found in oral cancers. The types of HPV found in cervical cancer are found in about 20 percent to 30 percent of oral cancers. The current view is that HPV may be a factor that contributes to the development of oral cavity and oropharyngeal cancers in around 20 percent of people (American Cancer Society, 2005). No cure exists at present for genital warts; however, there are treatments that decrease the size and the risk of spreading. Some of these include topical applications of Aldara TM cream, trichloracetic/bichloracetic acid (TCA/BCA), cryotheraphy (freezing with a probe or liquid nitrogen), and podophyllin. Other less common treatments include laser surgery and interferon (ACHA, 2005). Genital and anal HPV are an extremely common viral STI in the United States (Crooks and Baur, 2007). Approximately 20 million people in the United States are infected with HPV and each year 6.2 million more are infected (CDC, 2008) or www.cdc.gov/STD/HPV/STDFact-HPV.htm. Typical prevalence of HPV for women under the age of twenty-five is between 40 and 50 percent (CDC, 2004). www.cdc.gov/vaccines/recs/acip/downloads/mtg-slides-feb08/15-4-hpv.pdf

Hepatitis B

Hepatitis B is a potentially serious and, at times, fatal illness. Fortunately, this is one of the few viruses that can be eradicated. Ninety percent of people infected with hepatitis B eliminate the virus. This is done by developing antibodies, called immunoglobulins, which the body produces in response to the presence of the virus. These immunoglobulins (IgG and IgM) can be measured in the bloodstream and can detect whether someone has had a hepatitis B infection. However, the remaining 10 percent of individuals infected with hepatitis B become chronic carriers. Of this group, 15 to 25 percent will die prematurely from cirrhosis or liver cancer (CDC, 2005) or www.cdc.gov/vaccines/ed/ciinc/special-topics/downloads/Feb_06_HepB-JC.ppt#262,6,Modes of HBV Transmission in Early Childhood. There were approximately 60,000 new cases in 2004, down from 260,000 new cases in the 1980s due to the increased use of vaccinations (CDC, 2005) or www.cdc.gov/vaccines/ed/ciinc/specialtopics/downloads/Feb_06_HepB-JC.ppt#262,6,Modes of HBV Transmission in Early Childhood. One out of one hundred U.S. residents is an infectious asymptomatic chronic carrier of hepatitis B (Crowley, 2006).

The illness is transmitted through exposure to infected blood or secretions. The disease is primarily spread through sexual contact, followed by injecting drug use (IDU). The following summarizes the routes of transmission in the United States:

Heterosexual contact	41%
Homosexual contact	14%
IDU (Injecting drug use)	12%
Household contacts	4%
Health care workers	2%
Unknown	25%

The concentration of hepatitis B is high in blood and serum, and lower in semen, vaginal secretions, and saliva. It can be transmitted through bites, but transmission through kissing is unlikely. Exposure to blood from cuts, nosebleeds, menstrual bleeding, and blood present on IV needles or personal items such as toothbrushes, razors, and manicuring instruments may result in infection. Pregnant women pass the virus to their babies in 20 to 90 percent of pregnancies, dependent upon the presence or absence of certain viral components. Ninety percent of these infants become chronic carriers, and 15 to 25 percent die of liver failure (CDC, 2007). Other means of spreading hepatitis B include tattooing, body piercing, sharing straws for inhaling cocaine, and hemodialysis machines.

Hepatitis B is diagnosed by elevated liver enzymes (caused when liver cells are damaged and release their enzymes into the bloodstream), and the presence of hepatitis B surface antigen (pieces of the protein coat of the virus), which is the most common test for detecting an acute infection or carrier status. Hepatitis B surface antigen can be detected as early as one to two weeks and as late as eleven to twelve weeks after exposure. If this test is positive, the person is infectious.

Once infected, the incubation period is 25 to 180 days, with an average of approximately 120 days. Thirty percent of adults infected are asymptomatic (CDC, 2007). For those who are symptomatic, some or all of the following symptoms may be present. Initially (approximately two weeks after exposure) there may be diminished appetite with an approximately five to ten pound weight loss, fatigue, headache, nausea, vomiting, muscle aches, cough, low grade fever and right-sided upper abdominal pain. This is known as the 'prodrome' phase. Following the prodrome is the icteric phase, approximately one to two weeks later, which lasts two to six weeks. The urine darkens and the stools become a clay color. The liver becomes enlarged and tender. Itching is common. There may be a yellow cast to the skin or eyes. The recovery phase then follows about six to eight weeks after exposure, at which time the individual usually recovers, but may develop chronic disease.

If a person develops a chronic disease (infection longer than six months), treatment may be necessary to diminish the risk of permanent liver damage. Interferon, which is given in these cases, is made by the body to boost immunity. The interferon, which is used for treatment, is manufactured and given by injection for sixteen weeks to stimulate the immune system to attack the infected liver cells. The virus is completely eradicated in approximately 58 percent of these cases. However, even if there is not total elimination of the virus, the health of the liver is often improved by this treatment. New agents being currently studied are the antivirals ganciclovir and famciclovir, which appear to be promising treatments.

It is imperative that someone with chronic hepatitis B receive the vaccine for hepatitis A to reduce the risk of a very serious complication called acute fulminant hepatitis, in which the liver is rapidly destroyed. The death rate is 63 to 93 percent with this condition. Liver transplantation is rarely an option due to the high rate of reinfection and rapid progression of the disease after transplantation.

The CDC recommends vaccination against hepatitis B for newborns, infants, and non-immunized adolescents and adults.

To prevent risk of exposure, one should practice 'safer sex' as detailed in the STI prevention section, avoid IV drug usage, as well as sharing of toothbrushes, eating utensils, razors, nail files, and clippers. If there is exposure to hepatitis B, an immunoglobulin with a high concentration of antibody against hepatitis B should be given within two weeks of exposure.

Parasitic STIs

Pubic Lice and Scabies

Pubic lice (often called "crabs") and scabies (itch mites) are parasitic insects that live on the skin. They are sometimes spread sexually, but are also transmitted by contact with infected bed linens, clothes, or towels. Pubic lice infect hairy parts of the body, especially around the groin area and can be transmitted by fingers to the armpits or scalp (Crooks and Baur, 2007). With scabies, an itchy rash is the result of a female mite burrowing into a person's skin to lay her eggs. The eggs can be seen on the hair close to the skin, where they hatch in five to ten days. Some individuals infected with pubic lice have no symptoms, while others may experience considerable itching in the area infected. Yellowish-gray insects the size of a pinhead

Table 8.7

What Are the Common Sexually Transmitted Infections (STIs)?

STI	Transmission (Body Fluids and/or Direct Contact)	Symptoms
Chlamydia	**Fluids**—contact of mucous membranes (cervix, urethra) with infected person's fluids (semen and mucus). Most common with exposure through vaginal or anal sex. Casual contact considered to be safe.	Most patients have no symptoms. If present, they may be: *Women*—pain or dull aching in lower abdomen, heavy feeling in pelvic area, pain with urination or intercourse, heavier menstrual flow, breakthrough bleeding, heavy cervical discharge. *Men*—urethral discharge, pain with urination, pain in scrotum (epididymitis).
Human Papillomavirus (HPV)/Genital Warts/Precancerous Tissue Change (Intraepithelial Neoplasia)	**Contact**—touching (hands/genital, genital/genital, or ano-genital) an infected person's lesions can transmit cells containing the virus. Can be transmitted through non-penetrative sexual contact.	Usually no symptoms, but external lesions may itch. Lesions on the skin can be either raised or flat. Most lesions on the cervix can be seen only with the use of acetic acid and magnification.
Herpes Simplex (HSV) both types I and II	**Contact**—touching (hand/genital, genital/genital, oral/genital, or ano-genital) an infected person's lesions. Can be transmitted through non-penetrative sexual contact. Transmission commonly occurs in the absence of lesions.	Single or multiple fluid-filled blisters appear typically in the ano-genital area and mouth. They rupture, sometimes leaving extremely painful shallow ulcers, which heal in about twelve days.
Pelvic Inflammatory Disease (PID)	**Fluids**—contact of mucous membranes with infected person's body fluids (mucus, semen). Transmission most common with exposure through anal and vaginal sex, or rarely, oral sex. Casual contact considered to be safe.	There may be no symptoms, but PID is usually characterized by moderate to severe lower abdominal pain, fever, chills, and possibly bowel symptoms. May mimic appendicitis, ureteral stones, twisted or ruptured ovarian cyst, and other acute lower abdominal conditions.

Source: From *Sexually Transmitted Infections: What Everyone Should Know* by American College Health Association. Copyright © 2005 by American College Health Association. Reprinted by permission.

Potential Complications/ Course of Infection	Treatment	Prevention—For all STIs, abstinence is the best protection
In women, serious complications can occur if spread to fallopian tubes. May result in tubal scarring, infertility, and risk of tubal pregnancy.	A number of commonly used antibiotics are effective. Partners **must** be treated at the same time.	Condoms (latex or polyurethane) reduce but do not eliminate risk.
Cervix—Most cervical infections are invisible to the naked eye. Occasionally, visible cervical warts may be present. Cervical cancer can be prevented by detection and treatment of pre-cancerous changes. *External skin and anus of men and women, and the vagina*—warty lesions, flat or raised. Some may be pre-cancers, but natural history of lesions is not to become cancers until advanced age. Long-term complications are not yet known.	Many treatments are available. The most expensive does not necessarily mean the best. *Cervix*—cryo (freezing), laser, and LEEP. *External*—Aldara, cryo, laser, liquid N, TCA/BCA, podophyllin, and interferon. In some individuals, the virus is cleared from the body. In others, viral particles remain latent after treatment. Lesions can be eliminated. It is unlikely that the presence of latent viral particles without lesions can result in transmission.	Barrier methods reduce but do not eliminate risk. With condoms, for example, lesions may be present in uncovered areas. Only total absence of any touching of infected tissue will avoid transmission. When both partners are infected, they probably do not continue to transmit to each other.
Recurrent painful attacks. Infants infected at or before delivery may sustain severe neurological damage or death.	Antiviral drugs are effective if taken early in the infection or continuously in a preventive regimen. Topical anesthetics may be helpful in reducing discomfort.	Barrier methods reduce but do not eliminate risk. With condoms, for example, lesions may be present in uncovered areas.
May progress to abscesses and injury resulting in infertility, ectopic pregnancy, chronic pain, and even death.	Therapy with one or more antibiotics with broad coverage. Individuals must always be treated for chlamydia and gonorrhea; management sometimes requires hospitalization. Partners **must** be treated at the same time.	Condoms (latex or polyurethane) reduce but do not eliminate risk.

(continued)

Table 8.7
continued

STI	Transmission (Body Fluids and/or Direct Contact)	Symptoms
Human Immunodeficiency Virus (HIV)/AIDS	**Fluids**—contact of open skin or mucous membranes with infected person's body fluids (blood, mucus, semen). Most common with exposure through anal or vaginal sex, and, though uncommon, oral sex. Casual contact considered to be safe. Health care workers at risk through scalpel cuts and needle sticks.	Divided into four stages: *Infection* and *Seroconversion*—flu-like illness for approximately two weeks. *Symptom-Free*—few months to many years. *Early Symptoms*—fevers, shingles, yeast infections—few months to several years. *AIDS*—opportunistic infections, neoplasia (Kaposi's sarcoma, lymphoma, cervical cancer), dementia, and other neurological symptoms—few months to several years.
Gonorrhea	**Fluids**—contact of mucous membranes (cervix, urethra) with infected person's fluids (semen, mucus). Most common with exposure through vaginal or anal sex. Casual contact considered to be safe.	Very similar to chlamydia for both women and men.
Hepatitis B (HBV)	**Fluids**—contact with mucous membranes (cervix, urethra, anal area) with infected person's fluids (semen, saliva, blood, mucus). Most common with exposure through vaginal or anal sex. Casual contact considered to be safe. Health care workers at risk through scalpel cuts and needle sticks.	At first, usually no symptoms. If disease progresses, symptoms may occur—fatigue, nausea, and jaundice (yellowing of the skin and eyes) with dark urine.
Syphilis	**Fluids** and **Contact**—Also, 50% risk of transmission from mother to infant in utero.	Occurs in three stages: *Primary*—painless ulcer. *Secondary*—rash, condylomata lata, lymph node enlargement, spotty baldness. *Late/Latent*—vascular and neurological damage may be occurring.

Potential Complications/ Course of Infection	Treatment	Prevention—For all STIs, abstinence is the best protection
Signs and symptoms of AIDS, death (current medications lengthening survival). Treatment of pregnant women with HIV greatly reduces the risk of maternal-fetal transmission.	Antivirals and specific medications for complications.	Condoms (latex or polyurethane) reduce but do not eliminate risk. Avoid contact with needles, particularly IV drug use.
In women, serious complications can occur if spread to fallopian tubes. May result in tubal scarring, infertility, and risk of tubal pregnancy.	A number of commonly used antibiotics are very effective. Partners **must** be treated at the same time.	Condoms (latex or polyurethane) reduce but do not eliminate risk.
Cirrhosis, liver cancer, liver failure, death.	Antiviral medications are indicated in certain circumstances.	Vaccination of infants and non-immunized adolescents and adults is highly recommended. Avoid contact with blood, needles, etc.
Late complications include: severe neurologic dysfunction, aortic aneurysm.	Penicillin or doxycycline—based on darkfield or blood test. Very important that pregnant women with positive blood tests be treated to prevent congenital syphilis. **Must** treat all contacts.	Condoms, spermicides.

moving on the skin or oval eggs attached to body hair may be visible. The primary symptom of scabies is itching, especially at night. A rash may appear in the folds of skin between the fingers or on the wrists, elbows, abdomen, or genitals. If you think you may have pubic lice or scabies, see your physician. They can determine whether treatment is necessary or not. The most effective treatments include shampoos and creams that contain lindane or a related compound. Pubic lice can be treated at home with special creams, lotions, and shampoos that are available in drugstores without a prescription. Be certain to follow the instructions carefully and do not exceed the recommended applications. The infestation may be stubborn, requiring an additional treatment. Avoid close contact with others if you have pubic lice or scabies until it is treated. Wash clothes, bed linens, and any other materials that may have been infected in hot water and dry on the hottest setting. If you have pubic lice or scabies be sure to tell your sexual partner(s) or anyone with whom you have had close contact or who has shared your bed linens, clothes, or towels. These individuals should be seen by a physician even if they do not have an itch or rash. The best way to protect yourself is to know your partner's sexual history, don't share towels, swimsuits, or underwear and thoroughly wash any materials that you think may carry pubic lice or scabies in hot water.

Trichomoniasis

Trichomoniasis is caused by a protozoan parasite, *Trichomonas vaginalis*. The most common sites of infection are the vagina (in women) and the urethra (in men). The parasite is sexually transmitted through the penis to the vagina during intercourse or vulva to vulva contact with an infected partner. Most men infected with trichomoniasis are asymptomatic, but have the parasites and can infect their sexual partners. Some women will have signs or symptoms from the infection which include a yellowish-green vaginal discharge, a slight burning after urination, or itching in the genital area. These signs or symptoms typically appear five to twenty-eight days after exposure.

A health care provider must perform a physical exam and laboratory tests to diagnose trichomoniasis. The treatment for trichomoniasis is a prescription drug (either Metronidazole or Tinidazole) taken by mouth in a single dose. It is important for both partners to be treated at the same time to eliminate the parasite.

The best way to avoid contracting trichomoniasis is to abstain from vaginal, oral, or anal intercourse or have a mutually monogamous relationship with an uninfected partner. Utilizing male condoms consistently and correctly can reduce the risk of transmission of trichomoniasis.

STI Prevention

Preventing the spread of STIs requires responsibility in sexual relationships. The best way to prevent contraction of an STI is to practice sexual abstinence or have a mutually monogamous relationship with an uninfected person and do not share needles for any reason. If an individual chooses to be sexually active, limit the number of sexual partners and use condoms consistently and correctly (see Figure 8.9 on page 269). If you think you are infected, avoid any sexual contact until you visit your physician, a local STI clinic, or hospital for testing. Remember that many STIs are spread by those with no noticeable symptoms. It only takes one infected partner to contract a sexually transmitted infection.

A major problem for health care providers is persuading sexually active people to seek testing for STIs early after exposure. While some STIs such as genital herpes, HIV/AIDS, and genital warts are chronic with no cure, early diagnosis can help to prevent further transmission of the infections, and in the case of herpes, early treatment of the lesions can lessen the symptoms. Symptoms of STIs can be slow to develop or may not manifest themselves at all. Thus, an individual can be infected with a number of STIs with only minor or no symptoms. For these reasons, regular and accurate evaluations are necessary to prevent the spread of STIs. Methods of testing for STIs vary with the type of infection suspected. These tests fall loosely into three categories: visual inspection, blood or urine testing, and/or examination of the fluids within the sores themselves or smears of fluids from the vagina or urethra of the male. Symptomatic genital warts, herpes, and pubic lice can usually be identified during an examination by a health care provider. A blood test is used to test for hepatitis B, HIV, and syphilis. If the testing is done less than six months after contracting HIV and less than three weeks after contracting syphilis, there is a possibility the blood test will not be sufficiently sensitive to detect the presence of the infection. A urine test for chlamydia and gonorrhea are available at many health clinics. Often, chlamydia, gonorrhea, and herpes require fluid collection from the infected site for a conclusive diagnosis (Marr, 2007). The importance of testing cannot be overemphasized. As discussed earlier, many of these infections have dangerous complications and are easily cured. To decrease your risk of infection with an STI, you and your sexual partner(s) should know and communicate your sexual history. The only way to have adequate knowledge of your history is to be tested if there is a chance of a previous exposure regardless of the presence or absence of signs or symptoms.

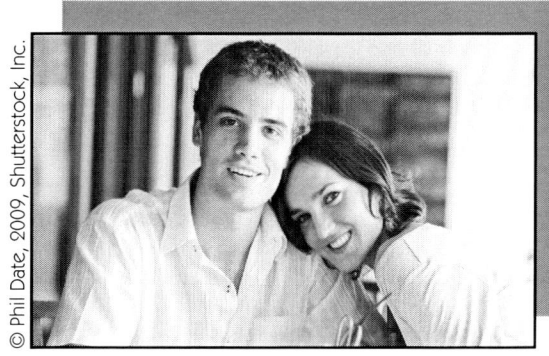

The best way to prevent STIs is to practice sexual abstinence, or have a mutually monogamous relationship with an uninfected person.

There is no single test that can be administered for all sexually transmitted infections. Listed below are the different STIs and the type of test that is required to determine if an individual is infected.

STI	Type of Test
Chlamydia	Urine test and/or culture
Genital Herpes	Visual inspection, culture and/or blood test
Gonorrhea	Urine test and/or culture
Hepatitis B	Blood test
HIV	Blood test
HPV	Visual inspection
Pubic Lice/Scabies	Visual inspection
Syphilis	Blood test

Most individuals at some point in their lives will strongly desire to have children. An STI can affect the ability to conceive and have children. Chlamydia and gonorrhea can cause both males and females to become sterile. Further complications can arise for pregnant women who are infected with STIs. Herpes and hepatitis B, for example, in rare instances can be fatal to the fetus. There is a very real risk of passing HIV to a newborn. Early treatment of STIs can reduce the risk of infertility, but fertility cannot be guaranteed.

REFERENCES

American Cancer Society. 2005.

American College Health Association (ACHA). *Sexually Transmitted Infections: What Everyone Should Know.* 2005.

American College Health Association (ACHA). 2004.

American College of Obstetricians and Gynecology (ACOG). 1998.

American Social Health Association (ASHA). 2004.

Association of Reproductive Health Pofessionals (ARHP). 2008. www.arhp.org

Centers for Disease Control and Prevention (CDC). 2008. www.cdc.gov/std/syphilis/STDFact-syphilis.htm
www.cdc.gov/std/herpes/STDFact-herpes.htm
www.cdc.gov/std/PID/STDFact-PID.htm

Centers for Disease Control and Prevention (CDC). *Youth Risk Behavior Survey.* 2007. www.cdc.gov/nchhstp/Newsroom/WADPressrelease-112408.htm

Centers for Disease Control and Prevention (CDC). *Guidelines for Treatment of Sexually Transmitted Infections.* 2006a.

Centers for Disease Control and Prevention (CDC). *HIV/AIDS Surveillance Report: Cases of HIV Infection and AIDS in the United States and Dependent Areas.* 2006b.

Crooks, R. and Baur, K. *Our Sexuality* (10th ed). Pacific Grove, CA: Brooks/Cole. 2007.

Crowley, L. *An Introduction to Human Disease: Pathology and Pathophysiology Correlations* (7th ed). Boston: Jones and Bartlett Publishers, Inc. 2006.

Donatelle, R. *Access to Health* (9th ed). San Francisco: Benjamin Cummings. 2006.

Ellertson, C. et al. Extending the Fine Limit for Starting the Yuzpe Regimen of Emergency Contraception to 120 Hours. *Obstetrics and Gynecology, 101,* 1168-1171. 2003.

ETR Associates. "Men's Health, What's Normal, What's Not." 2007a.

ETR Associates. "Not Ready for Sex, Talking with Your Partner." 2007b.

ETR Associates. "Women's Health, What's Normal, What's Not." 2007c.

ETR Associates. "Nine Sexually Responsible Behaviors." 2008.

Floyd, P. et al. *Personal Health: Perspectives & Lifestyles* (4th ed). Englewood, CO: Morton Publishing Co. 2007.

Herek, G. et al. Psychological Sequelae of Hate-Crime Victimization among Lesbian, Gay, and Bisexual Adults. *Journal of Consulting and Clinical Psychology, 67,* 6. 1999.

Ho, G. et al. Natural History of Cervix Vaginal Papillomavirus Infection in Young Women. *New England Journal of Medicine, 338*(7): 423-8. 1998.

Marr, L. *Sexually Transmitted Diseases: A Physician Tells You What You Need to Know.* (2nd ed). Baltimore: Johns Hopkins University Press. 2007.

Sexuality Information and Education Council of the United States (SIECUS). 2008. www.siecus.org/index.cfm?fuseaction=Page.viewPage+pageId=598+ParentID=477

Trussell, J. and Jordan, B. Mechanism of Action of Emergency Contraceptive Pills. *Contraception, 74,* 87-89. 2006.

U.S. Department of Health and Human Services. "Bone Health and Osteoporosis: A Report of the Surgeon General." 2004.

www.cdc.gov/STD/HPV/STDFact-HPV.htm

www.cdc.gov/vaccines/recs/acip/downloads/mtg-slides-feb08/15-4-hpv.pdf

www.cdc.gov/vaccines/ed/ciinc/specialtopics/downloads/Feb_06_HepB_JC.ppt#262,6 Modes of HBV Transmission in Early Childhood

www.fwhc.org/birth-control

CONTACTS

AIDS Treatment Information Service
800-HIV-0440
http://www.aidsinfo.nih.gov

American Social Health Association and CDC National Hotline
800-227-8922
http://www.ashastd.org

Brazos County Health Department
201 North Texas Avenue
Bryan, TX 77803
979-361-4440

CDC National AIDS Hotline
800-342-AIDS (2437)
http://www.ashastd.org

Centers for Disease Control and Prevention
http://www.cdc.gov

Emergency Contraception Hotline
800-584-9911

Gay and Lesbian Medical Association
459 Fulton Street, Ste 107
San Francisco, CA 94102
415-255-4547
www.glma.org

Gladney Center for Adoption
817-922-6000

Good Samaritan Gabriel Project Life Center
1314 E 29th St.
Bryan, TX 77802
979-822-9340

Healthfinder
http://www.healthfinder.gov

National Herpes Resource Center
800-227-8922

Hope Pregnancy Centers of Brazos County
205 Brentwood Drive
College Station, TX 77840
979-695-9193

International Childbirth Education Association
800-624-4934
http://www.ICEA.org

National Abortion Federation
800-772-9100

National Council For Adoption
703-299-6633
www.adoptioncouncil.org

National Directory of LGBT Community Centers
www.lgbtcenters.org

North American Council on Adoptable Children (NACAC)
651-644-3036

Parents, Families and Friends of Lesbians and Gays (PFLAG)
1726 M Street, NW, Suite 400
Washington, DC 20036
202-467-8180
979-694-2617 (College Station, TX)

Planned Parenthood
4112 East 29th
Bryan, TX 77802
979-846-1744
http://www.plannedparenthood.org

Shanti Project
(Counseling and assistance for persons with AIDS)
415-674-4700
http://www.shanti.org

Texas A&M University Student Health Services
979-458-8250
http://shs.tamu.edu/

TAMU A.P. Beutel Health Center Health Education Division
979-847-8910
http://healthed.tamu.edu/

TAMU Student Life Gender Issues Education Services (GIES)
979-845-1107

ACTIVITIES

In-Class Activities

Apply percent incidence of STIs, HIV, unplanned pregnancy, adoption, and abortion to class size.

Can We Make Ends Meet?

Parents

Notebook Activities

STI Attitudes

Hepatitis Risk Assessment

Name: _____ Section: _____ Date: _____

IN-CLASS ACTIVITY

Can We Make Ends Meet?

Concept/Description: Being a parent can drastically change a person's life socially, emotionally, physically, and financially.

Objective: To explore the financial strain that being a parent would cause the typical college student.

Materials:
Classified section of the newspaper
Parents sheet
Parents (2) sheet
Pens or pencils

Directions:
1. Divide the class into groups of four and give each group the Parents sheets.
2. Ask each group to choose a job from the classified section for which they would be qualified. Assuming that they got the job, they estimate how much money they would make in a year. (Call the company, if possible.)
3. Give students a few days to research the information on the sheets by asking people, calling various companies to get rates, and so on.
4. Have students fill in the sheets and figure out if "income" could cover "expenses."
5. Ask students to list the many difficulties parents face, besides financial strain.
6. Discuss.

Name: _____ Section: _____ Date: _____

IN-CLASS ACTIVITY

Parents

Directions: Being a parent can drastically change your life. Figure out the financial aspect of being a parent by filling in the information below:

HOUSING

1. Rent		$ _____	per month
2. Utilities	Gas	$ _____	per month
	Electricity	$ _____	per month
	Garbage	$ _____	per month
	Water	$ _____	per month
	Sewer	$ _____	per month
3. Approximate phone bill		$ _____	per month
4. Cable television		$ _____	per month
	TOTAL	$ _____	per month

AUTO

1. Car payment $ _____ per month
2. Gasoline $ _____ per month
3. Car repairs $ _____ per month
4. License and insurance $ _____ per month
                    TOTAL $ _____ per month

BABY

1. Day care $ _____ per month
2. Diapers $ _____ per month
3. Baby clothing $ _____ per month
                    TOTAL $ _____ per month

Name: _____ Section: _____ Date: _____

IN-CLASS ACTIVITY

Parents (2)

G E N E R A L

1. Food bill	$ _____ per month
2. Health care	$ _____ per month
3. Entertainment	$ _____ per month
4. Savings	$ _____ per month
5. Miscellaneous (gifts, toys, etc.)	$ _____ per month
TOTAL	$ _____ per month

TOTALS:

Housing	$ _____ _____
Auto	$ _____ _____
Baby	$ _____ _____
General	$ _____ _____
TOTAL MONTHLY COSTS	$ _____ _____

Do you think that a typical college student could make ends meet? Why or why not?

Name: _____ Section: _____ Date: _____

NOTEBOOK ACTIVITY

Hepatitis Risk Assessment

Check Your Risk of Hepatitis A	Yes	No
1. Do you believe you have been exposed to hepatitis A in the past 2 weeks?		
2. Do you live with someone currently ill with hepatitis A?		
3. Have you had sex with someone currently ill with hepatitis A?		
4. Do you currently live in a region of the United States where hepatitis A rates are very high?		
5. Do you travel or work in an area outside of the United States where hepatitis A is a problem? (This includes everywhere EXCEPT Australia, New Zealand, Western Europe, Japan, and Canada)		
6. If you are a man, do you have sex with other men?		
7. Are you an injecting or a non-injecting (snort cocaine) drug user?		

If you check yes to any of the questions, you are at risk and should see your doctor.

Check Your Risk of Hepatitis B	Yes	No
1. Is someone in your household infected with hepatitis B?		
2. Have you ever been diagnosed with a sexually transmitted infection?		
3. Have you had sex with more than one partner in a 6-month period?		
4. If you are a man, do you have sex with other men?		
5. Have you or any of your sex partner(s) ever injected illegal drugs?		
6. Have you ever shared equipment (needles, syringes, cotton, water, etc.) when injecting drugs with someone else?		
7. Have you ever received hemodialysis?		
8. Did your mother have hepatitis B when you were born?		
9. Have you worked in a health care job or other occupation where you had a needlestick injury or other sharps exposures on the job?		
10. Have you shared a toothbrush, razor, or any other item that might have blood on it (visible or not) with a person who has hepatitis B?		

If you check yes to any of the questions, you are at risk and should see your doctor.

Check Your Risk for Hepatitis C	Yes	No
1. Did you receive a blood transfusion or solid organ transplant (heart, lung, liver, pancreas, kidney) before July 1992?		
2. Did you receive clotting factor concentrates produced before 1987?		
3. Have you ever received hemodialysis?		
4. Have you had blood tests that showed a liver problem?		
5. Have you had a needlestick injury working in a health care setting?		
6. Did your mother have hepatitis C when you were born?		
7. Have you shared a toothbrush, razor, or any other item that might have blood on it (visible or not) with a person who has hepatitis C?		
8. Have you or any of your sex partner(s) injected illegal drugs, even if it was only one time many years ago?		

If you check yes to any of the questions, you are at risk and should see your doctor.

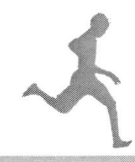

CHAPTER 9

Drugs

"First we form habits, then they form us. Conquer your bad habits, or they'll eventually conquer you."

—Dr. Rob Gilbert

OBJECTIVES

Students will be able to:
- Identify types of alcoholic beverages and the alcohol content for each.
- Identify the physiological and societal effects of alcohol.
- Identify penalties for alcohol-related offenses.
- Identify factors relating to binge drinking and alcohol poisoning.
- Identify risks of drinking and driving.
- Identify the adverse effects of tobacco use.
- Identify types of tobacco use.
- Identify the effects of environmental tobacco smoke.
- Identify types of psychoactive drugs and their physiological effects.
- Identify the types and risks of inhalant use.
- Identify the adverse effects of Rohypnol and gamma hydroxybutyrate (GHB).

Tobacco

The U.S. Surgeon General reported in 1970 that cigarette smoking is dangerous to your health. Over the years we have come to realize just how dangerous. Cigarette smoking is the leading preventable cause of death in the United States, responsible for one in five deaths annually. Through study after study, reports have proven that tobacco use is one of the biggest public health issues that faces the world today (CDC, 2006). Tobacco is a risk factor for six of the eight leading causes of death, with smokers dying thirteen to fourteen years earlier than non-smokers. Worldwide, there are 5.4 million deaths annually because of tobacco use with current trends estimating an increase to 8 million deaths by 2030 (CDC, 2006).

Tobacco Components

The toxic components of tobacco include tar, nicotine, and carbon monoxide. **Tar** is a by-product of burning tobacco. Its composition is a dark, sticky substance that can be condensed from cigarette smoke. Tar contains many potent carcinogens and chemicals that irritate tissue in the lungs and promote chronic bronchitis and emphysema. These substances paralyze and destroy the cilia that line the bronchi, causing "smoker's cough." Long-term exposure of extremely toxic tar to lung tissue can lead to the development of cancer.

Nicotine is a colorless, oily compound that is extremely poisonous in concentrated amounts. This highly addictive drug is a major contributor to heart and

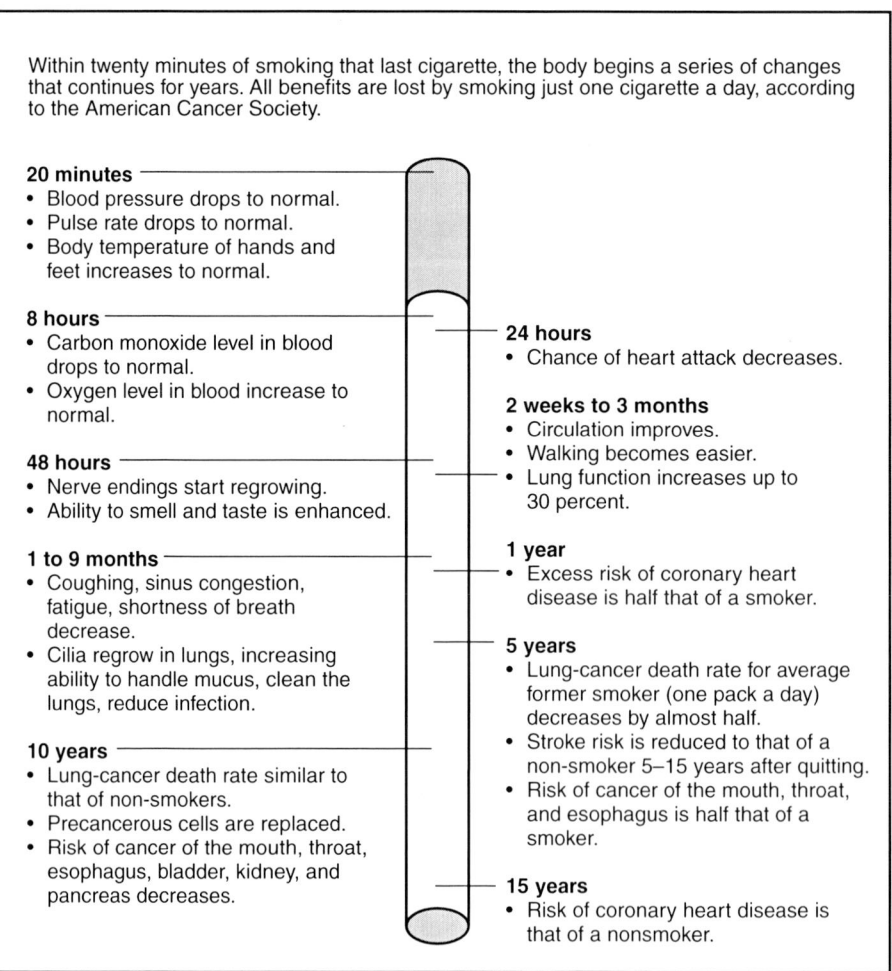

FIGURE 9.1 When Smokers Quit

respiratory diseases causing short-term increases in blood pressure, heart rate, and blood flow from the heart, resulting in narrowing of the arteries. A strong dependence on nicotine can occur after as little as three packs of cigarettes, and it is more addictive than cocaine or heroin. Because of its addictive effects, the Food and Drug Administration (FDA) has determined nicotine should be regulated.

At first, nicotine acts as a stimulant and then it tends to tranquilize the nervous system. The effects depend largely on how one chooses to smoke. Shallow puffs seem to increase alertness because low doses of nicotine facilitate the release of acetylcholine, which creates feelings of alertness. Long, deep drags tend to relax the smoker because high doses of nicotine block the flow of acetylcholine. Ninety percent of the nicotine inhaled while smoking is absorbed into the body, while 20 to 30 percent of nicotine is absorbed if the smoke is drawn only into the mouth, not the lungs.

Other side effects include inhibiting formation of urine, discoloration of the fingers, dulling the taste buds, and irritating the membranes in the mouth and throat. Because nicotine constricts blood vessels, it causes the skin to be clammy and have a pallid appearance, as well as reducing body temperature. The highly addictive nature of nicotine can cause withdrawal symptoms to occur quite suddenly. These symptoms include irritability, anxiousness, hostility, food cravings, headaches, and the inability to concentrate.

Carbon monoxide is an odorless, tasteless gas that is highly toxic. It reduces the amount of oxygen the blood can carry, causing shortness of breath. Carbon monoxide ultimately damages the inner walls of the arteries, thus encouraging a buildup of fat on the walls of the arteries; this is called atherosclerosis. Over time, this causes the arteries to narrow and harden, which may lead to a heart attack.

Approximately 1 percent of cigarette smoke and 6 percent of cigar smoke is carbon monoxide. It impairs normal function of the nervous system and is partially responsible for the increased risk of heart attacks and strokes in smokers.

Types of Tobacco Use

Smokeless tobacco comes in two forms: snuff and chewing tobacco. Snuff is a fine grain of tobacco, and chewing tobacco is shredded or bricked; either choice is placed in the mouth and the user sucks on the tobacco juices, spitting out the saliva. The sucking allows the nicotine to be absorbed in the bloodstream. It can be equally as dangerous and harmful as smoking. Smokeless tobacco is addictive. According to the Centers for Disease Control and Prevention (CDC) estimates, 8 percent of high school students are current smokeless tobacco users. Nationally, an estimated 3 percent of adults are current smokeless tobacco users.

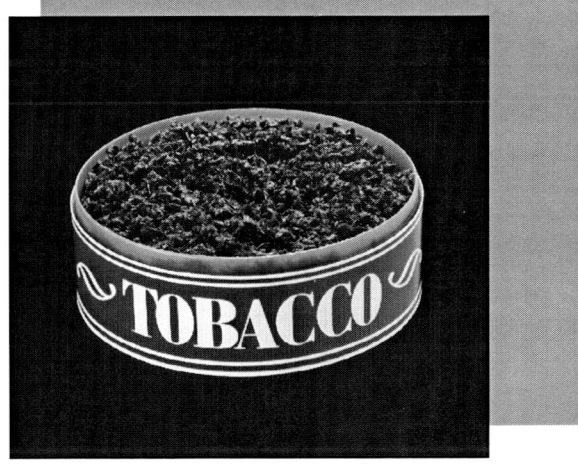

The National Cancer Institute reports there are three thousand chemical compounds in smokeless tobacco. Nicotine is the addictive drug in all forms of tobacco. Holding one pinch of smokeless tobacco in your mouth for thirty minutes delivers as much nicotine as three to four cigarettes (National Cancer Institute, 2008). There have been at least twenty-eight cancer-causing agents found in smokeless tobacco:

- Nitrosamines—20 to 43,000 more nitrosamines are found in smokeless tobacco. Other consumer products like beer or bacon only contain five parts per billion
- Polonium 210—radioactive particles that turn into radon
- Formaldehyde—embalming fluid

- Cadmium—metallic element; its salts are poisonous
- Arsenic—poisonous element

Immediate effects from chewing tobacco are bad breath and stains on your teeth. Mouth sores also accompany smokeless tobacco users. The complications of long-term use can be very serious. These complications include increased gum and teeth problems, increased heart rate, irregular heartbeat, heart attacks, and cancer. Oral cancer can occur in the mouth, lips, tongue, cheeks, or gums. Other cancer possibilities resulting from smokeless tobacco can be stomach cancer, bladder cancer, and cancer of the esophagus.

Another major problem caused by smokeless tobacco is **leukoplakia**, a precancerous condition that produces thick, rough, white patches on the gums, tongue, and inner cheeks. A variety of cancers such as lip, pharynx, larynx, esophagus, and tongue can be attributed to smokeless tobacco. Dental and gum problems are major side effects as well.

Cigarette smoking greatly impairs the respiratory system and is a major cause of chronic obstructive pulmonary diseases (COPD), including emphysema and chronic bronchitis.

Problems associated with cigarette smoking (see Figure 9.2) include mouth, throat, and other types of cancer, cirrhosis of the liver, stomach, and duodenal ulcers, gum and dental disease, decreased HDL cholesterol and decreased platelet survival and clotting time, as well as increased blood thickness.

Cigarette smoking increases problems such as heart disease, atherosclerosis, and blood clots. It increases the amount of fatty acids, glucose, and various hormones in the blood, cardiac arrhythmia, allergies, diabetes, hypertension, peptic ulcers, and sexual impotence. Smoking doubles the risk of heart disease, and those who smoke have only a 50 percent chance of recovery. Smokers also have a 70 percent higher

FIGURE 9.2

The Health Effects of Smoking

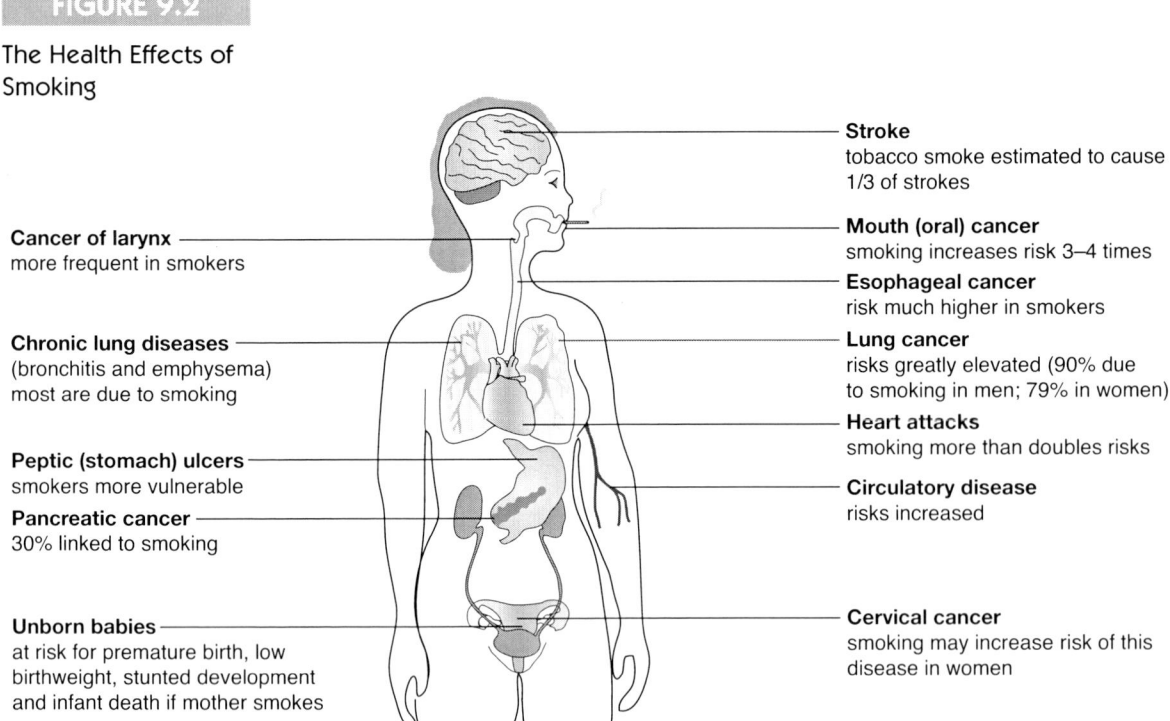

Source: Adapted from "The Health Effects of Smoking" *Lifetime Physical Fitness & Wellness* by Hoeger and Hoeger, Wadsworth Publishing.

death rate from heart disease than non-smokers (CDC, 2006). Smoking also causes cardiomyopathy, a condition that weakens the heart's ability to pump blood.

Life expectancy of smokers parallels smoking habits in that the younger one starts smoking and the longer one smokes, the higher the mortality rate. Also, the deeper smoke is inhaled and the higher the tar and nicotine content, the higher the mortality rate.

The risk and mortality rates for lip, mouth, and larynx cancers for **pipe and cigar smoking** are higher than for cigarette smoking. Pipe smoke, which is 2 percent carbon monoxide, is more irritating to the respiratory system than cigarette smoking, but for those who do not inhale, the risk for developing cancer is just as likely.

Cigars have recently gained popularity in the United States among younger men and women with approximately 4.5 billion cigars consumed yearly.

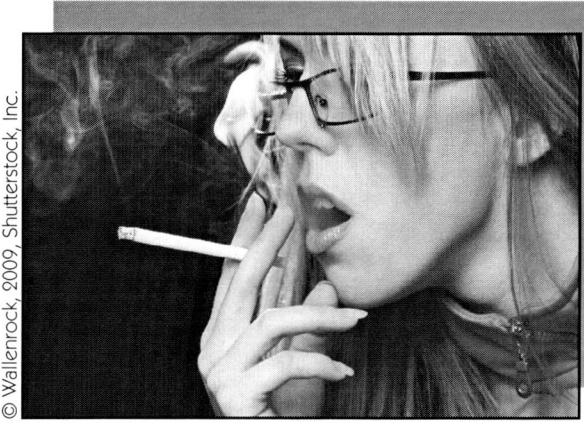

The younger someone is when they start smoking, and the longer they continue to smoke, the greater their chance of dying from a smoking-related illness.

Clove cigarettes are erroneously believed to be safer because they do not contain as much tobacco. In actuality, clove cigarettes are most harmful because they contain **eugenol**, which is an active ingredient of clove. Eugenol deadens sensations in the throat, which allows smokers to inhale more deeply and hold smoke in the lungs longer. Clove cigarettes also contain twice as much tar, nicotine, and carbon monoxide as most moderate brands of American cigarettes.

Once thought of as a less harmful way to smoke tobacco, **water pipes** have regained popularity in many cities across the United States. In 2005 the World Health Organization (WHO) published its findings emphasizing the harmful effects of waterpipe smoking, also known around the world as narghile, shisha, goza, and hookah. For centuries, smokers have been lead to believe that water pipe smoking is a

Smokeless Tobacco Users

Check Monthly for Early Signs of Disease

The early signs of cancer in the mouth and tongue may be detected by self-examination. Dr. Elbert Glover, director of the Tobacco Research Center at West Virginia University, and the American Cancer Society recommend that the following self-check procedures be conducted every month.

- Check your face and neck for lumps on either side. Both sides of your face and neck should be the same shape.
- Look at your lips, cheeks, and gums. Look for sores, white or red patches, or changes in your gums by pulling down your lower lip. Check your inner cheeks, especially where you hold your tobacco. Gently squeeze your lip and cheeks to check for lumps or soreness.
- Put the tip of your tongue on the roof of your mouth. Place one finger on the floor of your mouth and press up under your chin with a finger from your other hand. Feel for bumps, soreness, or swelling. Check around the inside of your teeth from one side of your jaw to the other.
- Tilt your head back and open your mouth wide. Check for color changes or bumps or sores in the roof of your mouth.
- Stick out your tongue and look at the top. Gently grasp your tongue with a piece of cloth and pull it to each side. Look for color changes. Feel both sides of your tongue with your finger for bumps.

If you use smokeless tobacco and find anything that looks or feels unusual, see your dentist or physician as soon as possible.

From *Decisions for Healthy Living* by Pruitt, Stein and Pruitt, Addison Wesley Longman Educational Publishers, Inc.

FIGURE 9.3
Comparison of Cigarette Smoking Session and Water Pipe Smoking Session

Cigarette Smoking Session	Water Pipe Smoking Session
8–12 puffs	50–100 puffs
5–7 minutes	20–80 minutes
0.5–0.6 liter of smoke inhaled	.015–1.0 liter of smoke inhaled

Note: Upon analysis, it is possible for a water pipe session to expose the smoker to the equivalent of up to one hundred cigarettes in a single session.

safer alternative to cigarette smoking, but research shows that this method exposes the smoker to high rates of lung cancer and heart disease, as well as other tobacco-related diseases. There is also a high risk of communicable diseases like tuberculosis and hepatitis because of shared mouthpieces (WHO, 2005).

When smoking tobacco through a water pipe, some nicotine is absorbed as it passes through a water bowl. Because most smokers stop when their nicotine craving has been satisfied, this may actually lead to longer smoking sessions, exposing the user to more smoke over a longer period of time (see Figure 9.3).

Some water pipe products and accessories are marketed and sold with claims of reducing the harmful effects of hookah, but according to the WHO, none have been shown to reduce the smoker's risk of exposure to toxins.

Environmental Tobacco Smoke

Environmental tobacco smoke (ETS), or secondhand smoke, contains at least 250 toxic chemicals and more than 50 carcinogens. Secondhand smoke exposure to non-smoking adults can cause heart disease, a 20–30 percent increased risk of lung cancer, and a 25–30 percent increased risk of heart attacks. Approximately 126 million non-smokers are exposed to secondhand smoke in homes, workplaces, and public places, resulting in an estimated 38,000 deaths and healthcare costs exceeding $10 billion annually. To those individuals with existing health issues, secondhand smoke exposure is an extremely high risk. There is no "risk-free" exposure to secondhand smoke; even brief exposure can be dangerous (CDC, 2006).

Secondhand smoke is especially dangerous to infants and children. In the United States, almost 22 million children are exposed to secondhand smoke. Globally almost half of the world's children breathe air polluted by tobacco smoke. This exposure can cause sudden infant death syndrome, acute respiratory infections, ear problems, slow lung growth, and severe asthma attacks. Each year in the United States, secondhand smoke is responsible for almost 300,000 new cases of bronchitis and pneumonia in children less than 18 months, resulting in nearly 15,000 hospitalizations annually (CDC, 2006).

There is no "risk-free" exposure to secondhand smoke.

Smoking Cessation

Each year an estimated 1.3 million smokers quit successfully. More than four out of five smokers say they want to quit (AHA, 2006). Although there are various pharmacological agents used to aid smokers in quitting, nicotine replacement therapy has been shown to be the most effective.

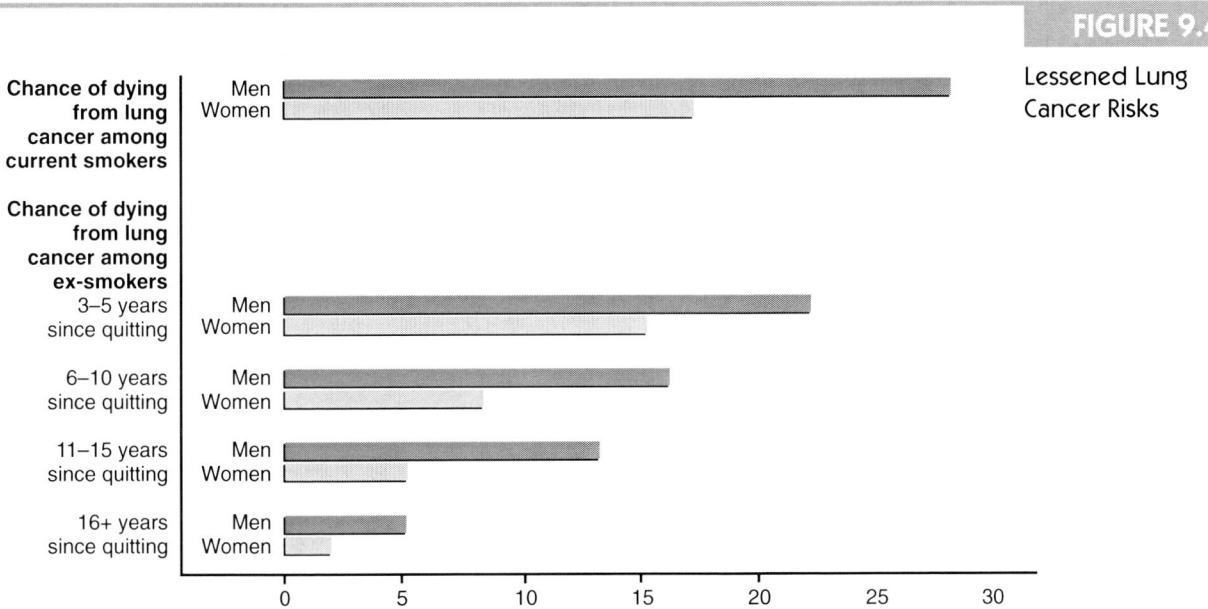

FIGURE 9.4 Lessened Lung Cancer Risks

The 1990 U.S. Surgeon General's report concludes that smokers who quit significantly reduce their risks of dying from lung cancer.

Source: Smoking and Health. (1990). Rockville, MD: Health and Human Services.

The transdermal nicotine patch is safe, as well as nicotine gum, although the patch appears to be preferred by most. In addition to the patch and gum, a nicotine nasal spray and nicotine inhalers are also available.

Of the 46 million Americans who currently smoke cigarettes, most are either actively trying to quit or want to quit (AHA, 2006). Since 1965, more than 49 percent of all adults who have ever smoked have quit. Quitting can bring a major reduction in the occurrence of coronary heart disease and other forms of cardiovascular diseases. Quitting reduces the risk for repeat heart attacks and death from heart disease by 50 percent or more (AHA, 2006). Quitting can also aid in the management of contributors to heart attacks such as atherosclerosis, thrombosis, and cardiac arrhythmia.

By choosing to quit smoking, the American Heart Association (AHA) reports that after one year off cigarettes, risk for heart attacks is reduced by 50 percent (see Figure 9.1). After fifteen years of abstinence from smoking, your risks are similar to that of a person who never smoked. In five to fifteen years of being smoke-free, the risk of stroke is the same as for non-smokers. Male smokers who quit between ages 35 to 39 add an average of five years to their lives, and females add three years to their lives (AHA, 2006; (see Figure 9.4).

The National Center for Chronic Disease Prevention and Control (part of the CDC) has shown that these five steps will help you quit and quit for good. You have the best chance if you use these together:

1. Get ready—set a quit date, get rid of all your cigarettes, do not let people smoke in your home; once you quit, do not smoke!
2. Get support and encouragement—tell family, friends, and co-workers. Ask them not to smoke around you.
3. Learn new skills and behaviors—change your routine, get busy with new tasks, reduce stress.

The Benefits of Quitting Smoking

Did you know that you could notice the health benefits in less than one hour after quitting smoking? If you were to quit smoking right now . . .

In 20 minutes

- Your blood pressure would decrease
- Your pulse rate would drop
- The body temperature of your hands and feet would increase.

In 8 hours

- The carbon monoxide level in your blood would drop to normal.
- The oxygen level in your blood would increase to normal.

In 24 hours

- Your chance of heart attack would decrease.

In 48 hours

- Your nerve endings would start regrowing.
- Your ability to smell and taste would enhance.

In 2 weeks to 3 months

- Your circulation would improve.
- Walking would become easier.
- Your lung function would increase.

In 1 to 9 months

- Coughing, sinus congestion, fatigue, and shortness of breath would decrease.

In 1 year

- You excess risk of coronary heart disease would decrease to half that of a smoker.

In 5 years

- From 5 to 15 years after quitting, your risk for stroke would be reduced to that of people who have never smoked.

In 10 years

- Your risk of lung cancer would drop to as little as one-half that of continuing smokers.
- Your risk of cancer of the mouth, throat, esophagus, bladder, kidney, and pancreas would decrease.
- Your risk of ulcer would decrease.

In 15 years

- Your risk of coronary heart disease would be similar to that of people who have never smoked.
- Your risk of death would return to nearly the level of people who have never smoked.

Source: Reprinted with permission © 2005 American Lung Association. For more information about the American Lung Association or to support the work it does, call 1-800-LUNG-USA (1-800-586-4872) or log on to www.lungusa.org

4. Get medication and use it correctly—ask your healthcare provider for advice; FDA approved medications:
   - Bupropion SR—prescription only
   - Nicotine gum—over the counter
   - Nicotine inhaler—prescription
   - Nicotine nasal spray—prescription
   - Nicotine patch—prescription and over the counter

5. Be prepared for relapse or difficult situations—most relapses occur within the first three months after quitting. Don't be discouraged, most people try several times before they finally quit. Keep trying!

There is some irreversible damage to virtually every organ system in the body. There are dangers from smoking that remain even after quitting. Although it is never too late to quit smoking, the damage that has been done may never entirely disappear. It is best to choose to never light up!

For more information on smoking and the health problems associated with tobacco products, contact these agencies:

- American Council on Science and Health (ACSH)
  www.acsh.org
  1995 Broadway, 2nd Floor
  New York, NY 10023-5860
  (212) 362-7044

- American Heart Association (AHA)
  www.aha.org
  National Center
  7272 Greenville Avenue
  Dallas, TX 75231
  1-800-AHA-USA1

- American Lung Association (ALA)
  www.lungusa.org/
  1740 Broadway
  New York, NY 10019-4274
  (212) 315-8700
  1-800-LUNG-USA

- American Medical Association (AMA)
  www.ama-assn.org/
  515 North State Street
  Chicago, IL 60610
  (312) 464-5000

- Centers for Disease Control and Prevention
  www.cdc.gov/tobacco

- U.S. Department of Health and Human Services
  Action on Smoking and Health (ASH)
  http://ash.org
  2013 H Street, N.W.
  Washington, D.C. 20006
  (202) 659-4310

- The Advocacy Institute (AI)
  http://www.advocacy.org/tobacco.htm
  1707 L Street, N.W.
  Washington, D.C. 20036-4505
  (202) 659-8475

- American Cancer Society (ACS)
  http://www.cancer.org
  1599 Clifton Road, N.E.
  Atlanta, GA 30329
  1-800-ACS-2345

- Americans for Nonsmoker's Rights (ANR)
  www.no-smoke.org/
  Suite J
  2530 San Pablo Avenue
  Berkley, CA 94702
  (510) 841-3032

- Association of State and Territorial Health Officials (ASTHO)
  www.astho.org/
  1275 K Street, NW
  Suite 800
  Washington, DC 20005
  (202) 371-9090

- Cancer Research Foundation of America (CRFA)
  www.preventcancer.org
  1600 Duke Street
  Alexandria, VA 22314
  (703) 836-4412
- Doctors Ought to Care (DOC)
  www.bcm.tmc.edu/doc/
  5615 Kirby Drive
  Suite 440
  Houston, TX 77005
  (713) 528-1487

Psychoactive Drugs

According to the Center on Addiction and Substance Abuse at Columbia University, the highest rate for illegal drug use is among the 18- to 25-year-old age group. People choose to take drugs for many reasons. Some choose to experiment while others try to escape from reality. Whatever the reason, the effects can be deadly.

Psychoactive drugs are classified into six categories according to their physiological effects on the body:

1. stimulants,
2. depressants,
3. hallucinogens,
4. cannabis,
5. narcotics,
6. inhalants.

All psychoactive drugs serve to disrupt the normal functioning of the central nervous system by interrupting the transfer of electrical impulses from neurotransmitters (chemical messengers) across the synapses between nerve cells (dendrites). Several different changes to the neurotransmitters may occur depending on the drug. The deactivation of the impulse may not occur, thus allowing for continuous stimulation, or the drug may allow for a continuous slow release of the neurotransmitter. An altered neurotransmitter can result from psychoactive drug use or the stimuli could be totally blocked. Neurotransmitters are important to the relay of information within this system. Substances that interrupt neurotransmitter function seriously disrupt the function of the nervous system.

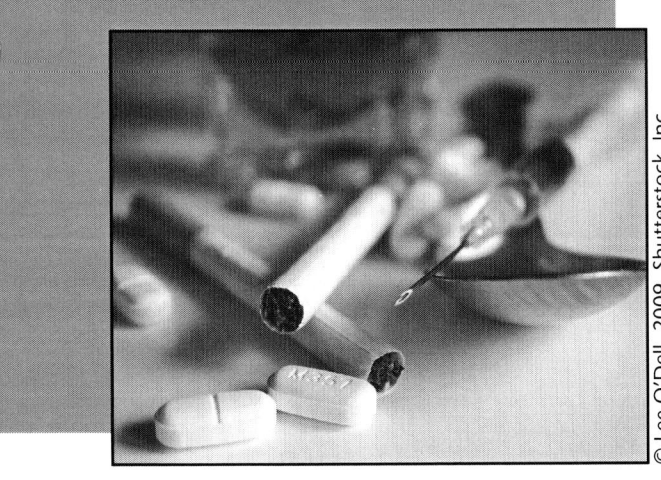

Psychoactive drugs are classified into six categories according to their physiological effects on the body.

Stimulants

Amphetamine

Amphetamines are drugs that speed up the nervous system. They do not occur naturally and must be manufactured in a laboratory. When used in moderation, amphetamines stimulate receptor sites for two naturally occurring neurotransmitters, having the effect of elevated mood, increased alertness, and feelings of well-being. In addition, the activity of the stomach and intestines may be slowed and appetite suppressed. When amphetamines are eliminated from the body, the user becomes fatigued. With abuse, the user will experience rapid tolerance and a strong psychological dependence, along with the possibility of impotence and episodes of psychosis. When use stops, the abuser may experience periods of depression.

Methamphetamines

An extremely addictive and powerful drug that stimulates the central nervous system is commonly known as "meth." In its smoked form, it is called "crystal," "crank," or "ice." It is chemically similar to amphetamines but much stronger. The effects from methamphetamine can last up to eight hours or in some cases even longer. It comes in many forms and can be injected, inhaled, orally ingested, or snorted.

Methamphetamine is considered to be the fastest growing drug in the United States. According to the director of the Substance Abuse and Mental Health Services Administration (SAMHSA), the growth and popularity of this drug is because of its wide availability, easy production, low cost, and highly addictive nature.

Methamphetamine is a psychostimulant but different than others like cocaine or amphetamine. Methamphetamine, like cocaine, results in an accumulation of dopamine. Dopamine is a neurotransmitter in regions of the brain that deal with emotion, movement, motivation, and pleasure. The large release of dopamine is presumed to help the drug's toxic effects on the brain. However, unlike cocaine, which is removed and metabolized quickly from the body, methamphetamine has a longer duration of action, which stays in the body and brain longer, leading to prolonged stimulant effects. The stimulated feeling from smoking methamphetamine can produce a "high" that can last up to twelve hours. After twelve hours, only 50 percent of the drug is removed from the body.

Methamphetamine abusers may display symptoms that include violent behavior, confusion, hallucinations, and possible paranoid or delusional feelings, also causing severe personality shifts. These feelings of paranoia can lead to homicidal or suicidal thoughts or tendencies.

The most serious problems associated with this drug are that it is so highly addictive and can be fatal. It is possible to become addicted after one time, and because it can be made from deadly ingredients such as antifreeze, drain cleaner, fertilizer, battery acid, or lantern fuel. The results when overused can cause heart failure and death. Long-term physical effects can lead to strokes, liver, kidney, and lung damage. Abuse can also lead to permanent and severe brain and psychological damage.

Cocaine

It is a naturally occurring psychoactive substance contained in the leaves of the South American coca plant. Crack cocaine, a rock-like crystalline form of cocaine made by combining cocaine hydrochloride with common baking soda, can be heated in the bowl of a pipe, enabling the vapors to be inhaled into the lungs. Cocaine is used occasionally as a topical anesthetic medicinally; however, more commonly it is inhaled (snorted), injected, or smoked illegally. The effects of cocaine use are rapid and short lived (from five to thirty minutes). Snorting enables only about 60 percent of the drug to be absorbed because the nasal vessels constrict immediately. Cocaine use causes dopamine and norepinephrine to be released into the brain, causing a feeling of euphoria and confidence; however, at the same time electrical impulses to the heart that regulate its rhythm are impaired. There is evidence that both psychological and physical dependence on cocaine occurs rapidly.

Today, the smoking of crack cocaine is more prevalent than inhalation. When smoked, the drug reaches the central nervous system immediately, affecting several neurotransmitters in the brain. The effects are short lived (usually around five to ten minutes), leaving the user with feelings of depression. Abuse of this drug can result in convulsions, seizures, respiratory distress, and sudden cardiac failure.

The relatively short-lived "high" from cocaine requires frequent use to maintain feelings of euphoria and is therefore quite costly for the addict. A single dose of crack sells for $30 or more, so to maintain a habit would cost hundreds of dollars a day. To pay for their habit, addicts will often turn to criminal activities such as dealing drugs, stealing, or prostitution. Crack houses are known for promoting the spread of HIV infection, and thousands of babies are born to crack-addicted mothers. These babies have severe physical and neurological problems, requiring significant medical attention. The cost of this drug is high, not just for the user, but for society as well.

Caffeine

Caffeine is a stimulant as well as a psychotropic (mind affecting) drug. Caffeine is generally associated with coffee, tea, and cola, but can also be found in chocolate, cocoa, and other carbonated beverages (see Table 9.1), as well as some medications, both prescription and non-prescription, i.e., Excedrin®. Approximately 65–180 mg of caffeine are found in one cup of coffee, compared to tea, which contains 40–100 mg per cup, and cola, which contains 30–60 mg per twelve ounce can. Caffeine is readily absorbed into the body and causes stimulation of the cerebral cortex and medullary centers in the brain, resulting in mental alertness.

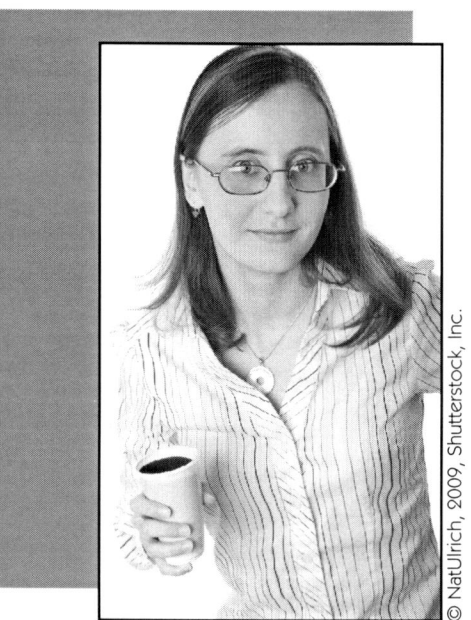

Moderation is the key when using caffeine.

Moderation is the key when using caffeine. Researchers agree that 300 mg of caffeine is considered moderate intake, which is equivalent to approximately three cups of coffee. Some individuals are more sensitive to caffeine than others and may feel the effects at smaller doses. According to research, caffeine in beverage form is not dehydrating, but if ingesting caffeine from food or tablets, be sure to rehydrate from the drug's diuretic action.

Excessive consumption of caffeine increases plasma levels of epinephrine, norepinephrine, and renin. It also can cause serious side effects, such as tremors, nervousness, irritability, headaches, hyperactivity, arrhythmia, dizziness, and insomnia. It can elevate the blood pressure and body temperature, increase the breathing rate, irritate the stomach and bowels, and dehydrate the body.

A study by researchers at Duke University Medical Center shows that caffeine taken in the morning has effects on the body that persist until bedtime and amplifies stress throughout the day. In addition to the body's physiological response in blood pressure elevations and stress hormone levels, it also magnifies a person's perception of stress. According to this study, caffeine enhances the effects of stress and can make stress even more unhealthy (Lane, Pieper, Phillips-Butte, Bryant, and Kuhn, 2002).

Excessive amounts of caffeine may increase the incidence of premenstrual syndrome (PMS) in some women and may increase fibrocystic breast disease (noncancerous breast lumps) as well. The U.S. Surgeon General recommends that women avoid or restrict caffeine intake during pregnancy. Withdrawal symptoms from caffeine may include headaches, depression, drowsiness, nervousness, and a feeling of lethargy.

Energy Drink Information:

In 2006, more than five hundred new energy drinks were released on the market worldwide. College students have been known to use caffeinated products like these for extra energy when studying, driving long distances, or needing more energy in general. A common practice of mixing energy drinks and alcohol is of special concern. Drinking large amounts of caffeine (a stimulant) combined with large amounts

Table 9.1
Caffeine Content of Energy Drinks, Carbonated Sodas, and Other Beverages

Beverage	Serving Size (oz)	Caffeine (mg/serving)
Energy Drinks		
Red Devil®	8.4	41.8
SoBe® Adrenaline Rush	8.3	76.7
SoBe® No Fear	16	141.1
Hair of the Dog®	8.4	none detected
Red Celeste™	8.3	75.2
E Maxx™	8.4	73.6
Amp™	8.4	69.6
Red Bull® Sugarfree	8.3	64.7
Red Bull®	8.3	66.7
KMX™	8.4	33.3
Carbonated Sodas		
Coca-Cola® Classic	12	29.5
Diet Coke®	12	38.2
Diet Coke® with Lime	12	39.6
Caffeine Free Diet Coke®	12	none detected
Vanilla Coke®	12	29.5
Pepsi®	12	31.7
Diet Pepsi®	12	27.4
Mountain Dew®	12	45.4
Mountain Dew® Live Wire™	12	48.2
Dr Pepper®	12	36.0
Diet Dr Pepper®	12	33.8
Sierra Mist™	12	none detected
Celeste™ Cola	12	19.4
Sprite®	12	none detected
Seagram's® Ginger Ale	12	none detected
Barq's® Root Beer	12	18.0
Pibb®Xtra	12	34.6
A&W® Root Beer	12	none detected
7-UP®	12	none detected
Other Beverages		
Nestea® Cool Lemon Iced Tea	12	11.5
Lipton® Brisk Lemon Iced Tea	12	6.5
Yoohoo® Chocolate Drink	9	< 2.7
Starbucks Doubleshot™	6.5	105.7
Starbucks Frappuccino® Mocha	9.5	71.8
Starbucks Frappuccino® Vanilla	9.5	63.8
Velda Farms® Chocolate Milk	16	< 3.8

Source: Reproduced from the *Journal of Analytical Toxicology* by permission of Preston Publications, a Division of Preston Industries, Inc.

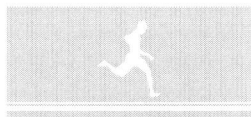

How can I reduce my caffeine consumption?

- Keep a log of how much caffeine you consume daily
- Limit your consumption to 200–300 mg/daily
- Substitute herbal tea or decaf coffee
- Stop smoking—caffeine and smoking often go together
- Remember coffee does not help sober up after drinking (McKinley, 2005)

of alcohol (a depressant) can cause people to misjudge their level of intoxication. The combination of drugs may mask symptoms such as headache, weakness, and muscle coordination, but in reality visual reaction time and motor coordination are still negatively affected by alcohol. Driving or making any other important decisions under these circumstances can be extremely dangerous.

Ephedrine

Ephedrine, ephedra, or Ma Huang are terms used for a substance from the plant ephedra. The active ingredients in ephedra are ephedrine and pseudoephedrine. These products are used for a variety of reasons, ranging from weight loss to increased energy.

According to the FDA, since 1994, over eight hundred injuries including fifty deaths have been attributed to the use of ephedra. "Consumers should be aware that just because a product is labeled 'natural' or from an herbal source, it is not guaranteed to be safe," said Dr. Michael Friedman, deputy commissioner of FDA. "The effects of ephedrine are potentially powerful ones" (FDA, 2005). Because these supplements are heart and nervous system stimulants, the side effects can be serious if not fatal. Adverse effects are high blood pressure, irregular heartbeat, headaches, insomnia, nervousness, heart attacks, strokes, and possibly death.

Depressants

Depressants are sedatives or anxiolytic (anti-anxiety) drugs that depress the central nervous system, reducing or relieving tension and/or anxiety, and inducing relaxation, drowsiness, or sleep.

Depressants can produce both a physical and psychological dependence within two to four weeks. Those with a prior history of abuse are at greater risk of abusing sedatives, even if prescribed by a physician. If there is no previous substance abuse history, one rarely develops problems if prescribed and monitored by a physician. Depressants can be very dangerous, if not lethal, if used in combination with alcohol, leading to respiratory depression, respiratory arrest, and death.

Cross-tolerance is a specific complication with sedatives. A person who is addicted to one sedative will likely develop a tolerance for other sedatives as well.

Some of the physiological effects of depressants include drowsiness, impaired judgment, poor coordination, slowed breathing, confusion, weak and rapid heartbeat, relaxed muscles, and pain relief.

A major health risk associated with the use of depressants is the development of a dependence to the drug, leading to serious side effects, such as stupors, coma, and death. The withdrawal symptoms from depressant use can cause fatal reactions as well. Symptoms can range from relatively mild discomfort to severe discomfort (with grand mal seizures), depending on the degree of dependence. Withdrawal symptoms can begin two to three days after stopping drug use and persist for several weeks. Individuals who have developed a dependency on depressants should seek medical attention when trying to quit or decrease the dosage.

Benzodiazepines

This is the most widely used group of depressants which are prescribed to relieve tension, muscle strain, sleep disturbances, panic attacks, anesthesia, or treatment for alcohol withdrawal and sometimes used to treat epileptic seizures. Examples include Librium, Valium, Serax, Ativan, Dalmand, and Xanax. All of these differ in action, absorption, and metabolism, but all produce similar intoxication and withdrawal symptoms.

Barbiturates

Barbiturates are used to induce relaxation, sleep, and relieve tension. They are usually taken orally in tablet, capsule, or liquid form, but when used as a general anesthetic, taken intravenously, they work as a serious respiratory depressant.

There are two types of barbiturates, short acting and long acting. The short-acting barbiturates are rapidly absorbed into the brain. Examples are Nembutal ("yellow jackets"), Secobarbital/Seconal ("reds"), and Thiopental (Pentothal). Long-acting barbiturates are taken orally and absorbed slowly into the bloodstream, lasting for several days. Examples are Amobarbital (Amytal—"blues," or "downers") and Phenobarbital (Luminal—"phennies").

Narcotics

Narcotics are drugs that relieve pain and often induce sleep.

Opium

Derived from poppy seeds, opium is the base compound used for all narcotics. Opiates, which are narcotics, include opium and other drugs derived from opium, such as morphine, codeine, and heroin. Methadone is a synthetic chemical that has a morphine-like action, and also falls into this category of drugs.

Morphine

This is the main alkaloid found in opium. It is ten times stronger than opium and brings quick relief from pain. It is most effectively used as an anesthetic during heart surgery, to relieve pain in post-operative patients, and sometimes used to relieve pain for cancer patients.

Codeine

A natural derivative of opium. Codeine is medically used as a mild painkiller or a cough suppressant. Although widely used, there is potential for physical dependence.

Heroin

Heroin is considered a semi-synthetic narcotic because it is derived from a naturally occurring substance in the Oriental poppy plant called opium. It is a highly effective, fast-acting analgesic (painkiller) if injected when used medicinally; however, its benefits are outweighed by its risk of toxicity and high dependence rate. When injected or "skin popped" (injected beneath the skin's surface), a dream-like euphoria is produced. Abuse is common because this drug creates a strong physical and psychological dependence and tolerance. Recently heroin has become more popular among young people. The risks of heroin use are increased due to the use of needles for injection. There is an increased likelihood of transmission of communicable diseases like HIV due to the practice of sharing needles. Although abrupt withdrawal from heroin is rarely fatal, the discomfort associated with going "cold turkey" is extremely intense.

Heroin accounts for 90 percent of the narcotic abuse in the United States. Anyone can become dependent, and life expectancy of the heroin addict who injects the drug intravenously is significantly lower than that of one who does not. Overdosing on heroin can result in death within minutes.

Withdrawal symptoms occur within four to six hours after the last injection. Full blown withdrawal symptoms such as shaking, sweating, vomiting, muscle aches, abdominal pains, and diarrhea may begin within twelve to sixteen hours of the last injection. The intensity of these symptoms is relative to the severity of the addiction.

Cannabis

Marijuana is a naturally occurring plant called *Cannabis sativa*, whose leaves and stems can be dried, crushed, and the mixture rolled in cigarettes (joints) and smoked. The fibers of this plant are also used to manufacture hemp rope and paper. The resins scraped from the flowering tops of the plant yield hashish, a form of marijuana that can be smoked in a pipe. The amount of the active ingredient, tetrahydrocannabinol (THC), determines the potency of the hallucinogenic effect. Because THC is a fat-soluble substance, it is absorbed and retained in the fat tissues of the body for up to a month. Drug tests can detect trace amounts of THC for up to three weeks after consumption. Medicinal uses include relief of the nausea caused by chemotherapy, improvement of appetite in AIDS patients, and the relief of pressure in the eyes of glaucoma patients. The effects of marijuana use vary from user to user, but usually result in some similar experiences. Users report food cravings, a relaxed mood, and a heightened sensitivity to music. The behavioral effects on users include an impairment of short-term memory, an overestimation of the passage of time, and loss of ability to maintain attention to a task.

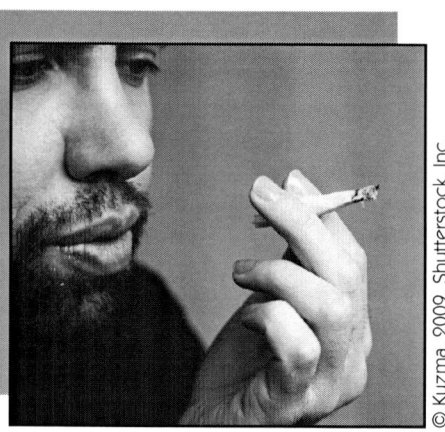

The behavioral effects on marijuana users include an impairment of short-term memory, an overestimation of the passage of time, and loss of the ability to focus on a task.

The long-term effects are still being studied; however, chronic abuse may lead to a motivational syndrome in some. Marijuana smoke is irritating to the lung tissues and may be more damaging than cigarette smoke. There are four hundred chemicals in marijuana linked to lung cancer development. In addition, the immune system and reproductive systems are damaged. There is an increase in birth defects among children whose mothers smoke marijuana during pregnancy. The drug distorts perception and therefore is very dangerous when used while driving. The biggest concern related to marijuana use is the perception that there is no risk or harm associated with occasional use.

Hallucinogens

Hallucinogens, also called psychedelics, are drugs that affect perception, sensation, awareness, and emotion. Changes in time and space and hallucinations may be mild or extreme depending on the dose, and may vary on every occasion. There are many synthetic as well as natural hallucinogens in use. Synthetic groups include LSD, which is the most potent; mescaline, which is derived from the peyote cactus, and psilocybin, derived from mushrooms, have similar effects.

Lysergic Acid Diethylamide (LSD)

LSD is a colorless, odorless, and tasteless liquid that is made from lysergic acid, which comes from the ergot fungus. It was first converted to lysergic acid diethylamide (LSD) in 1938. In 1943, its psychoactive properties accidentally became known (NIDA, 2007).

Hallucinations and illusions often occur, and effects vary according to the dosage, personality of the user, and conditions under which the drug is used. A flashback is a recurrence of some hallucinations from a previous LSD experience days or months after the dose. Flashbacks can occur without reason, occurring to heavy users more frequently. After taking LSD, a person loses control over normal thought process. Street LSD is often mixed with other substances and its effects are quite uncertain.

Phencyclidine Hydrochloride

Also known as PCP or angel dust, phencyclidine hydrochloride is sometimes considered a hallucinogen, although it does not easily fit into any category. First synthesized in 1959, it is used intravenously and as an anesthetic that blocks pain without producing numbness. Taken in small doses, it causes feelings of euphoria. The harmful side effects include depression, anxiety, confusion, and delirium. High doses of PCP cause mental confusion, hallucinations, and can cause serious mental illness and extreme aggressive and violent behavior, including murder.

Inhalants

Inhalants are poisonous chemical gases, fumes, or vapors that produce psychoactive effects when sniffed. When inhaled, the fumes take away the body's ability to absorb oxygen. Inhalants are considered delerients, which can cause permanent damage to the heart, brain, lungs, and liver. Common inhalants include model glue, acetone, gasoline, kerosene, nail polish, aerosol sprays, Pam™ cooking spray, Scotchgard™ fabric protectant, lighter fluids, butane, and cleaning fluids, as well as nitrous oxide (laughing gas). These products were not made to be inhaled or ingested. They were designed to dissolve things or break things down, which is exactly what they do to the body.

Inhalants reach the lungs, bloodstream, and other parts of the body very quickly. Intoxication can occur in as little as five minutes and can last as long as nine hours. Inhaled lighter fluid/butane displaces the oxygen in the lungs, causing suffocation. Even a single episode can cause asphyxiation or cardiac arrhythmia and possibly lead to death.

The initial effects of inhalants are similar to those of alcohol, but they are very unpredictable. Some effects include dizziness and blurred vision, involuntary eye movement, poor coordination, involuntary extremity movement, slurred speech, euphoric feeling, nosebleeds, and possible coma.

Health risks involved with the use of inhalants may include hepatitis, liver and/or kidney failure, as well as the destruction of bone marrow and skeletal muscles.

Table 9.2
Dependence or Abuse of Specific Substances among Past Year Users of Substances: 2003

Substance	Percent of Users with Dependence or Abuse of Specific Substance
Heroin	57.4
Cocaine	25.6
Sedatives	19.0
Marijuana	16.6
Stimulants	13.7
Pain Relievers	12.2
Alcohol	11.5
Tranquilizers	8.6
Hallucinogens	8.2
Inhalants	8.2

Source: www.oas.samhsa.gov

Respiratory impairment and blood abnormalities, along with irregular heartbeat and/or heart failure, are also serious side effects of inhalants. Regular use can lead to tolerance and the need for more powerful drugs.

Some specific signs of inhalant abuse can be a rash around the nose and mouth, nosebleeds, residue found on the face, hands, or clothing, as well as breath odors. Redness, tearing, or swelling of the eyes, irritation of the throat, lungs, and nose that may lead to gagging and coughing are also considered signs of inhalant abuse.

Club Drugs

MDMA

MDMA, also known as **ecstasy**, has a chemical structure similar to methamphetamines and mescaline, causing hallucinogenic effects. As a result, it can produce both stimulant and psychedelic effects. In addition to its euphoric effects, MDMA can lead to disruptions in body temperature and cardiovascular regulation causing panic, anxiety, and rapid heart rate. It also damages nerves in the brain's serotonin system and possibly produces long-term damage to brain areas that are critical for thought and memory (NIDA, 2001). Physical effects can include muscle tension, teeth clenching, nausea, blurred vision, and faintness. The psychological effects can include confusion, depression, sleep disorders, anxiety, and paranoia that can last long after taking the drug. It is most often available in tablet form and usually taken orally. Occasionally it is found in powder form and can be snorted or smoked, but it is rarely injected. An overdose can be lethal, especially when taken with alcohol or other drugs, for instance heroin ("H-bomb").

Rohypnol

Flunitrazepam is an illegal drug in the United States, but an approved medicine in other parts of the world where it is generally prescribed for sleep disorders. A 2-mg tablet is equal to the potency of a six-pack of beer. Rohypnol is a tranquilizer, similar to Valium, but ten times more potent, producing sedative effects including muscle relaxation, dizziness, memory loss, and blackouts. The effects occur twenty to thirty minutes after use and lasts for up to eight hours.

Rohypnol, more commonly known as "roofies," is a small, white, tasteless, pill that dissolves in food or drinks. It is most commonly used with other drugs, such as alcohol, ecstasy, heroin, and marijuana to enhance the feeling of the other drug. Although Rohypnol alone can be very dangerous, as well as physically addicting, when mixed with other drugs it can be fatal. It is also referred to as the "date rape" drug because there have been many reported cases of individuals giving Rohypnol to someone without their knowledge. The effects incapacitate the victim, and therefore they are unable to resist a sexual assault. It produces an "anterograde amnesia," meaning they may not remember events experienced while under effects of the drug (NIDA, 2001).

Gamma Hydroxybutyrate (GHB)

GHB is a fast-acting, powerful drug that depresses the nervous system. It occurs naturally in the body in small amounts. First synthesized in the 1960's, GHB was once sold in health food stores as a performance-enhancing additive in body building supplements.

Commonly taken with alcohol, it depresses the central nervous system and induces an intoxicated state. GHB is commonly consumed orally, usually as a clear liquid or a white powder. It is odorless, colorless, and slightly salty to taste. Effects from GHB can occur within fifteen to thirty minutes. Small doses (less than 1 g) of GHB act as a relaxant with larger doses causing strong feelings of relaxation, slowing heart

Table 9.3
Commonly Misused and Abused Substances

Category	Substances	Possible Effects
Stimulants	Caffeine Cocaine, crack cocaine Methamphetamines Amphetamines Dextroamphetamines Nicotine Over-the-counter diet aids Asthma treatments	Increase mental and physical activity, produce temporary feelings of alertness, prevent fatigue, suppress appetite.
Hallucinogens	LSD (lysergic acid diethylamide) PCP (phencyclidine) Mescaline Peyote Psilocybin	Cause changes in mood, sensation, thought, emotion, and self-awareness; alter perceptions of time and space; and may produce profound depression, tension, and anxiety, as well as visual, auditory, or tactile hallucinations.
Depressants	Barbiturates Narcotics Alcohol Antihistamines Sedatives Tranquilizers Over-the-counter sleep aids	Decrease mental and physical activity, alter consciousness, relieve anxiety and pain, promote sleep, depress respiration, relax muscles, and impair coordination and judgment.
Narcotics	Morphine Codeine Heroin Methadone Opium	Relieve pain, may produce stupor or euphoria, may cause coma or death, and are highly addictive.
Inhalants	Medical anesthetics Gasoline and kerosene Glues in organic cements Lighter fluid Paint and varnish thinners Aerosol propellants	Alter moods; may produce a partial or complete loss of feeling; may produce effects similar to drunkenness, such as slurred speech, lack of inhibitions, and impaired motor coordination. Can also cause damage to the heart, lungs, brain, and liver.
Cannabis products	Hashish Marijuana THC (tetrahydrocannabinol)	Produce feelings of elation, increase appetite, distort perceptions of time and space, and impair motor coordination and judgment. May irritate throat, redden eyes, increase pulse, and cause dizziness.
Other	MDMA (methylene-dioxymethamphetamine or ecstasy)	Elevates blood pressure and produces euphoria or erratic mood swings, rapid heartbeat, profuse sweating, agitation, and sensory distortions.
	Anabolic steroids	Enhance physical performance, increase muscle mass, and stimulate appetite and weight gain. Chronic use can cause sterility, disruption of normal growth, liver cancer, personality changes, and aggressive behavior.
	Aspirin	Relieves minor pain and reduces fever. Can impair normal blood clotting and cause inflammation of the stomach and small intestine.
	Laxatives	Relieve constipation. Can cause uncontrolled diarrhea and dehydration.
	Decongestant nasal sprays	Relieve congestion and swelling of nasal passages. Chronic use can cause nosebleeds and changes in the lining of the nose, making it difficult to breathe without sprays.

Source: From *American Red Cross First Aid: Responding to Emergencies,* 3rd Edition.

rate, and respiration. There is a very fine line to cross to find a lethal dose, which can lead to seizures, respiratory distress, low blood pressure, and coma.

According to the Drug Abuse Warning Network, The Drug Induced Rape Prevention and Punishment Act of 1996 was enacted into federal law in response to the abuse of Rohypnol. This law makes it a crime to give someone a controlled substance without his/her knowledge and with the intent to commit a crime. The law also stiffens the penalties for possession and distribution of Rohypnol and GHB. Used in Europe as a general anesthetic and treatment for insomnia, GHB is growing in popularity and is widely available underground. Manufactured by non-professional "kitchen" chemists, concerns about quality and purity should be considered.

2C-B

This is a psychedelic drug synthesized by a chemist in 1974 and is considered both a psychedelic and a drug similar to MDMA. 2C-B is a white powder found in tablets or gel caps and is taken orally. The visual effects can be more intense than those created by LSD and can cause nausea, trembling, chills, and nervousness.

Ketamine Hydrochloride

"Special K" or "K" was originally created for use in a medical setting on humans and animals. Ninety percent is legally sold for veterinary use. Ketamine usually comes in liquid form and is cooked into a white powder for snorting. Higher doses produce a hallucinogenic effect and may cause the user to feel far away from their body. This is called a "K-hole" and has been compared to near-death experiences. Low doses can increase heart rate and numbness in the extremities with higher doses depressing consciousness and breathing. This makes it extremely dangerous if combined with other depressants such as alcohol or GHB.

Anabolic Steroids

Anabolic androgenic steroids are man-made and very similar to male sex hormones. The word *anabolic* means "muscle building," and *androgenic* refers to masculine. Legally, steroids are prescribed to individuals to treat problems occurring when the body produces abnormally low amounts of testosterone and problems associated with delayed puberty or impotence. Other cases for prescribed steroids use would involve individuals with whom a disease has resulted in a loss of muscle mass (NIDA, 2005).

Although steroids are a banned substance in all professional and collegiate sports, most people who use steroids do so to enhance physical performance in sports or other activities. Some choose to use steroids to improve physical appearance or to increase muscle size and to reduce body fat. Some steroids can be taken orally or injected into the muscle. There are also some forms of steroid creams and gels that are to be rubbed into the skin. Most doses taken by abusers are ten to one hundred times the potency of normal doses used for medicinal purposes. Usually taken in cycles, the individual increases the dosage with each cycle, then slowly reduces the dosage during the second half of the cycle.

Consequences from steroid abuse can cause some serious health issues. There can be some problems with the normal hormone production in the individual, which can be very severe and irreversible. Major side effects of steroid abuse can lead to cardiovascular disease, high blood pressure, and stroke because it increases the LDL cholesterol levels while decreasing the HDL levels. There can also be liver damage, muscular and ligament damage, as well as stunted bone growth. In addition to these problems, the side effects for males can be shrinkage of the testes and a reduction in sperm count. For females, steroid use can cause facial hair growth and the cessation of the menstrual cycle.

Research also suggests some psychological and behavioral changes. Steroid abusers can become very aggressive and violent and have severe mood swings. Users are reported to have paranoid and jealous tendencies along with irritability and impaired judgment. Depression has also been linked to steroid use once the individual stops taking the drug, therefore leading to continued use. This depressed state can lead to serious consequences, and in some cases it has been reported to lead to suicidal thoughts (NIDA, 2005).

Prescription Drugs

One of the most commonly abused groups of prescription drugs is narcotics (see Table 9.3 on page 331). These drugs are used medicinally for pain relief but often abused by individuals. These drugs include morphine, codeine, Oxycodone, Vicodin, and Demerol. According to the National Institute on Drug Abuse (NIDA), approximately 9 million Americans misuse and abuse prescription drugs for non-medicinal purposes. To add to the severity of the problem, many of those who abuse prescription drugs abuse alcohol and other drugs as well.

It is not that these drugs should not be used for the purpose intended, as "they have an important place in the treatment of debilitating conditions," says Richard Brown, M.D., associate professor at the University of Wisconsin (FDA, 2005). It is generally uncommon for addiction to occur to patients using the drug as prescribed. It is the individuals abusing and misusing these drugs that can lead to problems. Some of these problems occur because prescription drugs are received through false prescriptions, overprescribing, and pharmacy theft. Sometimes problems arise because there is a lack of communication or information provided to the patient (FDA, 2005).

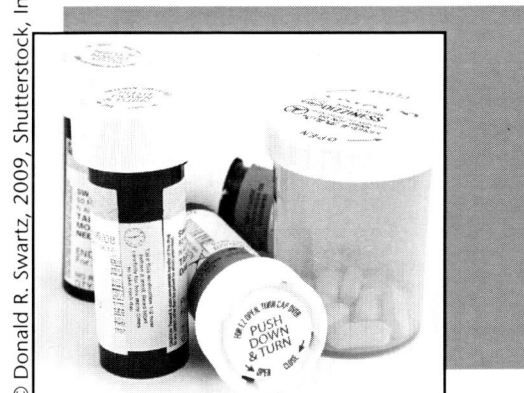

Some of the most commonly abused prescription drugs are pain killers such as morphine, codeine, Oxycodone, Vicodin, and Demerol.

Hydrocodone Information Hydrocodone is a narcotic used to relieve pain and suppress cough. This drug, which can lead to both physiological and psychological dependence, saw a dramatic increase in legal sales between 1990 and 2000 and with that, abuse increased as well.

Oxycodone, a drug used for moderate to severe pain relief, has a high potential for abuse. Tablets should be take orally, but when crushed and injected intravenously or snorted, a potentially lethal dose is released (FDA, 2004).

According to recent reports from the FDA, a highly abused stimulant among middle and high school students is methylphenidate, commonly known as **Ritalin.** This drug is more powerful than caffeine but not as potent as amphetamines and is prescribed for individuals with attention-deficit/hyperactivity disorders, ADHD, and sometimes to treat narcolepsy. Researchers speculate that Ritalin increases the slow and steady release of dopamine, therefore improving attention and focus for those in need of the increase. "Individuals abuse Ritalin to lose weight, increase alertness and experience the euphoric feelings resulting from high doses" (U.S. Dept. of Justice, 2006). When abused, the tablets are either taken orally or crushed and snorted; some even dissolve the tablets in water and inject the mixture. Addiction occurs when it induces large and fast increases of dopamine in the brain (DOJ, 2006).

Adderall is another stimulant used to treat ADHD as well as narcolepsy. Physical and psychological dependence may occur with this drug. Symptoms of Adderall overdose include dizziness, blurred vision, restlessness, rapid breathing, confusion, hallucinations, nausea, vomiting, irregular heartbeat, and seizures.

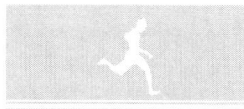

FDA Guidelines on How to Use Prescription Drugs Safely:

- Always follow medication directions
- Do not increase or decrease doses without consulting your physician
- Do not stop taking medication on your own
- Do not crush or break pills
- Be clear about the drug's effect on driving and other tasks
- Know the drug's potential interactions with alcohol and other drugs
- Inform your doctor if you have had past problems with substance abuse
- Do not use others' prescription medications, and do not share yours.

Prescription Drug Conclusion The danger from prescription and over-the-counter drugs is often underestimated by students. Many assume that if the drug is legal and prescribed by a physician, even if for someone else, it must be safe. However, what they fail to realize is that medications and dosages are tailored to each patient and may not be appropriate in the manner they intend to use them.

For more information:

National Institutes of Health
www.nih.gov

Substance Abuse and Mental Health Services Administration
www.samhsa.gov

Web of Addictions
www.well.com/user/woa.

National Institute on Drug Abuse
www.nida.gov

Alcohol

Prevalence

According to the National Institute on Alcohol Abuse and Alcoholism (NIAAA), more than 60 percent of adults are regular drinkers. Currently, there are eighteen million Americans experiencing problems with alcohol, and ten million are alcoholics. But, in addition to addiction and health issues, alcohol contributes to many other serious problems in our society. Some of these problems can be fatal. For example, according to the NIAAA, alcohol is a factor in:

- over 40 percent of all highway deaths
- 50 percent of all spousal abuse cases
- 30 percent of child abuse cases
- 65 percent of drownings
- 54 percent of those jailed for violent crimes were drunk
- 49 percent convicted of murder or attempted murder

What Is Alcohol?

Ethyl alcohol, or ethanol, has been prevalent in our society for centuries. Except for the Prohibition Era in the United States from 1917 to 1932 when alcohol was considered an illegal substance, it has become the legal and accepted drug of choice. There are three major types of alcoholic beverages:

1. beer,
2. distilled spirits or hard liquor,
3. wine or wine coolers.

Distilled spirits include scotch, gin, rum, vodka, tequila, and whiskey. The alcohol content varies according to the proof of the beverage, which is twice the percent of alcohol. For example, if whiskey is 80 proof, then that particular beverage is 40 percent alcohol by volume. The average mixed drink contains a one-ounce shot of hard liquor.

Wine usually averages 12 percent alcohol by volume, and wine coolers average approximately 5 percent alcohol by volume. The average glass of wine is four ounces, and wine coolers are usually served in twelve-ounce bottles.

Beer is usually served in twelve-ounce cans or bottles. The average alcohol content of beer is 4.5 percent by volume. To be considered a beer, the alcohol content must not exceed 5 percent by weight by volume. If the amount of alcohol is greater, it is considered an ale.

Blood alcohol concentration (BAC) is a measure of the concentration of alcohol in blood, expressed in grams per 100 ml. An example would be 100 mg of alcohol in 10 ml of blood would be reported as .10 percent. The higher the alcohol content of the drink, the higher BAC it will produce.

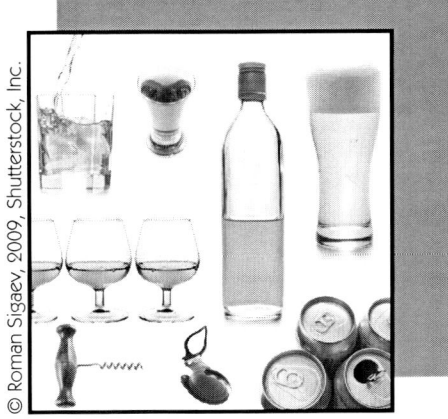

Alcoholic content varies according to the type of drink and the proof of the beverage.

```
12 oz. Beer          12 oz. Wine cooler
× .045               × .05
─────────            ─────────
.54 oz. Alcohol      .60 oz. Alcohol

1 oz. Whiskey        4 oz. Wine
× .40                × .12
─────────            ─────────
.40 oz. Alcohol      .48 oz. Alcohol
```

The alcoholic content of some other typical drinks:

one ounce shot 86 proof liquor	.43 oz.
Light beer 12 oz.	.46 oz.
Champagne 4 oz.	.58 oz.
Malt liquor 12 oz.	.75 oz.
Margarita	.75 oz.

Factors influencing a person's BAC are body weight, alcohol content of the drink, size of the drink, time spent drinking, and food (see Table 9.5 on page 339). Gender is also a factor in determining one's BAC. Women do not process alcohol as well as men because of the enzyme alcohol dehydrogenase, which breaks down alcohol. Men produce more alcohol dehydrogenase than women; therefore, men can eliminate alcohol at a slightly faster rate (Dennis and the Texas Commission on Alcohol and Drug Abuse, 2005). Women also have less water content, so a woman at the same weight as a man will have a higher BAC. The higher alcohol content of a drink, the higher BAC it will produce. For example, a one-ounce shot of a 100 proof beverage has more alcohol than a one-ounce shot of an 80 proof beverage. The larger an alcoholic drink, the more alcohol it will contain and produce a higher BAC. For example, a twenty-four ounce beer will have twice the amount of alcohol of a twelve-ounce beer. The liver begins to process alcohol shortly after it is absorbed into the bloodstream. The longer time factor will result in a lower BAC. For example, if a person drinks a six-pack in three hours, they will have a lower BAC than if they had consumed a six-pack in one hour. Having food in the stomach may coat the lining of the stomach, therefore slowing down the absorption of alcohol. Food will not absorb or soak up the alcohol, so the alcohol will eventually reach the bloodstream.

There are three ways that alcohol is removed or eliminated from the body. Ninety percent of alcohol is eliminated through the oxidation process of the liver at .015 percent per hour. The alcohol dehydrogenase then converts alcohol to acetaldehyde. Alcohol is then metabolized at approximately .25 to .30 ounces per hour, regardless of the blood alcohol concentration. The rate of metabolism is based on the activity of alcohol dehydrogenase, working at its own pace (Ray and Kisr, 1999).

Eight percent of alcohol is eliminated through breath, which is why a breath test is used to determine BAC. A small amount of alcohol, approximately 2 percent, is eliminated through sweat. For the average individual, elimination will reduce a given blood alcohol concentration by .015 per hour. Contrary to popular belief, cold showers, black coffee, aspirin, or exercise will not speed up this elimination process (see Figure 9.5).

Tolerance is when an individual adapts to the amount consumed so that larger quantities are needed to achieve the same effect. This basically means that a person needs to drink more alcohol to achieve the same effect. This can take place over several months or years of consuming alcohol, depending on the amount consumed and at what age the individual begins to drink. At some point, after a person's tolerance has increased over a period of time, it begins to drop, allowing the effects of alcohol to be felt after only a few drinks. This reverse tolerance is caused by the natural aging process or liver disease after years of abusive drinking (Dennis and the Texas Commission Alcohol and Drug Abuse, 2005).

Intoxication is defined as a transient state of physical and mental disruption due to the presence of a toxic substance, such as alcohol (Maisto, 2005). As BAC increases, the central nervous system alters behavior and physical function. Change can occur as low as .02 BAC in some people, while everyone is impaired to some degree at .05 BAC.

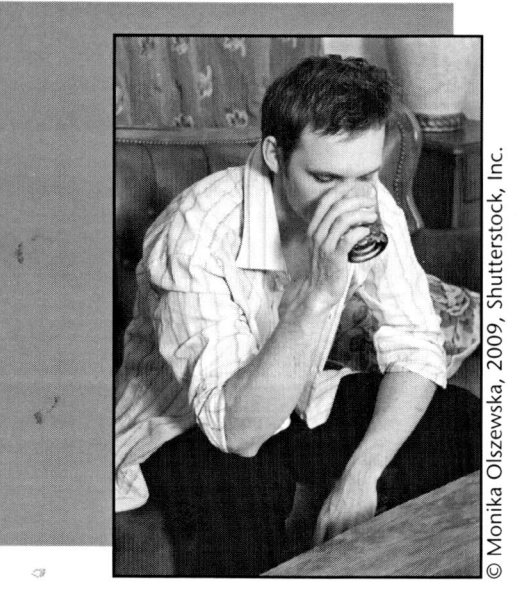

Alcohol slows down the nervous system, impairs vision, and increases the risk of certain cancers, heart and blood pressure problems.

Physiological Effects

Alcohol is a drug that has two major effects on the body. Being a depressant, it slows down the nervous system (respiratory and cardiovascular systems). Alcohol and its by-products also **irritate** the nerve endings and eventually **sedate** or deaden them. **Vision** is another sense that alcohol affects quickly. This is an important ability for driving because 90 percent of the information we receive is obtained through vision. Alcohol has a direct effect on our vision by causing the loss of fine muscle control in the eyes accounting for eye focus, visual acuity, peripheral vision, color distinction, night vision, distance judgment, and double vision (Dennis and the Texas Commission on Alcohol and Drug Abuse, 2005). Other physiological effects are impaired mental and physical reflexes, increased risk of diseases such as cancer of the brain, tongue, mouth, esophagus, larynx, liver, and the bladder. Heart and blood pressure problems are also associated with alcohol consumption.

Laws Relating to Alcohol

In every state in the United States, it is illegal for a person under the age of 21 to attempt to purchase, possess, or consume alcohol. In Texas, this violation is a **minor in possession** (MIP). This offense is punishable by fines, community service, loss of driver's license, alcohol awareness class, and possibly jail.

The **Zero Tolerance Law** prohibits the use of alcohol by a minor operating a motor vehicle. In Texas, it is illegal for a minor to operate a motor vehicle in a public place with *any* **detectable** amount of alcohol. This violation is referred to as **driving under the influence** (DUI). This may be determined by a blood/breath test or simply smelling alcohol on the minor's breath. The penalties are very similar to MIP with fine, loss of license, education courses, and community service.

By operating a motor vehicle in a public place, the driver has given consent to take a breath/blood test to determine alcohol in his/her system. Refusing or failing

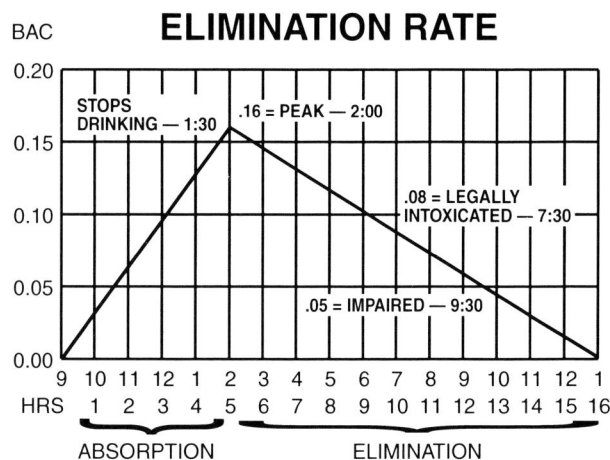

FIGURE 9.5

Alcohol Absorption and Elimination

Source: Texas Commission on Alcohol and Drug Abuse.

the test is considered a violation, and penalties will result in loss of license, regardless of the outcome of the violation.

In most states, the legal definition of **intoxication** is not having normal use of your mental or physical faculties because of alcohol or other drugs; or an alcohol concentration of .08 or more. It is, however, illegal in all states to drink and drive. In addition, in most states, it is also illegal for anyone in the vehicle to possess an open container of alcohol regardless of age.

When someone is injured in an alcohol-related motor vehicle accident, the intoxicated driver can be charged with **intoxication assault.** If there were a fatality in a drinking-and-driving accident, the offense would be elevated to **intoxication manslaughter.** Each state may have different terminology, but the offense is the same throughout the country. In Texas, both offenses are considered felonies.

Societal Problems

The dangers of alcohol consumption are a major problem in our society. Drinking too much alcohol can cause a range of very serious problems, in addition to the obvious health issues. Alcohol is a contributing factor in motor vehicle accidents, violence, and school/work problems, as well as family problems.

Drinking and Driving

Driving under the influence of alcohol is the most frequently committed and deadliest crime in America. In the Federal Bureau of Investigation's (FBI) Uniform Crime Report, more than 1.4 million people were arrested in 2003 for alcohol-impaired driving. The National Highway Traffic Safety Administration (NHTSA) reported in 2006 that more than 17,602 people were killed in alcohol-related highway crashes. This is 40 percent of the nation's total traffic fatalities for the year. The 17,602 deaths in 2006 represent an average of one alcohol-related fatality every thirty-one minutes (NHTSA, 2007).

Drivers 21 to 24 years old represent the highest percentage of drivers involved in fatal crashes with a BAC of .08 or higher (see Table 9.4 and Figure 9.6). More than half of the drivers killed had a BAC of .16 or greater (NHTSA, 2007). The average BAC of a driver killed in an alcohol related crash is .17.

Table 9.4
Driving under the Influence of Alcohol in the Past Year, by Age: 2003

Age in Years	Percent Driving under the Influence
16–17	9.7
18–20	20.1
21–25	28.7
26–29	23.8
30–34	19.1
35–39	17.5
40–44	17.0
45–49	14.2
50–54	11.9
55–59	9.6
60–64	4.1
65+	3.2

Males were nearly twice as likely as females (18.2 vs. 9.3 percent, respectively) to drive under the influence of alcohol.
Source: www.oas.samhsa.gov

The NHTSA reports the United States averages one death every thirty-three minutes due to alcohol and every two minutes someone is injured in alcohol-related crashes. These crashes in the United States cost the public more than $100 billion annually. The average alcohol-related fatality cost is $3 million, $1.2 in monetary cost and $1.8 million in quality of life loss (NHTSA, 2006).

Drunk driving is no accident; it is a crime. The greatest tragedy is that these crashes are preventable, predictable, and 100 percent avoidable. An estimated three in every ten Americans will be involved in an alcohol-related crash at some time in their lives. It is also estimated that every weekday night from 10:00 p.m. to 1:00 a.m., one in thirteen drivers are drunk. Between 1:00 a.m. and 6:00 a.m. on

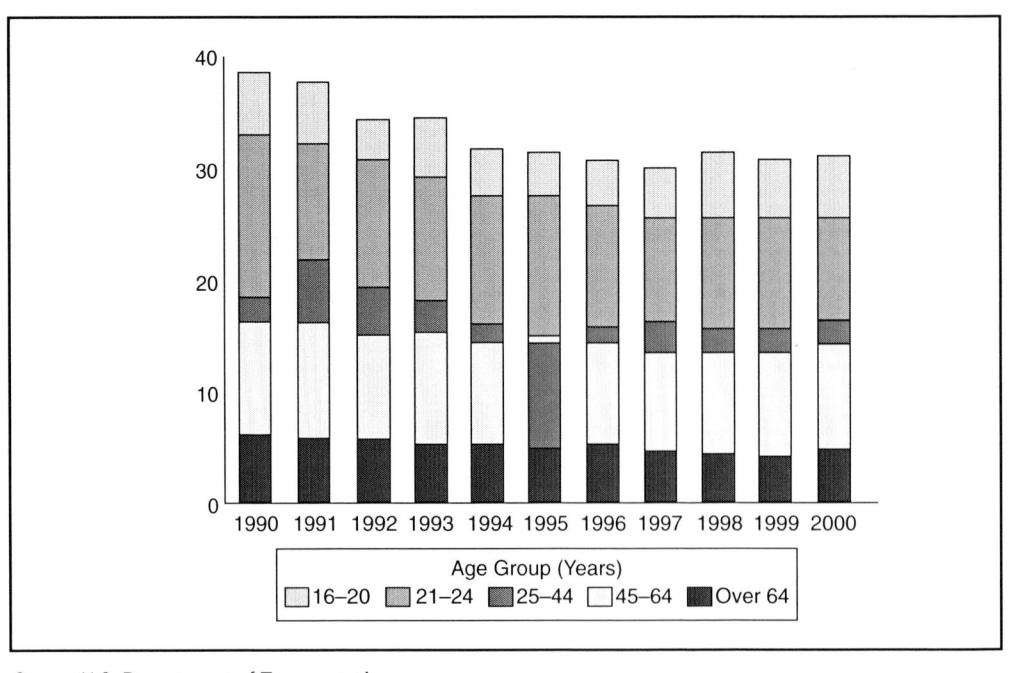

FIGURE 9.6
Percentage of Drivers with a Blood Alcohol Concentration of 0.10 or More

College students and other young adults are at a higher risk of dying in car accidents due to drunk driving than people in any other age group.

Source: U.S. Department of Transportation.

weekend mornings, one in seven drivers are drunk (Miller et al., 1996). Although more Americans have died in alcohol-related crashes than in all the wars the United States has been involved in, there has been a steady decrease in alcohol-related deaths since 1982.

As BAC increases, the likelihood of being involved in an alcohol-related crash increases significantly. A driver with a BAC of .15 is more than three hundred times more likely to be involved in a fatal crash. BAC levels as low as .02 affect driving ability and crash responsibility. The probability of a crash increases greatly at .05 BAC and begins a rapid increase at .08 BAC (Dennis, 2005).

Although most drivers involved in fatal crashes have no prior convictions for DUI, about one-third of all drivers arrested for DUI are repeat offenders, which greatly increases their risk of causing a drunk driving accident. As a nation, we have seen a downward trend in alcohol-related fatalities. Today, all states have lowered their legal level of intoxication to .08 BAC. All states have some form of the zero tolerance law, as well as an open container law. These laws, in addition to stricter enforcement of existing laws, have helped in changing behavior. High school and university education programs, such as non-alcoholic activities for prom nights and designated driver organizations, have also contributed in raising awareness to combat such a serious problem.

The NHTSA and the Advertising Council's Innocent Victims public service campaign stresses the need to get the keys from someone who is about to drive. Here are some tips:

- If it is a close friend, try to use a soft, calm approach. Suggest to them that they have had too much to drink and it would be better if someone else drove, or call a cab.
- Be calm. Joke about it. Make light of it.

Table 9.5

Blood Alcohol Concentration (BAC): A Measure of Drunk Driving

Within minutes after having a drink, the brain's normal functioning is changed. One measure of how your brain, vision, and decision-making might be impaired is how much alcohol is in your blood. This is called the blood alcohol concentration.

Your Weight	Number of drinks (over a two-hour period) 1.5 oz. 80 proof liquor or 12 oz. can of beer											
100	1	2	3	4	5	6	7	8	9	10	11	12
120	1	2	3	4	5	6	7	8	9	10	11	12
140	1	2	3	4	5	6	7	8	9	10	11	12
160	1	2	3	4	5	6	7	8	9	10	11	12
180	1	2	3	4	5	6	7	8	9	10	11	12
200	1	2	3	4	5	6	7	8	9	10	11	12
220	1	2	3	4	5	6	7	8	9	10	11	12
240	1	2	3	4	5	6	7	8	9	10	11	12
	Social Drive with caution BAC to 0.05%				Warning Driving impaired 0.05–0.09%				Intoxicated Do not drive 0.10% and up			

This table is only a guide. Information presented is based on averages and may vary according to particular circumstances or from individual to individual.
Source: U.S. Department of Transportation.

- Try to make it sound like you are doing them a favor.
- If it is somebody you do not know well, speak to their friends; usually they will listen.
- If it is a good friend, tell them if they insist on driving, you are not going with them.
- Locate their keys while they are preoccupied and take them away. Mostly they will think they lost them and will be forced to find another mode of transportation.
- Avoid embarrassing the person or being confrontational.

Alcohol Use in College

An estimated 4,441 lives were saved over the last five years by the minimum 21 year old drinking age law (NHTSA, 2006). The legal drinking age in all states is 21 years old, but that does not mean individuals under 21 do not consume alcohol. Studies suggest that substance use, including alcohol, tobacco, and other drug use, is common among college-aged youth. Students who use any of these substances are at significantly greater risk than non-substance using peers to: drive after drinking and with a driver who has been drinking, and are less likely to use a seatbelt. These consistently poor and risky choices increase their risk of being in a motor vehicle crash and having crash-related injuries (Everett, 1999). College students and administrators struggle with the problems associated with alcohol abuse, binge drinking, and drunk driving (see Figure 9.7). These actions put students at risk for many serious problems, such as date rape and possibly death.

The National Institute on Alcohol Abuse and Alcoholism (NIAAA) reports that 1,700 college students die annually from alcohol-related unintentional injuries, including motor vehicle crashes, with 2.1 million students driving under the influence of alcohol. Another 599,000 between the ages of 18 and 24 are injured, and approximately 696,000 students per year are assaulted by a drinking student. Also, approximately 400,000 students between 18 and 24 years old reported having unprotected sex as a result of drinking. More than 97,000 students are victims of alcohol-related sexual assault or date rape. More than 150,000 college students develop an alcohol-related health problem, with 1.5 percent attempting suicide because of alcohol (NIAAA, 2006).

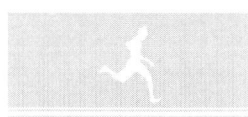

According to a report by the Center on Addiction and Substance Abuse at Columbia University:

- College students spend $5.5 billion dollars on alcohol per year, averaging $466/student/year.
- Alcohol is a factor in 40 percent of all academic problems and 28 percent of all dropouts.
- Sixty percent of college women diagnosed with STDs were drunk at the time of infection.

Binge Drinking

College presidents agree that **binge drinking** is the most serious problem on campus. It is defined as consuming five or more drinks at one sitting for men, and four or more for women. Binge drinkers usually experience more alcohol-related problems than their non-drinking counterparts. These problems affect their health, education, safety, and interpersonal relationships. According to the Harvard School of Public Health College Alcohol Study, these problems include driving after drinking, damaging property, getting injured, missing classes, and getting behind in school work. According to the same Harvard study, one in five students surveyed experienced five or more different alcohol-related problems and more than one-third of the students reported driving after drinking.

The study also found that the vast majority of non-binge drinking students are negatively affected by the behavior of binge drinkers. It was reported that four out of five students who were non-binge drinkers and who lived on campus experienced secondary effects of binge drinking such as being the victim of a sexual assault or an unwanted sexual advance, having property vandalized, and having sleep or study interrupted.

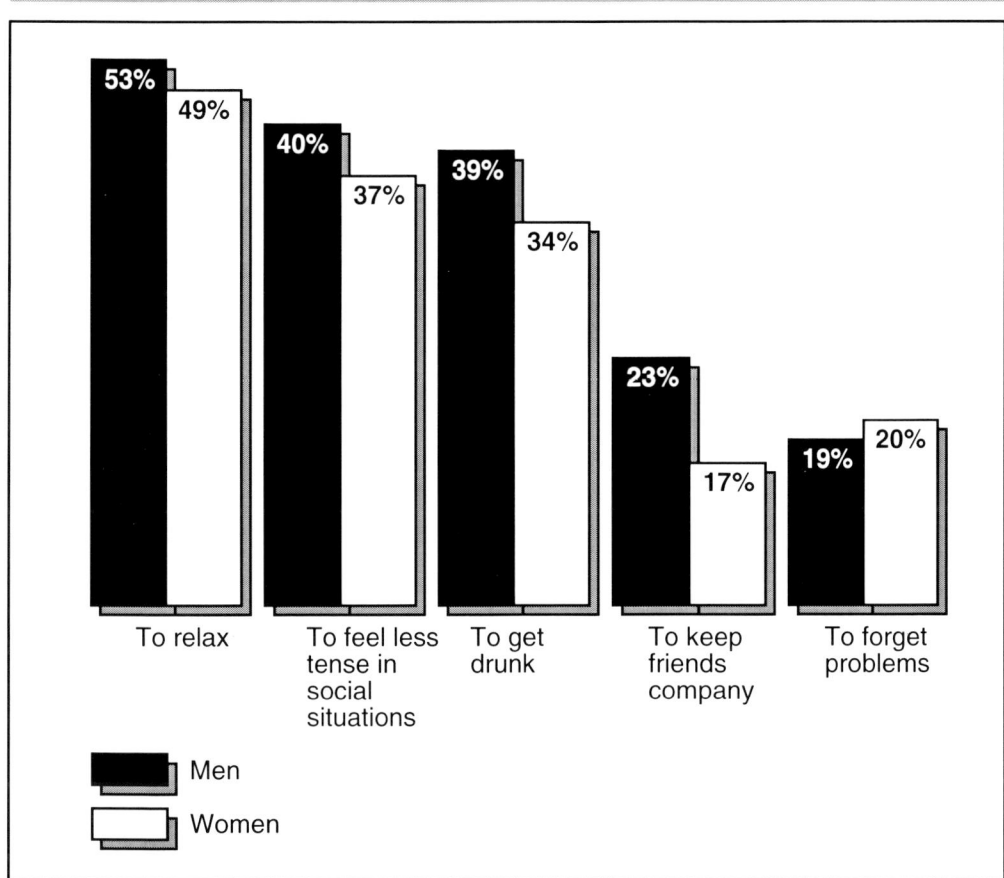

FIGURE 9.7
Why College Freshmen Drink

Source: Adapted from Weschler and McFadden for AAA Foundation for Traffic Safety. Survey of 1,669 college freshmen at 14 Massachusetts institutions.

Alcohol Poisoning

The most serious consequence of binge drinking is **alcohol poisoning.** This results when an overdose of alcohol is consumed. When excessive amounts of alcohol are consumed, the brain is deprived of oxygen, which causes it to shut down the breathing and heart rate functions. Many think that the only deadly mix is alcohol and driving, but an alcohol overdose can be lethal. It can happen to anyone.

Some symptoms of alcohol poisoning are:

- Person does not respond to talking, shouting, or being shaken.
- Person cannot stand up.
- Person has slow, labored, or abnormal breathing—less than eight breaths/minute or ten or more seconds between each breath.
- Person's skin feels clammy.
- Person has a rapid pulse rate and irregular heart rhythm.
- Person has lowered blood pressure.
- Vomiting.

If you think a friend is experiencing alcohol poisoning, seek medical attention immediately. Stay with the person until help arrives. Turn the victim onto one side in case of vomiting. Choking to death on one's own vomit after an alcohol overdose is quite common. Death by asphyxiation occurs when alcohol depresses and inhibits the gag reflex to the point that the person cannot vomit properly. **Do not**

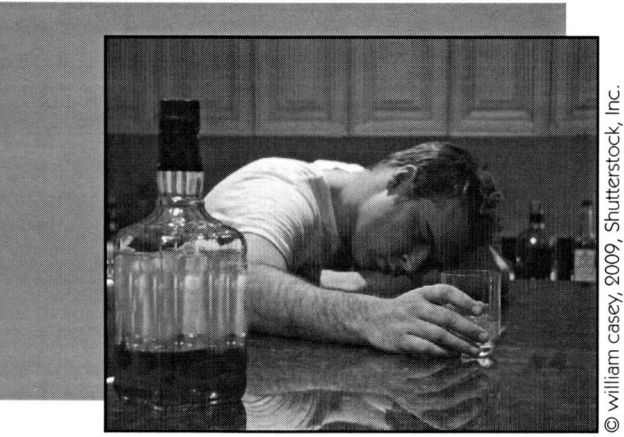

The most serious consequence of binge drinking is alcohol poisoning. Alcohol overdose can be lethal.

leave the victim alone. Be honest in telling medical staff exactly how much alcohol the victim consumed. This is an extreme medical emergency and one that is a matter of life and death.

Colleges are attempting to make progress in preventing some of these problems. Many sororities and fraternities as well as other student organizations have taken action by banning alcohol at many functions. By implementing alcohol awareness programs, stronger hazing policies, and tougher enforcements on drinking violations and alcohol restrictions on campus and with the student body, some of these tragedies may be prevented.

Drinking Problems

Nearly 14 million Americans, one in every thirteen adults, abuse alcohol or are alcoholics. Rates of alcohol problems are highest among young adults ages 18 to 29 and lowest in adults ages 65 and older (NIAAA, 2006).

The National Institute on Alcohol Abuse and Alcoholism (NIAAA) found that the earlier young people begin to drink alcohol, the more likely they are to become an alcohol abuser or alcoholic. According to the report:

- Young people who start drinking before age 15 are four times more likely to become an alcoholic than if they start after age 21.
- Forty percent who drink before age 15 become alcohol dependent; 10 percent if they wait until 21.
- Fourteen percent decreased risk of alcoholism for each year drinking is delayed until age 21.

Michael Wagener Story

On August 3, 1999, Michael Wagener, a student at Texas A&M University celebrating his 21st birthday, died as a result of alcohol poisoning. He was an intelligent and insightful young man with many friends and his whole life ahead of him. He was not an alcoholic, nor did he abuse alcohol. Michael was typically a responsible drinker.

On August 2nd, the eve of his 21st birthday, friends joined Michael at a local establishment. While having a few beers, some friends bought him a couple of shots for his birthday. His friends had bought him eight or nine (four-ounce) shots in a matter of thirty to forty-five minutes. Michael had many friends who wanted to share in his celebration; no one wanted him to die.

By the time he was taken home, Michael's body had begun to shut down. He could no longer move and had to be carried into the house. His friends thought they had taken all the precautions: designated driver, turn him on his side in case he vomits. They even stayed the night to ensure his safety.

At 7:00 a.m. his mother called to wish Michael a happy birthday. The call stirred his friends. At 7:10 a.m. the call was made to 911—Michael never woke up. One fun-filled night of celebration turned deadly.

This can happen to anyone. Consuming excessive amounts of alcohol, even one night, can kill you. We often think the only way alcohol can kill is if someone drinks and drives or abuses alcohol for many years. Educating yourself about alcohol will help you make informed decisions and hopefully prevent this tragedy from occurring again.

How can you tell if someone has a drinking problem? An individual does not have to be an alcoholic to have problems with alcohol. Problems linked to abuse are neglecting work, school, or family responsibilities. Legal issues such as alcohol violations and drinking-and-driving-related problems can also be a result of alcohol abuse. There are many "red flags" that can point to a problem with alcohol. One way is to answer these questions developed by Dr. John Ewing:

- Have you ever felt you should CUT down on your drinking?
- Have people ANNOYED you by criticizing your drinking?
- Have you ever felt bad or GUILTY about your drinking?
- Have you ever had a drink first thing in the morning to steady your nerves or to get rid of the hangover ("EYE OPENER")?

To help remember these questions, notice that the first letter of each key word spells CAGE. One "yes" answer suggests a possible alcohol problem. More than one "yes" means it is highly likely that a problem exists (Ewing, 1995).

Other signs and symptoms also could indicate that a person could be misusing or abusing alcohol or other drugs. One or two of them does not necessarily point to a problem, but several, combined with the right circumstances, need to be addressed. Some of these signs may include a grade decline or a sudden drop in grades, frequently missing class because of hangovers, binge drinking, legal problems associated with alcohol, or a significant increase in tolerance to alcohol. Other major signs of a drinking problem could be frequently drinking alone, drinking to forget about personal problems, or avoiding activities where alcohol is not available. Another more serious physical sign of alcohol abuse is a **blackout**. This occurs when an individual has amnesia about events after drinking, even though there was no loss of consciousness.

Alcoholism

Alcoholism, also known as alcohol dependence, is a chronic, progressive disease with symptoms that include a strong need to drink and continued drinking despite repeated negative alcohol-related consequences. There are four symptoms generally associated with alcoholism:

1. a craving or a strong need to drink,
2. impaired control or the inability to limit one's drinking,
3. a physical dependence accompanied by withdrawal symptoms such as nausea, sweating, shakiness, and anxiety when alcohol use is stopped, and
4. an increased tolerance.

Can alcoholism be hereditary? Alcoholism has a biological base. The tendency to become an alcoholic is inherited. Men and women are four times more likely to become alcoholics if their parents were (NIAAA, 2008). Currently, researchers are finding the genes that influence vulnerability to alcohol. A person's environment may also play a role in drinking and the development of alcoholism. This is not destiny. A child of an alcoholic parent will not automatically develop alcoholism, and a person with no family history of alcohol can become alcohol dependent.

There are ways to avoid becoming alcohol dependent. It is important to know your limit and stick to it. If choosing to drink, drink slowly and alternate an alcoholic beverage with a non-alcoholic beverage, eat while drinking, and most importantly find more effective ways of dealing with problems instead of turning to alcohol.

If you feel this is a problem, the sooner you stop the better the chances of avoiding serious psychological effects.

- Admit to your drinking—first step in avoiding serious problems.
- Change your lifestyle—try to stay out of situations where alcohol is prominent until you can control your drinking.
- Get involved in self-help groups.

Chronic Effects

Drinking too much alcohol can cause a wide range of chronic health problems including liver disease, cancer, heart disease, nervous system problems, as well as alcoholism (see Figure 9.8). The *Journal of the American Medical Association* (JAMA) suggested that moderate levels of alcohol consumption (one or two drinks per day) might reduce the risk of coronary heart disease (JAMA, 1994). However, researchers report in a more recent issue of JAMA that moderate consumption of alcohol decreases the risk of stroke but heavy consumption increases the risk of stroke. The National Stroke Association guidelines say that drinking one drink each day may actually lower the risk of stroke.

Although moderate amounts of alcohol may not be harmful, there are some major health issues associated with chronic alcohol use and abuse.

- *Liver disease* is commonly associated with alcohol abuse. The liver has many vital functions in the body. It is a common mistake for people to think that only those individuals who abuse alcohol can harm the liver. Individuals who are heavy social drinkers may run the risk of liver damage as well.
- *Hepatotoxic trauma* or "fatty liver" is the most common alcohol-related disorder causing enlargement of the liver. Some damage can be reversed if alcohol is completely avoided.

FIGURE 9.8

Long-term Risks Associated with Alcohol Abuse

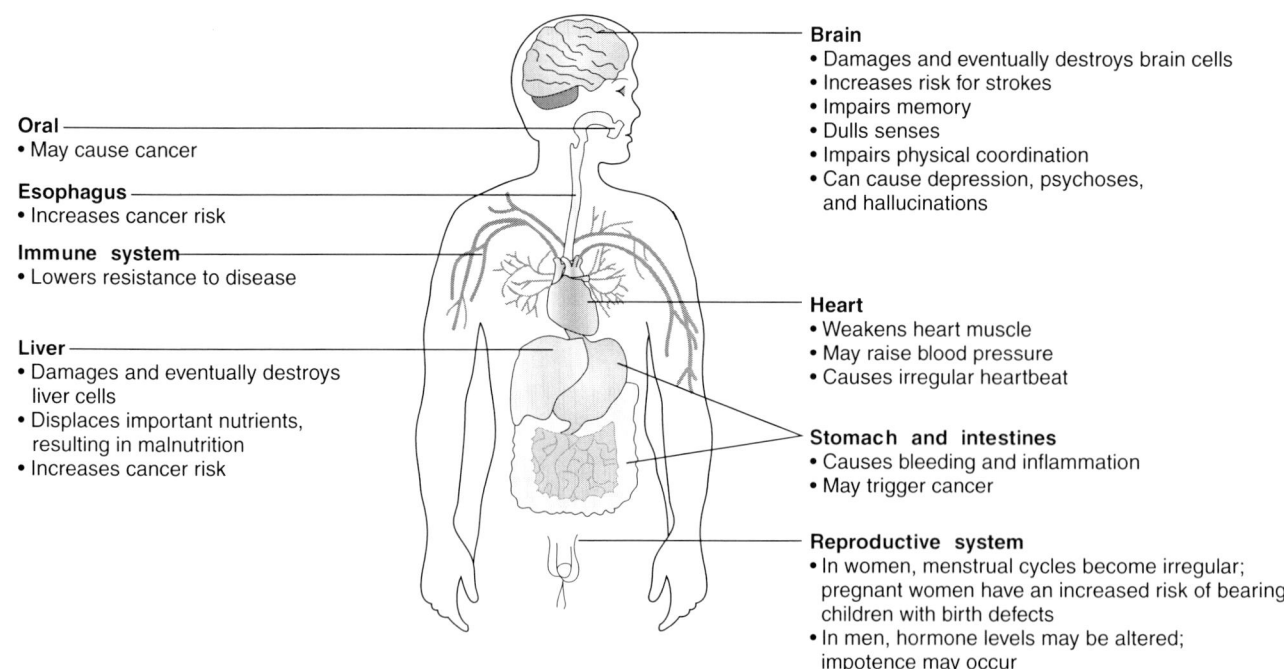

Source: Adapted from "Long-Term Risk Associated with Alcohol Abuse" *Lifetime Physical Fitness & Wellness* by Hoeger and Hoeger, Wadsworth Publishers.

- *Alcoholic hepatitis* is an enlarged and tender liver with an elevation of white blood cells. Symptoms can include nausea, vomiting, abdominal pain, fever, and jaundice. If alcohol use continues, this could progress to cirrhosis.
- *Alcohol cirrhosis* results from continued alcohol use and may cause permanent scar tissue to form when the liver cells are damaged. This problem usually occurs in 10 to 15 percent of people who consume large quantities and can develop in as little as five years of heavy drinking.
- *Alcohol pellagra* is a deficiency of protein and niacin. Symptoms may include skin inflammation, gastrointestinal disorders, diarrhea, and mental and nervous disorders.
- *Malnutrition* occurs from a lack of needed nutrients through prolonged alcohol consumption, by depressing the appetite and attacking the lining of the stomach. Heavy drinkers do not get the calories they need, which triggers increased mineral loss and increases fatty acids because of the interference of the transfer of glucose into energy.
- *Polyneuritis* is a condition caused by thiamin deficiency, which causes inflammation of several nerves and causes the drinker to become weak and have a tingling sensation.
- *Cancers*—It is established that 2 to 4 percent of all cancer cases could be caused by alcohol use. Cancer of the upper digestive tract such as mouth, esophageal, pharynx, and larynx can be attributed to alcohol use. Liver cancer as well as breast cancer may be caused by excessive alcohol consumption. Studies indicated that a woman's risk of developing breast cancer increases with age and alcohol consumption (JAMA, 1995).
- *Fetal alcohol syndrome.* The alcohol crosses the placenta but experts don't know exactly how drinking causes problems for the fetus. It may directly affect the fetus or it may be acetaldehyde, the metabolic by-product of alcohol that is harmful to the fetus. Some researchers believe that alcohol effects on the placenta cause blood flow and nutrient deficiencies. Whatever the reason, drinking during pregnancy clearly puts infants at risk for birth defects (Herman, 2003).

Neurological disorders associated with alcohol use are:

- *Wernickes disease* is caused by a thiamine deficiency. Some symptoms include decreased mental functions, double vision, and involuntary oscillation of the eyeballs.
- *Korsakoff's syndrome* is caused by a B complex vitamin deficiency. Symptoms are amnesia, personality alterations, and a loss of reality. This person may become apathetic and have difficulty walking.

Organizations   For information regarding alcohol use and abuse contact:

- National Institute on Alcohol Abuse and Alcoholism (NIAAA) www.niaaa.org
- *Alcoholics Anonymous (AA)* is an organization designed to support and help individuals become sober and stay sober. AA has over 19,000 affiliated groups and more than 350,000 members across the United States AA (212) 870-3400 www.alcoholic-anonymous.org
- *Al-Anon* and *Alateen* are organizations designed to help family members of alcoholics to cope with problems. 800-344-2666 www.al-anon-alateen.org

REFERENCES

American Heart Association (AHA). *Annual Report.* 2006.

Center on Addiction and Substance Abuse at Columbia University. Commission on Substances Abuse at Colleges and Universities.

Department of Justice. National Drug Intelligence Center. Ritalin Fast Facts, 2006.

Everett, S. A., Lowry, R., Cohen, L. R., Dellinger, A. M. Unsafe motor vehicle practices among substance-using college students. *Accident Analysis,* 1999.

Ewing, J. Detecting Alcoholism: the CAGE Questionnaire. *Journal of the American Medical Association,* 1984.

Dennis, M. E. and the Texas Commission on Alcohol and Drug Abuse. *Instructor Manual, Alcohol Education Program for Minors.* Austin: TCADA. 2005.

Galizio, Mark and Maisto, Stephen A. Determinants of substance abuse: biological, psychological, and environmental factors. Springer Publisher, 1985.

Herman, A., et al. In an ongoing search to understand the mechanisms of fetal alcohol syndrome. National Institute on Alcohol Abuse and Alcoholism, 2003.

Hoeger, W. and Hoeger, S. *Principles and Labs for Fitness and Wellness* (5th ed). Englewood, CO: Morton Publishing Company. 1999.

Journal of the American Medical Association. Moderate alcohol intake and lower risk of coronary heart disease, 1994.

Journal of the American Medical Association. Lifetime alcohol consumption and breast cancer risk among postmenopausal women in Los Angeles, 1995.

Lane, J., Pieper, C., Phillips-Butte, B, Bryant, J., and Kuhn, C. Caffeine's Effects Are Long-Lasting and Compound Stress. *Psychosomatic Medicine.* National Institutes of Health, July /August, 2002.

McCusker, R., Goldberger, B., and Cone, E. The Content of Energy Drinks, Carbonated Sodas, and Other Beverages. *Journal of Analytical Toxicology,* Vol. 30, March 2006.

McKinley Health Center. University of Illinois at Urbana-Champaign, 2005.

Miller, W., Tonigan, J., Longabaugh, R. Drinking Inventory of Consequences. An instrument for assessing adverse consequences of alcohol abuse. Test manual. Rockville, MD: National Institute on Alcohol Abuse and Alcoholism, 1995.

Miller, E. K., Erickson, C. A., & Desimone, R. Neural mechanisms of visual working memory in prefrontal cortex of the macaque. *Journal of Neuroscience,* 1996.

National Cancer Institute, U.S National Institutes of Health, 2008.

National Highway Traffic and Safety Administration (NHTSA). *Annual Report.* 2007.

National Institute on Alcohol Abuse and Alcoholism. National Institutes of Health. Statistic Snapshot of College Drinking, 2006.

National Institute on Alcohol Abuse and Alcoholism (NIAAA). College Drinking—Changing the Culture. "A Snapshot of Annual High-Risk College Drinking Consequences." 2007.

National Institute on Alcohol Abuse and Alcoholism. National Institutes of Health. Integrative Genetic Analysis Of Alcohol Dependence Using the Genenetwork Web Resources, 2008.

National Institute of Drug Abuse (NIDA). U.S. Dept. of Health and Human Services, 2008.

National Institute on Drug Abuse. The Science of Drug Abuse & Addiction. NIDA Info Facts: Hallucinogens, 2007.

National Institute on Drug Abuse. The Science of Drug Abuse & Addiction. NIDA Info Facts: Anabolic Steroids, 2005.

National Institute of Drug Abuse (NIDA). Update on Ecstacy. *NIDA Notes,* Volume 16, Number 5, Dec. 2001.

National Traffic Safety Administration. Traffic Safety Facts. Annual Assessment of Alcohol Related Fatalities, 2006.

Ray, O. and Ksir, C. *Drugs, Society, and Human Behavior* (8th ed). New York: WCB McGraw-Hill. 1999.

SAMHSA, National Clearinghouse for Alcohol and Drug Abuse; www.health.org

Centers for Disease Control and Prevention (CDC). Smoking and Tobacco Use. Fast Facts. Atlanta: Author. 2006.

U.S. Food and Drug Administration. Prescription Drug Use and Abuse: Complexities of Addiction, 2005.

U.S. Food and Drug Administration. Oxycodone. FDA Statement. Statement on Generic Oxycodone Hydrochloride Extended Release Tablets, 2004.

U.S. Food and Drug Administration, Department of Health and Human Services. FDA Issues Regulation Prohibiting Sale of Dietary Supplements Containing Ephedrine Alkaloids and Reiterates Its Advice That Consumers Stop Using These Products, 2005.

World Health Organization (WHO). *Waterpipe Tobacco Smoking: Health Effects, Research Needs and Recommended Actions by Regulators.* Geneva: Author. 2005.

ACTIVITIES

In-Class Activities

The Physical Effects of Smoking

Notebook Activities

Are You Addicted to Nicotine?

"Why Do You Smoke?" Test

"Do You Want to Quit?" Test

Addictive Behavior Questionnaire

Alcohol Screening Self-Assessment

Making Changes

Name: _____ Section: _____ Date: _____

IN-CLASS ACTIVITY

The Physical Effects of Smoking

This test consists of twenty statements about the effects of smoking. Put a check to show whether you think each statement is true or false. If you don't know whether a statement is true or false, put a check under "Don't know."

	True	False	Don't know
1. Smoking low-tar and low-nicotine cigarettes reduces the risk of all smoking-related diseases.	___	___	___
2. Carbon monoxide is inhaled when a person smokes.	___	___	___
3. How deeply a smoker inhales is not related to his or her chance of developing lung cancer.	___	___	___
4. Most experts agree that the harmful effects of smoking on health are not as great for women as for men.	___	___	___
5. Cigarette smoking increases the risk of developing breathing problems.	___	___	___
6. Cigarette smoke can increase air pollution in homes and offices.	___	___	___
7. Cigarette smoking increases the health dangers associated with taking birth control pills.	___	___	___
8. Frequent pipe and cigar smokers are more likely than nonsmokers to develop lung cancer.	___	___	___
9. The average life expectancy of a smoker is the same as that of a non-smoker.	___	___	___
10. People who smoke filter cigarettes inhale less carbon monoxide than do people who smoke nonfilter cigarettes.	___	___	___
11. Most people gain weight when they quit smoking.	___	___	___
12. Smokers have an increased risk of developing a lung infection after an operation.	___	___	___
13. Smoking during pregnancy does not increase a baby's risk of death.	___	___	___
14. Pipe smokers have a greater risk of developing cancer of the mouth than do cigarette smokers.	___	___	___
15. Smoking causes the heart to beat more slowly.	___	___	___
16. The health risks due to smoking do not change even after a person stops smoking.	___	___	___
17. The more a person smokes, the greater the chance of developing heart disease.	___	___	___
18. Cigarette smoke in the air can cause eye soreness in nonsmokers.	___	___	___
19. On average, babies born to mothers who smoke during pregnancy are smaller than babies born to nonsmokers.	___	___	___
20. Nicotine does not cause dependence similar to other addictive drugs.	___	___	___

Source: U.S. Department of Health and Human Services.

Answers

1 F; 2 T; 3 F; 4 F; 5 T; 6 T; 7 T; 8 T; 9 F; 10 F; 11 T; 12 T; 13 F; 14 T; 15 F; 16 F; 17 T; 18 T; 19 T; 20 F

Name: _____ Section: _____ Date: _____

NOTEBOOK ACTIVITY

"Why Do You Smoke?" Test

	Always	Frequently	Occasionally	Seldom	Never
A. I smoke cigarettes to keep myself from slowing down.	5	4	3	2	1
B. Handling a cigarette is part of the enjoyment of smoking it.	5	4	3	2	1
C. Smoking cigarettes is pleasant and relaxing.	5	4	3	2	1
D. I light up a cigarette when I feel angry about something.	5	4	3	2	1
E. When I have run out of cigarettes, I find it almost unbearable until I can get them.	5	4	3	2	1
F. I smoke cigarettes automatically without even being aware of it.	5	4	3	2	1
G. I smoke cigarettes for the stimulation, to perk myself up.	5	4	3	2	1
H. Part of the enjoyment of smoking a cigarette comes from the steps I take to light up.	5	4	3	2	1
I. I find cigarettes pleasurable.	5	4	3	2	1
J. When I feel uncomfortable or upset about something, I light up a cigarette.	5	4	3	2	1
K. I am very much aware of the fact when I am not smoking a cigarette.	5	4	3	2	1
L. I light up a cigarette without realizing I still have one burning in the ashtray.	5	4	3	2	1
M. I smoke cigarettes to give me a "lift."	5	4	3	2	1
N. When I smoke a cigarette, part of the enjoyment is watching the smoke as I exhale it.	5	4	3	2	1
O. I want a cigarette most when I am comfortable and relaxed.	5	4	3	2	1
P. When I feel "blue" or want to take my mind off cares and worries, I smoke cigarettes.	5	4	3	2	1
Q. I get a real gnawing hunger for a cigarette when I haven't smoked for a while.	5	4	3	2	1
R. I've found a cigarette in my mouth and didn't remember putting it there.	5	4	3	2	1

Source: U.S. Department of Health and Human Services.

Scoring Your Test

Enter the numbers you have circled on the test questions in the spaces provided below, putting the number you circled for question A on line A, for question B on line B, etc. Add the three scores on each line to get a total for each factor. For example, the sum of your scores for lines A, G, and M gives you your score on "Stimulation," lines B, H, and N give the score on "Handling," etc. Scores can vary from 3 to 15. Any score 11 and above is high; any score 7 and below is low.

A _____ + G _____ + M _____ = _____ Stimulation

B _____ + H _____ + N _____ = _____ Handling

C _____ + I _____ + O _____ = _____ Pleasure/Relaxation

D _____ + J _____ + P _____ = _____ Crutch: Tension Reduction

E _____ + K _____ + Q _____ = _____ Craving: Psychological Addiction

F _____ + L _____ + R _____ = _____ Habit

Name: _____ Section: _____ Date: _____

NOTEBOOK ACTIVITY

"Do You Want to Quit?" Test

	Strongly Agree	Mildly Agree	Mildly Disagree	Strongly Disagree
A. Cigarette smoking might give me a serious illness.	4	3	2	1
B. My cigarette smoking sets a bad example for others.	4	3	2	1
C. I find cigarette smoking to be a messy kind of habit.	4	3	2	1
D. Controlling my cigarette smoking is a challenge to me.	4	3	2	1
E. Smoking causes shortness of breath.	4	3	2	1
F. If I quit smoking cigarettes, it might influence others to stop.	4	3	2	1
G. Cigarettes damage clothing and other personal property.	4	3	2	1
H. Quitting smoking would show that I have willpower.	4	3	2	1
I. My cigarette smoking will have a harmful effect on my health.	4	3	2	1
J. My cigarette smoking influences others close to me to take up or continue smoking.	4	3	2	1
K. If I quit smoking, my sense of taste or smell would improve.	4	3	2	1
L. I do not like the idea of feeling dependent on smoking.	4	3	2	1

Scoring Your Test

Write the number you have circled after each statement on the test in the corresponding space to the right. Add the scores on each line to get your totals. For example, the sum of your scores A, E, I gives you your score for the Health factor. Scores can vary from 3 to 12. Any score of 9 or over is high, and a score of 6 or under is low.

A _____ + E _____ + I _____ = Health

B _____ + F _____ + J _____ = Example

C _____ + G _____ + K _____ = Aesthetics

D _____ + H _____ + L _____ = Mastery

Source: U.S. Department of Health and Human Services.

Name: _____ Section: _____ Date: _____

NOTEBOOK ACTIVITY

Addictive Behavior Questionnaire

Could You Be an Addict?

I. Recognizing Addictive Behavior*

Instructions. The following test, designed by Dr. Lawrence J. Hatterer, is not a way to diagnose whether you are in the early, middle, or chronic stages of addictive disease. It is meant merely to help you understand addictive behavior better so you can recognize it in yourself or perhaps in people you know.

1. I am a person of excesses. I can't regulate what I do for pleasure and often use a substance or indulge in a an activity heavily to get high.
2. I am an extremely self-involved person. People tell me I am into myself too much.
3. I am compulsive. I must have what I want when I want it, regardless of the consequences.
4. I am excessively dependent on or independent of others.
5. I am preoccupied. I spend a lot of time thinking or fantasizing about a particular activity or substance. Also, I will work my day around doing it or go to pains to make sure it's available.
6. I deny that I do this and lie about it to others who ask me.
7. I have been involved in this behavior for a least a year.
8. I've told myself I could easily stop, even though I've shown no signs of slowing down.
9. Once I start indulging in this behavior or substance, I find I have trouble stopping.
10. One or more members of my family are also involved in some kind of excessive behavior or substance abuse.
11. I find I gravitate mostly toward people who have the same behavior or take the same substance as I do.
12. I seem to be developing a tolerance of the behavior or substance. I have had a need to steadily increase the amounts I take or the time I spend doing it.
13. I have found that my excessive use of highs has, in fact, only made my problems worse.
14. If someone tries to keep me from obtaining the substance or practicing the activity, I get angry and reject or abuse that person.
15. I experience withdrawal symptoms if I cannot indulge in the substance or activity.
16. This has gotten in the way of my functioning. I have missed something important—days at work or time with my friends, family, children—because of it.
17. The substance/activity is destroying my home life. I know I am hurting those closest to me.
18. I have failed in many goals in life, lost money, given up many social and occupational contracts, all because of my excessive behavior.
19. I have tried to stop or cut down on my excesses but have been unsuccessful.
20. I have physically endangered myself or others in accidents that were a direct result of my excessive behavior.

Evaluation: If you answer "yes" to half or more of the questions, you may have a problem with addictive disease and should seek immediate professional help. For a referral, contact your local mental health clinic (look in the Yellow Pages) or speak to your doctor.

Source: From *McCall's* magazine, 1986.

II. Stage of Change for Addictive Behavior

If chemical dependency is a problem in your life, use Figure 2.4 (page 41) and Table 2.3 (page 41) to identify your current stage of change for participation in a treatment program for addictive behavior.

III. Changing Addictive Behavior

On a separate sheet of paper indicate the steps that you are going to take to correct addictive behavior(s) and identify people or organizations that you will contact to help you get started.

Name: _____ Section: _____ Date: _____

NOTEBOOK ACTIVITY

Making Changes

Breaking the Habit

Here's a six-point program to help you or someone you love quit smoking. (Caution: Don't undertake the quit-smoking program until you have a two- to four-week period of relatively unstressful work and study schedules or social commitments.)

1. *Identify your smoking habits.* Keep a daily diary (a piece of paper wrapped around your cigarette pack with a rubber band will do) and record the time you smoke, the activity associated with smoking (after breakfast, in the car), and your urge for a cigarette (desperate, pleasant, or automatic). For the first week or two, don't bother trying to cut down; just use the diary to learn the conditions under which you smoke.

2. *Get support.* It can be tough to go it alone. Phone your local chapter of the American Cancer Society, or otherwise get the names of some ex-smokers who can give you support.

3. *Begin by tapering off.* For a period of one to four weeks, aim at cutting down to, say, twelve or fifteen cigarettes a day; or change to a lower-nicotine brand, and concentrate on not increasing the number of cigarettes you smoke. As indicated by your diary, begin by cutting out those cigarettes you smoke automatically. In addition, restrict the times you allow yourself to smoke. Throughout this period, stay in touch, once a day or every few days, with your ex-smoker friend(s) to discuss your problems.

4. *Set a quit date.* At some point during the tapering-off period, announce to everyone—friends, family, and ex-smokers—when you're going to quit. Do it with flair. Announce it to coincide with a significant date, such as your birthday or anniversary.

5. *Stop.* A week before Q-day, smoke only five cigarettes a day. Begin late in the day, say after 4:00 p.m. Smoke the first two cigarettes in close succession. Then, in the evening, smoke the last three, also in close succession, about fifteen minutes apart. Focus on the negative aspects of cigarettes, such as the rawness in your throat and lungs. After seven days, quit and give yourself a big reward on that day, such as a movie or a fantastic meal or new clothes.

6. *Follow-up.* Stay in touch with your ex-smoker friend(s) during the following two weeks, particularly if anything stressful or tense occurs that might trigger a return to smoking. Think of the person you're becoming—the very person cigarette ads would have you believe smoking makes you. Now that you're quitting smoking, you're becoming healthier, sexier, more sophisticated, more mature, and better looking—and you've earned it!

Sources: American Cancer Society; National Cancer Institute.

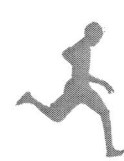

CHAPTER 10

Safety Awareness

"This above all, to refuse to be a victim."
—Margaret Atwood

OBJECTIVES

Students will be able to:
- Identify the four classes of accidents.
- Identify risks associated with drowsy driving.
- Identify elements of a crime.
- Identify steps in preventing a sexual assault.
- Become aware of the prevalence of acquaintance rape.
- Become aware of the prevalence of domestic violence.
- Identify organizations that provide assistance to victims of violent crime.

The purpose of this chapter is to provide information to help students make informed choices on personal safety and awareness issues. Being aware of possible hazardous situations may prevent accidents from occurring and save lives.

The National Safety Council (NSC) defines an accident as "that occurrence in a sequence of events which usually produces unintended injury, death, or property damage" (Bever, 1995). Accidents are the fifth leading cause of death in the United States after heart disease, cancer, stroke, and chronic obstructive pulmonary diseases. For people between the ages of 1 and 39, unintentional injuries are the leading cause of death. In the United States in 2006, there were 120,000 deaths due to unintentional injuries and over 26,200,000 disabling injuries.

In the United States alone, we average 14 unintentional injury deaths and 2,990 disabling injuries every hour (NSC, 2008).

Classes of Unintentional Injuries

Motor Vehicle Crashes

The leading cause of unintentional death is motor vehicle crashes. In 2006, over 44,000 individuals died in motor vehicle crashes in the United States. The 15–24 year-old age group had nearly 11,000 deaths for that year.

One of the leading factors in motor vehicle crashes is driver inattention. According to the National Highway Traffic Safety Administration (NHTSA), nearly 80 percent of crashes involve some form of driver inattention. This signifies the importance of the driving task and that the need for attention is critical.

Cell Phone Usage

Research has shown that using a cell phone while driving can create serious distractions and can decrease driving performance. The NHTSA estimates that driver distraction contributes to 25 percent of all reported traffic accidents. Drivers using cell phones are four times more likely to get into crashes causing injuries. Records indicate that cell phone users are over-involved in rear-end collisions. The hands-free models do little to increase safety—engaging in the conversation whether its business or personal appears to be the problem associated with the distractions. The National Highway Traffic Safety Administration's policy on cell phones while driving: "The primary responsibility of the driver is to operate a motor vehicle safely. The task of driving requires full attention and focus. Cell phone use can distract drivers from this task, risking harm to themselves and others. Therefore, the safest course of action is to refrain from using a cell phone while driving" (NHTSA, 2007).

Drowsy Driving

Fatigue on the road can be a killer. It happens frequently on long trips, especially long night drives. There is no test to determine sleepiness and no laws regarding drowsy driving; therefore, it is difficult to attribute crashes to sleepiness. According to the NHTSA, drowsy driving accounts for approximately 100,000 accidents each year, injuring 71,000 and producing 1,550 fatalities. In a 2006 poll conducted by the National Sleep Foundation (NSF, 2007) 62 percent of adults surveyed reported driving a vehicle while feeling drowsy during the prior year with 27 percent reporting that they actually dozed off while driving. Seventy-two percent between the ages of 18 and 24 have driven drowsy. It is equally as dangerous if not more dangerous to drive when you are drowsy than intoxicated. Some drivers abstain from alcohol but no one can resist the need to sleep. People are less likely to admit that they are feeling fatigued and therefore continue to drive when drowsy, leaving it up to self-regulation. Results from a recent study by the Stanford Sleep Disorders Clinic, performed by Dr. Nelson Powell, concluded that the sleepy drivers performed the same as the drunk drivers on basically all skills tested.

The NSF has created the "Drive Alert . . . Arrive Alive" campaign to help people become aware of the dangers of drowsy driving. One very important detail pointed out by this campaign is that people fall asleep more often on high-speed, long, boring, and rural highways. The more monotonous the drive, the more likely the driver will suffer some fatigue. According to the NSF, drivers who pose a greater risk for drowsy driving are those who are sleep deprived, drive long distances without breaks, drive through the night, drive alone, or those drivers with undiagnosed sleep disorders. Shift workers also pose a greater threat because they typically have non-traditional work schedules. Young people are more prone to sleep-related crashes because they typically do not get enough sleep, stay up late, and drive at night. NSF has a few warning signs to indicate that a driver may be experiencing fatigue. These include not remembering the last few miles driven, drifting from their lane, hitting rumble strips, yawning repeatedly, having difficulty focusing, and having trouble keeping the head up. The NSF also offers these tips for staying awake while driving:

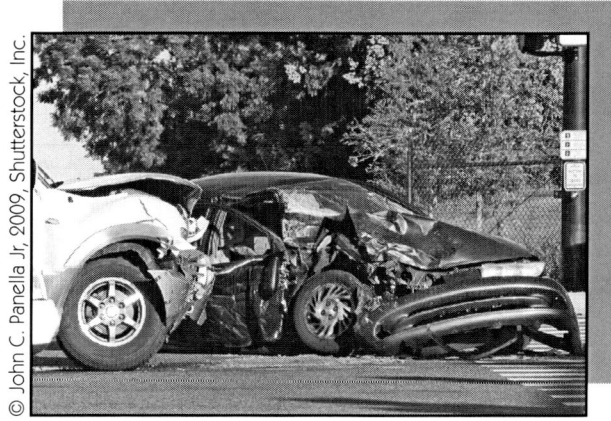

The leading cause of accidental death is motor vehicle accidents.

- Get a good night's sleep.
- Schedule regular stops.
- Drive with a companion.
- Avoid alcohol.
- Avoid medications that may cause drowsiness.

If anti-fatigue measures do not work, of course the best solution is sleep. If no motels are in sight and you are within one to two hours of your destination, pull off the road in a safe area and take a short twenty- to thirty-minute nap.

Most drowsy driving crashes involve males under the age of 30. Results of a recent poll by the NSF state that 72 percent of the people between the ages of 18 and 24 admitted to drowsy driving. Because of this growing problem, many colleges and universities, such as Texas A&M University, are providing awareness programs to try to prevent this tragedy from occurring.

In any kind of motor vehicle crash, a seat belt may save your life! The lap/shoulder safety belts reduce the risk of fatalities to front seat passengers of cars by 45 percent and for trucks by 60 percent. They also reduce the severity of injuries by 50 percent for cars and 65 percent for trucks (NSC, 2008). In 2006 seat belts saved an estimated 15,383 lives (NSC, 2008).

An additional 5,441 would have been saved if they had been wearing a seat belt (NSC, 2008). In crashes involving a fatality, only 1 percent of restrained passengers were ejected compared to 31 percent ejections of unrestrained occupants. A passenger involved in a motor vehicle crash is less likely to be seriously injured if they remain in the vehicle as opposed to being thrown from the vehicle involved in an accident.

Air bags combined with safety belts offer the best protection. There has been an overall 14 percent reduction in fatalities since adding air bags to vehicles, saving an estimated 2,796 lives in 2006 (NSC, 2008).

Motorcycles

There are almost five million motorcycles registered in the United States. The increasing popularity with motorcycles is attributed to the initial low cost of purchase compared to automobiles, and good fuel efficiency, which is very important with the rising cost of gas. Motorcycles represent only 3 percent of registered vehicles but they represent 11 percent of the fatalities. Of the 44,700 occupant deaths in motor vehicle crashes, nearly 5,000 fatalities were motorcycle riders. Approximately 80 percent of the motor vehicle crashes result in death or serious injury. One of the main reasons motorcyclists are killed or injured is that an estimated 33 percent of motorcycle riders are not licensed or they are improperly licensed to operate a motorcycle. Most states require an education course uniquely for motorcycles to ensure riders have the knowledge and the skill to safely ride (NSC, 2008).

Another significant factor is protection. Because there is no protection provided by the motorcycle, the rider must rely on clothing, eye protection, and of course a helmet. Motorcycle helmets are estimated to be 37 percent effective in preventing fatal injuries, saving the lives of almost 1,658 motorcyclists in 2001 (NSC, 2008). According to the National Safety Council, as of 2006, twenty states have mandatory helmet requirements for all motorcyclists. Another twenty-seven states require only riders less than 18 years of age to wear helmets. And there are three states with no laws involving helmet usage.

As in motor vehicle accidents, riding a motorcycle while under the influence of alcohol can decrease a rider's ability to operate the motorcycle safely. Almost 50 percent of riders killed annually are alcohol impaired. Alcohol diminishes reaction time, decision-making ability, and visual acuity. As with motor vehicles, all drivers or riders are impaired at .05 blood alcohol count (BAC).

Bicycle Safety

According to the National Safety Council, bicycle-related head injuries in 2004 resulted in 843 deaths. Wearing a helmet reduces the risk of serious head injuries by as much as 85 percent and the risk of brain injury by as much as 88 percent (NHTSA, 2007). Helmets have also been shown to reduce injuries to upper and mid-face by 65 percent.

If each rider wore a helmet, an estimated 500 bicycle-related fatalities and 151,000 non-fatal head injuries would be prevented each year (Thompson, 1996).

Helmet Laws

According to the Bicycle Helmet Safety Institute, in 2007, twenty-one state laws and more than 145 local governments had enacted some form of bicycle helmet legislation, most dealing with children or adolescents.

Ensuring that helmets provide real protection, U.S. Consumer Product Safety Commission (CPSC) issued a new safety standard for bike helmets in 1999. The new standard ensures that bike helmets will adequately protect the head and that chinstraps will be strong enough to prevent the helmet from coming off in a crash, collision, or fall. All bike helmets in the United States must meet the CPSC standard.

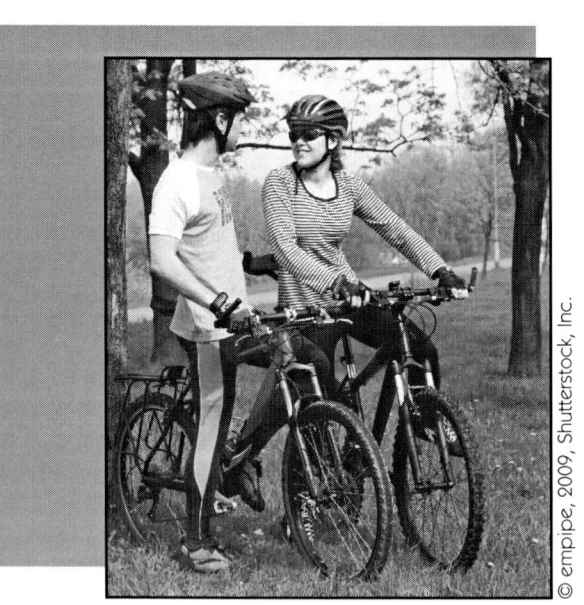

By wearing helmets, these bicyclists significantly reduce the risk of serious head injuries.

Prevention

According to the National Center for Injury Prevention and Control:

- Wear your helmet correctly. A helmet should fit snugly and not rock forward, backward, or side-to-side.
- Only buy a helmet if it meets or exceeds CPSC standards.
- Obey all traffic laws! Bicycles must adhere to all motor vehicle traffic laws.
- When riding at night, you must have a white front reflector or bright headlight and red rear reflector.

Home Accidents

Poisoning

The leading cause of death in the home is poisoning. Poisonings account for almost 20,000 deaths annually. Children under 5 years of age are especially susceptible to household poisons, such as cleaning agents and medications.

Poisoning by gases and vapors causes an average of 400 deaths each year. The primary cause of gas poisoning is carbon monoxide (odorless and colorless gas) due to incomplete combustion involving heating equipment, cooking stoves, and motor vehicle exhaust.

Hundreds of people die each year from improperly or malfunctioning fuel-burning appliances. It is important to have your heating system checked each year for any possible leaks. Carbon monoxide poisoning can also come from motor-vehicle exhaust, exhaust from a motorboat, or a generator:

- Don't use any gas-powered engines in an enclosed area.
- Don't use a gas oven to heat your home.
- Don't run the car in the garage.
- Don't sleep in an enclosed room with a gas or kerosene heater.

The symptoms of CO poisoning are severe headache, mental confusion, dizziness, and other flu-like symptoms. If you experience these symptoms, get to a place with fresh air immediately and seek medical attention.

Falls

There are over 40,000 deaths each year in the United States that occur at home, as well as almost a million disabling injuries. The second leading cause of death due to injuries in the home is falls, resulting in over 11,000 deaths per year. The age groups most prone to death from falls are the elderly (65 and over) and the very young (between 0 and 4 years old) (NSC, 2008). The National Safety Council estimates over eight million hospital visits were because of injuries resulting from falls.

Fires and Burns

Fires and burns account for between 2,000 and 3,000 deaths each year and are the third leading cause of unintentional death in the home (NSC, 2008). The United States has more fire deaths each year than any other industrialized country. According to the U.S. Fire Administration, cigarette smoking is the leading cause of residential fire deaths.

Three factors can be effective in preventing injuries and fatalities from fires:

1. Take responsibility and view fire as a personal threat. We sometimes feel that fires happen to "someone else," not us.

2. Take precautions and preventative measures, such as installing smoke detectors, carbon monoxide detectors, and having fire extinguishers in the home.
3. Implement a plan of action for escaping a fire to save valuable time as well as your life.

Work Accidents

The National Safety Council estimates that over 5,000 people each year die as a result of work-related accidents, and almost 4,000,000 are injured. The Occupational Safety and Health Act was passed in 1970 to assure safe working conditions for every man and woman in the United States. The Occupational Safety and Health Administration (OSHA) is the governing body established to enforce safety rules and regulations.

The leading cause of occupational death is *motor vehicle accidents*. According to the National Safety Council, motor vehicle accidents account for over 20 percent of the occupational deaths, which primarily involve the transportation industry; 14 percent of the deaths are due to *assaults on the job* (workplace violence), 9 percent are due to *falls*, and 9 percent come from being *struck by an object*.

Occupational illnesses are conditions caused by repeated exposure to factors associated with employment, such as *repetitive strain injury* (RSI), or repeated trauma. An example of RSI, *carpal tunnel syndrome* (CTS) is inflammation in the tendons of the wrist, damaging nerves in the hand and can be caused by typing, computer use, or any repeated use of the hands. Certain occupations pose a higher risk for CTS, such as computer technicians, clerical workers, electricians, carpenters, and those in the manufacturing field.

Public Accidents

These accidents include deaths in public places and non-motor vehicle accidents. Fatalities consist of water and air transportation accidents, railroad accidents, recreational boating and drowning fatalities, sports injuries and deaths, as well as fatalities as a result of natural disasters.

According to data from the U.S. Coast Guard, deaths associated with recreational boating average about 700 each year. Alcohol is involved in approximately 34 to 40 percent of the deaths due to boating accidents. The U.S. Coast Guard estimates that in eight out of ten boating fatalities, the victims were not wearing life jackets. Injuries associated with personal watercraft (PWC), have increased, accounting for over 1,800 deaths annually.

With regard to sports injuries, data from the NSC indicate that basketball and bicycle riding account for more than half a million emergency room visits each year.

Tornadoes are the most destructive of all storms, causing almost ninety deaths each year. According to data from the National Climatic Data Center (NCDC), Texas has the greatest number of tornadoes, with 132 during an average year.

Over the last thirty-eight years, lightning has accounted for an average of eighty-nine deaths per year according to the NCDC. States with the greatest numbers of lightning deaths during these years were Florida, Texas, and North Carolina.

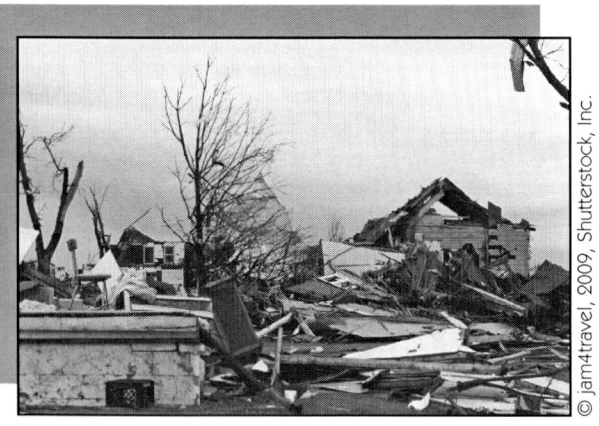

Educate yourself about community disaster plans and procedures.

Disaster Planning

You never know where you might be when a natural disaster occurs. They can occur with little warning, and you could be at home, school, or work. What will you do if basic services like water and electricity are cut off? What if communication with family and loved ones is difficult? What will you do if you are asked to evacuate your home or are required to be confined there? You need to have a plan to effectively cope with the difficulties that come when a natural disaster takes place.

FEMA, the Federal Emergency Management Agency, and the American Red Cross have created a four-step disaster planning program:

1. get informed,
2. make a plan,
3. assemble a kit,
4. maintain your plan and kit.

First, **get informed**. Be aware of high-risk hazards for your local area. Do you live in an area known to be at high risk for tornadoes, earthquakes, or hurricanes? Educate yourself about community disaster plans and ask about disaster plans and procedures for schools, places of employment and other areas that you frequent. Understand community warning systems. How will your community warn its citizens of possible risks and how will communication occur after a disaster?

Second, **make a plan.** Include the entire family in this process, especially children. Allow them to ask questions, offer input and practice this plan with them frequently. Include all caregivers who may be responsible for family members during a disaster as well. The focus of this plan is communication. If family members are separated during an emergency choose an out-of-town contact for family members to call, if possible, to report their location and status. It is often easier to make a long-distance call from a disaster area than a local call. If you experience a disaster such as a fire, choose a location where all family members can meet in the immediate vicinity. A page of sample cards has been included in the notebook activities from www.ready.gov. Each member of the family should have this information handy. Next, discuss escape routes and safe places in the event of a natural disaster. Include plans for family members or guests with special needs, children, and pets to be protected during disasters.

Next, **assemble a disaster kit.** These are supplies that may be used by your family to stay safe and more comfortable, during and after a disaster. This kit should be assembled, stored in easy-to-carry containers, and reviewed at least once per year, or as your needs change. Figure 10.1 contains a list of common items.

Last, you must **maintain your plan.** Make sure you review your plan on a regular basis. Conduct drills to work out any foreseeable problems. Restock food supplies. Check expiration dates and replace medications, food, and water as needed. Also, check batteries in smoke detectors, flashlights, and radios.

During and after a natural disaster, the local, state, and federal governments and disaster relief agencies work to restore normal activity as soon as possible. It is your responsibility, as a citizen, to be prepared to take care of your family and loved ones until normal conditions are restored.

Environmental Safety

We have spent time discussing ways to protect people. Next we will cover suggestions on protecting our environment.

FIGURE 10.1

Disaster Planning

The following is a list of items recommended by FEMA and the American Red Cross that you may find helpful during and after a natural disaster. A disaster supply kit should be readily available in your home. Also consider preparing a modified version for your place of employment and vehicle.

- Three-day supply of nonperishable food and manual can opener
- Three-day supply of water (one gallon of water per person, per day)
- Portable, battery-powered radio or television and extra batteries
- Flashlight and extra batteries
- First-aid kit and manual
- Sanitation and hygiene items (hand sanitizer, moist towelettes, and toilet paper)
- Matches in waterproof container
- Whistle
- Extra clothing and blankets
- Kitchen accessories and cooking utensils
- Photocopies of identification and credit cards
- Cash and coins
- Special needs items such as prescription medications, eyeglasses, contact lens solution, and hearing aid batteries
- Items for infants, such as formula, diapers, bottles, and pacifiers
- Tools, pet supplies, a map of the local area, and other items, to meet your unique family needs

If you live in a cold climate, you must think about warmth. It is possible that you will not have heat during or after a disaster. Think about your clothing and bedding needs. Be sure to include one set of the following for each person:

- Jacket or coat
- Long pants and long-sleeved shirt
- Sturdy shoes
- Hat, mittens, and scarf
- Sleeping bag or warm blanket

Source: FEMA and the American Red Cross. *Preparing for a Disaster*, 2008.

Reduce, Reuse, Recycle

The Environmental Protection Agency (EPA) defines sustainability as meeting the needs of the present without compromising the ability for future generations to meet their own needs. Easy ways to live green are to reduce, reuse, and recycle.

The best way to have a positive effect on your environment is to get involved with programs through your campus or community. Simple things can make big differences. Here are some suggestions made by The Office of Sustainability at Texas A&M University:

- Bring your own bags to the grocery store. It saves paper/plastic and the bags are reusable.
- When printing, use both side of the paper. It saves money.
- Think before you print—fewer copies save paper. Also consider using recycled paper.

- Drive less. Reduce your short trips around town and combine them for one day. Or better yet, ride your bike. It saves gas and money, and you get some exercise.
- Don't use paper or Styrofoam. Use reusable plates, cups, and water bottles. Make sure you use BPA-free plastic. Exposure to bisphenol A (BPA) may cause negative health effects.
- Conserve water by spending less time in the shower or turning off the water while brushing your teeth.
- Turn off your lights and computer. Unplug your phone charger and appliances when not in use. Lower your thermostat during the winter months and raise air conditioning temperatures in the summer, especially during the day when you are not home.
- Use fluorescent light bulbs—they use 50 percent less energy and last longer. However, remember to dispose of them properly because they do contain mercury.
- Carpool when you can or use the transit system, if available.
- Recycle, recycle, recycle—the amount of garbage we create is increasing. Our landfill sites are filling up fast. Waste has a negative effect on the environment and recycling helps to reduce the need for raw materials as well as using less energy. Locally you can recycle plastics, aluminum, clear and brown glass, and newspapers. Check your local community for pick-up or deposit stations.
- Properly dispose of your used electronic devices such as cell phones and computers. A growing form of toxic waste is e-waste. With technology, e-waste now makes a significant portion of our waste. That waste contains heavy metals like mercury and lead, which can leach out of the landfills. Nearly 70 percent of all waste in our landfills comes from electronic equipment.
- Recycling your old phone keeps it and its (likely toxic) battery out of the landfill. Most phones contain metals like copper and silver. If these are recycled, it lessens the demand for mining new metals. The EPA states that recycling a million phones may reduce greenhouse gases by the same amount as taking 1,368 cars off the road for a year.
- Bringing your lunch to work or school can save money and save on the use of plastic and Styrofoam containers. If you spend about $7–8 each day on lunch, that can add up to almost $2,000 a year. Instead, make your lunch at home and use reusable containers. Bringing your coffee from home in a reusable container can save you money as well.
- Buying used goods and selling your old goods can help save the landfills and save you money. Looking online is an easy way to find great items for less money. Selling your used items such as phones, furniture, or electronics online or in a garage sale could bring you some extra cash and save the landfills. You can also donate your items to a local charity to help others and keep the landfills clear.

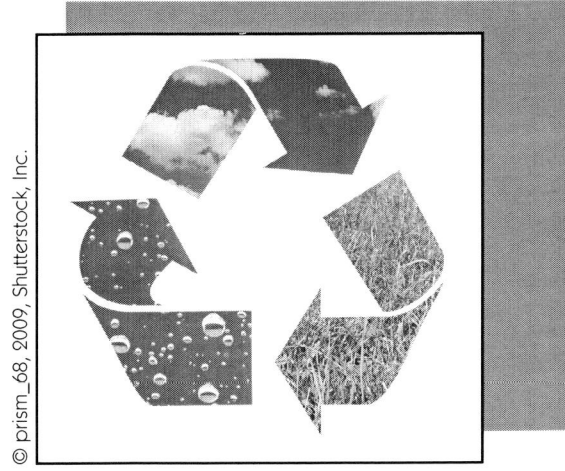
Reduce, reuse, recycle. Your efforts make a difference.

These are just a few ideas that you can use to make your environment a safer, greener place. Get educated! To find out how you can reduce carbon emissions or your carbon footprint, go to www.carbonfootprint.com.

Personal Safety

Personal safety is something that affects our everyday lives, regardless of who we are or where we live. Crime can happen to anyone at anytime, and it is essential to take certain precautions for protection. Being aware of your surroundings and learning to avoid certain situations can reduce the likelihood of becoming a victim.

In order for a crime to take place, three elements must exist:

1. the ability of the criminal,
2. the desire of the criminal,
3. an opportunity for the crime to be committed.

As individuals, we can only control one of the above elements, the most important—opportunity. If a criminal does not have the opportunity to commit a crime, the likelihood of the crime occurring diminishes.

Statistically, four out of five individuals will be victims of violence, whether simple assault or armed robbery. Contrary to what most believe, the typical crime victim is a single, unemployed young male. Young people in general, ages 16 to 24, are more than ten times as likely to be victims of violence as compared to older individuals.

Despite declining crime rates over the past few years, one in eight Americans say they are more fearful of walking in their neighborhood compared to the last year. These findings from the National Crime Prevention Survey, sponsored by the National Crime Prevention Council (NCPC), state that a large percentage of Americans feel less than "safe" at work, commuting, shopping, or engaging in leisure activities.

Although this fear has prompted many individuals to become more aware of preventative steps, the survey indicates that a substantial portion of Americans do not take simple prevention measures. Many Americans are unintentionally putting themselves at risk because they refuse to practice simple safety tips on a daily basis. According to the survey, 25 percent do not park in well-lighted areas; 34 percent do not lock their cars and roll up the windows whether driving or parked. Nearly 50 percent of those surveyed are targeted for crime by carrying large amounts of cash or valuable jewelry, and more than 50 percent frequently take short cuts and walk through poorly lighted areas. Another surprising finding is that only about half of American homes have deadbolt locks.

The following are a few simple safety tips and precautions to lower your risk of becoming a victim of violent crime.

Safety Tips

The National Crime Prevention Council (2003) produces an information sheet that includes tips for staying safe. They include:

Home

- Always keep doors and windows locked.
- Have adequate lighting around your home or apartment (notify manager if additional is needed).
- Do not open the door to strangers—always ask for credentials from maintenance or repair personnel.
- Do not give out any personal information over the telephone.
- Prepare records of personal items.
- Avoid being in isolated areas such as laundry rooms or parking garages by yourself.

- List your initials instead of your first name on your mailbox.
- Always have your keys ready for quick entrance into your residence.
- Have peepholes, deadbolt locks, and bars to lock sliding glass doors installed in your home or apartment.

Car

- Keep doors and windows locked.
- Always park in well-lighted areas.
- If being followed, do not go home. Go to a police station or well-populated area.
- Be aware of your surroundings at all times.

Campus

- Avoid walking alone.
- Do not leave personal possessions unattended.
- Always notice other people—make eye contact.
- Avoid taking shortcuts through campus.
- Do not walk like a victim. Walk like you are on a mission.
- Always be aware of your surroundings.
- **Trust your instincts.** If someone or something makes you feel uncomfortable, get out of the situation.
- Use well-lighted stops if taking a bus.
- Have key in hand before reaching your room or car.
- Avoid jogging or walking alone.
- Hang up immediately once you realize the nature of a harassing call.
- Call a campus escort when on campus late at night.

College Campuses

Many of the crimes on college campuses are crimes of opportunity. Theft is the most frequent crime on campus, yet it is the toughest challenge to convince students that their property can be taken. College students are typically very trusting, leaving their belongings unattended or inside vehicles in open view. Properly identifying your personal property such as backpacks, laptops, CD players, and textbooks becomes extremely important. If you consider the amount of valuables you carry with you in a backpack, including wallet, cell phones, and possibly credit cards, the need for protection against theft becomes crucial. Reducing the opportunity and using common sense is the key to most crime prevention on college campuses.

It is also important to be cautious with the amount of personal information that you make available to the public whether it is on campus or over the Internet. Social networking sites like Facebook and MySpace have become very popular, but they are not without safety concerns. With 140 million active users on Facebook alone, the risk of being victimized is very real. Choose the sites you post on carefully. Two main crimes can occur by using these types of sites: identity theft and unwanted attention/stalking.

To protect yourself from identity theft choose strong passwords. Passwords that are lengthy, contain letters, numbers, and symbols and use the entire keyboard are ideal. Always type the address directly into your browser or use personal bookmarks

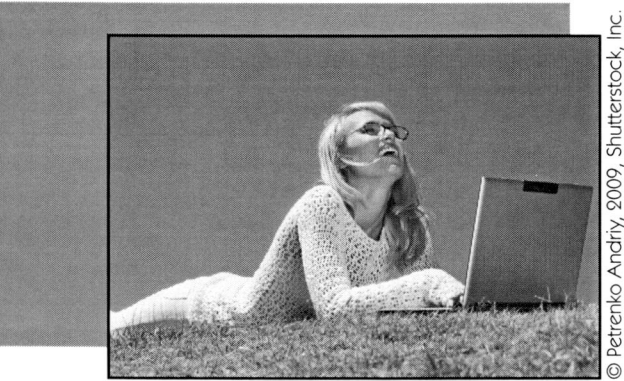

When you post information on the Internet, assume it is permanent. Consider limiting the information you include on your profile.

instead of accessing the site through an email or other Web page; you might be inadvertently typing your password into a fake site. Protect your personal information: your name, birthdate, and/or social security number can be used to create numerous kinds of accounts in your name.

When you post information on the Internet, assume that it is permanent. Even if you remove it, the possibility exists that someone else has copied it to another location. Consider limiting the information you include on your profile. Information that can be used to locate you, such as your address, phone number, work, or class schedule, may be found and used by someone you don't want to see. And always use the privacy settings available with any site you choose to use. The less information given out, the less likely it will be used to harm you.

Stalking

Stalking is a very common crime on college campuses across the United States, as well as the rest of society. Most stalkers are acquaintances, some with a previous connection to the target. Others can be classmates, neighbors, and co-workers. In a few cases, the stalker may be completely unknown to the target. The victim typically feels powerless, isolated, and confused. Whatever the situation, stalkers can be dangerous. It is estimated that 3.4 million people, age 18 or older, are victims of stalking each year (Department of Justice, 2006). Victims usually range in age between 19 and 39 years of age, but that does not mean it does not occur in other age groups.

If you know you are being stalked:

- Be very direct and tell the individual to leave you alone and never contact you again.
- Tell family, friends, co-workers that you are being stalked.
- Record everything that happens—every phone call, incident, or contact.
- Get an answering machine and keep all messages.
- Break old routines, change your normal patterns.
- Get a cell phone and keep it with you at all times.

Crime Awareness and Campus Security Act of 1990 The Clery Act was named for Jeanne Clery, a 19-year-old freshman who was raped and murdered in her dorm room at Lehigh University in 1986. Her parents were later informed that there had been thirty-eight violent crimes on this campus and the students were unaware of this problem. As a result, her parents, Connie and Howard Clery, along with other campus crime victims, convinced Congress to enact the law known as the "Crime Awareness and Campus Security Act of 1990." The law was amended in 1992 and 1998 to include rights to victims of campus sexual assault and to expand the reporting requirements of the colleges and universities. In 1998, the law was officially named the "Clery Act."

The Clery Act requires all colleges and universities to accurately report the number of campus crimes per category to the campus community and prospective students. College campuses have often been the site for criminal activity. These offenses include sex offenses, robbery, aggravated assault, burglary, arson, and motor vehicle theft. Hate crimes as well as hazing issues can be included in the reports as well as alcohol and weapons violations. Approximately 80 percent of the crimes that take place on college campuses are student-on-student, with nine out of ten felonies involving alcohol or other drugs.

As of 2002, the Clery Act also requires all states to register sex offenders, under Megan's Law, if they are students or employees of the college or university. This information is available to the campus police as well as students who request such information.

Under this law, colleges and universities can be fined for failure to report campus crimes. Omission of this information is not only illegal but it poses a threat to students' safety. The fines send a strong message for schools to take the obligation of reporting crimes and protecting students seriously.

Sexual Assault

Sexual assault is a serious, violent, and frightening crime committed against women, men, and children. It is an act of violence. Sexual assault is not about sex, it is about power. It is an attempt to control a person using sex as a weapon. Rape can happen to anyone at anytime, and rapists can be anyone. Most rape victims are women, but that does not exclude men as victims. According to the National Crime Victimization Survey, sexual assault is the fastest growing violent crime in the United States. It occurs with increasing frequency but remains the crime least often reported to the police. It is estimated that only about 10 to 15 percent of rape cases are reported and that in one out of seven reported rapes, the male is the victim. Forcible rape is comprised of three elements:

1. the use of force (not necessarily physical),
2. absence of the victim's consent,
3. and oral, penile/vaginal penetration.

Rape can happen to anyone at any age. Ages of reported cases range from 6 months to 90 years old, with the majority of victims under the age of 25 and the majority of their attackers also under the age of 25 (Weinberg, 1994).

On college campuses, 90 percent of sexual assaults occur when the victim or attacker is under the influence of alcohol. The National Institute of Alcohol Abuse and Alcoholism (NIAAA) estimated that drinking by college students contributes to an estimated 70,000 sexual assaults/date rapes each year and also contributes to 500,000 injuries and 1,400 deaths.

What does this mean? Impairment by alcohol or other drugs places an individual in a situation where their safety could be compromised. Alcohol affects the higher learning centers of the brain, making it difficult to focus on important information. This also makes it difficult for the individual to respond to negative situations in appropriate ways. The more aware and in control of your surroundings, the less likely you will become a victim.

The Department of Justice estimates that for every sexual assault, there are at least two attempts made on someone. Most rapists plan their attack by familiarizing themselves with the victim's surroundings. In all rape cases, the attacker has the advantage from a surprise standpoint. By being aware and avoiding compromising situations, you can reduce the likelihood of becoming a victim, but this does not mean that all rapes can be prevented. Rapists commit the crime, not victims.

Studies by the Department of Justice have shown that women who used physical resistance at the beginning of the attack were two times more likely to escape rape than those who did not resist. Although choosing to resist increases your chances of injuries, you will have a higher probability of avoiding rape. All studies show that *active resistance* works in most attack situations. One study commissioned by the National Center for the Prevention and Control of Rape showed that women who are the most aggressive and use the most aggressive methods of resistance are the ones most likely to escape rape and serious injury. Are you capable of using physical force? If so, then do it. Learning basic self-defense maneuvers can be extremely helpful in gaining self-confidence. Take advantage of anything that you can use as a weapon: pens, keys, umbrella. Punching, kicking, screaming—whatever it takes, use what you can to survive the situation. If you are inside a building, pull the fire alarm!

How you respond to the situation has a lot to do with where you are, for instance, in a mall parking lot, or in a deserted park. The best defense against an attack is to have a plan, an idea of what you would do if you were ever in a situation that called for a response. This certainly does not mean that in every situation, if you fight back you will survive. It is a good idea to have several plans to choose from. What works in one situation may not work in another—there are no guarantees!

Passive resistance could be effective in some situations. Examples of passive resistance are verbal persuasion, pleading, or submission. This sometimes can be helpful in regaining your stability and possibly giving you a chance to think through the situation and plan a defense. However, research has shown that passive resistance is not as effective as active resistance and does not seem to reduce the chance of victim injury (Bever, 1995). But the bottom line is, if it works it is successful.

Self-defense experts suggest reasons why individuals are easy targets for random violent acts. These reasons include: lack of awareness, body language, and being in the wrong place. Always be aware of your surroundings and walk like you are "on a mission"—making eye contact with everyone you pass. Psychologists have known for years that perpetrators select their victims based on signs and signals given off by the potential victim. Studies have shown that stride length and speed, walking too slow as if you are afraid, and jerky or independent arm swing, as well as slumped posture all play a role in "looking" like a victim (Grayson, 1981).

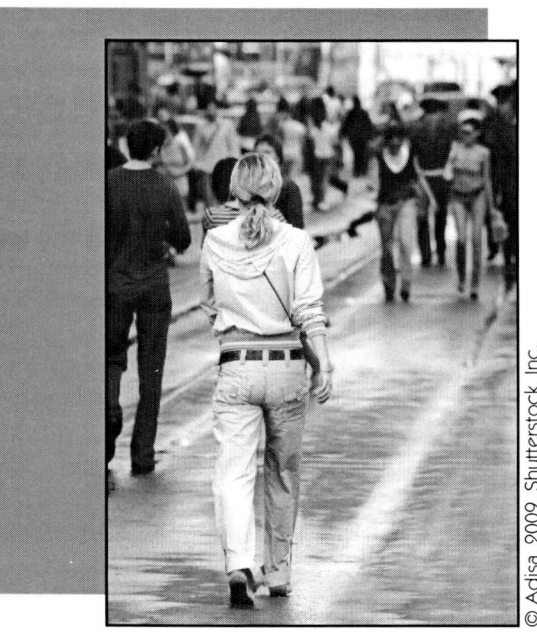

Always be aware of your surroundings and walk like you are "on a mission." Make eye contact with everyone you pass.

Avoid being alone in an isolated area. If you feel like you are being followed, cross the street and go to a populated area. If an attacker approaches you, utilize the first rule of self-defense—run! Most people feel that they cannot escape. Even if the attacker has a gun, if you are not under their control, then run. If you do find yourself in a violent situation, react immediately. Do not allow the attacker to take you to a second location. You have a better chance of surviving by doing whatever it takes at the original site. Do not hesitate to take action. Remember, you are responsible for your own safety, do not rely on someone else to take care of you or protect you from harm!

Acquaintance Rape/Intimate Violence

Acquaintance rape or date rape can be defined as interaction that begins between two people at a social event or on a date and ends with one forcing the other to participate in sexual activity (Sawyer, Desmond, and Gabrielle, 1993). This is a particularly volatile issue on college campuses. The prevalence of date rape on campus is difficult to determine because victims are even less likely to report a rape by someone that they know. Studies indicate that as many as one in eight college women will be raped while in college and 84 to 90 percent of the victims knew their attacker, a classmate, friend, previous partner, or acquaintance. Most date rapes occur at either the victim's home or the home of the attacker, with 57 percent occurring on an actual date.

Women ages 16 to 24 experience the highest per capita rates of *intimate violence* (intimate is defined as current/former spouse or boyfriends/girlfriends). Alcohol also plays a role in intimate violence. The Bureau of Justice Statistics estimates about three million violent crimes occur each year in which the offenders have been drinking alcohol at the time of the offense. Two-thirds of victims who suffered violence by an intimate reported that alcohol had been a factor. Approximately 31 percent of stranger victimizations were alcohol related.

Safety Tips

- When at a party or club, do not leave beverages unattended or accept a drink from someone you do not know.
- When going to a party or club, go with friends and leave with friends.
- Be aware of your surroundings at all times.
- Do not allow yourself to be isolated with someone you do not know.
- Know the level of intimacy you want in a relationship and state your limits.
- Trust your instincts—if you are uncomfortable, get out of the situation.
- Have your own transportation—if you need to end the date, end it.
- When meeting someone new, meet in a public place.

Steps to Take if Rape Occurs

- Go to a friend's house or call someone you know to come over. You do not need to be alone!
- DO NOT shower or make any attempt to clean yourself; do not change clothes or remove any physical evidence of the attack.
- Call your local Rape Crisis Center for assistance and counseling. A counselor can also accompany you to the hospital.
- Seek immediate medical attention and notify the police.

Domestic Violence

Another form of violence affecting our society is **domestic violence.** This includes partner violence, family violence, spouse abuse, child abuse, and battering. Domestic violence does not always have to be physical. Psychological abuse can be equally as harmful and can progress into physical abuse. A few examples of domestic violence are name calling or put downs, isolation from family and friends, withholding money, threatening or physical harm, sexual assault, disrespect, abusing trust, and harassment.

Battering focuses on control of a relationship through violence, intimidation, or psychological abuse in an attempt to create fear in the victim. The violence may not happen often, but the fear of it happening is a terrorizing factor (FBI, 1990). Approximately 95 percent of the victims are women; however, in a small number of cases the victims are men. According to the Surgeon General, domestic violence is the leading cause of injury to women between the ages of 15 and 44, and approximately 70 percent of men who abuse their female partners also abuse their children. Every day in America, intimate male partners kill at least four women, and more than 50 percent of all women in the United States are battered at sometime in their lives (FBI, 1991). If you or a friend is the victim of domestic violence, seek help. Call the police or go to a shelter. Realize that the violence could even result in death, so action must be taken immediately.

REFERENCES

Bever, D.L. *Safety—A Personal Focus* (3rd ed). St. Louis, MO: Mosby Year Book, 1995.

Department of Justice. Bureau of Justice Crime and Victims Statistics. Stalking Victimization in the United States. 2006.

Driver Electronic Device Use in 2007. *Traffic Safety Facts*. National Highway Traffic Safety Administration, 2008.

Federal Bureau of Investigation (FBI). *Uniform Crime Reports*, 1990, 1991.

Federal Emergency Management Agency and American Red Cross. Preparing for Disaster. U.S Department of Homeland Security, 2008.

Grayson, Betty and Stein, Morris I. Attracting Assault: Victims' Nonverbal Cues *Journal of Communication,* Volume 31, 1981.

Glassbrenner, D. and Ye, T. Driver Cell phone Use in 2006. *Traffic Safety Facts*. National Highway Traffic Safety Administration, 2007.

Help Make Sustainability an Aggie Tradition. Office of Sustainability, Texas A&M University, 2008.

National Crime Prevention Council, *2003 National Crime Victimization Survey*. U.S. Department of Justice, Bureau of Justice Statistics.

National Institute of Mental Health, National Center for the Prevention and Control of Rape. www.fullpower.org

National Safety Council: *Injury Facts, 2008 Edition*, Itasca, IL. 2008.

National Sleep Foundation. *State of the States Report.* National Highway Traffic Safety Administration, 2007.

Sawyer, R., Desmond, S., and Gabrielle, M. Sexual Communication and the College Student: Implications for Date Rape. *Health Values: The Journal of Health Behavior, Education and Promotion,* 8/31/1993.

The TerraPass. (n.d.). http://terrapass.com

Thompson, D., Rivara, F., Thompson, R. Effectiveness of bicycle safety helmets in preventing head injuries. A case-control study. *JAMA,* 1996.

Travisano, J. The Dangers of Drowsy Driving. *Current Health* 2, March 1998.

Weinberg, C. *The Complete Handbook of College Women.* New York: New York University Press. 1994.

Williams, B. K. and Knight, S. M. *Healthy for Life—Wellness and the Art of Living.* Pacific Grove, CA: Brooks/Cole Publishing Co. 1997.

CONTACTS

Most communities have a Rape Crisis Center, as well as centers for domestic violence. National Information Hotlines are also available.

For help contact:

Rape Abuse & Incest National Network
1-800-656-HOPE
www.rainn.org

National Coalition against Domestic Violence
P.O. Box 34103
Washington, D.C 20043-4103
202-638-6388

National Coalition against Sexual Assault
P.O. Box 21378
Washington, D.C. 20009
202-483-7165

VOICES in Action
P.O. Box 148309
Chicago, IL 60614
312-327-1500

National Domestic Violence Hotline
1-800-799-SAFE

National Resource Center on Domestic Violence
1-800-537-2238

Family Violence Prevention Fund
383 Rhode Island St. Suite 302
San Francisco, CA 94103-5133
endabuse.org

National Victim Center
1-800-FYI-CALL

ACTIVITIES

Notebook Activities

Family Emergency Plan
Checklist of Rape Prevention Strategies

Name: _____ Section: _____ Date: _____

NOTEBOOK ACTIVITY

Family Emergency Plan

 Family Emergency Plan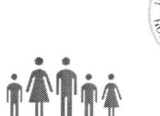

Prepare. Plan. Stay Informed.

Make sure your family has a plan in case of an emergency. Before an emergency happens, sit down together and decide how you will get in contact with each other, where you will go and what you will do in an emergency. Keep a copy of this plan in your emergency supply kit or another safe place where you can access it in the event of a disaster.

Out-of-Town Contact Name: _____ Telephone Number: _____
Email: _____
Neighborhood Meeting Place: _____ Telephone Number: _____
Regional Meeting Place: _____ Telephone Number: _____
Evacuation Location: _____ Telephone Number: _____

Fill out the following information for each family member and keep it up to date.

Name: _____ Social Security Number: _____
Date of Birth: _____ Important Medical Information: _____

Name: _____ Social Security Number: _____
Date of Birth: _____ Important Medical Information: _____

Name: _____ Social Security Number: _____
Date of Birth: _____ Important Medical Information: _____

Name: _____ Social Security Number: _____
Date of Birth: _____ Important Medical Information: _____

Name: _____ Social Security Number: _____
Date of Birth: _____ Important Medical Information: _____

Name: _____ Social Security Number: _____
Date of Birth: _____ Important Medical Information: _____

Write down where your family spends the most time: work, school and other places you frequent. Schools, daycare providers, workplaces and apartment buildings should all have site-specific emergency plans that you and your family need to know about.

Work Location One
Address:
Phone Number:
Evacuation Location:

Work Location Two
Address:
Phone Number:
Evacuation Location:

Work Location Three
Address:
Phone Number:
Evacuation Location:

Other place you frequent
Address:
Phone Number:
Evacuation Location:

School Location One
Address:
Phone Number:
Evacuation Location:

School Location Two
Address:
Phone Number:
Evacuation Location:

School Location Three
Address:
Phone Number:
Evacuation Location:

Other place you frequent
Address:
Phone Number:
Evacuation Location:

Important Information	Name	Telephone Number	Policy Number
Doctor(s):			
Other:			
Pharmacist:			
Medical Insurance:			
Homeowners/Rental Insurance:			
Veterinarian/Kennel (for pets):			

Dial 911 for Emergencies

 # Family Emergency Plan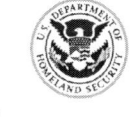

Prepare. Plan. Stay Informed.

Make sure your family has a plan in case of an emergency. Fill out these cards and give one to each member of your family to make sure they know who to call and where to meet in case of an emergency.

< FOLD HERE >

ADDITIONAL IMPORTANT PHONE NUMBERS & INFORMATION:

Family Emergency Plan

EMERGENCY CONTACT NAME:
TELEPHONE:

OUT-OF-TOWN CONTACT NAME:
TELEPHONE:

NEIGHBORHOOD MEETING PLACE:
TELEPHONE:

OTHER IMPORTANT INFORMATION:

DIAL 911 FOR EMERGENCIES

Ready

Name: _____ Section: _____ Date: _____

NOTEBOOK ACTIVITY

Checklist of Rape Prevention Strategies

The final test of your learning about rape is how your attitudes and beliefs affect your behavior. There are a number of things you can do to keep from being involved in a rape situation. Complete the following "Checklist of Rape Prevention Strategies" to see if you are doing everything you can to reduce your risk of involvement in a rape situation.

Circle the number that best describes how often you do each of the items below:

Never	Sometimes	Frequently	Always
1	2	3	4

For Everyone

Awareness

1 2 3 4   Think about what you really want to do with a sexual partner.

1 2 3 4   Be aware of stereotypes that prevent you from acting as you want to (such as a woman not being able to initiate sexual activity or a man not being able to say "no").

1 2 3 4   Observe how the environment is changing (such as being left at a party by your friends and having no way home).

Assertiveness

1 2 3 4   Believe and act as if you come first, without exploiting others.

1 2 3 4   Do not allow yourself to be put in vulnerable situations.

Control

1 2 3 4   Watch your use of alcohol or other substances so that you do not lose your self-control. Drug intoxication can both diminish the capacity to prevent and escape from assault as well as reduce inhibition from engaging in assaultive behavior.

1 2 3 4   Watch how others are using alcohol and other drugs and how this is affecting their self-control.

Interpersonal Relations

1 2 3 4   When dating someone for the first time, do so in a group situation or public place so that you can assess your date's behavior.

1 2 3 4   Pay attention to nonverbal cues as well as verbal cues. Do they match?

1 2 3 4   Treat others as equals. For example, share expenses so no one feels that something is "sexually owed."

Communication

1 2 3 4   Directly communicate what you are really thinking and what you want.

1 2 3 4   Ask, rather than assume, what would be most enjoyable together.

1 2 3 4   Listen to what your partner is really saying, and pay attention to the words (such as "no" means "no.").

1 2 3 4   Respect your partner's responses.

Source: From *Exploring Our Sexuality* by Patricia Koch. Copyright © 1995 by Patricia Barthalow Koch. Reprinted by permission of the author.

| 1 2 3 4 | Set clear limits for acceptable behavior (such as "I would like to invite you back to my apartment to listen to music and talk. However, I do not want to do anything sexual, except kissing."). |
| 1 2 3 4 | Find out what is wanted and unwanted sexual behavior for both you and your partner. |

Especially for Women

Awareness

| 1 2 3 4 | Trust your instincts when you are fearful (listen to that little voice inside you). Then act in ways to make yourself safer. |

Control

1 2 3 4	Dress so you can move easily, freely, and quickly.
1 2 3 4	Yell "fire" (rather than "rape" or "help") if you need help.
1 2 3 4	Get out of a dangerous situation as soon as you sense danger.
1 2 3 4	Always have an alternative way to get home.
1 2 3 4	Take assertiveness training and self-defense courses.
1 2 3 4	Carry a device for making a loud noise, like a whistle or small air horn. Sound the noise alarm at the first sign of danger.
1 2 3 4	Avoid putting yourself in known high-risk situations, such as walking alone in dark, deserted areas or hitchhiking.

Where you live:

1 2 3 4	Have and use secure locks on all doors and windows.
1 2 3 4	Have lights in all entrances and have keys in hand when you approach your entrance.
1 2 3 4	If you live by yourself or with other women, do not use your first name on mailboxes, answering machines, or in the phonebook.
1 2 3 4	Know and avoid dangerous places (e.g., under stairs, alleys).
1 2 3 4	Know neighbors you could trust in an emergency.
1 2 3 4	Ask salespeople, repair persons, public officials, etc. for physical identification before opening the door. (Have people call ahead.)
1 2 3 4	Have an escape plan from your home.

On the street:

1 2 3 4	Walk confidently at a steady pace and be aware of your surroundings.
1 2 3 4	Keep your hands free—don't overload yourself with packages, purses, books.
1 2 3 4	Avoid dark, unlighted areas.
1 2 3 4	Walk or jog with a companion.
1 2 3 4	Walk or jog in the open, not near bushes or cars where someone can hide.

While using private transportation:

1 2 3 4	Keep your car locked and check the back seat before getting in.
1 2 3 4	Keep your car doors locked when driving.
1 2 3 4	Do not stop for anyone you do not know or does not show you official identification, like a police officer.
1 2 3 4	If your car breaks down while you're alone, attach a white cloth to the antenna and lock yourself in until a police officer arrives. If anyone else stops to help, have them call the police or garage for you.

While using public transportation:

1 2 3 4	Keep your hands free while securing purses and packages.
1 2 3 4	While sitting or standing, look aware.
1 2 3 4	If you are not sure of where you are going, ask the driver and sit near her or him.

Communication

1 2 3 4   Practice your communication and assertiveness skills in a comfortable environment to prepare you for the times you need them to protect yourself.

1 2 3 4   Use assertive verbal confrontation if you need to (such as "I feel uncomfortable when you don't listen to me or when you touch me like that").

Interpersonal

1 2 3 4   Watch for indications that a date may hold negative, stereotyped attitudes toward women.

1 2 3 4   Watch for indications that a date may be a controlling or dominating person who may try to control your behavior.

1 2 3 4   Do not allow others to violate your personal space.

1 2 3 4   Do not assume that someone who has been nonviolent in the past will be nonviolent in the future.

1 2 3 4   Reject the activity, and let the person clearly know this, if you do not like what someone is doing to you.

1 2 3 4   Do not play games. Passivity, coyness, and submissiveness (sometimes parts of flirting) are dangerous and can support a climate of sexual aggression.

1 2 3 4   Use rape prevention strategies with everyone, since you can't tell who has the potential for rape by their appearance.

Especially for Men

Awareness

1 2 3 4   Realize that sexual relations are not "all or nothing" choices. There are many ways to give and receive pleasure. Kissing, touching, and even nudity do not mean that a person wants or expects to have genital relations.

1 2 3 4   Do not choose to involve yourself with negative influences, such as media that depict violence against women or peers who espouse negative attitudes toward women.

1 2 3 4   Ask yourself if you really want to have sexual relations with someone who does not want to have such sexual relations with you? How will you feel about your sexual behavior later, especially if the person indicated discomfort or resistance?

1 2 3 4   Consider the motivations behind your actions. Are you pursuing shared pleasure or self-gratification and power?

1 2 3 4   Consider acquaintance rape and other forms of sexual assault as crimes. An acquaintance rape happens if you have intercourse with a partner against her or his will and without consent.

1 2 3 4   Know that sexual desires are natural and spontaneous, but your actions are always within your control.

Interpersonal

1 2 3 4   Use peer pressure positively to help stop abusive behaviors which may lead to acquaintance rapes (for example, condemn rather than condone the behavior of a peer who has taken advantage of a sexual partner).

1 2 3 4   Realize that being turned down for some type of sexual interaction is not necessarily a personal rejection; it may just mean not wanting to participate in a certain act at a certain time.

1 2 3 4   Assume that "no" means "no" and do not continue. Allow your partner to take the initiative for what he or she wants.

1 2 3 4   Do not use sex for your self-gratification at the expense of others.

1 2 3 4   Do not think that you always have to initiate sexually.

1 2 3 4   Do not initiate sex if you don't want to.

1 2 3 4   Join with other men and women in taking action in eliminating negative sexual experiences, such as creating safer public environments.

1 2 3 4   Be alert to anyone who may be suffering a verbal or physical assault. Help in any way you can, such as speaking up for someone who is being harassed at a party.

Communication

1 2 3 4   Clarify others' motivations. This will eliminate confusing friendliness with sexual invitation.

1 2 3 4   Voice your needs and feelings but realize you do not have the right to take away the freedom of choice from someone else.

1 2 3 4   Do not assume that previous permission for sexual contact applies to the current situation. ALWAYS ASK.

You should always be trying to do each of the items described on this checklist. If you are not currently using each of these as frequently as you could, explore the reasons why you are not. See if you can make the changes necessary to reduce your risk of being in a rape situation. What change will you try to make?

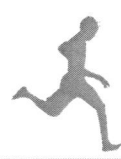

CHAPTER 11

Human Diseases

"Habits are to the soul what the veins and arteries are to the blood, the courses in which it moves."

—Horace Bushnell

OBJECTIVES

Students will be able to:
- Differentiate between communicable and non-communicable diseases.
- Discuss strategies to avoid contraction of communicable diseases and identify the symptoms and treatment for each disease.
- Know the risk factors for cancer and describe the cancer warning signs represented in the CAUTION acronym.
- Identify four cancers that affect young adults; discuss prevention and risk factors.
- Describe early detection exams and list treatment options.
- Differentiate between Type I and Type II diabetes.
- List three risk factors for Type II diabetes.

The purpose of this chapter is to inform individuals regarding symptoms, methods of transmission, precautions, and treatments of communicable and noncommunicable diseases most common to the college-aged population.

Communicable Diseases

Communicable diseases are those diseases that are transmitted from person to person. These diseases can be transmitted directly by physical contact, which can include coughing or sneezing, or indirectly by contaminated water or infected insects.

HIV/AIDS (Non-Sexual Contraction)

HIV/AIDS can be contracted through blood transfusions, sharing needles, and/or the exchange of blood or breast milk from a mother to her unborn or newborn child. The groups that have been found to be at higher risk include IV drug users and those individuals who received a blood transfusion before 1985.

Tuberculosis

Tuberculosis (TB) is a communicable disease that primarily affects the lungs and was responsible for a large number of deaths and disabilities until the middle of the twentieth century. There was a sharp decline in the devastation caused by this illness from 1950 to 1980 due to the discovery of effective medications.

TB is caused primarily by the bacillus (or rod-shaped) microorganism *Mycobacterium tuberculosis*; other mycobacteria strains are responsible for some cases, particularly with coexistent HIV infection. The disease is transmitted by airborne droplets when someone with the active disease coughs, talks, or sneezes. Those at risk for contracting TB are persons who spend a lot of time, particularly indoors, with individuals who have active infectious tuberculosis.

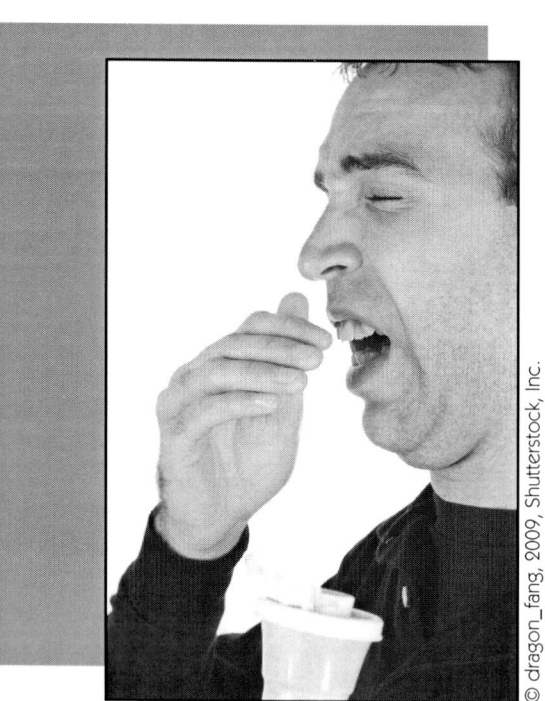

Communicable diseases are diseases that are transmitted from person to person.

The mycobacterium is covered with protective waxes and fatty substances, and is thus more durable and difficult to eradicate than many other infectious organisms. The bacteria lodge in the lungs, particularly the upper lobe, then migrate to the lymph nodes where an immune response occurs, mobilizing defenses which wall off the bacteria. Most individuals infected with TB are successful in "locking away" the bacillus organisms, which are then incapable of growing and multiplying. Those with 'latent' (inactive) TB are not ill and cannot infect others. However, there is an overall lifetime risk of one in ten of developing active TB later in life, particularly when immunity declines. Someone with latent TB will have a positive skin (Mantoux) test, which is a test for the presence of antibodies against the mycobacterium organism. Many physicians recommend that someone with a reactive skin test receive preventative (prophylactic) antibiotic treatment to destroy the TB bacilli and minimize the risk of developing active TB later in life. The most common prophylactic treatment is a six- to twelve-month course of the medication isoniazid.

Those at greatest risk are infants, adolescents, and young adults. Common symptoms of the illness include fatigue, weight loss, lethargy, decreased appetite, low-grade fever, and night sweats. A cough generally develops slowly. Eighty-five percent of TB infections involve the lung (pulmonary tuberculosis), destroying healthy tissue in the process; however, the disease can be spread through the bloodstream to many other parts of the body including the central nervous system, bones, joints, kidneys, uterus, heart, intestines, and skin. In progressive pulmonary TB, approximately one-half of untreated individuals will die. Overall, 5 to 10 percent of patients die despite treatment due to drug-resistant disease, poor medication compliance, or improper drug therapy.

As mentioned previously, the rates of TB infection have risen over the past decade. Reasons for the increased incidence of this disease in the United States include HIV infection, which attacks the immune system and allows a latent infection to reactivate, the emergence of drug-resistant forms of mycobacteria, immigration into the United States from countries with a high prevalence of TB infection, and social conditions that foster increased risk of transmission such as poverty, drug and alcohol abuse, and homelessness.

Active TB is diagnosed with a chest X-ray, culture, and microscopic examination of sputum samples. The sputum culture not only identifies the causative organism, but also allows for determination of drug sensitivity or resistance.

Treatment for the active form of tuberculosis consists of a combination of medications due to the difficulty in destroying the organisms and the presence of drug-resistant forms. The combination of choice for treatment of active disease includes the medications isoniazid, rifampin, pyrazinamide, and ethambutol or streptomycin for six to nine months (McCance and Huether, 2005). If the organism is resistant to isoniazid, then ethambutol or streptomycin is added. If HIV infection is present, a longer course of treatment is often required.

Treatment failure is usually due to irregularity in taking medications, which can foster the development of drug-resistant strains. Nationwide, 15 percent of active TB cases are resistant to one medication, and 3 percent are resistant to two medications. Therefore, it is imperative that those who are treated take their full course of medication as prescribed. It is also important to be cautious when exposed to someone with active TB while they remain contagious.

Mononucleosis

Mononucleosis, also known as "the kissing disease" because it is transmitted by saliva exchange, is primarily a self-limited (one that does not need treatment and will go away on its own) infection of young adults. The majority of cases occur in the 15 to 30 age range. This disease is most frequently caused by the Epstein-Barr virus (EBV); however, other viruses including cytomegalovirus (CMV) and the bacterium *Toxoplasma gondii* have been implicated (McCance and Huether, 2005). The virus attacks lymphocytes (cells found in blood and lymph tissues), which causes proliferation of cells in the immune system. This results in swelling of the lymph nodes, which is a prominent feature of this illness. After infection, there is an incubation period of thirty to fifty days (McCance and Huether, 2005). Initially, there are mild symptoms of headache and fatigue. This is followed by fever, lymph node enlargement (primarily those in the neck), and sore throat, which is the most common symptom and can be quite severe.

Enlargement of the spleen (splenomegaly) can occur in up to one-half of affected individuals. Rarely, this enlargement leads to the rupture of the spleen, which can be a life-threatening medical emergency. Other rare but possible complications include meningitis, encephalitis, and Bell palsy (McCance and Huether, 2005). By far, however, the most common course is a self-limiting illness with sore throat, fatigue, and fever as the principal manifestations and recovery within a few weeks.

Diagnosis is made with a blood test called the monospot agglutination test, which is specific for infection with the Epstein-Barr virus. There is also an elevation of white blood cells with a relative increase in the percentage of lymphocytes and monocytes (types of white blood cells), as well as the presence of large, irregular shaped cells called atypical lymphocytes. Up to 95 percent of infected persons have elevated liver function tests as well.

Treatment is non-specific, including bed rest, adequate hydration, and non-aspirin analgesics for pain relief. Aspirin should be avoided due to an association with Reye's syndrome, a potentially serious complication. Sore throat pain can be decreased with saltwater gargle. Participation in contact sports should be avoided for up to one month after recovery to reduce the risk of spleen rupture. Fifteen to 20 percent of EBV antibody positive healthy adults become long-term carriers (Benenson, 1995).

Hepatitis

Hepatitis means "inflammation of the liver." There are various causes, such as alcohol or drug-induced inflammation; however, the most common cause of hepatitis is infection with a virus. At the current time, there are six types of viruses known to cause hepatitis (A, B, C, D, E, and G). Descriptions of hepatitis have been found by Hippocrates as far back as the fifth century B.C. The first recorded cases were believed to be transmitted by the smallpox vaccine contaminated with infected human lymph tissue given to German shipyard workers in 1883.

The liver is the largest internal organ, with a weight of approximately three pounds. Essential to life, the liver performs multiple important functions, one of which is to clear various substances from the blood. These include medications and potential toxins, either ingested (i.e., alcohol) or manufactured in the body (such as ammonia). The liver also manufactures proteins necessary for bodily functions and stores sugar, fats, and vitamins.

The course of hepatitis can vary from asymptomatic infection (which is completely cleared by the immune system and unknown to the infected person) to rapid liver failure and death, or a slower process with cirrhosis and/or liver cancer. In early hepatitis there is an inflammation of the liver due to the response of the immune system in an attempt to eradicate the virus. The damaged liver produces scar tissue as it attempts to heal itself, which can lead to cirrhosis (causing the liver to shrink and harden). This makes the liver unable to perform its life-sustaining functions. The individual who is chronically infected with hepatitis B or C is at a higher risk for the development of liver cancer. Unfortunately, chronic hepatitis is often asymptomatic until irreversible liver damage has occurred.

As mentioned previously, there are six known types of viral hepatitis. Hepatitis A, B, and C are the most common and will be covered in more depth (see Table 11.1), whereas hepatitis D, E, and G are not as common and will only be briefly discussed. Hepatitis A and B are more likely to cause symptoms, whereas the B and C types are more likely to contribute to long-term health problems.

Hepatitis A

Hepatitis A poses the least serious threat to the long-term health of infected individuals. Infection is almost always acute, and the virus is generally cleared from the body by the immune system within three to four months. There is very little risk of long-term liver damage. There are no chronic carriers of hepatitis A, as there are with B and C (Crowley, 2006).

Hepatitis A is transmitted by contact with food or water that has been contaminated with infected human waste or by direct person-to-person transmission in settings such as daycare centers or institutional settings (for instance, group homes for mentally retarded individuals), where there is frequent close contact among clients and caretakers. After exposure, the incubation period is four to six weeks (McCance and Huether, 2005). An infected person is contagious during the ten to fourteen days prior to symptoms and during the first week of symptoms. Antibodies develop four weeks after infection (McCance and Huether, 2005).

Table 11.1

Comparison of the Three Major Types of Viral Hepatitis

	Hepatitis A	Hepatitis B	Hepatitis C
Type of virus	RNA	DNA	RNA
Incubation period	2–6 weeks	6 weeks–4 months	3–12 weeks
Method of transmission	Fecal–oral: contaminated food or water	Blood or body fluids	Blood or body fluids
Prevention	Good hygiene and proper sanitation	Use condom if sexually active; do not share razors or toothbrushes; consider the risks if you are thinking about getting a tattoo or body piercing; do not share needles or reuse	Same as hepatitis B
Antigen-antibody test results	anti-HAV (confers immunity)	Infected persons are HbsAg positive and lack anti-HBs Immune persons lack HbsAg and have anti-HBs	HCV RNA in blood indicates virus in blood and active infection Anti-HCV denotes infection (does not confer immunity)
Signs & symptoms	Jaundice, fatigue, abdominal pain, loss of appetite, nausea, diarrhea, and fever	30 percent have no signs or symptoms Same as A and vomiting and joint pain	80 percent have no signs or symptoms Same as A and dark urine
Complications	No carriers or chronic liver disease	10 percent become chronic carriers and may develop chronic liver disease	70 percent become carriers and many develop chronic liver disease
Treatment	Treatment of the symptoms	Adeforir dipivoxil, alpha interferon, lamivudine, and entecavir	Interferon and ribavirin
Immunization available	Yes (age 2 and older)	Yes	No

Source: CDC, 2005. www.cdc.gov/hepatitis

There may be no symptoms at all, but more commonly there is a "flu-like" syndrome with fatigue, nausea, vomiting, and upper right side abdominal pain. The course of illness varies from mild symptoms lasting one to two weeks to severe symptoms that last for several months, although severe prolonged illness is rare. Less often an infected person may experience fever, darkening of the urine, and light-colored stools. Those at higher risk for contracting hepatitis A are household or sexual contacts of infected individuals, children in day care settings and their adult caretaker, patients and caretakers in institutionalized settings, as well as recent travelers to developing countries.

Diagnosis is made by testing the blood and finding elevated liver enzymes and detecting antibodies against hepatitis A. There is no specific treatment other than symptomatic, such as giving analgesics for pain and intravenous fluids in the presence of excessive vomiting to prevent dehydration. Alcohol consumption should be avoided to reduce the risk of liver damage.

A vaccine is available for this disease. The CDC recommends that persons who plan to travel to a country with poor sanitation be vaccinated approximately one month prior to travel, and repeated every four to six months if exposure continues.

Prevention consists of proper sanitation, including careful hand washing, proper sewage disposal, and effective water treatment present in developed countries. Close contacts of infected persons can help prevent infection if given immune globulin (concentrated antibodies) within two weeks of exposure (Benenson, 1995).

Hepatitis B

See Chapter 8 for more information on hepatitis B.

Hepatitis C

Hepatitis C is the most serious viral hepatitis to date, as mentioned earlier, affecting 3,200,000 Americans. There are 19,000 new cases per year in the United States (CDC, 2006) www.cdc.gov/hepatitis/statistics.htm. The disease was contracted through blood transfusions given prior to 1992 (prior to the development of techniques to detect the presence of the virus in donor blood). IV drug abuse is an

FIGURE 11.1 Ways in Which Hepatitis A, B, and C Are Contracted

■ Frequent　　▲ Common　　● Uncommon/Rare

Source of Infection	Form of Hepatitis		
	A	B	C
Food/water	■	●	▲
Household contact	■	●	●
Needlestick injuries		▲	●
IV drug use (shared needles)	●	▲	■
Transfusions	●	■	■
Hemodialysis		▲	▲
Vaginal intercourse		■	●
Anal/oral sex	■	■	●
Mother to child at birth		■	●
Body piercing/tatooing (contaminated needles)		●	●
Within certain institutions			
Day care		▲	●
Prison		●	▲	■
Organ transplant		●	●
Occupational exposure (e.g., medical workers)		●	▲

Source: American Liver Foundation, "Getting Hip to Hep: What You Should Know about Hepatitis A, B, and C," 2002. www.liverfoundation.org (75 Maiden Lane, Suite 603, New York, NY 10038, 1–800–GO–LIVER).

important risk factor for transmission of this virus; hepatitis C transmission is very similar to that of the hepatitis B virus. The incubation period is six to eight weeks (McCance and Huether, 2005) and antibodies may not appear for several months.

Most individuals who contract the virus have no symptoms. Some will have the typical "flu-like" symptoms discussed in the previous section. Seventy-five to eighty-five percent of those infected will develop a chronic infection (www.cdc.gov/hepatitis/Resources/Professionals/PDFs/ABCTable.pdf), which, if untreated, places the infected person at a high risk of cirrhosis, liver failure, and liver cancer.

Diagnosis is made by testing liver enzyme levels and for the presence of hepatitis C antibodies, which indicates exposure, but does not ascertain whether the infection is current. The hepatitis C virus RNA test detects the presence of the virus in the blood.

If the infection continues beyond six months, medical treatment may be begun to decrease the risk of liver damage. Interferon and ribavirin are given for six to twelve months and are effective in approximately 40 to 80 percent of cases (www.cdc.gov/hepatitis/HCV/HCVfac.htm#section4). Hepatitis C virus is eliminated with this treatment in a number of patients.

There is currently no vaccine available for hepatitis C. There is some evidence that treatment with immune globulin may prevent infection after exposure.

Hepatitis D, E, and G

Hepatitis D is a viral parasite, or incomplete virus, which is active only in the presence of a coexistent hepatitis B infection. Hepatitis E is spread through contaminated food and water, much like hepatitis A, but is not seen in the United States. Hepatitis G has been recently identified, and there will likely be additional types characterized in future years.

After infection, individuals can become contagious to others in as little as two weeks. As individuals with hepatitis are often without symptoms, it is important to be tested if exposed to the viruses. The diseases can only be correctly identified with blood tests.

A diagnosis of hepatitis is, of course, alarming. However, with advances in treatment, there can be optimism for recovery, particularly if treatment is begun early in the course of the illness. Responsibility for one's health in following through with testing and receiving treatment can reduce the menace posed to public health by these illnesses. It is also important that responsible action be taken in one's conduct with others, either with self-protection to prevent acquiring the disease or taking measures to protect the health of one's friends and family members with the precautions discussed previously.

Meningitis

Meningitis is an inflammation of the membranes that cover the spinal cord and the brain. Meningitis is usually caused by a viral (the most common type) or bacterial infection. It is important to determine which type of infection is causing the meningitis. If the meningitis is from a viral source, typically it will be less severe and resolve on its own. The best course of action if you have contracted viral (aseptic) meningitis is bed rest, drink plenty of fluids, and take medicine to relieve fever and headaches. If the meningitis is from a bacterial source, it can result in blindness, deafness, permanent brain damage, learning disability, or even death. Most often bacterial meningitis can be treated successfully with antibiotics if caught early. Many times these individuals need to be hospitalized to receive intravenous antibiotics and to be watched closely. Some of the classic symptoms associated with all types of meningitis in anyone over the age of 2 years include high fever, severe headache, a stiff neck, and a skin rash that looks like small, purplish red spots. Other

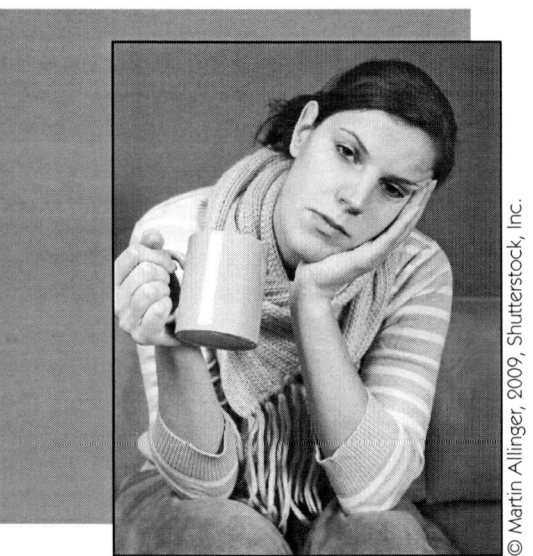

Some of the classic symptoms associated with meningitis include high fever, severe headache, stiff neck, and a skin rash.

symptoms might include nausea, vomiting, discomfort looking into bright lights, confusion, and sleepiness. After close exposure to someone with meningitis, symptoms can take anywhere from two to ten days to develop, with the average being three to four days. Some of the classic symptoms listed above may be absent in individuals under the age of 2. The main symptoms to look for in newborns and small infants include: appearing slow or inactive, irritability, vomiting, loss of appetite, or not easily wakened.

Diagnosis of meningitis is typically done with a sample of spinal fluid. The spinal fluid is obtained by performing a spinal tap, in which a needle is inserted into an area in the lower back where fluid in the spinal canal is readily accessible. Then a culture is grown from the fluid to determine which type (viral or bacterial) of infection is causing the meningitis.

Meningitis is spread by direct contact through respiratory and throat secretions (for instance, coughing, sneezing, kissing, and immediate sharing of unwashed eating utensils). Fortunately, none of the bacteria that cause meningitis are as contagious as the viruses of the common cold or flu. Meningitis is not spread by casual contact or by simply breathing the air where a person with meningitis has been (www.cdc.gov/meningitis/bacterial/faqs.htm#contagious). There should be special concern if someone in your household or dorm, daycare, or intimate partner has contracted meningitis. In some cases a prophylactic course of antibiotics will be given to lessen the chances of contracting the illness. If an epidemic is occurring, a widespread use of vaccines may be enacted. It is important to realize that in most cases it takes the vaccine two weeks to become protective. So, it is not helpful for treatment of individuals who have already been in contact with an individual infected with meningitis.

The best ways to decrease infection rates include:

1. Covering your nose and mouth when sneezing or coughing,
2. Frequent hand washing,
3. Not sharing common eating utensils,
4. Avoiding overcrowded conditions.

The CDC recommends that college freshman living in dormitories be immunized against the meningococcal disease to reduce the risk of infection.

Common Cold

The common cold is caused by several different viruses that are spread by droplets from sneezing or coughing, or touching surfaces where the virus is present such as hands, money, or door handles. Symptoms include congestion, sneezing, sore throat, coughing, and a low-grade fever (see Table 11.2). There is no treatment for the common cold; however, the symptoms can be treated to help the infected individual feel more comfortable until the virus has run its course. Gargle with saltwater at the onset to relieve symptoms and possibly reduce the severity of the illness.

Table 11.2
Is It a Cold or the Flu?

Symptoms	Cold	Flu
Fever	Rare	Characteristic, high (102–104°F); lasts 3–4 days
Headache	Rare	Prominent
General Aches, Pains	Slight	Usual; often severe
Fatigue, Weakness	Quite mild	Can last up to 2–3 weeks
Extreme Exhaustion	Never	Early and prominent
Stuffy Nose	Common	Sometimes
Sneezing	Usual	Sometimes
Sore Throat	Common	Sometimes
Chest Discomfort, Cough	Mild to moderate; hacking cough	Common; can become severe
COMPLICATIONS	Sinus congestion or earache	Bronchitis, pneumonia; can be life-threatening
PREVENTION	None	Annual vaccination; antiviral medicines–see your doctor
TREATMENT	Only temporary relief of symptoms	Antiviral medicines–see your doctor

Source: From the National Institute of Allergy and Infectious Diseases, www.niaid.nih.gov Nov 2008

Influenza

Influenza (flu) is a viral infection of the nose, throat, bronchial tubes, and lungs. The flu is spread in a similar manner as the common cold. Symptoms include high fever, chills, headache, muscle and joint ache, coughing, and fatigue (see Table 11.2). As with the common cold, there is no treatment for the flu; however, medication can be taken to ease the symptoms.

The following reduce the risk of contracting colds and/or flu:

- Wash hands often.
- Keep hands away from your eyes, nose, and mouth.
- Drink at least eight glasses of water a day.
- Get enough rest (six to eight hours a day).
- Use Kleenex instead of handkerchiefs.
- Get enough vitamin C.
- Receive a flu shot.

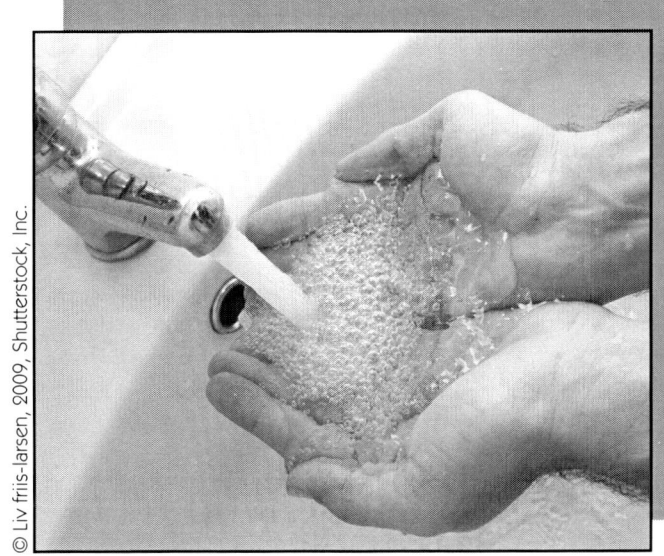

Reduce the risk of contracting a cold or the flu by washing your hands often.

Non-Communicable Diseases

Non-communicable diseases are not transmitted person to person. These diseases can develop from many sources, some of which include genetic predisposition, behaviors such as excessive sun exposure, smoking, unhealthy eating habits, and/or lack of exercise.

Cancer

Cancer is characterized by the spread of abnormal cells that serve no useful purpose. Tumors can be either benign, having a slow and expanding type of growth rate, remaining localized, and being well differentiated; or malignant, growing rapidly, infiltrating (crowding out and replacing normal cells), metastasizing (spreading to other parts of the body via the circulatory or lymphatic system) and being poorly differentiated. There are four classifications of cancers according to the type of cell and organ of origination:

1. *Carcinoma* cancers originate in epithelium (layers of cells that cover the body and line organs and glands). These are the most common.
2. *Sarcomas* begin in the supporting or connective tissues including bones, muscles, and blood vessels.
3. *Leukemias* arise in the blood-forming tissues of bone marrow and spleen.
4. *Lymphomas* form in the lymphatic system.

Risk factors include a family history, race and culture, viruses, environmental and occupational hazards, cigarette smoking, alcohol consumption, poor dietary habits, and psychological factors that compromise the immune system. Heredity or family history is thought to account for 10 percent of all cancers with the most likely sites for inherited cancers involving the breast, brain, blood, muscles, bones, and adrenal gland (see Figure 11.2). Research has revealed a variety of internal and external agents that are believed to cause cancer. These agents are termed carcinogens and include occupational pollutants (nickel, chromate, and asbestos), chemicals in food and water, certain viruses, and radiation (including the sun).
The seven warning signs of cancer are:

1. Change in bowel or bladder habits,
2. A sore that does not heal,
3. Unusual bleeding or discharge,
4. Thickening or lump in the breast, testes, or elsewhere,
5. Indigestion or difficulty swallowing,
6. Obvious change in a wart or mole,
7. Nagging cough or hoarseness.

Be certain to contact a physician if you experience any of these signs.

With any cancer, early detection is the key to treatment and survival. A common misconception is that cancer is a death sentence. However, the forms of cancer with the highest incidence and mortality rates are those directly related to lifestyle factors that can be changed or eliminated (see Table 11.3). Due to dramatic improvements in diagnosis and treatment, more cancer patients are being cured and their quality of life is greatly improved (see Tables 11.4 and 11.5 on page 399). Treatment usually involves one or the combination of the following procedures:

- *Surgery*—removal of the tumor and surrounding tissue
- *Radiation*—X-rays that are aimed at the tumor to destroy or stop the growth

FIGURE 11.2

Leading Sites of New Cancer Cases and Deaths—2007 Estimates

Estimated New Cases*		Estimated Deaths	
Male	**Female**	**Male**	**Female**
Prostate 218,890 (29%)	Breast 178,480 (26%)	Lung & bronchus 89,510 (31%)	Lung & bronchus 70,880 (26%)
Lung & bronchus 114,760 (15%)	Lung & bronchus 98,620 (15%)	Prostate 27,050 (9%)	Breast 40,460 (15%)
Colon & rectum 79,130 (10%)	Colon & rectum 74,630 (11%)	Colon & rectum 26,000 (9%)	Colon & rectum 26,180 (10%)
Urinary bladder 50,040 (7%)	Uterine corpus 39,080 (6%)	Pancreas 16,840 (6%)	Pancreas 16,530 (6%)
Non-Hodgkin lymphoma 34,200 (4%)	Non-Hodgkin lymphoma 28,990 (4%)	Leukemia 12,320 (4%)	Ovary 15,280 (6%)
Melanoma of the skin 33,910 (4%)	Melanoma of the skin 26,030 (4%)	Liver & intrahepatic bile duct 11,280 (4%)	Leukemia 9,470 (4%)
Kidney & renal pelvis 31,590 (4%)	Thyroid 25,480 (4%)	Esophagus 10,900 (4%)	Non-Hodgkin lymphoma 9,060 (3%)
Leukemia 24,800 (3%)	Ovary 22,430 (3%)	Urinary bladder 9,630 (3%)	Uterine corpus 7,400 (3%)
Oral cavity & pharynx 24,180 (3%)	Kidney & renal pelvis 19,600 (3%)	Non-Hodgkin lymphoma 9,600 (3%)	Brain & other nervous system 5,590 (2%)
Pancreas 18,830 (2%)	Leukemia 19,440 (3%)	Kidney & renal pelvis 8,080 (3%)	Liver & intrahepatic bile duct 5,500 (2%)
All sites 766,860 (100%)	All sites 678,060 (100%)	All sites 289,550 (100%)	All sites 270,100 (100%)

*Excludes basal and squamous cell skin cancers and in situ carcinoma except urinary bladder.
Source: American Cancer Society. *Cancer Facts and Figures 2008*. Atlanta: American Cancer Society, Inc. Used with permission.

- ■ *Chemotherapy*—an intravenous administration of fifty or more drugs combined to kill the cancerous cells
- ■ *Immunotherapy*—activating the body's own immune system with interferon injections to fight the cancerous cells

Eighty to 90 percent of all cancers are thought to be caused by environmental factors that could be prevented by either avoiding certain substances or using protective substances or devices. Healthy lifestyle practices such as not smoking [30 percent of all cancer deaths are attributed to smoking (Donatelle, 2006); those smoking two or more packs a day are fifteen to twenty-five times more likely to die of cancer than nonsmokers (Hales, 2006)], exercising regularly, and avoiding sun exposure are simple yet essential ways to decrease your risk of cancer. A diet low in fat (less than 30 percent of total calories) but high in fruits, vegetables (at least five servings per day),

Table 11.3
Preventing Cancer through Diet and Lifestyle

Type	Decreases Risk	Increases Risk	Preventable by Diet
Lung	Vegetables, fruits	Smoking; some occupations	33–50%
Stomach	Vegetables, fruits; food refrigeration	Salt and salted food	66–75%
Breast	Vegetables, fruits	Obesity; alcohol	33–50%
Colon/rectum	Vegetables; physical activity	Meat; alcohol; smoking	66–75%
Mouth/throat	Vegetables, fruits; physical activity	Salted fish; alcohol; smoking	33–50%
Liver	Vegetables	Alcohol; contaminated food	33–66%
Cervix	Vegetables, fruits	Smoking	10–20%
Esophagus	Vegetables, fruits	Deficient diet; smoking; alcohol	50–75%
Prostate	Vegetables	Meat or meat fat; dairy fat	10–20%
Bladder	Vegetables, fruits	Smoking; coffee	10–20%

Here are some tips issued by a panel of cancer researchers:
- Avoid being underweight or overweight, and limit weight gain during adulthood to less than eleven pounds.
- If you don't get much exercise at work, take a one-hour brisk walk or similar exercise daily, and exercise vigorously for at least one hour a week.
- Eat eight or more servings a day of cereals and grains (such as rice, corn, breads, and pasta), legumes (such as peas), roots (such as beets, radishes, and carrots), tubers (such as potatoes), and plantains (including bananas).
- Eat five or more servings a day of a variety of other vegetables and fruits.
- Limit consumption of refined sugar.
- Limit alcoholic drinks to less than two a day for men and one a day for women.
- Limit intake of red meat to less than three ounces a day, if eaten at all.
- Limit consumption of salted foods and use of cooking and table salt. Use herbs and spices to season foods.

Sources: World Cancer Research Fund; American Institute for Cancer Research, 2003.

and whole grains are the best nutritionally for reducing cancer risk. Avoid smoke-filled areas. Secondhand or environmental tobacco smoke (ETS) can increase the risk among nonsmokers. Researchers have found the risk of cancer to increase threefold with as little as three hours of exposure per day. Avoid environmental carcinogens whenever possible. Follow safety precautions if employed in or living near factories that create smoke or dust.

Skin Cancer

Overexposure to the ultraviolet (UV) rays of the sun is the primary culprit in these cases. Ninety percent occur on parts of the body not usually covered with clothes, including the face, hands, forearms, and ears. The two most common types of skin cancers are basal cell carcinoma and squamous cell carcinoma (non-melanomas). Both are usually treated successfully with surgery, especially if detected early. Subsequent tumors are likely in persons previously treated for these types of cancer. The fatality rate for these cancers is less than 1 percent.

A less prevalent but much more serious type of skin cancer is malignant melanoma, and its incidence is rising 3 to 4 percent each year (Hales, 2006). This type of cancer affected approximately 62,000 and killed approximately 10,710 Americans in 2006 (Floyd, Mimms, and Yelding-Howard, 2007). Although the overall risk is 1 in 120, individuals with any of the following characteristics are at greater risk:

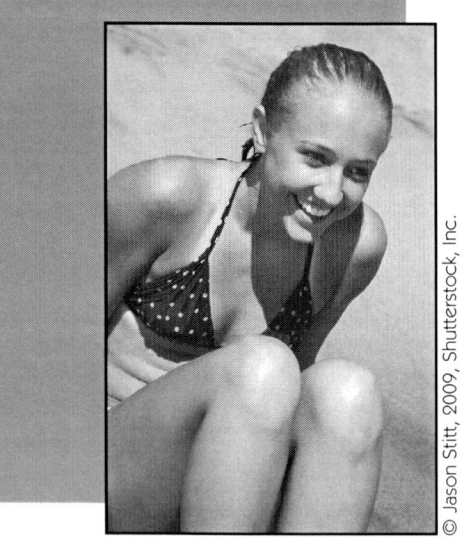

Overexposure to the UV rays of the sun is the primary cause of skin cancer.

Table 11.4
Five-Year Relative Survival Rates* by Stage at Diagnosis, 1992–1999

Site	All Stages %	Local %	Regional %	Distant %	Site	All Stages %	Local %	Regional %	Distant %
Breast (female)	86.6	97.0	78.7	23.3	Ovary	53.0	94.7	72.0	30.7
Colon & rectum	62.3	90.1	65.5	9.2	Pancreas	4.4	16.6	6.8	1.6
Esophagus	14.0	29.1	13.1	2.2	Prostate†	97.5	100.0	–	34.0
Kidney	62.6	89.9	60.0	9.1	Stomach	22.5	59.0	21.7	2.5
Larynx	64.7	82.6	47.9	20.0	Testis	95.5	99.1	95.0	73.1
Liver	6.9	16.3	6.0	1.9	Thyroid	95.8	99.3	95.5	59.9
Lung & bronchus	14.9	48.7	16.0	2.1	Urinary bladder	81.8	94.4	48.2	5.8
Melanoma	89.6	96.7	60.1	13.8	Uterine cervix	71.3	92.2	50.9	16.5
Oral cavity	57.2	82.1	47.9	26.1	Uterine corpus	84.4	96.2	64.7	26.0

*Rates are adjusted for normal life expectancy and are based on cases diagnosed from 1992–1999, followed through 2002. †The rate for local stage represents local and regional stages combined.

Local: An invasive malignant cancer confined entirely to the organ of origin. **Regional:** A malignant cancer that 1) has extended beyond the limits of the organ of origin directly into surrounding organs or tissues; 2) involves regional lymph nodes by way of lymphatic system; or 3) has both regional extension and involvement of regional lymph nodes. **Distant:** A malignant cancer that has spread to parts of the body remote from the primary tumor either by direct extension or by discontinuous metastasis to distant organ, tissues, or via the lymphatic system to distant lymph nodes.

Source: American Cancer Society. *Cancer Facts and Figures 2008.* Atlanta: American Cancer Society, Inc. Used with permission.

Table 11.5
Trends in Five-year Relative Survival (%)* Rates, US, 1975-2003

Site	1975-1977	1984-1986	1996-2003
All sites	50	54	66
Breast (female)	75	79	89
Colon	51	59	65
Leukemia	35	42	50
Lung and bronchus	13	13	16
Melanoma	82	87	92
Non-Hodgkin lymphoma	48	53	64
Ovary	37	40	45
Pancreas	2	3	5
Prostate	69	76	99
Rectum	49	57	66
Urinary bladder	74	78	81

*Five-year relative survival rates based on follow up of patients through 2004.

Source: American Cancer Society. *Cancer Facts and Figures 2008.* Atlanta: American Cancer Society, Inc. Used with permission.

How to Examine Your Skin

It's important to check your own skin, preferably once a month. Self-examination is best done in a well-lit room in front of a full-length mirror. A handheld mirror can be used for areas that are hard to see. A spouse or close friend or family member may be able to help you with these exams, especially for those hard-to-see areas like the lower back or the back of your thighs.

The first time you inspect your skin, spend a fair amount of time carefully going over the entire surface of your skin. Learn the pattern of moles, blemishes, freckles, and other marks on your skin so that you'll notice any changes. Any trouble spots should be seen by a doctor. Follow these step-by-step instructions to perform your skin self-exam:

1. Face the mirror:
Check your face, ears, neck, chest, and belly. Women will need to lift breasts to check the skin underneath.

Check both sides of your arms, the tops and palms of your hands, and your fingernail beds.

2. Sit Down:
You will need a hand mirror for your thighs, back, and scalp.

First checking one leg, then the other, now look at the bottoms of your feet, your calves, and the backs of your thighs.

3. What to Look For
Non-melanomas: The most common non-melanoma skin cancers are basal cell cancers and squamous cell cancers. Look for new growths, spots, bumps, patches, or sores that don't heal after two to three months.

Basal cell carcinomas often look like flat, firm, pale areas or small, raised, pink or red, translucent, shiny, waxy areas that may bleed following minor injury. They may have one or more irregular blood vessels, a lower area in their center, and/or blue, brown, or black areas. Large basal cell carcinomas may have oozing or crusted areas.

Squamous cell carcinomas may look like growing lumps, often with a rough, scaly, or crusted surface. They may also look like flat reddish patches in the skin that grow slowly. Squamous cell carcinoma is linked to too much exposure to the sun.

Both of these types of non-melanoma skin cancer may develop as a flat area, showing only slight changes from normal skin.

Actinic keratosis, also known as solar keratosis, is a precancerous skin condition caused by too much sun exposure. Actinic keratoses are small (usually less than 1/4 inch) rough spots that may be pink-red or flesh-colored. Usually they develop on the face, ears, back of the hands, and arms of middle-aged or older people with fair skin, although they can arise on other sun-exposed areas of the skin. People with one actinic keratosis usually develop many more. Some can grow into squamous cell cancers, but others may stay the same or even shrink. Because they can turn cancerous, such areas should be regularly examined by a doctor. The doctor can then decide whether these areas should be removed.

Melanomas: The "ABCD rule" is an easy guide to the usual signs of melanoma. Be on the look out and notify your doctor about any spots that match the following description:
- **A** is for **ASYMMETRY:** One half of a mole or birthmark does not match the other.
- **B** is for **BORDER:** The edges are irregular, ragged, notched, or blurred.
- **C** is for **COLOR:** The color is not the same all over and may include shades of brown or black, sometimes with patches of red, white, or blue.
- **D** is for **DIAMETER:** The spot is larger than 6 millimeters across (about 1/4 inch—the size of a pencil eraser) or is growing larger.

Other important signs of melanoma include changes in size, shape, or color of a mole or the appearance of a new spot. Some melanomas do not fit the ABCD rule described above, so it is particularly important for you to notice changes in skin markings or new spots on your skin.

Other warning signs are:
- A sore that does not heal
- A new growth
- Spread of pigment from the border of a spot to surrounding skin
- Redness or a new swelling beyond the border
- Change in sensation—itchiness, tenderness, or pain
- Change in the surface of a mole—scaliness, oozing, bleeding, or the appearance of a bump or nodule.

Source: Copyright © 2004. American Cancer Society, Inc. www.cancer.org. Reprinted with permission.

- Lighter natural skin color
- Blue or green eyes
- Blond or red hair
- Marked freckling on upper back
- Rough red bumps on the skin (actinic keratoses)
- Family history of melanoma
- Three or more blistering sunburns during the teenage years
- Three or more years at an outdoor summer job during the teenage years
- Living in the southern United States

A person's risk increases three to four times with one or two of the factors listed previously. With three or more, the risk is increased to twenty to twenty-five times (Marwick, 1995).

Occupational exposure to carcinogens and inherited skin disorders are risk factors as well. Malignant melanomas are highly curable if detected early; however, the chance of recurrence is high. To help prevent skin cancer: avoid the sun anytime your shadow is shorter than you are, cover up when in the sun (wear

Distinguishing Benign Moles from Melanoma

To prevent melanoma, it is important to examine your skin on a regular basis, and become familiar with moles and other skin conditions in order to better identify changes. According to recent research, certain moles are at a higher risk for changing into malignant melanoma. Moles that are present at birth, and atypical moles, have a greater chance of becoming malignant. Recognizing changes in your moles, by following this ABCD Chart, is crucial in detecting malignant melanoma at its earliest stage. The warning signs are:

Normal Mole/Melanoma	Sign	Characteristic
	Asymmetry	when half of the mole does not match the other half
	Border	when the border (edges) of the mole are ragged or irregular
	Color	when the color of the mole varies throughout
	Diameter	if the mole's diameter is larger than a pencil's eraser

Photographs used by permission: National Cancer Institute.

Melanomas vary greatly in appearance. Some melanomas may show all of the ABCD characteristics, while others may only show changes in one or two characteristics. Always consult your physician for a diagnosis.

wide-brimmed hats, long sleeves, and pants), use a sunscreen with a Sun Protection Factor (SPF) of at least 15; beware of cloudy days (when burning is still possible), water (the sun's rays can reach three feet deep), and snow (which reflects sunlight). Avoid use of tanning beds or sunlamps. "Tanning beds are potentially even more dangerous than the actual sun because of the concentrated effect of the bulbs. The concentrated UV radiation from the bulbs makes a few minutes in a tanning bed equal to several hours in the sun" (Spence, 1998). Observe your skin for changes in size, color, number, and thickness of moles, or pigmented growths, spots, or changes in birthmarks.

Monthly skin self-exam (SSE) can reveal cancerous changes at an early stage. Use a systematic approach. During this exam, look for abnormal growth of cells.

If you notice any of these warning signs see your physician immediately.

Lung Cancer

Lung cancer is the number one cause of cancer deaths in the United States (American Cancer Society, 2004). The major cause of lung cancer is cigarette smoking, accounting for 85 percent of all lung cancer deaths, making it one of the most preventable forms of cancer. Smoking cessation decreases the death rate of lung cancer in half. Other risk factors include asbestos exposure, secondhand smoke, radiation exposure, and radon exposure. Early detection of lung cancer is difficult, resulting in only 15 percent of cases being discovered early. With early detection, there is a 43 percent chance of surviving twelve months; however, the overall five-year relative survival rate is only 16 percent. Symptoms include a nagging or persistent cough, blood in the sputum, chest pain, shortness of breath, recurring bronchitis or pneumonia, weight loss, loss of appetite, and/or anemia.

Breast Cancer

One in eight women will develop breast cancer in her lifetime (American Cancer Society, 2008). Risk factors include: age 40 years or older (see Table 11.6), family history or personal history of breast cancer, early onset of menstruation (before age 12), having no children, having a first child at a late age (after age 30), late menopause (after age 55), exposure to radiation, obesity, and certain types of benign breast disease (premenopausal women). Early detection is the best way to reduce the mortality rate among breast cancer patients. It is recommended by the American Cancer Society that women 20 years of age and older perform a breast self-examination once a month. Any persistent lumps, swelling, thickening or distortion of the breast, pain or tenderness of the nipple, or discharge of blood or fluid from the nipple should be reported immediately. A diagnostic X-ray, called a mammogram, can detect a tumor two or three years before it can be detected by a self-exam. The American Cancer Society recommends all women begin routine mammograms by the age of 40, and physicians recommend that women at high risk (with a family history) have mammograms every six to twelve months beginning between the ages of 25 and 35 (see Table 11.7). With early diagnosis and a localized tumor, there is an 89 percent chance of surviving five years.

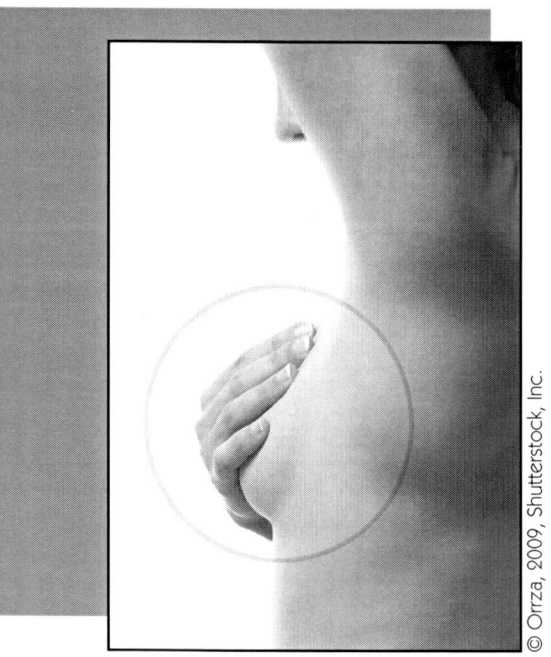

A monthly breast self-exam helps women detect changes in the breast tissue.

Breast self-exam (BSE) is a method utilized in an effort to promptly detect lumps located in the breast. Early detection increases survival. During this exam, one looks for masses within the soft tissue of the breast or changes in the breast appearance. Due to the varying texture, size, and sensitivity of

Table 11.6
Probability of Developing Invasive Cancers Over Selected Age Intervals by Sex, US, 2002-2004*

		Birth to 39 (%)	40 to 59 (%)	60 to 69 (%)	70 and Older (%)	Birth to Death (%)
All sites†	Male	1.42 (1 in 70)	8.58 (1 in 12)	16.25 (1 in 6)	38.96 (1 in 3)	44.94 (1 in 2)
	Female	2.04 (1 in 49)	8.97 (1 in 11)	10.36 (1 in 10)	26.31 (1 in 4)	37.52 (1 in 3)
Urinary bladder ‡	Male	0.02 (1 in 4,477)	0.41 (1 in 244)	0.96 (1 in 104)	3.50 (1 in 29)	3.70 (1 in 27)
	Female	0.01 (1 in 9,462)	0.13 (1 in 790)	0.26 (1 in 384)	0.99 (1 in 101)	1.17 (1 in 85)
Breast	Female	0.48 (1 in 210)	3.86 (1 in 26)	3.51 (1 in 28)	6.95 (1 in 15)	12.28 (1 in 8)
Colon & rectum	Male	0.08 (1 in 1,329)	0.92 (1 in 109)	1.60 (1 in 63)	4.78 (1 in 21)	5.65 (1 in 18)
	Female	0.07 (1 in 1,394)	0.72 (1 in 138)	1.12 (1 in 89)	4.30 (1 in 23)	5.23 (1 in 19)
Leukemia	Male	0.16 (1 in 624)	0.21 (1 in 468)	0.35 (1 in 288)	1.18 (1 in 85)	1.50 (1 in 67)
	Female	0.12 (1 in 837)	0.14 (1 in 705)	0.20 (1 in 496)	0.76 (1 in 131)	1.06 (1 in 95)
Lung & bronchus	Male	0.03 (1 in 3,357)	1.03 (1 in 97)	2.52 (1 in 40)	6.74 (1 in 15)	7.91 (1 in 13)
	Female	0.03 (1 in 2,964)	0.82 (1 in 121)	1.81 (1 in 55)	4.61 (1 in 22)	6.18 (1 in 16)
Melanoma of the skin	Male	0.15 (1 in 656)	0.61 (1 in 164)	0.66 (1 in 151)	1.56 (1 in 64)	2.42 (1 in 41)
	Female	0.26 (1 in 389)	0.50 (1 in 200)	0.34 (1 in 297)	0.71 (1 in 140)	1.63 (1 in 61)
Non-Hodgkin lymphoma	Male	0.13 (1 in 760)	0.45 (1 in 222)	0.57 (1 in 174)	1.61 (1 in 62)	2.19 (1 in 46)
	Female	0.08 (1 in 1,212)	0.32 (1 in 312)	0.45 (1 in 221)	1.33 (1 in 75)	1.87 (1 in 53)
Prostate	Male	0.01 (1 in 10,553)	2.54 (1 in 39)	6.83 (1 in 15)	13.36 (1 in 7)	16.72 (1 in 6)
Uterine cervix	Female	0.16 (1 in 638)	0.28 (1 in 359)	0.13 (1 in 750)	0.19 (1 in 523)	0.70 (1 in 142)
Uterine corpus	Female	0.06 (1 in 1,569)	0.71 (1 in 142)	0.79 (1 in 126)	1.23 (1 in 81)	2.45 (1 in 41)

*For people free of cancer at beginning of age interval. † All sites exclude basal and squamous cell skin cancers and in situ cancers except urinary bladder. ‡ Includes invasive and in situ cancer cases.

Source: American Cancer Society. *Cancer Facts and Figures 2008*. Atlanta: American Cancer Society, Inc. Used with permission.

Table 11.7
Recommended Breast Exam Schedule

Procedure	Risk	Age	Frequency
Breast Self-Exam (BSE)	Average	20 & Over	Once a Month
	High*	20 & Over	Once a Month
Clinical Breast Examination (CBE)	Average	20 to 39	Every 3 Years
	Average	40 & Over	Every Year
	High*	20 to 39	Every Year
Mammography	Average	40 & Over	Once a Year
	High*	Begin between 25 & 35	Once Every 6-12 Months

*Personal history of breast cancer or family history of premenopausal breast cancer in mother or sister.

one's breast, it is important to do the self-exam at the same time each month. The following is a guideline to determine the proper timing:

- *Women with menstrual cycles*—one week after the beginning of the menstrual period when the breasts are usually not tender
- *After menopause or hysterectomy*—choose a day that is easy to remember, such as the first day of the month.

How to Examine Your Breasts

- Lie down and place your right arm behind your head. The exam is done while lying down, and not standing up, because when lying down the breast tissue spreads evenly over the chest wall and it is as thin as possible, making it much easier to feel all the breast tissue.
- Use the finger pads of the three middle fingers on your left hand to feel for lumps in the right breast. Use overlapping dime-sized circular motions of the finger pads to feel the breast tissue.
- Use three different levels of pressure to feel all the breast tissue. Light pressure is needed to feel the tissue closest to the skin; medium pressure to feel a little deeper; and firm pressure to feel the tissue closest to the chest and ribs. A firm ridge in the lower curve of each breast is normal. If you're not sure how hard to press, talk with your doctor or nurse. Use each pressure level to feel the breast tissue before moving on to the next spot.
- Move around the breast in an up and down pattern starting at an imaginary line drawn straight down your side from the underarm and moving across the breast to the middle of the chest bone (sternum or breastbone). Be sure to check the entire breast area going down until you feel only ribs and up to the neck or collar bone (clavicle).
- There is some evidence to suggest that the up and down pattern (sometimes called the vertical pattern) is the most effective pattern for covering the entire breast and not missing any breast tissue.
- Repeat the exam on your left breast, using the finger pads of the right hand. While standing in front of a mirror with your hands pressing firmly down on your hips, look at your breasts for any changes of size, shape, contour, or dimpling. (The pressing down on the hips position contracts the chest wall muscles and enhances any breast changes.)
- Examine each underarm while sitting up or standing and with your arm only slightly raised so you can easily feel in this area. Raising your arm straight up tightens the tissue in this area and makes it very difficult to examine.
- This procedure for doing breast self-exam is different than previous procedure recommendations. These changes represent an extensive review of the medical literature and input from an expert advisory group. There is evidence that the woman's position (lying down), area felt, pattern of coverage of the breast, and use of different amounts of pressure increase the sensitivity of BSE as measured with silicon models, and for CBE using patient models with known small non cancerous lumps in their breasts.

Source: American Cancer Society. *Cancer Facts and Figures 2008.* Atlanta: American Cancer Society, Inc. Used with permission.

Cervical Cancer

Cervical cancer is representative of abnormal growth and maturation of the cervical squamous epithelium. Typically there are no symptoms in the early stages (see Figure 11.3). Eventually individuals with cervical cancer will have uterine bleeding, cramps, infections, and pain in the abdominal region. Risk factors include: first vaginal intercourse at an early age, multiple sexual partners, cigarette smoking, and infections with certain types of human papilloma viruses. See information on the Gardasil vaccine in chapter 8. The Pap smear is a screening test a physician

FIGURE 11.3

Screening Guidelines for the Early Detection of Cancer in Asymptomatic People

Site	Recommendations
Breast	• Yearly mammograms are recommended starting at age 40 and continuing for as long as a woman is in good health. • Clinical breast exam should be part of a periodic health exam, about every three years for women in their 20s and 30s, and every year for women 40 and older. • Women should know how their breasts normally feel and report any breast change promptly to their health care providers. Breast self-exam is an option for women starting in their 20s. • Women at increased risk (family history, genetic tendency, past breast cancer) should talk with their doctors about the benefits and limitations of starting mammography screening earlier, having additional tests (breast ultrasound and MRI), or having more frequent exams.
Colon and rectum	Beginning at age 50, men and women should follow one of the examination schedules below: • A fecal occult blood test (FOBT) every year • A flexible sigmoidoscopy (FSIG) every five years • Annual fecal occult blood test and flexible sigmoidoscopy every five years* • A double-contrast barium enema every five years • A colonoscopy every ten years *Combined testing is preferred over either annual FOBT, or FSIG every five years, alone. People who are at moderate or high risk for colorectal cancer should talk with a doctor about a different testing schedule.*
Prostate	The PSA test and the digital rectal examination should be offered annually, beginning at age 50, to men who have a life expectancy of at least ten years. Men at high risk (African American men and men with a strong family history of one or more first-degree relatives diagnosed with prostate cancer at an early age) should begin testing at age 45. For both men at average risk and high risk, information should be provided about what is known and what is uncertain about the benefits and limitations of early detection and treatment of prostate cancer so that they can make an informed decision about testing.
Uterus	**Cervix:** Screening should begin approximately three years after a woman begins having vaginal intercourse, but no later than 21 years of age. Screening should be done every year with regular Pap tests or every two years using liquid-based tests. At or after age 30, women who have had three normal test results in a row may get screened every two to three years. However, doctors may suggest a woman get screened more often if she has certain risk factors, such as HIV infection or weak immune system. Women 70 years and older who have had three or more consecutive normal Pap tests in the last ten years may choose to stop cervical cancer screening. Screening after total hysterectomy (with removal of the cervix) is not necessary unless the surgery was done as a treatment for cervical cancer. **Endometrium:** The American Cancer Society recommends that all women should be informed about the risks and symptoms of endometrial cancer, and strongly encouraged to report any unexpected bleeding or spotting to their physicians. Annual screening for endometrial cancer with endometrial biopsy beginning at age 35 should be offered to women with or at risk for hereditary nonpolyposis colon cancer (HNPCC).
Cancer-related checkup	For individuals undergoing periodic health examinations, a cancer-related checkup should include health counseling, and depending on a person's age, might include examinations for cancers of the thyroid, oral cavity, skin, lymph nodes, testes, and ovaries, as well as for some nonmalignant diseases.

American Cancer Society guidelines for early cancer detection are assessed annually in order to identify whether there is new scientific evidence sufficient to warrant a re-evaluation of current recommendations. If evidence is sufficiently compelling to consider a change or clarification in a current guideline or the development of a new guideline, a formal procedure is initiated. Guidelines are formally evaluated every five years regardless of whether new evidence suggests a change in the existing recommendations. There are nine steps in this procedure, and these "guidelines for guideline development" were formally established to provide a specific methodology for science and expert judgment to form the underpinnings of specific statements and recommendations from the Society. These procedures constitute a deliberate process to insure that all Society recommendations have the same methodological and evidence-based process at their core. This process also employs a system for rating strength and consistency of evidence that is similar to that employed by the Agency for Health Care Research and Quality (AHCRQ) and the US Preventive Services Task Force (USPSTF).

Source: American Cancer Society. *Cancer Facts and Figures 2008.* Atlanta: American Cancer Society, Inc. Used with permission.

performs in order to check for pre-cancerous cells or early cancer of the cervix. The physician obtains a sampling of tissue from inside the cervix and sends the specimen to a lab to be analyzed. Due to early detection with the Pap smear, cancer of the cervix is rare and easily treated in women who have regular exams. It is recommended that all women begin Pap tests no later than three years after first intercourse or starting at age 21, whichever comes first. This procedure should continue until an individual reaches the age of 70, at which point the physician may recommend discontinuing Pap smears. The best time to schedule a Pap smear is fourteen days after the start of a period. Do not have intercourse for twenty-four hours or any substances in the vagina for forty-eight hours before the exam.

Testicular Cancer

Although testicular cancer accounts for only 3 percent of cancers of the male genitals and urinary tract, it is one of the most common cancers in young males, with the majority of cases identified between the ages of 20 and 54 (American Cancer Society, 2007) or www.cancer.org/docroot/CRI/Content/CRI_2_2_2x_What_Causes_Testicular_Cancer_41.asp?rnav=cri. Men with undescended testicles in childhood seem to be at greatest risk. Other risks may include: family history, inguinal hernia, testicular trauma, mumps orchitis, elevated testicular temperature, vasectomy, or exposure to electromagnetic fields. Testicular self-exams should be performed monthly to detect any enlargement or thickening of the testes. The cure rate if detected early is close to 80 percent.

How to Examine Your Genitals

1. **Roll each testicle between the thumbs and fingers of both hands.** A normal testicle is firm, smooth, egg-shaped, about 1-1/2 inches long. One testicle may be a little larger or hang lower in the scrotum. This is normal.
2. **Feel the epididymis behind the testicle on each side.** It should feel soft, rope-like and tender.
3. **Check the skin on your scrotum and penis for sores and little rough bumps.** These could be signs of STI, such as herpes, syphilis, or genital warts.
4. **If you are not circumcised, be sure you pull back the foreskin.** Check the glans and the inside of the foreskin.
5. **Look at the opening at the tip of the penis.** It should not be red or painful. A yellow or white discharge could be a sign of an STI.
6. **Feel your groin area on both sides** for any lumps or swollen glands.

It Isn't Normal:

- If you feel a lump or hard area in the testicle
- If the whole testicle feels harder than usual
- If one side of your scrotum is very swollen

These could be signs of cancer, even if there is no pain.

What if I Find Something?

Any lumps in your testicles or groin, any skin sores, bumps, or other changes in your genitals that do not seem normal should be checked right away by your health care provider.
Don't wait. Your health depends on getting care as soon as you can.

After age 50, every man should talk with his health
care provider about a prostate examination.

Testicular self-exam (TSE) can detect cancer in early stages when disease is more curable. Exams should begin at age 15. Self-examination should be performed every month in order to detect any changes. The best time to perform the exam is after taking a warm bath or shower when the skin of the scrotum is relaxed.

Colon and Rectum Cancers

Colon and rectum cancers are the third leading types of cancer in men and women, claiming about 60,000 lives a year (Hales, 2006). The majority of cases occur in men and women over the age of 50. Risk factors include a family or personal history of colorectal cancer or polyps (growths) and ulcerative colitis. High fat, low-fiber diets have also been shown to increase the risk. Symptoms include bleeding from the rectum, blood in the stool, or a change in bowel habits (recurring constipation or diarrhea). Digital rectal exams, stool blood tests, and proctoscopic exams can detect early stages of colorectal cancer. It is recommended that a digital rectal exam is performed annually after age 40, a stool blood test performed every year after age 50, and a proctosigmoidoscopy performed every three to five years after age 50. Regular exercise has been shown to reduce the risk in both men and women (Payne, Hahn, and Lucas, 2008). Hormone replacement therapy in postmenopausal women may significantly lower the risk of colon cancer.

Oral Cancers

Each year, more than 30,000 new cases of cancer of the oral cavity and pharynx are diagnosed and over 8,000 deaths due to oral cancer occur. The five-year survival rate for these cancers is only about 50 percent (CDC, 2007) www.cdc.gov/OralHealth/Topics/Cancer.htm. Oral cancer is related directly to a person's behavior. The major behavioral risk factors include cigarette, pipe, or cigar smoking, excessive alcohol use, and chewing tobacco use. Particularly vulnerable are persons who drink and smoke. Early symptoms include: a bleeding sore that will not heal, a lump or thickening, a red or white patch (lesion) that will not go away, a persistent sore throat, difficulty chewing, swallowing, or moving of the tongue or jaws. A cure is often achieved easily with early detection.

Asthma

Asthma is a respiratory disorder that involves difficulty breathing, wheezing, and/or coughing due to the constriction of the bronchial tubes. An individual will typically notice a wheezing sound when they are trying to breathe, while coughing and/or when experiencing difficulty breathing. In some cases those who suffer from asthma can stop an attack by simply removing themselves from an irritant such as cigarette smoke. Most of the time asthma attacks require some type of medical intervention, and, in rare cases, death can result from lack of treatment. Antihistamines, corticosteroids, and bronchodilating drugs are usually successful in reducing the bronchospasm. Reducing exposure to allergens, such as air pollution, pollen, dust, secondhand smoke, animal fur, bee venom, and specific foods, as well as non-allergens such as stress or intense exercise, can help prevent further asthma attacks. In the event that one must encounter an irritant, prescription drugs are available that help prevent asthma attacks. Some individuals are more likely to have difficulties with asthma: those with a family history, presence of atopy (the predisposition to respond to environmental allergens with specific IgE antibody production), and exposure to allergens, certain viral infections, and cigarette smoke. Children whose mothers smoke at least half a pack of cigarettes a day are twice as likely to have asthma as children of nonsmoking mothers (University of California, Berkley, 1990). More children than adults suffer from asthma, because many children outgrow this condition.

Diabetes

Diabetes is becoming more common in the United States. From 1980 through 2006, the number of Americans with diabetes has more than tripled (from 5.6 million to 16.8 million; see Figure 11.4) (CDC, 2008) www.cdc.gov/diabetes/Statistics/prev/national/figpersons.htm. Diabetes is the result of insufficient insulin production or the body's inability to utilize insulin readily produced by the pancreas. Insulin has two major functions: to move glucose from the blood to the cells of the body where it is used as energy and to convert excess glucose to glycogen, for storage as an energy reserve in the liver and the muscles for later use (Floyd et al., 2007). There are three types of diabetes, Type I, Type II, and gestational.

Type I or insulin-dependent diabetes is typically associated with childhood or adolescent onset. In this form of diabetes the pancreas does not produce insulin, and the individual requires regular injections. The signs and symptoms of Type I diabetes appear suddenly and dramatically. Symptoms include fatigue, irritability, abnormal hunger and thirst, frequent urination, and weight loss (Floyd et al., 2007). This type of diabetes is only seen in about 5 percent of all diabetics and is considered the more serious of the two forms.

FIGURE 11.4

Number (in Millions) of Persons with Diagnosed Diabetes, United States, 1980–2006

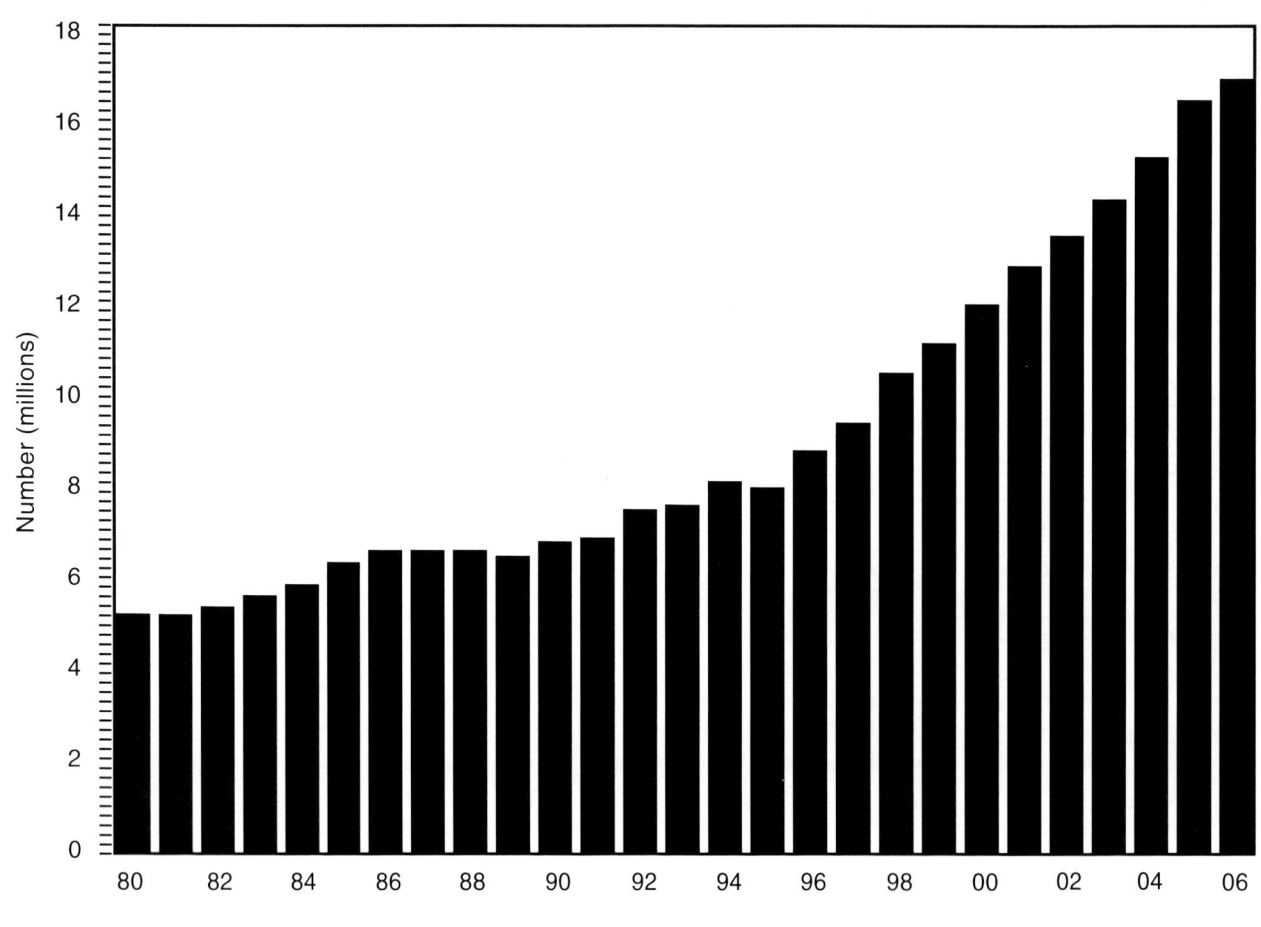

Source: www.cdc.gov.

Type II or non-insulin-dependent diabetes is typically associated with adult onset and obesity. In this form of the disease the pancreas produces insulin, but the cells of the body are not able to use it effectively. The onset of Type II diabetes is more gradual than Type I. Some symptoms include drowsiness, blurred vision, itching, slow healing of cuts, skin infections, and numbness of fingers or toes (Floyd et al., 2007).

Gestational diabetes is a form of glucose intolerance or insulin resistance that is typically diagnosed in some women late in pregnancy. This type of diabetes affects about 4 percent of all pregnant women in the United States each year (ADA, 2005) or www.diabetes.org/gestational-diabetes.jsp. Gestational diabetes can cause dangerously high blood sugar levels to occur in the pregnant female. This type of diabetes occurs more frequently among African Americans, Hispanic/Latino Americans, and Asians (Dabelea, Snell-Bergeon, Heartsfield, et al, 2005). (See also Figure 11.5) It is also more common among obese women and women with a family history of diabetes.

Gestational diabetes can be managed by eating healthy foods, exercising regularly, and in some cases, by taking medication to normalize maternal blood glucose levels to avoid complications in the mother and infant. Taking good care of yourself can help ensure a healthy pregnancy for you and a healthy start for your baby. After a pregnancy with gestational diabetes, 5 to 10 percent of women are found to have Type II diabetes. If a female has had gestational diabetes, there is a 66 percent chance that it will return in future pregnancies (www.diabetes.org/gestational-diabetes.jsp).

If an individual suffering from diabetes is not treated, the illness can progress into a diabetic coma. If too much insulin is taken or inadequate food is eaten, an insulin reaction may occur, which, if serious, can result in a seizure (convulsions).

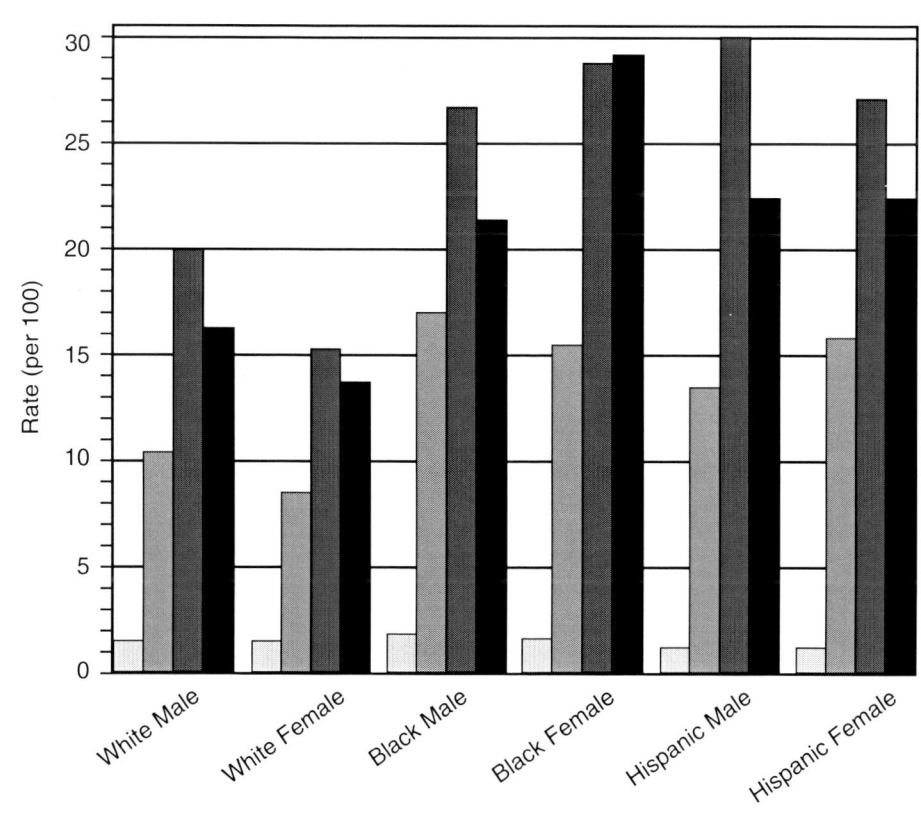

FIGURE 11.5

Age-Specific Prevalence of Diagnosed Diabetes, by Race/Ethnicity and Sex, United States, 2005

Source: www.cdc.gov.

From Head to Toe

Diabetes strikes nearly every part of the body. But studies show that treating diabetes aggressively can curb the damage.

BRAIN

People with diabetes are more likely to be diagnosed with dementia. Researchers don't know if the dementia is due to diabetes or to multiple mini-strokes (common in people with diabetes) that gradually impair mental function over time. If it's mini-strokes, lowering blood pressure might protect the brain.

HEART and BRAIN

The risk of heart attack or stroke is two to four times higher in people with diabetes.

Lowering high cholesterol can reduce heart attack and stroke by 20% to 50%.

Lowering high blood pressure can reduce the risk of heart attack and stroke by 33% to 50%.

FEET

Diabetes causes more than 60% of foot and leg amputations that are not caused by accidents.

Proper foot care (trim nails, check feet daily for red spots, cuts, swelling, blisters, etc.) can reduce the risk of amputation by 45% to 85%.

EYES

Diabetes is the leading cause of blindness among adults ages 20 to 74.

Every 1% reduction in A1C (from 8% to 7%, for example) lowers the risk of eye, kidney, and nerve disease by 40%.
Treating eye disease with laser therapy can reduce severe vision loss by 50% to 60%.

KIDNEYS

Diabetes is the leading cause of end-stage kidney disease.

Detecting early diabetic kidney disease (by testing urine for protein each year) and treating it can curb the loss of kidney function by 30% to 70%.

NERVES

An estimated six out of ten people with diabetes have nerve damage that can cause problems like numbness or pain in the feet or hands, carpal tunnel syndrome (in the wrist), and delayed digestion of food.

Lowering high blood pressure can reduce the risk of nerve, eye, and kidney damage by 33%.

Source: www.cdc.gov.

Image © clipart.com

Patients with diabetes have a higher incidence of arteriosclerosis and the associated complications such as strokes, heart attacks, and gangrene of the lower extremities due to poor circulation, as well as degenerative effects of the small blood vessels supplying oxygen to the retina of the eye, which can lead to blindness.

The goal for those who have this condition is to balance blood sugar levels. Normal blood sugar ranges from 70 to 110 mg/dL. This can be done with insulin regimens, a structured diet, and regular exercise. With Type I diabetes, the individual usually can achieve this by monitoring the blood glucose level and adjusting the amount of insulin injected each day. In Type II diabetes, this can be accomplished with a controlled diet and regular exercise alone; in some instances oral hypoglycemic medication or insulin is required as well. The risk of developing diabetes can be reduced with regular activity, which reduces body weight and fat levels, and increases insulin sensitivity and glucose tolerance. Healthy dietary habits also decrease the fat levels as well as obesity, therefore enhancing the body's ability to transport glucose into the muscles.

Approximately 8 percent of Americans have diabetes (www.diabetes.niddk.nih.gov/dm/pubs/statistics/index.htm#allages). Diabetes is the leading cause of blindness among adults and accounts for about half of all amputations annually.

Anemia

Anemia means "without blood." It is a condition in which the quantity or quality of red blood cells is insufficient. Normal red blood cells contain hemoglobin, which carries oxygen to organs and tissues. Anemic individuals have a reduced oxygen-carrying capacity. Anemias can be the result of too little iron, loss of blood (including heavy menstrual bleeding or frequent blood donations), insufficient red cell production or genetic abnormalities. Symptoms include fatigue, infection, and/or trouble healing. There are four types of anemias known:

1. *Iron-deficiency anemia*—develops with inadequate iron intake in the diet or excessive loss of iron, which can result from heavy menses. This is the most common form of anemia and can be corrected with iron supplements.

2. *Pernicious anemia*—caused by deficiency of vitamin B12, which decreases the production of red blood cells. The deficiency is due to an inability of the body to absorb B12 and is treated with vitamin B12 injections.

3. *Aplastic anemia*—stems from bone marrow failure resulting in a decreased number of red blood cells. Injury to bone marrow usually results from ingesting a toxic drug or chemical. Treatment is primarily with blood transfusions; however, the condition is most often fatal.

4. *Sickle-cell anemia*—an inherited trait caused by abnormal hemoglobins. These abnormal hemoglobins cause the red blood cells to be sickle-shaped, which impedes the flow of oxygen-carrying blood. Signs and symptoms include episodes of severe pain, swelling in hands or feet, susceptibility to infection due to a weakened immune system, and possible premature death. There is no cure for sickle-cell anemia, although the cancer drug hydroxyurea has proved to be successful in alleviating the pain. Sickle-cell anemia affects approximately 72,000 African Americans and one out of every 1,000–1,500 Latinos in the United States (Floyd et al., 2007). This type of anemia is a recessive trait-inherited condition, so there are many asymptomatic carriers without the disease. Because of this and the fact that there is no cure, the emphasis is shifting to prevention through education and genetic counseling.

Lupus

Lupus is a chronic inflammatory disease that occurs when your body's immune system attacks your own tissues and organs. There are four different types of lupus. They are: **systemic lupus erythematosus** (SLE), **cutaneous lupus erythematosus** (CLE), **drug-induced lupus,** and **neonatal lupus.**

SLE is an autoimmune disease that can affect various parts of the body including the skin, joints, heart, lungs, blood, kidneys, and brain. CLE is confined to the skin, but can evolve into SLE in approximately 10 percent of CLE cases (Lupis Foundation of America, 2008). Drug-induced lupus may develop after taking certain prescription medications. Symptoms associated with drug-induced lupus typically only last a few days to a few months. With an autoimmune disease the body cannot tell the difference between foreign substances such as viruses and bacteria and its own cells and tissues. When this happens the body begins attacking itself with auto-antibodies. This causes inflammation, pain, and damage in different parts of the body. Signs of inflammation include swelling, redness, pain, and warmth. If this inflammation is chronic, as with SLE, it can cause long-term damage. Signs and symptoms of a lupus flare include: aching all over, swollen joints, loss of appetite, recurring nose bleeds, sores on the skin, headache, nausea or vomiting, puffy eyelids, persistent fever over 100 degrees, prolonged fatigue, skin rashes, anemia, pain in the chest with deep breaths, excessive protein in urine, sensitivity to sun, hair loss, abnormal blood clotting problems, seizures, or mouth ulcers which last more than two weeks.

Lupus flares are highly variable as are the remission periods. Flare and remission periods can last a few days to a few years. Lupus affects people in varying degrees; most do not experience significant organ involvement and can lead a relatively normal life. Others have more flares and more discomfort associated with the disease and have to make changes in their previous lifestyle. More than 90 percent of people with lupus are women. Symptoms and diagnosis occur most often when women are in their child-bearing years, between the ages of 15 and 45.

In the United States, lupus is more than three times as common in African Americans as it is in Caucasians (LFA, 2008). Because diagnosis of lupus is relatively difficult, a rheumatologist is the best medical specialist to see if lupus is suspected. Because of the difficulty in diagnosing lupus, many individuals have been misdiagnosed and actually have had thyroid disease, fibromyalgia, rheumatoid arthritis, multiple sclerosis, or another disease. There is no cure for lupus, but depending upon the severity of the disease, treatment may consist of non-steroidal anti-inflammatory drugs such as ibuprofen or naproxen; corticosteroids such as prednisone or cortisone; anti-malarials such as hydroxychloroquine; or immunosuppressants for individuals who have the most severe flares of lupus.

Gastrointestinal Disorders

Ulcers, which are open sores, can develop in the lining of the stomach (gastric ulcers) or small intestine (duodenal ulcers) and are due to the corrosive effect of excessive gastric juices. Conventional theory blames lifestyle factors such as stress and diet. However, new research has identified a link between the bacterium *Helicobacter pylori* (*H. pylori*) and the formation of ulcers. One theory suggests that an infection caused by this bacterium leads to an inflammation of the stomach lining, which results in increased susceptibility of the stomach to stressors such as smoking, alcohol, high-fat diets, and/or anxiety. The most prominent symptom is a burning pain in the upper abdomen that is related to the digestive cycle. A bleeding ulcer, although not common, can be fatal. Excessive weight loss and anemia can result from an untreated ulcer. Medications that reduce stomach acid and relieve symptoms, lifestyle changes such as eating small, frequent meals, avoiding high-fat foods, cigarettes, alcohol, caffeine, and taking antacids can all reduce the effects of ulcers. One in five men and one in ten women suffer from peptic ulcers. Risk factors include: a stressful lifestyle, cigarette smoking, heavy use of alcohol, caffeine, or painkillers containing aspirin or ibuprofen, advanced age, and family history.

Irritable bowel syndrome (IBS) (spastic colon or irritable colon) is a common problem resulting from intestinal spasms. Symptoms include episodes of abdominal cramping, nausea, pain, gas, loud gurgling bowel sounds, and disturbed bowel function. No biochemical or structural abnormalities have been identified as the cause; therefore, no standard medical treatment exists for IBS. Common interventions include reducing emotional stress, eating high-fiber diets, or taking stool softeners, laxatives, and drugs to reduce intestinal spasms.

REFERENCES

American Cancer Society. 2004. www.cancer.org

American Cancer Society. *Cancer Facts and Figures 2008*. Atlanta: Author. 2008.

American Diabetes Association (ADA). 2005. www.diabetes.org/gestational-diabetes.jsp

Benenson, A. *Control of Communicable Diseases in Man* (16th ed). Washington, DC: American Public Health Association. 1995.

Centers for Disease Control and Prevention (CDC). 2003. www.cdc.gov/meningitis/bacterial/faqs.htm#contagious

Centers for Disease Control and Prevention (CDC). 2005. www.cdc.gov/hepatitis

Centers for Disease Control and Prevention (CDC). 2006. www.cdc.gov/hepatitis/statistic/htm

Centers for Disease Control and Prevention (CDC). 2007. www.cdc.gov/OralHealth/Topics/cancer.htm

Crowley, L. *An Introduction to Human Disease: Pathology and Pathophysiology Correlations* (7th ed). Boston: Jones and Bartlett Publishers, Inc. 2006.

Donatelle, R. *Access to Health* (9th ed). San Francisco: Benjamin Cummings. 2006.

Floyd, P., Mimms, S. and Yelding, C. *Personal Health: Perspectives & Lifestyles* (4th ed). Englewood, CO: Morton Publishing Co. 2007.

Hales, D. *An Invitation to Health* (12th ed). Pacific Grove, CA: Brooks/Cole Publishing Co. 2006.

Lupus Foundation of America. 2008.

Marwick, C. New light on skin cancer mechanisms. *Journal of the American Medical Association*, 274 (6). 1995.

McCance, K. and Huether, S. *Pathophysiology: The Biologic Basis for Disease in Adults and Children* (5th ed). St. Louis, MO: Mosby-Year Book, Inc. 2005.

Payne, W., Hahn, D., and Lucus, E. *Understanding Your Health* (10th ed). Boston: McGraw-Hill. 2008.

Dabelea, D., Snell-Bergeon, J. K., Heartsfield, C. L., et al. Increasing Prevalence of Gestational Diabetes Mellitus (GDM) Over Time and by Birth Cohort. *Diabetes Care* 28:579–584, 2005.

Schering Corporation. 1999. *Detection and Referral: The Primary Care Physician Guide to Chronic Viral Hepatitis*. Kenilworth, NJ. 1999.

Spence, W. "Skin Cancer: The Bare Facts." Health Edco. 1998.

University of California, Berkley. *Wellness Letter*. November, 1990.

www.cancer.org/docroot/CRI/content/CRI_2_2_2x_What_Causes_Testicular_Cancer_41.asp?rnav=cri

www.cdc.gov/diabetes/Statistics/prev/national/figpersons.htm

www.cdc.gov/hepatitis/HCVfac.htm#section4

www.cdc.gov/hepatitis/Resources/Professionals/PDFs/ABCTable.pdf

www.diabetes.niddk.nih.gov/dm/pubs/statistics/index.htm#allages

www.niaid.nih.gov

CONTACTS

American Cancer Society
800-ACS-2345
http://www.cancer.org

American Diabetes Association
800-342-2383
http://www.diabetes.org

American Institute for Cancer Research
http://www.aicr.org

American Liver Foundation
75 Maiden Lane, Suite 603
New York, NY 10038
212-668-1000
www.liverfoundation.org

Asthma and Allergy Foundation of America
800-7-ASTHMA
www.AAFA.org

National Cancer Institute
800-4-CANCER
www.cancer.gov

Centers for Disease Control and Prevention
800-232-4636
www.cdc.gov

Juvenile Diabetes Research Foundation
800-533-2873

National Headache Foundation
888-NHF-5552
www.headaches.org

National Institute of Diabetes & Digestive & Kidney Diseases
www.niddk.nih.gov

ACTIVITIES

Notebook Activities

Family Health Portrait (www.hhs.gov/familyhistory/)
Are You at Risk for Diabetes?

Name: _____ Section: _____ Date: _____

NOTEBOOK ACTIVITY

Family Health Portrait

In order to do this project you must first research your family history. You may do an oral history or written correspondence with a family member, or you may research old records. Identify your source or sources of information. Record diseases and afflictions of all known family members through your great-grandparents. Pay particular attention to genetic disorders and the age of onset. Go to www.hhs.gov/familyhistory/ and enter your information. Once you are done, print out your Family Health Portrait. Have you inherited cardiac risk factors? Common factors to consider are family history of heart disease, diabetes, high blood pressure, high cholesterol, and some forms of cancer. What, if any, diseases are you at risk for due to your family history? What can you do now to have an impact on your long-term health for the future? How do you intend to avoid becoming "at-risk" in the future?

Please turn in your Family Health Portrait, as well as a typed (double-spaced) paragraph on how you can live your lifestyle now to best ensure you have a long and healthy life.

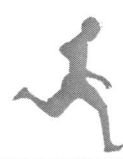

CHAPTER 12

Alternative and Complementary Medicine

"The doctor of the future will give no medicine, but will interest his patients in the care of the human frame, in diet, and in the cause and prevention of disease."

—Thomas Edison

OBJECTIVES

Students will be able to:
- Identify components of holistic self-care.
- Define key terms related to complementary and alternative medicine (CAM).
- Become familiar with the therapies contained in each major CAM domain.
- Identify pros and cons associated with each major CAM practice.
- Identify benefits of mindfulness in everyday life.
- Participate in a self-guided relaxation/meditation practice.

Introduction

by Amy V. Nowak, Ph.D. TAMU

As an adult, making informed healthcare decisions is key to achieving higher levels of health and wellness. To become an informed healthcare consumer, it is important to be aware of the many choices available to you in healthcare today. Learning about each form of healthcare, as well as its risks and benefits, will allow you to make the best choices that meet the needs of your health situation.

Americans value choice in any venue and healthcare is no different. When buying a car, you want a quality vehicle to meet your needs, a company that can give you a good product, and a salesperson that you trust, and who is dedicated to helping you meet your goals. The same goes for healthcare. You want to find a healthcare option that fits with your healthcare needs, a treatment which will be effective, and a healthcare provider whom you trust and who is dedicated to helping you. With healthcare, you have the option of choosing one or a combination of healthcare approaches and providers to best meet your needs.

There are two main camps of healthcare today. You are probably very familiar with what is called conventional medicine. When you go to a conventional clinic or hospital, doctors and nurses work to diagnose an illness and then treat the symptoms with medication, surgery, or radiation. The roots of conventional medicine date back to the mid-1800's with the discovery of the germ and its relationship to illness. While this is the main form of healthcare used in the United States and similar developed nations around the world, more and more people are turning to other types of healthcare that do not fit in the mainstream of conventional medicine.

The other main category of medicine is a group of traditional systems and practices, which are currently called complementary and alternative medicine (CAM). The terms complementary and alternative are actually designations of how traditional medical practices, some of which developed thousands of years ago, are used in relation to conventional care. Systems and practices are considered *complementary* when used in conjunction with conventional care and *alternative* when used instead of conventional care. The emphasis in CAM is holistic, in the sense that its purpose is to treat the whole person and support the body's natural ability to heal itself. The increasing use of CAM is expected to continue as people seek out options in healthcare to best meet their needs.

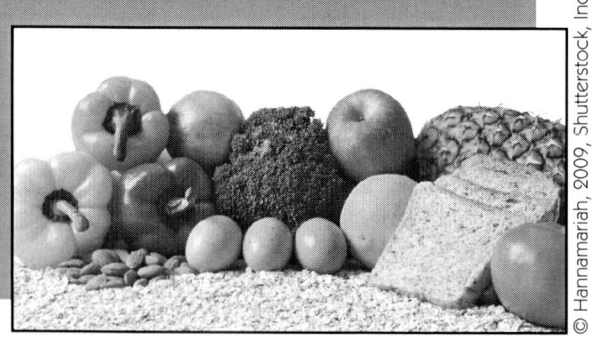

Alternative practitioners emphasize a wholesome diet rich in organic fruits, vegetables, nuts, seeds, fiber, pure water, and organically raised meat products.

Medicine has come a long way since the days of the snake-oil salesmen of the early nineteenth century. In the 1800's, homeopaths, midwives, naturopaths, and an assortment of lay healers used herbs and nostrums to combat illness. Thanks to the wonders of modern conventional and emergency medicine, many of the ill and injured can survive what fifty years ago would have meant certain death. This is surely being played out in the modern landscape of war-torn Iraq. Due to improved body armor, field medical procedures, and medevac capabilities, wounded soldiers are surviving what they would not have survived in the Vietnam War or World War II. Conventional medicine can work mini-miracles in acute trauma care, the treatment of bacterial infections and life-threatening diseases. Life saving antibiotics and other drugs have revolutionalized the medical field. What conventional medicine has failed to do is prevent the lifestyle-related hypokinetic diseases that plague Western society. Conventional (also called Western, allopathic, or biomedical) medicine developed from the evidence-based scientific method. Traditionally, alternative medicine (also called natural, unconventional, or unorthodox in the past) has been based on anecdotal evidence, word of mouth, testimonials, or even the placebo effect. Scientists in the bio-medical research community are recognizing that more and more Americans are choosing complementary and alternative medicine (hereafter referred to as CAM), and therefore funding to test the safety and efficacy of CAM approaches is increasing. Part of the attraction of the CAM modalities may be their identification with prevention rather than cure, and consequently CAM has come to be identified with wellness and self-care.

Today, alternative medicine is also called holistic, complementary, or integrative. Refer back to the wellness dimensions from Chapter 1; a holistic practitioner considers the physical, emotional, mental, social, occupational, environmental, and spiritual factors associated with the individual as a "whole person." "Practitioners of alternative medicine approach healing from a holistic perspective whose primary goal is the creation and maintenance of optimum health in body, mind, and spirit. In addition to the comprehensive care they provide to achieve that goal, they also serve as teachers, instructing their patients in effective methods of self-care. Such methods not only assist patients in their journey back to wellness, but also help them prevent disease from occurring in the first place "(Goldberg, 2002).

Alternative practitioners emphasize **holistic self-care.** A wholesome **diet** minimizing intake of processed food with foods rich in organic fruits and vegetables, nuts, seeds, fiber, pure water, and organically raised meat products is recommended. **Exercise** is critical to maintaining physical health. Adequate **sleep** is necessary to allow the regenerative processes in the body to work. Keeping the **environment** at home and work healthy may mean adding indoor plants, air filters, humidifiers, and avoiding toxic chemicals and secondhand smoke. Peace of mind and contentment are part of **good mental health.** Spiritual health is also considered an important part of self-care. **Spiritual health** can be gained through prayer, meditation, or even giving of yourself through volunteerism. *In alternative or holistic care, the patient takes an active role and is responsible for looking at all aspects or his/her health.*

How many Americans are using CAM? According to a 2007 National Health Interview Study (NHIS) four out of ten adults use some form of CAM therapy on a regular basis. Twelve percent of children (ages 0–18 years) use CAM (see Figure 12.1). Native Alaskan and American Indians were the most likely to use some form of CAM, followed by white adults. Caucasian college-educated women in a higher income bracket use CAM more than other segments of the population. However, CAM is practiced by all types of people across racial, cultural, and socioeconomic lines (see Figure 12.2). The most commonly used CAM therapies are non–vitamin, non–mineral, natural products (for instance, fish oil, echinacea, DHA, glucosamine, and ginseng), deep breathing, meditation, yoga, massage, chiropractic care, and diet-based therapies (see Figure 12.3). Chiropractic is used the most by patients with back pain.

Note: The 2007 NHIS did not include folk medicine practices (i.e., covering a wart with a penny and then burying it) or religious healing, as in prayer for oneself or for others. The 2002 NHIS did include prayer in its survey.

Figure 12.4 shows several accepted and widely used treatments that are rooted in CAM. Indeed, even exercise prescribed as a healing modality was once considered "alternative." "In an age of M.R.I. scans and spinal fusion surgery, a treatment as low tech as exercise can seem to some patients rudimentary or even dangerously illogical" (Ryzik, 2005). Cardiovascular exercise helps with increased circulation

FIGURE 12.1

CAM Use by U.S. Adults and Children

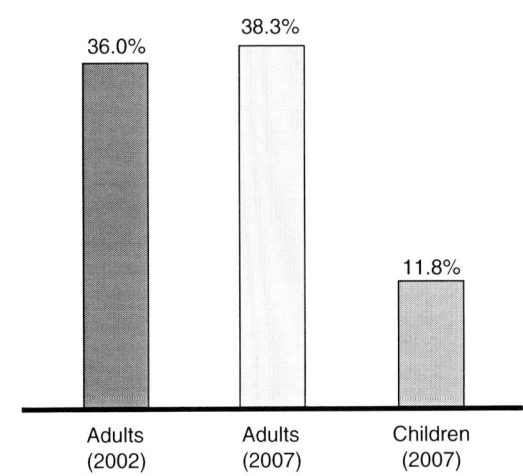

Source: National Institute of Health.

FIGURE 12.2

CAM Use by Race/Ethnicity among Adults - 2007

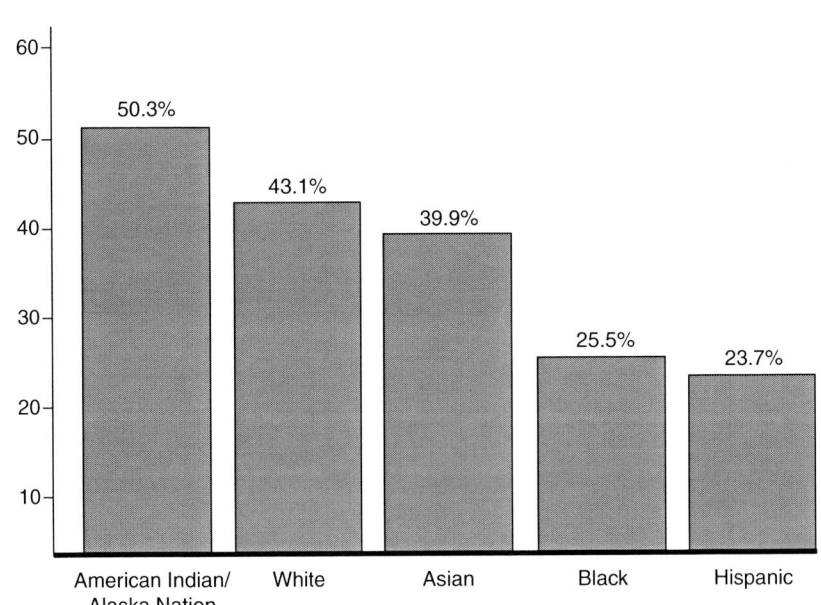

Source: National Institute of Health.

FIGURE 12.3

Ten Most Common CAM Therapies among Adults - 2007

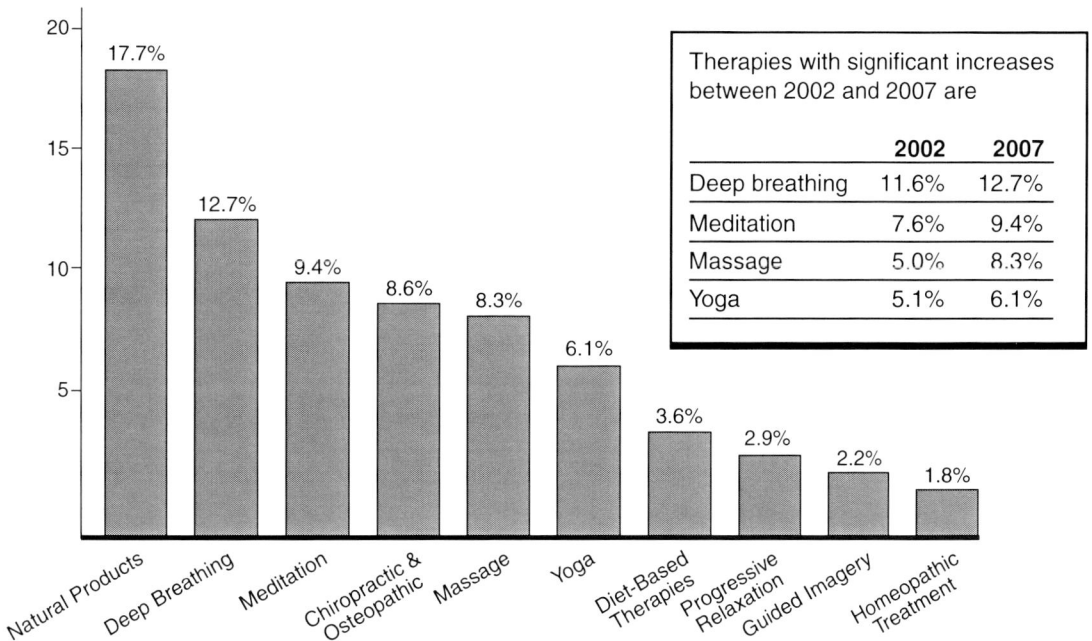

Therapies with significant increases between 2002 and 2007 are

	2002	2007
Deep breathing	11.6%	12.7%
Meditation	7.6%	9.4%
Massage	5.0%	8.3%
Yoga	5.1%	6.1%

Source: Center for Disease Control.

FIGURE 12.4

CAM Domains and Their Related Pratices

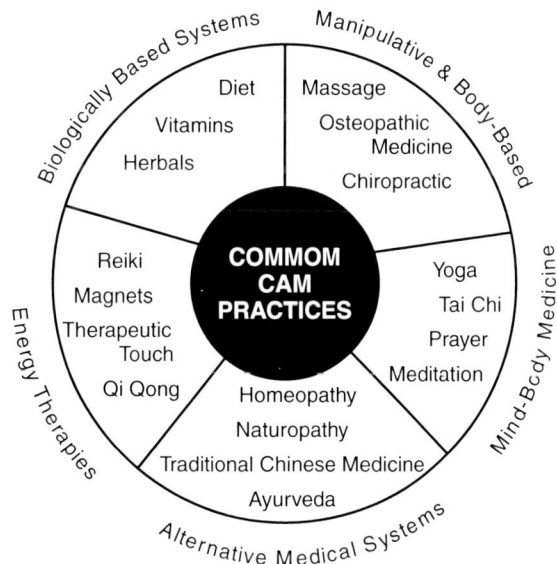

Source: White House Commission on Complementary and Alternative Medicine Policy (2008)

and flexibility, and core muscle strength focuses on supporting the spine which can help prevent future pain. Perhaps in the future many more CAM modalities will become mainstream (see Table 12.1).

Alternative Healthcare Systems

Alternative healthcare systems are holistic "whole person" systems. Whole person systems refer to treating more than just a patient's symptoms. The CAM practitioner often interviews the patient in an attempt to determine the patient's history, eating habits, lifestyle choices, and so on. Some patients report that they appreciate the fact that their practitioner often regards self-care, positive lifestyle habits, behaviors, quality of life, and the combined role of the mind, body, and spirituality in health, disease, and healing as being very important (WHCCAMP, 2002). Typically the CAM practitioner works out of a small facility and spends a fair amount of time with their patient, which may be more attractive to the patient than the short fifteen-minute appointment most people get with their busy conventional doctor. Included in the Alternative Healthcare System domain of CAM is ayurvedic medicine, homeopathic medicine, Native American medicine, and traditional Chinese medicine (including acupuncture and Chinese herbal medicine). Interestingly, the CAM therapies with the most acceptance by the medical community are some of the most infrequently used by patients—hypnotherapy, acupuncture, and biofeedback.

Ayurveda is thought to be the oldest medical system known. In Hindu mythology Ayurveda is considered the medicine of the gods. In Sanskrit, ayurveda is "knowledge of life," with life being defined as mind, body, and spiritual awareness. "Ayurveda is based on the belief that the natural state of the body is one of balance. We become ill when this balance is disrupted, with specific conditions or symptoms indicating a particular disease or imbalance. Ayurveda emphasizes strengthening and purifying the whole person, whereas in conventional medicine, the focus is on a set of symptoms or an isolated region of the body" (Alternative Medicine Foundation, 2005).

Ayurvedic teaching states that every living thing in the universe is made of these five elements: earth, water, fire, air, and space. The elements combine to determine a dosha, or metabolic type. A person's personality and character determine which of three doshas they are: Vata, Pitta, or Kapha. The practitioner can determine which dosha a patient is, then prescribe botanics, exercise, yoga, and scash or massage therapy according to the person's particular dosha type. Ayurvedic practitioners mainly diagnose by observation and by touch. Caution with botanicals

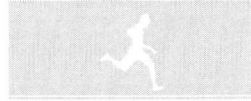

"The competent physician, before he attempts to give medicine to the patient, makes himself acquainted not only with the disease, but also with the habits and constitution of the sick man."
—Cicero

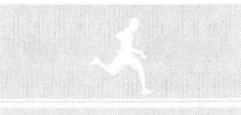

"The art of healing comes from nature and not from the physician. Therefore, the physician must start from nature with an open mind."
—Paracelsus

Table 12.1
Currently Used CAM Modalities

CAM Modalities Now in Mainstream Medicine
Codeine for pain
Digitalis for heart failure
Quinine for malaria
Aspirin for fever
Behavioral therapy for headache
Hypnosis for smoking cessation
Exercise for diabetes
Support groups for breast cancer
Low-fat, low-cholesterol diets

is advised as a 2008 study determined that a type of ayurveda that uses Rasa shastra (herbal medicines mixed with minerals and metals) may be cause for concern. Twenty-one percent of the medicines tested (obtained from the Internet) had unsafe levels of lead, arsenic, and mercury (Saper, Phillips, Sehgal, et al., 2008).

Homeopathy is based on a three pronged theory that *like cures like,* treatment is very individualized, and less is more. Homeopathic practitioners give very diluted forms of the substance that causes the symptoms of the disease in healthy people to the ill in the hopes that it will help support the body's natural healing power. The World Health Organization (WHO) has cited homeopathy as one of the systems of traditional medicine that should be integrated worldwide with conventional medicine in order to provide adequate global care in the twenty-first century (Goldberg, 2002). Homeopaths use low-cost herbals, chemicals, and minerals.

Naturopathy is based on the motto "Vis Medicatrix Naturae," which is Latin for *helping nature heal.* Naturopaths emphasize restoring health rather than curing disease. Naturopaths utilize many different healing "tools" found in nature, such as magnets, water, heat, crystals, the sun, herbal medicine, manipulation, light therapy, electrical currents, and more. Naturopaths argue that Americans should return to a more natural and to a simpler way of life. Some naturopaths contend that we should go so far as to cease fluoridation of water and eliminate the addition of preservatives to food. There are three naturopathic training schools in the United States and one in Canada. Although these schools have a four year program emphasizing humanistic medicine, the naturopath is not an M.D.

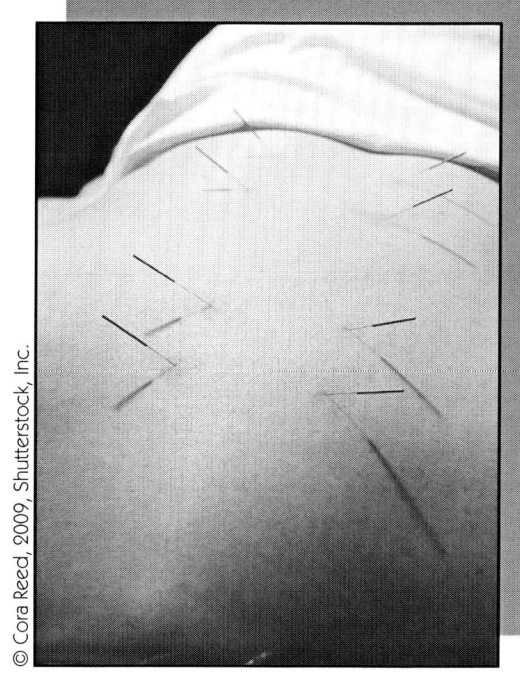

Acupuncture is an ancient medical art using the insertion of very fine needles into the body.

Traditional oriental medicine (TOM) is a comprehensive system that dates back to the Stone Age. Also called traditional Chinese medicine (TCM), it includes acupuncture, acupressure, herbal medicine (discussed under Biological-Based Therapies), oriental massage, and qi gong (discussed under Energy Therapies). **Acupuncture** is an ancient medical art using the insertion of very fine needles on the body in order to affect physiological functioning in the body. The needles are placed on the body at points that correspond to twelve meridians throughout the body. Manipulation of the needles, electrical stimulation, heat, and burning herbs (moxibustion) can be used in acupuncture. Before making a diagnosis, the practitioner talks with, and asks questions about, the patient. Typically the acupuncturist will check the pulse and the tongue of the patient to help diagnose the problem. A reputable acupuncturist will use disposable needles or sterilize reusable needles in an autoclave. With the millions of people treated with acupuncture, there have been

Can acupuncture give the athlete an edge in competition? It is possible that acupuncture treatment can be a positive adjunct to training, just like massage or physical therapy. Needles placed at sites of inflammation may reduce time out of training due to injury or swelling of tissue. There is little research, but Whitfield Reaves (2008) has used pre-performance needling and found personal benefit. Ear (auricular) acupuncture has been used during an athlete's competition, with small "tacks" kept in the ear. Acupuncture points don't work for everyone, but perhaps some sports acupuncture can make your next run a little more enjoyable.

relatively few complications reported to the U.S. Food and Drug Administration (FDA). Acupuncturists have a Master of Traditional Oriental Medicine and are required to be state-licensed.

All TOM recognizes an energy force that flows through the body called qi (pronounced chi). Qi consists of the spiritual, physical, mental, and emotional aspects of life. Yin and yang are the vital forces of life that run throughout the twelve meridians within the body. Stimulation of points on the meridians is thought to activate the qi, which restores the body's equilibrium and allows the free flow of qi. The body is considered a flowing, self-healing system. Pain and discomfort can be the result of stagnation of energy which needs to be brought back into balance. Patients may experience calm and peacefulness as well as rejuvenation when their qi has been restored.

U.S. medical doctors became more interested in acupuncture in 1971 when James Reston, a well respected New York Times columnist, had to undergo emergency surgery while in China. Doctors there eased his post-surgery pain with acupuncture. There have been numerous studies done in the United States on the effectiveness of acupuncture. In December 2004 results of the largest randomized, controlled phase III clinical trial of acupuncture ever conducted were published in the *Annals of Internal Medicine*. The study was conducted on 570 patients with osteoarthritis of the knee. The results showed that "acupuncture reduces pain and functional impairment of osteoarthritis of the knee" (NIH, 2004). Dr. Brian M. Berman, M.D. of the University of Maryland School of Medicine directed the study and concluded that acupuncture is an effective complement to conventional arthritis treatment. According to a CDC 2002 survey, 2.1 million Americans have used acupuncture.

Acupressure is similar to acupuncture, but without the needles. The practitioner applies pressure to critical points along the meridian lines to balance yin and yang. There are different pressure points corresponding to specific parts of the body. The pressure releases muscular tension and promotes circulation of blood and qi to promote healing. Gradual steady penetrating pressure for up to three minutes is common (Gach, 1990). Simple acupressure techniques can be practiced on oneself. For example, between the forefinger and thumb is an acupressure point for headaches. **Shiatsu** is a type of acupressure massage using fingers, elbows, fists, and so on to apply pressure to restore the flow of energy in the body.

Manipulative and Body-Based Therapies

Manipulative and body-based therapies in CAM use movement or manipulation of part of the body (see Figure 12.5).

Chiropractic is a medical treatment defined as the science of spinal manipulation. Chiropractic is the most commonly used form of CAM in the United States with 18 million Americans visiting the chiropractor each year. A June 2005 Consumer Reports Survey of 34,000 readers reported that of those interviewed with back pain, more went to the chiropractor than used prescription drugs. Practiced in earnest in the United States since 1895, chiropractic can trace its roots back to Galen and Hippocrates who laid their hands on patients for manipulation. Chiropractic is considered to be the oldest indigenous CAM practices in the United States (NIH Lecture Series, 2002). Chiropractic has been seen in the past to be in competition with conventional medical treatment. Early in the last century, state medical boards used their power to restrict chiropractic practice. The chiropractors successfully brought an antitrust suit against the American Medical Association for allegedly trying to eliminate chiropractic practice in the United States. Today the medical doctors and the doctors of chiropractic enjoy a better working relationship. Chiropractors train for up to six years with in-depth courses in anatomy, physiology, nutrition, and pathology. They also have clinical training.

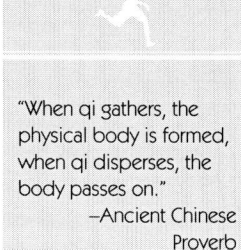

"When qi gathers, the physical body is formed, when qi disperses, the body passes on."
—Ancient Chinese Proverb

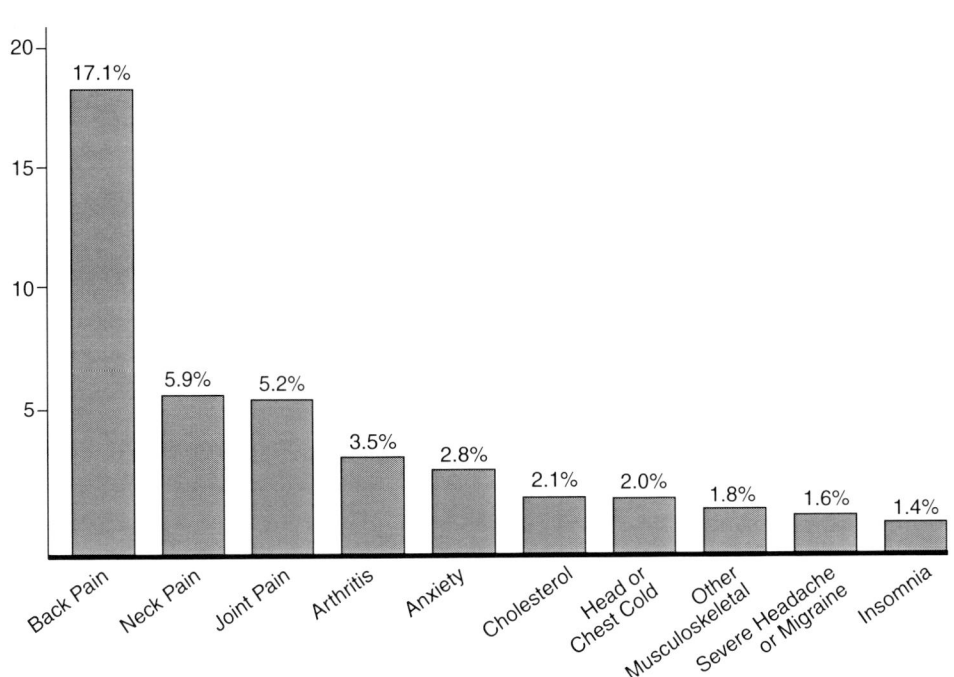

FIGURE 12.5

Diseases/Conditions for Which CAM Is Most Frequently Used among Adults - 2007

Source: Center for Disease Control.

Chiropractors manipulate the spine, often with high-velocity, low-amplitude spinal adjustments, to align the spine in order to let energy flow through the nervous system. It is unclear exactly how chiropractic works, however scientific evidence supports the use of chiropractic to treat acute or chronic back pain (NIH Lecture Series, 2002). Safety is always a concern, and the apparent risk for lumbar vertebrae adjustment is one in 1 million. Back and head complaints are the most common reason patients visit the physician or chiropractor, which results in $100 billion annually in lost productivity.

Massage involves manipulation of muscle and connective tissue to enhance function of those tissues and to promote relaxation and well-being. Massage is growing in popularity as the use and acceptance of massage therapy increases. Many Fortune 500 companies are including massage as a benefit for their employees. Even small companies that offer on-site fifteen-minute massage are seeing the benefit in lower employee absenteeism due to headache, fatigue, and back pain (AMTA, 2005). Deep tissue, Swedish, myofascial release, petressage (kneading), sports massage, and trigger point therapy are just a few of the popular types of massage today.

Reflexology is based on the fact that the feet and hands represent a microcosm of the body and that specific parts of the foot and hand correspond or "reflex" to other parts of the body. Working with the feet has been used in many ancient medical practices; however William Fitzgerald developed modern reflexology in the early 1900's in England.

Craniosacral therapy has its origins in the 1800's with Andrew Still M.D. The current form of craniosacral therapy was developed by osteopathic physician John E. Upledger at Michigan State University as a therapy that uses gentle touch to evaluate the physiological functioning of the craniosacral system. The craniosacral system is comprised of the membranes and the cerebrospinal fluid

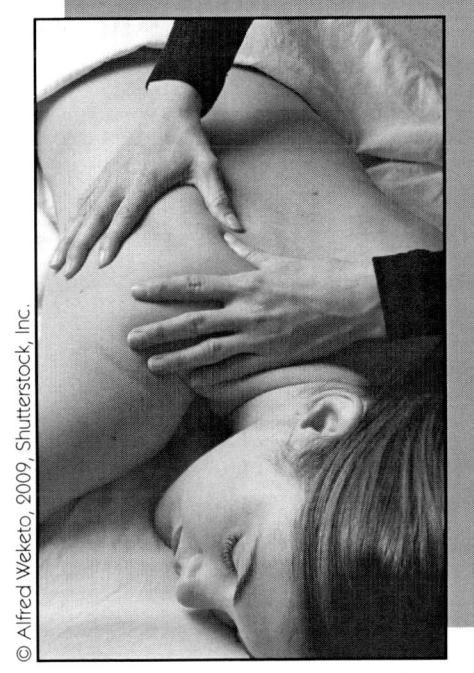

Massage involves manipulation of muscle and connective tissue to enhance function and promote relaxation and well-being.

that surrounds and protects the spinal cord. Imbalance in the cerebral and spinal systems may cause sensory or motor dysfunction (IAHE, 2005). As relaxing as a massage, this therapy is typically used by people experiencing chronic pain who have not found relief with other therapies.

Biological-Based Therapies

Biological-based therapies use substances found in nature such as food, vitamins, minerals, herbal products, animal-derived products, probiotics, amino acids, whole diets, and functional foods. Some biological-based therapies are evidenced-based. For example, the FDA now fortifies some foods with folic acid to deter potential neural tube defects in developing fetuses. There are other biological-based therapies that are as of yet unproven. An example is the use of shark cartilage as a treatment for cancer. The consumer should be informed and use common sense and do a little research before spending money and making important decisions regarding healthcare. Drugs are monitored by the FDA, but biological-based systems are measured for truth in advertising by the Federal Trade Commission (FTC). The following biological-based therapies are just a few of the options for consumers today.

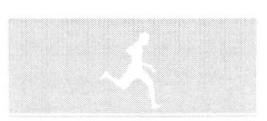

"Let thy food be thy medicine and thy medicine be thy food."
—Hippocrates
(460-377 B.C.)

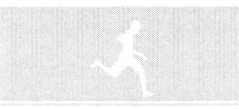

"No illness which can be treated by the diet should be treated by any other means."
—Moses Maimonides
(1135-1204)

Macrobiotics is more than a diet, it is a discipline based on a philosophy of balance in accordance with the universe. It involves managing or changing diet to enhance health or for spiritual benefit. Macrobiotics is characterized by excluding meat and concentrating heavily on whole grains. Besides modifying diet, basic macrobiotic practices emphasize an active life, a positive mental outlook, and regularly eating small portions. There are numerous testimonials from cancer patients that have recovered from a stage IV cancer diagnosis using the macrobiotic diet. The National Cancer Institute has funded a clinical study to determine the effects of a macrobiotic diet on cancer therapy (www.clinicaltrials.gov/ct/gui/c/alb/show/NCT00010829). As you recall, evidence-based science needs clinical trials to provide scientific evidence in order for a therapy or treatment to have wide acceptance.

Herbals and dietary supplements are a hot trend in the industry, making manufacturers four billion dollars richer each year. Herbal therapy has been around for several thousand years. It is likely the oldest and most widely used therapy with roots in traditional Oriental medicine and the ayurvedic tradition. Herbs are substances derived from trees, flowers, plants, seaweed, and lichen. Herbs are prepared in several different forms: tinctures which contain grain alcohol for preservation, freeze-dried extracts, and standardized extracts. Herbs are contained in some manufactured drugs; drugs can also contain a synthetic copy of the herb. *Many plant extracts can be very beneficial, however it is prudent to remember that herbs are drugs and should be consumed only as prescribed.* Even if the consumer is using the herbal remedy correctly, there may be an adverse interaction with food, over-the-counter drugs (OTC), vitamins and minerals, or prescriptions drugs. Recent studies done by NCCAM (NIH, 2002) found that St. John's wort reduces the action of a common AIDS drug called Indinavir (see Figure 12.6). St. John's wort, commonly used for mild to moderate depression, also clears 50 percent of all pharmaceutical drugs from the human body (Markowitz et al., 2003).

An herbalist is a practitioner who bases most of his therapy on the medicinal qualities of plant and herbs. Herbs are prescribed so much in some parts of Europe that they might not

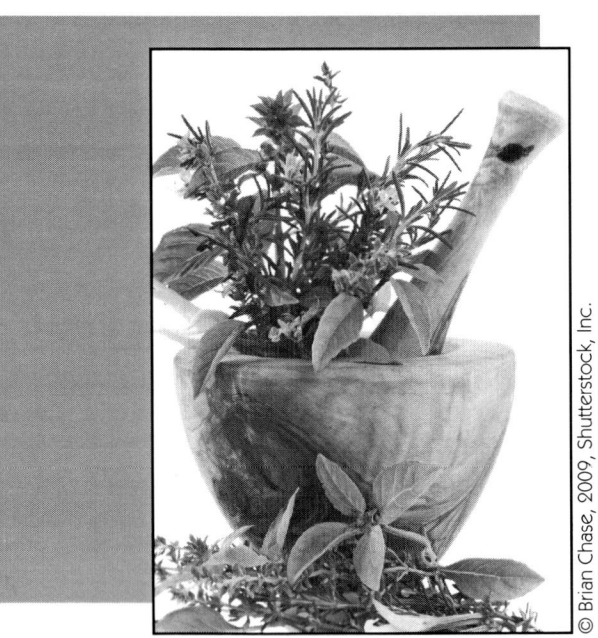

Many plant extracts can be beneficial, however it is prudent to remember that herbs are drugs and should be consumed only as prescribed.

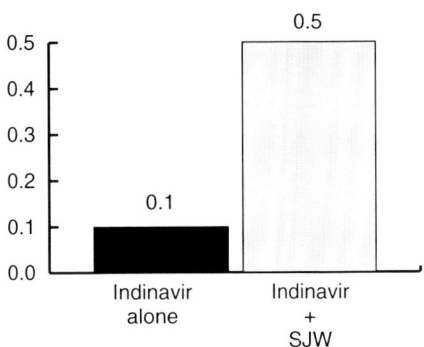

FIGURE 12.6

Biologically Based Systems: St. John's Wort Lowers Blood Levels of HIV Protease Inhibitor Indinavir

Note: HIV Inhibition threshold = 0.1.
Indinavir Level (ug/ml)

even be considered alternative. There are volumes of testimonials, lots of anecdotal evidence, and many cultural traditions supporting herbal therapy. Gingko biloboa is purported to help with memory. St. John's wort helps with depression (some studies support this, some refute it). Saw palmetto helps manage an enlarged prostate. Butterbur, bee pollen, and stinging nettle may help with allergy symptoms. Evening primrose oil helps to manage PMS. The list is endless! When working with an experienced herbalist it is important to try and regulate the quality of the product you are getting. Using caution, especially when self-prescribing, is important because: safety is assumed, not proven; products are not standardized; products can be contaminated; you may have an allergic reaction, some herbs or certain amounts of the herb can be toxic, and the herbs can interact with drugs. Purity, standardization, and quality of the herbs can be an issue in consistency and the amount of the herb in the product. Another reason to use caution is that sometimes we get the sense that if a little works, perhaps a little more will work better. Toxic levels of drugs and herbs can be dangerous. If your friend takes 200 mg of a drug or herb, then you might do the same with disastrous consequences. You may be a nonresponder for that substance and get no result, or you may tolerate the substance and need a larger amount. Another issue is the amount of product actually contained in the packaging. See Figure 12.7 on ginseng.

Did You Know?

National Consumers League Food and Drug Interaction Brochure

NCL is your consumer healthcare advocate.

Medicines are powerful. The drugs your physician prescribes to you can help your health. A drug's effectiveness can be rendered ineffective or enhanced by food, drink, herbs (botanicals), and other drugs in your diet. Log on to this Web site, write, or call the NCL to obtain this important food and drug interaction brochure.

www.nclnet.org
National Consumers League (nonprofit membership organization)
1701 K Street, NW, Suite 1200
Washington DC 20006
(202) 835-3323

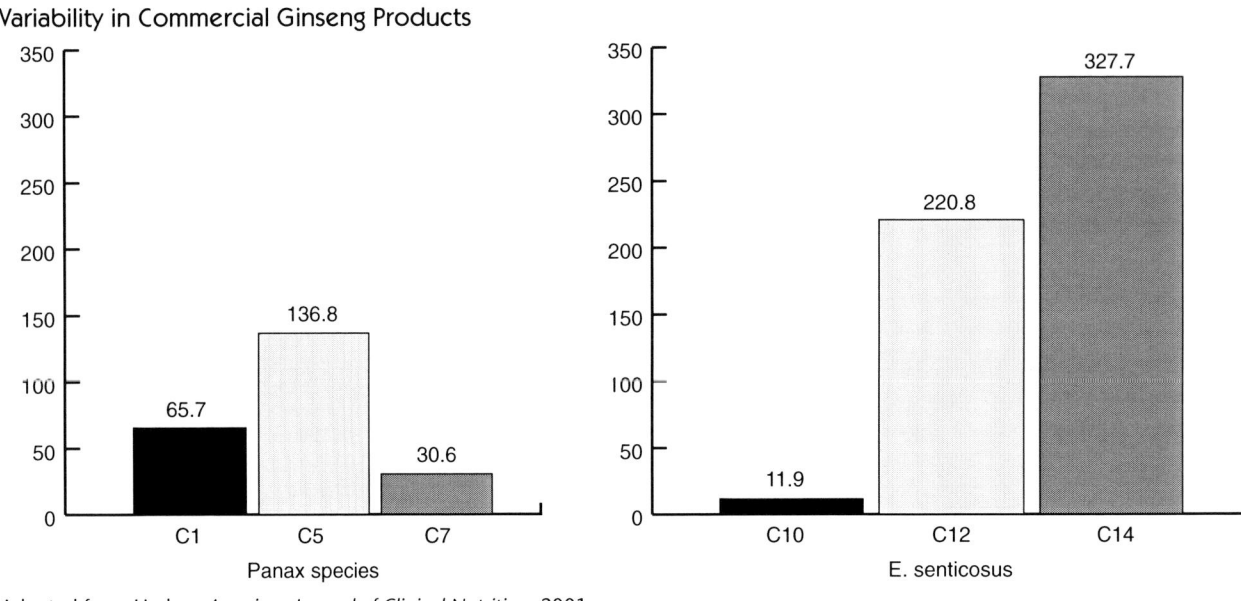

FIGURE 12.7
Variability in Commercial Ginseng Products

Adapted from Harkey, *American Journal of Clinical Nutrition*, 2001.

An example of an unsafe drug is ephedra, derived from the Chinese herb Ma Huang. Traditionally Ma Huang has been used in China to treat asthma and other ailments associated with respiration. Ephedra was confirmed to be a factor in the death of Orioles pitching prospect Steve Belcher in February of 2003. Steve was taking ephedra to give him energy and to assist him with weight loss. The facts that Steve used ephedra, it was hot, and he was exercising combined to cause his death. The FDA has since banned the use of ephedra. If you are wondering about the safety of a particular herb, a very informative website that contains warnings and safety information is the USFDA Center for Food Safety and Applied Nutrition's Dietary Supplements: Warnings and Safety Information (www.cfsan.fda.gov/~dms/ds-warn.html).

Functional foods are foods that contain compounds like phytochemicals that are beneficial beyond basic nutrition, especially when eaten on a regular basis as part of a varied diet. This is a relatively new classification of foods and the specific benefits are still being determined. It is possible that functional foods act synergistically with other foods and antioxidants. See Table 12.2 for examples of functional foods and potential benefits. Isoflavones in soy products, omega-3 fatty acids in cold water fish, essential fatty acids and fiber in ground flaxseed, and probiotic yeasts found in some yogurts are examples of other functional foods. If you eat a wholesome diet with plenty of fruits and vegetables and whole grains, then most likely you are getting functional foods in your diet (Corbin et al., 2009).

Vitamins and minerals are two of the six essential components for life in the human diet. As with herbs, a little is good but more is not always better. Use caution when megadosing on vitamins and minerals to avoid toxicity and health risks. As always, it is good to consult your physician or an educated CAM practitioner. We will not discuss the particulars of vitamins and minerals here; however, remember that often the best way to get vitamins and minerals is through a daily balanced diet. For those that have chronically deficient diets, a multivitamin and mineral supplement is most likely a good recommendation. For evidence-based information on herbal and supple ments, log onto *HerbMed* for herbal information or to *Medline Plus* for other supplement information; the address is found at the back of the chapter in the list of resources.

> "The revolution we call mind-body medicine was based on this simple discovery: Wherever thought goes, a chemical goes with it. This insight has turned into a powerful tool that allows us to understand, for example, why recent widows are twice as likely to develop breast cancer, and why the chronically depressed are four times more likely to get sick. In both cases, distressed mental states get converted into the bio-chemicals that create disease."
> —Deepak Chopra, M.D. (1993)

Table 12.2
Examples of Functional Foods and Potential Benefits

Carotenoids	Potential Benefits
Beta-carotene: found in carrots, pumpkin, sweet potato, cantaloupe	May bolster cellular antioxidant defenses
Lutein, zeaxanthin: found in kale, collards, spinach, corn, eggs, citrus	May contribute to healthy vision
Lycopene: Found in tomatoes, watermelon, red/pink grapefruit	May contribute to prostate health
Flavonoids	**Potential Benefits**
Anthocyanins: found in berries, cherries, red grapes *Flavanones*: found in citrus foods *Flavonols*: found in onions, apples, tea, broccoli	May bolster antioxidant defenses; maintain brain function and heart health
Isothiocyanates	**Potential Benefits**
Proanthocyanidins: found in cranberries, cocoa, apples, strawberries, grapes, peanuts	May contribute to maintenance of urinary tract health and heart health
Sulforaphane: found in cauliflower, broccoli, brussels sprouts, cabbage, kale, horseradish	May enhance detoxification of undesirable compounds; bolsters cellular antioxidant defenses
Phenolic Acids	**Potential Benefits**
Caffeic/ferulic acids: found in apples, pears, citrus fruits, some vegetables, coffee	May bolster cellular antioxidant defenses; may contribute to maintenance of healthy vision
Sulfides/Thioles	**Potential Benefits**
Sulfides: found in garlic, onions, leeks, scallions *Dithiolthiones*: found in cruciferous vegetables	May enhance detoxification of undesirable compounds; may contribute to maintenance of heart health and healthy immune function

Source: From *Concepts of Physical Fitness,* 15th Edition, by Charles Corbin et al. Copyright © 2009 by McGraw-Hill Companies. Reprinted by permission of The McGraw-Hill Companies, Inc.

Mind-Body Medicine

Mind-body medicine taps into the connection between the physical body and the very powerful mind. Mind-body therapies are designed to enhance the mind's capacity to influence the body. Creative therapy involving dance, art, and music, as well as prayer and mental healing, are considered to be in the mind-body category.

Meditation is a way to deal with the effects of chronic stress. The person meditating is able to let go by focusing primarily on taking time (twenty minutes is great) to relax, shutting out external stimuli. There are numerous meditative techniques, and there really is no "right" way to meditate. Almost all techniques involve focus on breathing. The most important factor is to commit the time to just do nothing. This can be a challenge in our busy lives today. Try simply to find a quiet place, eliminate distractions, close your eyes, repeat a

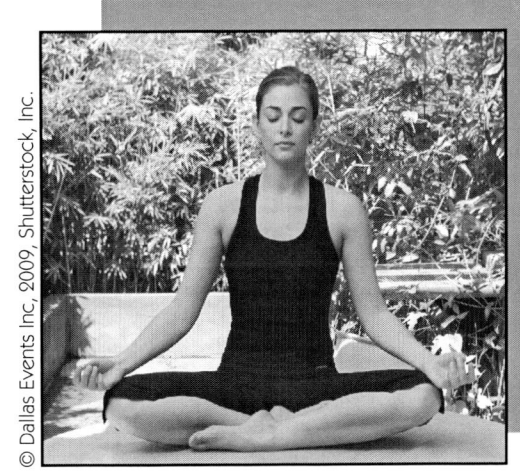

There are numerous meditative techniques. Almost all techniques involve focus on breathing.

Meditation Exercise

The most important thing is to allow yourself to do nothing.

Easy steps to meditation:

1. Eliminate distractions.
Turn off the cell phone, decide not to answer the door, let family or friends know you are unavailable for the next ten or fifteen minutes. Go to the bathroom, get a drink of water, and generally take care of any physical distractions that might arise. You might find it helpful to set a timer.

2. Just sit.
Get comfortable—consider sitting on a folded blanket to allow for less stress on the knees. Take a deep breath and allow your spine to extend and your ribs to lift. Maintain a tall posture as you soften your shoulders. Dim lights, a candle, incense, and appropriate music are nice but not necessary.

3. Let go.
Practice silence. Close your eyes and quietly observe the thoughts that come to your mind. Acknowledge them and then let them go. Let go of the outside stimuli so you can focus inward.

4. Listen.
Listen to the sounds of life in and around you. Become receptive to the sounds that are obvious, but also to the sounds that you normally don't hear because your attention is elsewhere. Hear without judgment; just observe. Notice your awareness of the present as it deepens.

5. Use your senses.
Cultivate an awareness of the present moment through sensations. Be attentive to where your body is connecting to the earth. What do you feel? Softness, hardness, coolness, warmth, pressure, and ease. How does your body change with each inhalation and exhalation? Settle into the present moment using your breath and your senses. Begin to focus on your inner self.

6. Simply breathe.
Attend to your breath. Try not to change your breath, just observe it how it is. Use all of your senses to increase awareness of how your body responds to your breath. Relax into your breath. Follow the rhythm of your breath with each inhalation and exhalation. When your mind wanders, just refocus and come back to the breath.

7. Mantra.
Saying a simple word, a phrase, a prayer, or anything meaningful to you over and over again as a mantra can coax you into a contemplative state. Repeat the mantra softly and slowly in an undulating rhythm with your breath, like riding a wave.

8. Practice kindness.
In your quiet state, consider someone who might be in need of some understanding and goodwill. Focus on this person. "In your mind's eye, send this person love, happiness, and well-being. Soften your skin, open the floodgates of your heart, and let gentle goodwill pour forth."

With consistent practice, meditation can make a difference in your life.

Adapted from Meditation 101 by Claudia Cummins, *Yoga Journal*. www.yogajournal.com/practice, 2009

word or phrase that is meaningful for you, and say that word over and over with each exhalation. Allow yourself to just let go. "For 30 years, research has told us that meditation works beautifully as an antidote to stress," says Daniel Goleman, author of *Destructive Emotions* (2003). More and more conventional health professionals are recommending meditation as a way to deal with chronic stress as well as chronic pain. Experiencing the calming effect of meditation, if only for ten minutes each day, creates a period of physical relief that can enhance immune function. Over time, the benefits of meditation can have a cumulative effect, improving the well-being of the meditator (Heistand, 2005). With practice, it can calm the body and quiet the mind. The benefits are numerous. Try committing to the above Meditation Exercise technique daily for one week to see if it has a positive effect on your life.

Meditation practice can alter brain activity. Andrew Newberg is a University of Pennsylvania neurologist who has studied changes in brain activity during meditation. Using radioactive dye with functional brain imaging, Newberg demonstrated

Beginning Your Own Spiritual Journey

Whether a person's quest for spiritual health takes the form of a love for nature, a weekly visit to a place of religious worship, or some other guise, it is clear that spirituality benefits overall health. While it is possible to achieve spiritual health in many ways, the following ideas have helped a number of people on their spiritual path:

Relaxation and Meditation

"There is no greater source of strength and power for me in my life now than going still, being quiet, and recognizing what real power is," says Oprah Winfrey on the segment of her daily television show called "Remembering Your Spirit." Many people take the time to sit quietly and to meditate; for example, more than five million people worldwide practice transcendental meditation, one popular relaxation technique.

Time in Nature

For Henry David Thoreau, who fled civilization to live on Walden Pond, nature was the temple of God and the perennial source of life. A powerfully spiritual moment—and one we have all experienced–is the instant we are confronted with earth's perfection and are filled with awe. The scientist Carl Sagan wrote about his time-in-nature experience: "The wind whips through the canyons of the American Southwest, and there is no one to hear it but us." The crisp, clean smell of the woods after rainfall, the soothing rhythm of crickets on a summer night, the beauty of freshly fallen snow—these experiences inspire unspeakable awe and humility because of the small but rich part that we, as individuals, play in the larger scheme of the universe.

Intimacy with Others

Loving selflessly is part of spiritual experience. Living life with passion and allowing ourselves to "feel" may be the greatest element of the spiritual journey. Experiencing emotion through a poignant musical passage, feeling the grief of a lost love, and surrendering to love's beauty are all part of human spirituality. By giving, sharing, and loving, we become whole and experience all that we are capable of feeling.

Spiritual Readings

Ranging from inspirational self-help books available at the local bookstore to traditional religious works, the written word has provided insight and guidance throughout human history, during its times of joy and darkest moments. For some it's the Bible; for others, it may be the Quran; and for still others, it may be a contemporary book such as *Spiritual Healing: Scientific Validation of a Healing Revolution* by Daniel J. Benor, M.D. (Vision Publications, 2001). To find books that will foster your personal growth a healing, listen to what others recommend and then search for whatever will move you or speak to you.

Prayer

Prayer may be the oldest spiritual practice and the most popular one in America. Almost all world religions include a form of prayer. Says George Lucas, who plays on religious themes such as good and evil in his blockbuster *Star Wars* series, "Religion is basically a container for faith. And faith is a very important part of what allows us to remain stable, remain balanced." The mental and emotional release, along with a sense of connection to a transcendent dimension, may be at the heart of prayer's effectiveness.

From *Psychology Today* (September/October 1999), 48; The Transcendental Meditation Program (see http://www.tm.org).

that the brains of Tibetan Buddhist monks blocked out information from the part of the brain that orients the body in space and time. The monks focused their energy inward, while blocking out any external stimuli (Pure Insight, 2005).

Applied psycho-neuro-immunology is based on research into psycho-neuro-endocrino-immunolgy, the science of how our experiences are encoded neurologically and about how this affects our immune and hormonal systems. How our bodies' encounter, adapt, and react to stress directly affects our immune system. This approach treats the whole body. Our minds can keep us in a dark hole of hopelessness and helplessness with a condition like depression, which can cause a breakdown of our immune system. The reverse can be true as well. "The profound power of the mind that causes this rundown and eventual loss of resistance can also naturally be used positively to tune-up and boost the immune system to maximum level: to repel viruses, bacterium and other micro-organisms and to speed up healing" (AAAPNI).

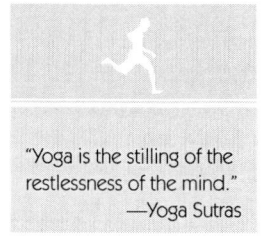

"Yoga is the stilling of the restlessness of the mind."
—Yoga Sutras

Prayer and Spirituality—*Newsweek* recently did a cover story on the growth of spirituality in America today (Adler, 2005). The article greatly contrasts with the cover story of a 1966 *Time* article entitled "Is God Dead?" Spirituality is experiencing resurgence among Americans: 55 percent of Americans consider themselves spiritual and religious, and 24 percent consider themselves spiritual but not religious. Young people especially seem to be searching for greater meaning in a rigorous form of faith and prayer. Wanting more than what traditional religious services offer, they want to experience God in their daily lives. Many are drawing on the influence of Eastern religions to enhance their traditional doctrines. Meditations, centering prayer, silent contemplation, as well as disciplines like yoga, are often used in addition to traditional church services (Adler, 2005).

More than half of the medical schools in the country now offer an elective course on "Spirituality and Medicine". Questions abound about the role of prayer in healing the sick. Eighty-four percent of Americans polled believe praying for the sick can improve their chance of recovery (Kalb, 2004). Anecdotal evidence says prayer works. Science demands concrete evidence; however, prayer is hard to measure.

Yoga is a mind/body/spiritual discipline that is rooted in the ancient Hindu religion traced back 5,000 years. Yoga has become popular in the United States in the last several decades. According to the *New York Times*, 16 million Americans currently practice yoga. There are many different styles of yoga—gentle, meditative, powerful, and relaxing yoga to name of few. Movement in yoga can be rigorous and intense, or gentle and calming. Physicians are recognizing the benefits that a yoga practice can have on strengthening the physical body and quieting the mind. In addition to the many physical benefits, the practice of yoga with emphasis on breathing can be a great stress management tool. Movement, breathing, chanting, and sound are a prelude to meditation and conscious relaxation that regular yoga practice can provide. Conscious relaxation gives our minds a break from the daily chatter and unending stimuli to which we are continuously exposed.

Guided imagery is a concept that has been used successfully with people suffering from post-traumatic stress disorder. Psychologist Kathleen Reyntjiens, Ph.D., reports that imagery was an integral part of her recovery efforts with those recently traumatized by Hurricane Katrina. "As our previous research with imagery has indicated, these simple self-regulation techniques—especially imagery and conscious breathing—are helping to minimize distress, anxiety, hypervigilance, anger, sadness, and insomnia, and allow all of us to be more effective, efficient, kind and caring neighbors in our survival and clean-up efforts" (Naparstek, 2005).

Mindfulness is a concept that includes strategies and activities that help us be more in the present moment. This helps us connect more intently with ourselves, others, and with nature. Peacefulness can be the result of being mindful throughout the day. Mindfulness is often thought of in conjunction with spirituality.

Feldenkrais method is "a form of somatic education that uses gentle movement and directed attention to improve movement and enhance human functioning. Through this method, you can increase your ease and range of motion, improve your flexibility and coordination, and rediscover your innate capacity for graceful, efficient movement" (The North American Feldenkrais Guild). Feldenkrais is excellent for dancers, athletes, and others, as well as those limited by neuromuscular pain or neurological dysfunction. Moshe Feldenkrais, an Israeli engineer, developed this technique.

Somatic movement re-educates the neuromuscular system toward greater health and well-being. Through hands-on movement work by the somatics practitioner, "people can learn to manage stress, relieve back pain, breathe more freely, heal from trauma to the neuromuscular system, and speed recuperation after illness or surgery" (Brockport, 2005). The Feldenkrais method is a type of somatic movement education. Meditation, visualization, craniosacral therapy, and myofascial release techniques are often practiced by the somatic movement practitioner.

Animal-assisted therapy is the use of companion animals to help people with special needs. Evidence is mounting that spending time with a loved pet not only has emotional and psychological benefits, but physiological benefits as well. The act of petting and caring for a loved animal can reduce blood pressure and heart rate and improve survival rates from heart disease (Arkow, www.animal therapy). Close to half of the psychologists responding to a survey indicated prescribing a pet to combat loneliness or depression. According to Phil Arkow, instructor of the Animal Assisted Therapy course at Camden County College in Blackwood, New Jersey, elderly people who have pets visit physicians 16 percent less than those who do not; dog owners in particular make 21 percent fewer visits. "A pet is an island of sanity in what appears to be an insane world. Friendship retains its traditional values and securities in one's relationship with one's pet. Whether a dog, cat, bird, fish, turtle, or what have you, one can rely upon the fact that one's pet will always remain a faithful, intimate, non-competitive friend-regardless of the good or ill fortune life brings us" (Dr. Boris Levinson, child psychologist).

Energy Therapies

Energy therapies engage the use of energy fields that surround the body and penetrate the body. The science behind energy fields has yet to be proven.

Qi gong combines movement, meditation, and regulation of breathing to enhance the flow of vital energy (qi), improve blood circulation, and enhance immune function (Donatelle, 2004). Qi gong literally means the skill of attracting vital energy. Those that practice qi gong call it a "self-healing art" that uses visualization and imagery with movement and meditation.

Reiki (pronounced ray-key) is a type of energy work that utilizes touch and visualization. Reiki is based on ancient Tibetan teachings and is said to date back thousands of years. Today reiki is practiced using the Eastern concept of the five chakras in the body, as well as using the organs and glands from Western anatomy.

Therapeutic touch is purported to induce the relaxation response, alleviate pain, and to speed the healing process. In therapeutic touch, the patient is not actually touched. In one study people were wounded on their arms. The control group had conventional therapy, while the other group experienced therapeutic touch. The entire second group experienced quicker healing (Wirth, 1990).

Bioenergy practitioners use psychotherapy, grounding exercise, and deep breathing to assist in releasing muscular tension, pain, and illness. Pain and illness are thought to be caused by suppressed emotions and behaviors (AMFI, 2005).

Ultimately the responsibility lies with the patient to secure quality health care. As time goes on, more CAM modalities will be studied and the results will help guide consumers to which therapies are best for each individual person.

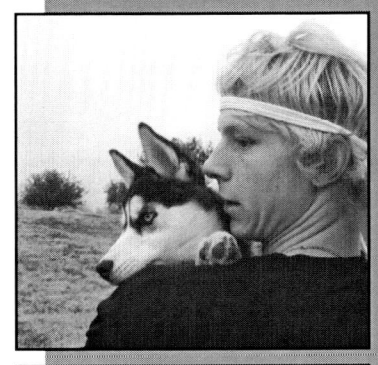
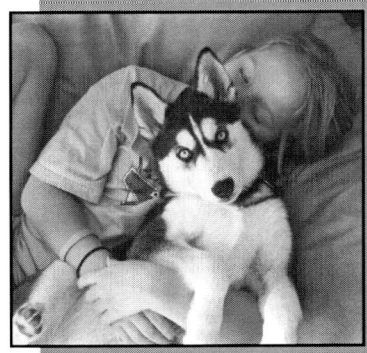
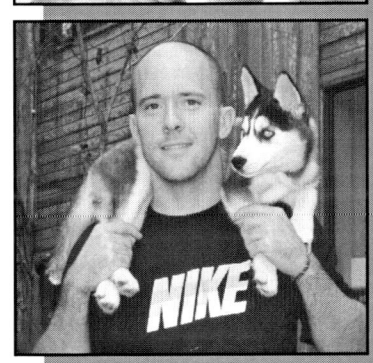
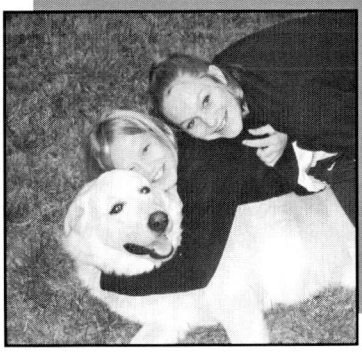

Evidence is mounting that spending time with a loved pet has emotional, psychological, and physiological benefits.

There are many more CAM therapies than are mentioned in this chapter. Conventional physicians and those they work closely with want the same things as most CAM practitioners—for patients to have good health and wellness. "The effectiveness of the healthcare delivery system in the future will depend upon its ability to make use of all approaches and modalities that provide a sound basis for promoting optimal health. People with better health habits have been shown to survive longer and to postpone and shorten disability" (WHCCAMP, 2002). Certainly many CAM practices will be useful in contributing to the nation's health goals. The modern patient is more informed and involved in his or her own health. Most likely the marriage of essential conventional practices with complementary and alternative therapeutics will be the way of the future.

Mindfulness in Everyday Life

Being mindful means focusing attention on what you're experiencing from moment to moment. It's a daunting challenge in a hectic world, but science has begun to establish that it's a worthwhile habit to cultivate. You can start by getting a sense of how much time you spend not being mindful. See if you recognize any of these statements from a questionnaire developed at the University of Rochester:

- I find it difficult to stay focused on what's happening in the present.
- I snack without paying much attention to what I'm eating.
- It seems I'm "running on automatic" without much awareness of what I'm doing.
- I rush through activities without being really attentive to them.
- I tend to walk quickly to get where I'm going without paying attention to what I experience along the way.
- I find myself listening to someone with one ear and doing something else at the same time.
- I tend not to notice physical tension or discomfort until they really grab my attention.

If these sound familiar, there's plenty of room for increasing mindfulness in your daily life. Take note of times when your thoughts are creating stress or distracting you from the present moment. The Mind/Body Medical Institute suggests that you slow down as you go about everyday activities, doing one thing at a time and bringing your full awareness to both the activity and your experience of it. Here are some tips for integrating mindfulness:

- Make something that occurs several times during the day, such as answering the phone or buckling your seat belt a reminder to return to the present—that is, think about what you're doing and observe yourself doing it.
- Pay attention to your breathing or your environment when you stop at red lights.
- Before you go to sleep, and when you awaken, take some "mindful" breaths. Instead of allowing your mind to wander over the day's concerns, direct your attention to your breathing. Feel its effects on your nostrils, lungs and abdomen. Try to think of nothing else.
- If the present moment involves stress—perhaps you're about to speak in public or undergo a medical test—observe your thoughts and emotions and how they affect your body.
- Find a task you usually do impatiently or unconsciously (standing in line or brushing your teeth, for example) and do it mindfully.

Being mindful doesn't mean you'll never "multitask," but you can make multitasking a conscious choice. It doesn't mean you'll never be in a hurry, but at least you will be aware that you are rushing. Although upsetting thoughts or emotions won't disappear, you will have more insight into them and become aware of your choices in responding to them.

From *Harvard Women's Watch*, Vol. 11, #6, February 2004.

Using the Internet for Credible Medical Information

You may find the Internet a valuable resource for researching potential CAM therapies. Using a typical search engine could net you thousands, if not more, hits. This information is intended as a resource to help you sift through the "junk mail" of sorts and to determine what is actual credible information.

Distinguish between different sorts of Web resources:

Information sites—have a domain ending .edu (education), .gov (government), .org (nonprofit organization), .net (technical services)—typically very reliable.

Advice and referral sites—look for the credentials, reputation, or experience to see if the source is credible.

Activist sites—typically promoting a particular cause rather than providing information.

Chat groups—can be unreliable but also a valuable extension of your community; a great way to connect with others sharing the same experience, such as a rare disease.

Individual testimonials—interesting but not always reliable or authoritative.

Commercial sites—the majority of Web sites are commercial and typically set up to sell products, therefore the information is usually biased.

TIP: You can avoid commercial Web sites by including "NOT .com" in your search string.

Other questions to consider:
Who is the group providing the Web site?
How is the Web site funded?
How is the information selected and presented? What are the qualifications of the author?
Does the site follow ethical practices? (The Web site should be current; check their privacy policy if they ask information from you.)

Reference: The Alternative Medicine Foundation

REFERENCES

Acupuncture Relieves Pain and Improves Function in Knee. *Osteoarthritis NIH News*, December 20, 2004 press release.

Adler, J. In Search of the Spiritual. *Newsweek*, August 29, 2005.

Alternative Medicine Foundation www.amfoundation.org

American Massage Therapy Association. www.amtamassage.org Phone (847) 864-0123

Arkow, P. *Animal Assisted Therapy: A Premise and a Promise.* http://www.animaltherapy.net/Premise%20%26%20Promise.html

Association for the Advancement of Applied Psychoneuroimmunology. http://hometown.aol.com/AAAPNI

Barnes, P. M., Bloom, B., and Nahin, R. *CDC National Health Statistics Report #12. Complementary and Alternative Medicine Use Among Adults and Children: United States, 2007.* December 10, 2008.

Chopra, D. *Ageless Body, Ageless Mind.* Harmony Books. 1993.

ClinicalTrials.gov; US National Library of Medicine, US National Institute of Health. www.clinicaltrials.gov/ct/gui/c/alb/show/NCT00010829

Corbin, C. et al. *Concepts of Physical Fitness* (15th ed). Dubuque, IA: McGraw Hill. 2009.

International Alliance of Healthcare Educators (IAHE). Craniosacral Therapy/Somatoemotional Release: Education for better patient care. 2005. http://www.iahe.come/html/therapies.cst.jsp

Donatelle, R. J. *Access to Health* (8th ed). Pearson/Benjamin Cummings. 2004.

Feldenkrais Educational Foundation of North America (FEFNA) 3611 SW Hood Ave. Suite 100 Portland, OR 97239, USA http://www.feldenkrais.com

Gach, M. R., *Acupressure's Potent Points.* Bantam Books. 1990.

Goldberg, B. *Alternative Medicine, The Definitive Guide* (2nd ed). Berkeley, CA: Celestial Arts. 2002.

Goleman, D. *Destructive Emotion: A Scientific Dialogue with the Dalai Lama.* 2003.

Alternative Medicine Foundation Information. How to Assess Credibility on the Web. 2009. www.amfoundation.org/assess.htm

Information on Clinical Trials being conducted; www.clinicaltrials.gov/ct/gui/c/alb/show/NCT00010829

Kalb, C. Faith and Healing, *Newsweek*, November 10, 2004.

Markowitz, J. et al. Effect of St John's Wort on Drug Metabolism by Induction of Cytochrome P450 3A4 Enzyme. *JAMA,* (290),1500–1503. 2003.

Naparstek, B. *Health Journeys.* 2005.

National Institutes of Health. NCCAM Online Continuing Education Lecture Series, Manipulative and Body-Based Therapies: Chiropractic and Spinal Manipulation. 2002. http://nccam.org/main.php

Psych-Neuro-Immunology http://hometown.aol.com/AAAPNI/

Pure Insight. 2005. http://pureinsight.org/PI/index/html

Saper, R. B., Phillips, R. S., Sehgal, A., et al. Lead, mercury, and arsenic in U.S. and Indian-manufactured Ayurvedic medicines sold via the Internet. *Journal of the American Medical Association*, 300(8):915–923. 2008.

Somatic Movement Studies http://www.brockport.edu/~dance/somatics/techniques.htm, 2005.

Reaves, W. Acupuncture and the Athlete, *ACSM Fit Society*, Fall 2008.

Ryzik, M. Z. Exercising That Back Pain Away. *New York Times*, September 15, 2005.

Wirth, D. P. The Effects of Non-Contact Therapeutic Touch on the Healing Rate of Full Thickness Dermal Wounds. *Subtle Energies*, Vol. 1, No. 1, 1990.

USFDA Center for Food Safety and Applied Nutrition's Dietary Supplements: Warnings and Safety Information. www.cfsan.fda.gov/~dms/ds-warn.html

White House Commission on Complementary and Alternative Medicine Policy (WHCCAMP). Final Report. 2002. *(electronic version)*

CONTACTS

Acupuncture and Oriental Medicine Alliance
www.acupuncturealliance.org

Alternative Medicine: Health Care Information Resources http://hsl.mcmaster.ca/tomflem/altmed.html This is an extremely thorough resource of alternative medicine for the informed consumer.

Alternative Medicine Foundation
www.amfoundation.org

American Massage Therapy Association
www.amtamassage.org
Phone (847) 864-0123

American Yoga Association
www.americanyogaassociation.org

The Art of Living Foundation www.artofliving.org Information on the science of the breath and it's healing qualities. Worldwide organization.

Center for Mindfulness in Medicine, Health Care, and Society; University of Massachusetts Medical School www.umassmed.edu/cfm

Complementary and Alternative Medicine: From Promises to Proof. NIH

Craniosacral Therapy Association of North America

FDA/Center for Food Safety and Applied Nutrition
http://www.cfsan.fda.gov/~dms/ds-warn.html Warnings and safety information regarding dietary supplements.

Heistand, C. http://www.orgsites.com/ca/acco/_pgg4.php3 very thorough site using CAM with cancer patients.

HerbMed http://www.herbmed.org Evidence-based herbal resource
http://nccam.nih.gov/news/images/cam-practice.htm (CAM category picture)

Medline Plus http://medlineplus.gov/ An excellent resource that is a service of the U.S. Library of Congress and the National Institute of Health.

MedWatch The FDA Safety Information and Adverse Event Reporting Program
http://www.fda.gov/medwatch

Mind/Body Medical Institute
www.mindbody.harvard.edu

Movement Educators www.movement-educators.com This site features a free Mindful Movement Lesson in the Fledenkrais method.

National Institute of Ayurvedic Medicine (NIAM)
www.niam.com

National Association of Chiropractic Medicine (NACM)
www.chiromed.org

National Institutes for Health National Center for Complementary and Alternative Medicine (NCCAM)
http://nccam.org/main.php

Nutrition Science News
http://exchange.healthwell.com/nutritionsciencenews/ information and research on natural medicine

Psych-Neuro-Immunology
http://hometown.aol.com/AAAPNI/

Psycho-Neuro-Immunolgy http://www.alpha-cs.co.za/PsychoNeurolmm.htm source of CD's to listen to harness the power of the mind to help health and well-being.

Qigong Association of America
http://www.qi.org/

Resources for Body, Mind and Spirit
www.healthjourneys.com Bellaruth Naparstek's very informative site. Ms. Napastek is a guided imagery pioneer and creator of desktopspa.com, (800) 800-8661.

Shiatsu: Japanese Massage
http://www.rianvisser.nl/shiatsu/e_index.htm This site includes a "do-in" link where you can learn specific exercises.

Somatic Movement Studies
http://www.brockport.edu/~dance/somatics/techniques.htm

Core movement patterning, Somatic Release and Contact Unwinding-educational/therapeutic techniques developed in East-West Somatics.

Tips for the Savvy Supplement User: Making Informend Decisions and Evaluating Information
http://www,cfsan.fda.gov/~dms/ds-savvy.html Dietary supplement info

University of Michigan Integrative Medicine
http://www.med.umich.edu/umim/
Source of the Healing Foods Pyramid.

USFDA Center for Food Safety and Applied Nutrition's Dietary Supplements: Warnings and Safety Information.
www.cfsan.fda.gov/~dms/ds-warn.html

White House Commission on Complementary and Alternative Medicine Policy, March 2002.

WHO Guidelines on Developing Consumer Information on Proper Use of Traditional, Complementary and Alternative Medicine.

Yoga Journal Periodical and online at www.yogajournal.com Excellent resource for all things related to yoga, relaxation, stress management and meditation.

RECOMMENDED BOOKS FOR FURTHER READING

Ageless Body, Timeless Mind. By Deepak Chopra (Harmony Books, 1993)

Awakening the Spine. By Vanda Scaravelli (HarperCollins Publishers, 1991)

Peace Is Every Step: The Path of Mindfulness in Everyday Life. By Thich Nhat Hanh (Bantam Books, 1992)

Relax and Renew By Judith Lasater (Rodmell Press, 1995)

Wherever You Go There You Are: Mindfulness Meditation in Everyday Life. By Jon Kabat-Zinn (Hyperion, 1995)

The Spectrum: A Scientifically Proven Program to Feel Better, Live Longer, Lose Weight, and Gain Health. By Dean Ornish (Ballantine Books, 2007)

Name: _____ Section: _____ Date: _____

APPENDIX

Health and Fitness Notebook Tally Sheet

Instructions: Please place this at the front of your notebook and mark all of the activities that you completed.

5-Point Activities

Personal Fitness
    Developing an Exercise Program for Cardiorespiratory Endurance   _____

Nutrition
    Food Processor   _____

Human Diseases
    Family Health Portrait   _____

3-Point Activities

Introduction
    Behavior Change and Goal Setting and Self-Evaluation Paper   _____

2-Point Activities

Introduction
    If I Had It to Do Over   _____

Stress and Psychological Health Chapter
    Stress Journal   _____

Personal Fitness
    Assessing Your Current Level of Muscular Endurance   _____
    Assessing Your Current Level of Muscular Strength   _____
    Karvonen Formula   _____

Lifestyle Choices and Hypokinetic Conditions
    Self-Assessment of Cardiovascular Fitness   _____
    Healthy Back Test   _____
    Body Fat Percentage (skin calipers or water weighing)   _____

Nutrition
    Cholesterol Level Measured   _____
    Beginning Now   _____
    Forbidden Foods   _____
    Ways I Sneak   _____

Relationships
    Relationship Report Card   _____

Human Diseases
    Blood Glucose Level   _____

1-Point Activities

Introduction
    Lifestyle Assessment Inventory   _____

Personal Fitness
    Par-Q and You   _____
    Calculating Your Activity Index   _____

Lifestyle Choices and Hypokinetic Conditions
    Blood Pressure Reading   _____

Relationships
    Relationship Readiness Assessment for Singles (Internet)   _____
    How Strong Is the Communication and Affection in Your Relationship?   _____
    Interactive Relationship Assessment Scale (Internet)   _____
    Are You in an Abusive Relationship?   _____

Sexuality
    STI Attitudes   _____
    Hepatitis Risk Assessment (Internet)   _____

Drugs
    Are You Addicted to Nicotine?   _____
    Alcohol Screening Self-Assessment   _____

Safety Awareness
    Checklist of Rape Prevention Strategies   _____

Human Diseases
    Are You at Risk for Diabetes?   _____

    TOTAL   _____

Name: _____ Section: _____ Date: _____

APPENDIX

Health and Fitness Notebook

Be certain to complete each activity for full credit.

5-Point Activities

Personal Fitness
Developing an exercise program for cardiorespiratory endurance—Complete the assignment on page 95.

Nutrition
Food Processor—Write down three days worth of food/drink in great detail (e.g. one cup of fruity pebbles with one-half cup of skim milk, six oz. orange juice, two oz. plain M&M's) before you go to Read 150, Blocker, Student Computing Center or West Campus to do the assignment. Be sure to include at least one weekend day and one weekday, not all three weekdays. Eat as normally as you can! You need to have a labs access account number if you do not already have one (e.g., to check email). Bring your ID with you to whichever computing center you choose to use. Pick up the instructions from the help desk, labeled "The Food Processor." Follow the instructions and you will have four printouts. Allow approximately one hour to complete this assignment.

Human Diseases
In order to do this project you must first research your family history. You may do an oral history or written correspondence with a family member or you may research old records. Identify your source or sources of information. Record diseases and afflictions of all known family members through your great-grandparents. Pay particular attention to genetic disorders and the age of onset. Go to www.hhs.gov/familyhistory/ and enter your information. Once you are done, print out your Family Health Portrait. Have you inherited cardiac risk factors? Common factors to consider are family history of heart disease, diabetes, high blood pressure, high cholesterol, and some forms of cancer. What, if any, diseases are you at risk for due to your family history? What can you do now to have an impact on your long-term health for the future? How do you intend to avoid becoming "at-risk" in the future? Please turn in your Family Health Portrait as well as a typed (double-spaced) paragraph on how you can live your lifestyle now to best ensure you have a long and healthy life.

3-Point Activities

Introduction
Behavior Change and Goal Setting and Self-Evaluation Paper—Complete the form on page 19.

2-Point Activities

Introduction
If I Had It to Do Over—Complete the form on page 21.

Stress and Psychological Health
Stress Journal—Complete the form on page 45.

Personal Fitness
Assessing Your Current Level of Muscular Endurance—Complete the form on page 97.

2-Point Activities (cont.)

Assessing Your Current Level of Muscular Strength—Complete the form on page 97.

Karvonen Formula—Complete the form on page 93.

Lifestyle Choices and Hypokinetic Conditions
Self-Assessment of Cardiovascular Fitness—Complete the form on page 137.

Healthy Back Test—Complete the form on page 139.

Body Fat Percentage (skin calipers or water weighing)—Performed by a licensed individual, turn in actual results from test.

Nutrition
Cholesterol Level Measured—Performed by a licensed individual, turn in actual results from test.

Beginning Now—Complete the form on page 51.

Forbidden Foods—Complete the form on page 47.

Ways I Sneak—Complete the form on page 49.

Relationships
Relationship Report Card—Complete the form on page 249.

Human Diseases
Blood Glucose Level—Performed by a licensed individual, turn in actual results from test.

1-Point Activities

Introduction
Lifestyle Assessment Inventory—Complete the form on page 17.

Personal Fitness
Par-Q and You—Complete the form on page 89.

Calculating Your Activity Index—Complete the form on page 91.

Lifestyle Choices and Hypokinetic Conditions
Blood Pressure Reading—Performed by a licensed individual, turn in actual results from test.

Relationships
Relationship Readiness Assessment for Singles (http://www.changeassociatescoaching.com/relassessment.htm). Go to the Web site, complete the questionnaire, and print your results. Turn in your answers to the questions along with the result printout for credit.

How Strong Is the Communication and Affection in Your Relationship?—Complete the form on page 245.

Interactive Relationship Assessment Scale (http://www.selfcounseling.com/help/relationships/interactiveassessment.html). Go to the Web site, complete the questionnaire, and print your results. Turn in your answers to the questions along with the result printout for credit.

Are You in an Abusive Relationship?—Complete the form on page 253.

Sexuality
STI Attitudes—Complete the form on page 309. Be sure to tally up your score for credit.

Hepatitis Risk Assessment (http://www.health.state.ny.us/nysdoh/hepatitis/en/assessment.htm). Go to the Web site, complete the questionnaire, and print your results. Turn in your answers to the questions along with the result printout for credit.

Name: _____ Section: _____ Date: _____

1-Point Activities (cont.)

Drugs
   Are You Addicted to Nicotine?—Complete the form on page 351.

   Alcohol Screening Self-Assessment—Complete the form on page 359.

Safety Awareness
   Checklist of Rape Prevention Strategies—Complete the form on page 383.

Human Diseases
   Are You at Risk for Diabetes?—Complete the form on page 417.

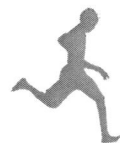

GLOSSARY

Abortion—any expulsion from the uterus of a fetus before it is able to survive.

Abstinence—refraining from something, e.g., certain foods, alcoholic beverages, or sexual intercourse.

Abuse—to mistreat or insult.

Accident—that occurrence in a sequence of events that produces unintended injury, death, or property damage.

Acquired immune deficiency syndrome—a reliably diagnosed disease that is at least moderately indicative of an underlying cellular immune deficiency, for example Kaposi's sarcoma in a patient aged less than sixty years or opportunistic infection where there is no known underlying cause of cellular immune deficiency nor any other cause of reduced resistance reported to be associated with the disease.

Activity nervosa—a condition where the individual suffers from an ever-present compulsion to exercise, regardless of illness or injury.

Acupuncture—traditional Chinese practice of inserting fine needles through the skin at specific points especially to cure disease or relieve pain (as in surgery).

Adenosine triphosphate (ATP)—high energy compound formed from oxidation of fat and carbohydrate and used as an energy supply.

Adoption—to take legally into one's own family and raise as one's own child.

Aerobic—means "in the presence of oxygen," and is used synonymously with cardiovascular.

Alcohol poisoning—an overdose of alcohol, which may lead to death.

Alcoholism—a chronic progressive disease that includes a strong need to drink alcohol despite the negative consequences.

Alimentary—pertaining to food.

Alternative healthcare systems—personalized holistic "whole person" healthcare emphasizing patient interview, history, eating habits, lifestyle choices, and so on.

Alveoli—tiny air sacs in the lungs through whose walls gases such as oxygen and carbon dioxide diffuse in and out of blood.

Amino acids—organic compounds containing carbon, hydrogen, nitrogen, and oxygen. They are the building blocks of protein.

Amphetamines—drugs that stimulate the nervous system.

Anaerobic—occurring in the absence of oxygen.

Anemia—a condition in which the blood is low in red cells or in hemoglobin, resulting in paleness and weakness.

Angina pectoris—insufficient blood flow to the heart muscle that results in severe chest and arm pain.

Anorexia nervosa—a state of starvation and emaciation usually resulting from severe dieting and excessive exercise.

Antibiotic—any of certain substances, such as penicillin or streptomycin, produced by various microorganisms and capable of destroying or weakening bacteria.

Antioxidants—compounds that come to the aid of every cell in the body facing an ongoing barrage of damage resulting from daily oxygen exposure, environmental pollution, chemicals and pesticides, additives in processed foods, stress hormones, and sun radiation.

Anus—the opening located just behind the perineum at the lower end of the alimentary canal that allows for elimination of solid waste.

Aorta—the large artery that receives blood from the left ventricle and distributes it to the body.

Arrhythmia—an irregularity in the rhythm of the heartbeat that often precedes a heart attack.

Arteriosclerosis—hardening of the arteries.

Asthma—a respiratory disorder that involves difficulty breathing, wheezing, and/or coughing due to the constriction of the bronchial tubes.

Asymptomatic—without symptoms.

Atherosclerosis—long-term buildup of fatty deposits and other substances such as cholesterol, cellular waste products, calcium, and fibrin on the interior walls of arteries.

Atria—the two upper chambers of the heart in which blood collects before passing to the ventricles.

BAC (Blood Alcohol Concentration)—the ratio of alcohol measured in the blood to total blood volume.

Bacteria—microorganisms that have no chlorophyll and multiply by simple division: some bacteria cause diseases, but others are necessary for fermentation.

Barbiturates—depressants used to induce sleep and relaxation.

Benign—non-invasive, non-cancerous (of a growth). Describes a condition or illness that is not serious and does not usually have harmful consequences.

Binge drinking—consuming five or more alcoholic beverages in one sitting for men, four for women.

Bingeing—consuming an excessive amount of food in a short period of time.

Blackout—individual has amnesia about events after drinking, though there was no loss of consciousness.

Blood pressure—the force exerted by the blood on the walls of the blood vessels; 120/80 is considered average.

Body composition—measures percentage of body fat in relation to the percentage of lean body mass (muscle, bone, and internal organs).

Breast—the mammary gland.

Bulimia nervosa—a process of bingeing and purging.

Caffeine—mild stimulant found in cola, coffee, chocolate.

Camaraderie—loyalty and warm, friendly feeling among companions.

Cancer—a disease characterized by the spread of abnormal cells that serve no useful purpose.

Carbohydrates—the body's main source of fuel. Between 55–60 percent of an individual's diet should be composed of carbohydrates.

Carbon Monoxide—odorless, tasteless gas that is highly toxic and contains carcinogens.

Carcinoma—any of several kinds of epithelial cancer.

Cardiovascular—pertaining to the heart and blood vessels.

Cardiovascular endurance—the ability of the body to perform prolonged, large-muscle, dynamic exercise at moderate-to-high levels of intensity. In order for this process to occur, the heart, lungs, and blood vessels must deliver oxygen to working muscles and the body's metabolic system must use oxygen to process fuels for sustained activity.

Cardiovascular exercise—when performed within certain guidelines, develops higher levels of cardiovascular endurance by improving the efficiency and strength of the cardiovascular system. Cardiovascular exercise uses large muscle groups in a continuous, rhythmic nature for an extended period of time.

Cervix—the neck of the uterus.

Cesarean section—delivery of the fetus through an abdominal incision.

Chemotherapy—use of a specific chemical agent to arrest the progress of, or eradicate, disease in the body without causing irreversible injury to healthy tissues.

Chiropractic—a health care approach that focuses on the relationship between the body's structure—mainly the spine—and its functioning.

Chlamydia—a sexually transmitted infection caused by a bacteria-like intracellular parasite called chlamydia trachomati, which can infect humans and birds.

Cholesterol—a crystalline substance of a fatty nature found in the brain, nerves, liver, blood, and bile. It is not easily soluble and may crystallize in the gallbladder and along arterial walls.

Clitoral hood—consists of inner lips, which join to form a soft fold of skin, or hood, covering and connecting to the clitoris.

Clitoris—a small erectile organ of the female genitalia.

Cocaine—psychoactive substance found in the leaves of the coca plant; stimulant.

Codeine—narcotic commonly found in cough suppressant.

Coercion—to restrain by force.

Cold—viral infection of the respiratory tract, causing congestion, sneezing, sore throat, coughing, and a low-grade fever.

Colon—the large bowel extending from the cecum to the rectum.

Coma—deep, prolonged unconsciousness caused by injury or disease.

Communicable—transmissible directly or indirectly from one person to another.

Communication—giving or exchanging information or messages.

Compatible—getting along or going well together.

Complex carbohydrates—provide the body with a steady source of energy for hours. The best sources of complex carbohydrates are breads, cereals, pastas, and grains.

Compromise—a settlement in which each side makes concessions.

Concede—to admit as true, valid, or certain.

Conception—the creation of a state of pregnancy; impregnation of the ovum by the sperm.

Condom (female)—a sheath, made of latex, placed into the vagina before sexual intercourse. Condoms help protect both partners against sexually transmitted infection.

Condom (male)—a rubber sheath used as a male contraceptive. Condoms help protect both partners against sexually transmitted infection.

Conviction—a strong belief.

Coronary arteries—two arteries branching from the aorta that provide blood to the heart muscle.

Cowper's glands—responsible for depositing a lubricant fluid in the semen to help with sperm motility.

Culture—a growth of bacteria or plant in a prepared substance.

Cyber—Internet.

Depo-Provera—a hormone shot injected into the arm or buttocks every twelve weeks.

Depressants—category of drugs that depress the nervous system.

Depression—a hollow or low place.

Diabetes—the result of insufficient insulin production or the body's inability to utilize insulin readily produced by the pancreas.

Diaphragm—a rubber cap that encircles the cervix to act as a contraceptive. It should be used with a spermicidal jelly or cream.

Diastolic blood pressure—the lowest arterial pressure attained during the heart cycle.

Dietary fiber (roughage or bulk)—a type of complex carbohydrate that is present mainly in leaves, roots, skins, and seeds. Dietary fiber is the part of the plant that is not digested in the small intestine, and it helps decrease the risk of cardiovascular disease, cancer, and may lower an individual's risk of coronary heart disease.

Disease—any deviation from or interruption of the normal structure and function of any part of the body. It is manifested by a characteristic set of signs and symptoms and in most instances the origin, route of transmission, and prognosis is known.

Distress—negative stress. It is a physically and mentally damaging response to the demands placed upon the body.

Divorce—to dissolve the marriage with one's spouse.

Duration—the length of time in which an activity or exercise is performed. Duration is generally expressed in minutes.

Economic—the management of income and expenditures.

Ecstasy—a drug that is chemically similar to mescaline and methamphetamines.

Ejaculation—the sudden emission of semen from the erect penis at the moment of male orgasm.

Emotion—any specific feeling, as love, hate, fear, anger, and so on.

Epidemic—a disease spreading rapidly among many people in a community.

Epididymis—a small, oblong body attached to the posterior surface of the testes. Mature sperm are stored in the epididymis until they are released during ejaculation.

Epithelium—cellular tissue covering external body surfaces or lining internal surfaces.

Essential amino acid—amino acids that the body cannot produce; thus, they must be supplied through an individual's diet.

Estrogen—a generic term referring to ovarian hormones.

Ethyl alcohol—a colorless liquid that depresses the nervous system. Made by the fermentation process and found in alcoholic beverages.

ETS (Environmental Tobacco Smoke)—secondhand smoke inhaled by the non-smoker.

Eustress—a positive stress that produces a state of well-being.

Exercise—a subcategory of physical activity that is planned, structured, repetitive, and purposive in the sense that the improvement or maintenance of one or more components of physical fitness is the objective. "Exercise" and "exercise training" frequently are used interchangeably and generally refer to physical activity performed during leisure time with the primary purpose of improving or maintaining physical fitness, physical performance, or health.

Exercise prescription—individualization of an exercise program on the basis of the exercise duration, frequency, intensity, and mode.

Exercise stress test—a test that involves analysis of the changes in electrical activity from the heart from an electrocardiogram taken during exercise.

Extravagant—going beyond the reasonable limits; wasteful or spending too much.

Fallopian tubes—tubes extending from beside the ovaries to the uterus that transport developed ovum. Fertilization usually takes place within the fallopian tubes.

Fat-soluble vitamins—vitamins transported by the body's fat cells and by the liver. They include vitamins A, E, D, and K.

Fats—the body's primary source of energy. Fat has many essential functions, including: providing the body with stored energy, insulating the body to preserve body heat, contributing to cellular structure, and protecting vital organs by absorbing shock.

Fear of obesity—an over-concern with thinness.

Fertilization—the impregnation of an ovum by a sperm.

Fetal Alcohol Syndrome—a group of physical and behavioral defects in a newborn caused by the mother's alcohol use during pregnancy.

Fibrin—insoluble blood protein formed in blood clots.

Flexibility—a health- and performance-related component of physical fitness that is the range of motion possible at a joint. Flexibility is specific to each joint and depends on a number of specific variables, including but not limited to the tightness of specific ligaments and tendons. Flexibility exercises enhance the ability of a joint to move through its full range of motion.

Foreskin—the prepuce or skin covering the glans penis.

Frequency—the number of times an exercise or activity is performed. Frequency is generally expressed in sessions, episodes, or bouts per week.

Gastrointestinal—pertaining to the stomach and intestine.

GHB (Gamma Hydroxybutrate)—a fast acting, powerful drug that depresses the nervous system.

Glucose—a simple sugar that circulates in the blood and can be used by cells to fuel ATP production.

Glycogen—a complex carbohydrate stored principally in the liver and skeletal muscles that is the major fuel source during most forms of intense exercise.

Gonorrhea—a sexually transmitted infection caused by the bacteria called Neisseria gonorrhea.

Hallucinogens—drugs that affect perception, sensation, and awareness.

Hazard—conditions or set of conditions that have the potential to produce injury and/or property damage.

Health—a state of complete physical, mental, and social well-being and not merely the absence of disease or infirmity.

Healthy—having good health.

Heart attack—when an artery that provides the heart muscle with oxygen becomes blocked or flow is decreased.

Hepatitis—inflammation of the liver in response to toxins or infective agents.

Heroin—a very strong narcotic.

Herpes—a lifelong, viral, sexually transmitted infection that can cause small blisters on the skin and mucous membranes.

High-density lipoprotein—a plasma protein relatively high in protein, low in cholesterol. HDL helps eliminate cholesterol from the body.

Honest—truthful and trustworthy.

Human chorionic gonadotropin (HCG)—a hormone produced by the placenta during pregnancy.

Human immunodeficiency virus (HIV)—a retrovirus that infects human T cells causes acquired immune deficiency syndrome.

Human papilloma viruses (HPV)—viruses that cause genital warts, some of which have a high correlation with cervical cancer.

GLOSSARY

Hymen—the thin mucous membrane that closes part or sometimes all of the opening of the vagina.

Hypertension—abnormally high blood pressure.

Hypokinetic—too little activity.

Immunotherapy—any treatment used to produce immunity.

Implantation—the insertion of living cells or solid materials into the tissues, e.g., implantation of the fertilized ovum into the endometrium.

Infection—the successful invasion, establishment, and growth of microorganisms in the tissues of the host.

Infidelity—unfaithfulness especially in marriage.

Influenza—an acute, contagious viral disease, characterized by inflammation of the respiratory tract, fever, and muscular pain.

Inhalants—chemicals that produce vapors having psychoactive effects.

Insoluble fiber—dietary fiber that does not dissolve easily in water; therefore, it cannot be digested by the body.

Insomnia—abnormal inability to sleep.

Intensity—refers to how much work is being performed or the magnitude of the effort required to perform an activity or exercise.

Intimate—very close or familiar.

Intimidate—to make afraid as with threats.

Intoxication—a transient state of physical and mental disruption due to the presence of a toxic substance such as alcohol.

Intrauterine device—a small plastic device that is inserted into the uterus to impede conception or prevent implantation of a fertilized egg.

Intravenous—directly into a vein.

Irrevocably—that which cannot be undone.

Irritable bowel syndrome—unusual motility of both small and large bowel which produces discomfort and intermittent pain, for which no organic cause can be found.

Ischemia—reduced blood flow.

Isolation—to set apart from others.

Jealous—resentfully suspicious of rivalry.

Labia majora—two longitudinal folds of skin that extend on both sides of the vulva and serve as protection for the inner parts of the vulva.

Labia minora—the delicate inner folds of skin that enclose the urethral opening and the vagina.

Lactic acid—a metabolic acid resulting from the metabolism of glucose and glycogen. Accumulation will produce fatigue.

Lactovegetarians—individuals who eat dairy products, fruits, and vegetables but do not consume any other animal products (meat, poultry, fish, or eggs).

Legume—a pod, such as that of a pea or bean that splits into two halves with the seeds attached to one of the halves.

Leukemia—a disease characterized by an abnormal increase in the number of leukocytes.

Leukoplakia—pre-cancerous condition that produces thick, rough, white patches on the gums, tongue, and inner cheek.

Lice—plural form of louse. Small, wingless parasite found on humans and some animals.

Lifestyle activities—term frequently used to encompass activities that a person carries out in the course of daily life and that can contribute to sizeable energy expenditure. Examples include taking the stairs instead of using the elevator, walking to do errands instead of driving, getting off a bus one stop early, or parking farther away than usual to walk to a destination.

Love—a passionate affection of one person for another.

Low-density lipoproteins—major cholesterol carriers that bind to receptors in various tissues, including the liver, muscle, and arteries. High levels of LDL are likely to lead to atherosclerosis.

Loyal—faithful to one's friends and ideals.

LSD (Lysergic Acid Diethylamide)—a hallucinogenic drug that distorts reality.

Lung—either of the two spongelike breathing organs in the thorax of vertebrates.

Lymphoma—any of a group of diseases resulting from the proliferation of malignant lymphoid cells.

Macrominerals—the seven minerals the body needs in relatively large quantities (100 mg or more each day).

Macronutrients—provide energy in the form of calories. They include carbohydrates, fats, and proteins.

Malignant—cancerous; a growth that tends to spread into nearby normal tissue and travel to other parts of the body.

Marijuana—from the cannabis sativa plant where the leaves and stems are dried and rolled into cigarettes.

Marriage—a close union.

Maximal oxygen consumption (VO$_2$ Max)—the highest rate of oxygen consumption an individual is capable of during maximum physical effort. Measured in ml/kg/min.

Meditation—a conscious mental process using certain techniques—such as focusing attention or maintaining a specific posture—to suspend the stream of thoughts and relax the body and mind.

Melanoma—a tumor arising from the pigment-producing cells of the deeper layers in the skin.

Meninges—the three membranes that envelop the brain and spinal cord.

Meningitis—inflammation of the meninges.

Menstruation—the flow of blood from the uterus once a month in the female. It commences about the age of thirteen years and ceases at about forty-five years of age.

MET—refers to metabolic equivalent, and one MET is the rate of energy expenditure while sitting at rest. It is taken by convention to be an oxygen uptake of 3.5 milliliters per kilogram of body weight per minute. Physical activities frequently are classified by their intensity using the MET as a reference.

Metabolism—the sum of all the vital processes by which food energy and nutrients are made available to and used by the body.

Microminerals—minerals that are essential to healthy living. They are needed in small quantities (less than 100 mg per day).

Micronutrients—regulate many bodily functions such as metabolism, growth, and development. They include vitamins and minerals.

Microorganisms—a microscopic cell. Often synonymous with bacterium but includes virus, protozoan, rickettsia, fungus, alga, and lichen.

Minerals—inorganic substances that are critical to many enzyme functions in the body.

Moderate-intensity physical activity—On an absolute scale, physical activity that is done at 3.0 to 5.9 times the intensity of rest. On a scale relative to an individual's personal capacity, moderate-intensity physical activity is usually a 5 or 6 on a scale of 0 to 10.

Mononucleosis—a self-limiting viral infection causing a sore throat, fatigue, fever, and possible spleen enlargement.

Monounsaturated fats—fats found in foods such as olives, peanuts, and canola oil, peanut oil, and olive oil.

Mons pubis—the soft fatty tissue covering the pubic symphysis on the female genitalia.

Morphine—a narcotic used for quick pain relief.

Muscle-strengthening activity (strength training, resistance training, or muscular strength and endurance exercises)—physical activity, including exercise that increases skeletal muscle strength, power, endurance, and mass.

Myocardial infarction (MI)—heart attack.

Narcotics—drugs used to relieve pain.

Nicotine—a highly addictive compound that is extremely poisonous.

Non-essential amino acids—amino acids that are manufactured in the body if food proteins in a person's diet provide enough nitrogen.

Obesity—the deposition of excessive fat around the body, particularly in the subcutaneous tissue.

Occlusion—the closure of an opening, especially of ducts or blood vessels.

Occupational illness—conditions caused by repeated exposure associated with employment.

Opium—the base substance for all narcotics.

Oral contraceptive (the pill)—a prescription medication containing the hormones estrogen and/or progestin.

Oral—pertaining to the mouth.

Osteoporosis—a disease characterized by a loss of bone density.

Ovary—female reproductive gland where eggs are produced and released usually once a month.

Over-training—a condition caused by training too much or too intensely.

Overweight—weighing in excess of the normal for one's age, height, and build; *overweight* adults typically have a body mass index of 25 to 30.

Ovolactovegetarians—a type of vegetarian who eats eggs as well as dairy products, fruits, and vegetables, but does not consume meat, poultry, and/or fish.

Parasite—one who lives at others' expense without making any useful return.

Parent—a person in relation to his or her offspring; a mother or father.

Partner—someone with whom you spend a lot of time and possibly the rest of your life.

PCP (Phencyclidine hydrochloride)—a hallucinogenic drug that blocks pain and produces numbness.

Penis—the male organ through which semen and urine pass. It has three main sections: the root, shaft, and glans penis.

Perineum—the smooth skin located between the labia minora and the anus.

Peripheral vascular disease—any abnormal condition arising in the blood vessels outside the heart, the main one being atherosclerosis, which can lead to thrombosis and occlusion of the vessel resulting in gangrene.

Pernicious—causing great injury or destruction.

Physical activity—any bodily movement produced by the contraction of skeletal muscle that increases energy expenditure above a basal level. In these Guidelines, physical activity generally refers to the subset of physical activity that enhances health.

Physical fitness—the ability to carry out daily tasks with vigor and alertness, without undue fatigue, and with ample energy to enjoy leisure-time pursuits and respond to emergencies. Physical fitness includes a number of components consisting of cardiorespiratory endurance (aerobic power), skeletal muscle endurance, skeletal muscle strength, skeletal muscle power, flexibility, balance, speed of movement, reaction time, and body composition

Polyunsaturated fats—fats found in margarine, pecans, corn oil, cottonseed oil, sunflower oil, and soybean oil.

Praise—to communicate worth or value.

Pregnancy—being with child, e.g., gestation from last menstrual period to delivery, normally 40 weeks or 280 days.

Probiotics—live microorganisms (in most cases, bacteria) that are similar to beneficial microorganisms found in the human gut. They are also called "friendly bacteria" or "good bacteria."

Progression—the process of increasing the intensity, duration, frequency, or amount of activity or exercise as the body adapts to a given activity pattern.

Prophylactic—preventive or protective; esp., preventing disease.

Prostate—a small gland at the base of the male bladder and surrounding the urethra.

Protein—essential "building blocks" of the body. They are needed for the growth, maintenance, and repair of all body tissues.

Psychoactive—mind-altering.

Psychoactive drugs—any agent that has the ability to alter moods, behavior, and perception.

Pubic—in the region of the genitals.

Pulmonary circulation—the part of the circulatory system that moves blood between the heart and lungs.

Purging—self-induced vomiting or elimination of food.

Ratings of perceived exertion—a system of monitoring exercise intensity based on assigning a number to the subjective perception of target intensity.

Rectum—the lowest or last segment of the large intestine.

Relationship—connection by blood or marriage.

Repetitions—the number of times a person lifts a weight in muscle-strengthening activities. Repetitions are analogous to duration in aerobic activity.

Respiratory system—deals with gaseous exchange. Comprises the nose, nasopharynx, larynx, trachea, bronchi, and lungs.

Reye's syndrome—consists of cerebral edema without cellular infiltration. Presents with vomiting, lethargy, confusion, rapid heartbeat, and respiration. May progress into a coma. There is an association with aspirin administration and viral infections.

Risk—the probability that a hazard will be activated and produce injury and/or property damage.

Rohypnol—a drug prescribed for sleep disorders; potent tranquilizer; "date rape drug."

Sacrifice—to give up one thing for the sake of another.

Sarcoma—a malignant growth of the connective tissue including muscles and bones.

Saturated fats—fats found primarily in animal products such as meats, lard, cream, butter, cheese, and whole milk.

Scabies—a highly contagious, itching skin disease caused by a mite that burrows under the skin to lay its eggs.

Scrotum—the pouch in the male that contains the testes.

Secretion—a fluid or substance formed or concentrated in a gland and passed into the alimentary tract, the blood, or to the exterior.

Self-esteem—belief in oneself.

Self-worth—the value placed upon oneself.

Semen—the fluid secreted from the testicles and accessory male organs, e.g., prostate.

Semivegetarian—a person who eats fruits, vegetables, dairy products, eggs, and a small selection of poultry, fish, and other seafood. These individuals do not consume any beef or pork.

Sexually transmitted infection—an infection (bacterial, parasitic, or viral) that is transmitted during vaginal, oral, or anal sexual activity, or in some cases by simply touching an infected area.

Sickle-cell anemia—an inherited chronic anemia found chiefly among African Americans, in which red blood cells become sickle-shaped due to defective hemoglobin.

Simple carbohydrates—sugars that have little nutritive value beyond their energy content.

Soluble fiber—dietary fiber that dissolves in water.

Sperm—an abbreviated form of the word spermatozoon or spermatozoa.

Spermicide—an agent that kills spermatozoa.

Sterilization—an operation performed on the female (tubal ligation) or male (vasectomy) to permanently prevent conception.

Strength—a health and performance component of physical fitness that is the ability of a muscle or muscle group to exert force.

Stress—the nonspecific response to demands placed on the body. "Nonspecific response" alludes to the production of the same physiological reaction regardless of the type of stress placed on the body.

Stroke volume—the amount of blood pumped with each heartbeat.

Stroke—the vessels that supply the brain with nutrients become damaged or occluded and the brain tissue dies.

Symphysis—joint of the pubic bones in the female.

Symptom—any circumstance or condition that indicates the existence, as of a particular disease.

Synthesize—the combining together of parts to form a whole.

Syphilis—a serious bacterial infection caused by the spirochete Treponema pallidum. This sexually transmitted infection can have three stages and be fatal.

Systemic circulation—the part of the circulatory system that moves blood between the heart and the rest of the body.

Systolic blood pressure—the highest arterial blood pressure attained during the heart cycle.

Tar—by product of burning tobacco; dark sticky substance which contains carcinogens.

Target heart rate zone—the range of heart rates that should be reached and maintained during cardiovascular endurance exercise to obtain training effects.

Testes—the reproductive glands inside the scrotum, which are also referred to as testicles. Sperm and hormone production are the two main functions of the testes.

THC (Tetrahydrocannabinol)—the active ingredient in marijuana.

Threat—an expression of intention to hurt, destroy, or punish.

Thrifty—not wasteful.

Thrombosis—the intravascular formation of a blood clot.

Tolerance—a condition in which an individual adapts to the amount of drug consumed to experience the same effects, e.g., alcohol use, and so on.

Triglyceride—an ester derived from glycerol, the chief component of fats and oils.

Trust—a firm belief in the honesty, reliability of another.

Tuberculosis—an infectious disease characterized by the formation of tubercles in body tissue; primarily affecting the lungs.

Ulcer—an open sore on the skin or some mucous membrane, discharging pus.

Unsaturated fats—fats derived primarily from plant products.

Urethra—the passage from the bladder through which urine is excreted.

Uterus—the hollow, pear-shaped muscular organ into which the ovum is received from the fallopian tubes and where it is retained during fetal development. When a female is not pregnant, it is about the size of a fist.

Vaccine—any preparation used to produce immunity to a specific disease.

Vagina—a sheath; the canal from the cervix to the vulva.

Values—beliefs or standards.

Vas deferens—a long tube through which sperm travel during ejaculation.

Vegans—true vegetarians. Their diets contain absolutely no meat, chicken, fish, eggs, or milk products.

Venae cavae—the large veins through which blood is returned to the right atrium of the heart.

Ventricles—the two lower chambers of the heart from which blood flows through arteries to the lungs and other parts of the body.

Vigorous-intensity physical activity—on an absolute scale, physical activity that is done at 6.0 or more times the intensity of rest. On a scale relative to an individual's personal capacity, vigorous-intensity physical activity is usually a 7 or 8 on a scale of 0 to 10.

Viral—involving, or caused by a virus.

Virus—tiny, infective agents that can multiply in plants and animals, causing various diseases.

Vitamins—organic substances that are necessary for normal body metabolism, growth, and development.

Vulva—the external female genitalia.

Water-soluble vitamins—vitamins not stored in the body for a significant amount of time. Amounts that are consumed and not used relatively quickly by the body are excreted through urine and sweat. Examples include the B vitamins and vitamin C.

Wellness—a process of making informed choices that will lead one, over a period of time, to a healthy lifestyle that should result in a sense of well-being.

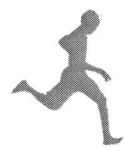

INDEX

Note: Page numbers followed by "f" indicate figures; those followed by "t" indicate tables.

A

Abdominal wall, 71
Abortion, 279–280
Abstinence, 268
Abusive relationships, 238–239
    explosion phase, 238
    honeymoon phase, 238
    tension phase, 238
Accident causes
    bicycle, 366–367
    cell phone usage, 364
    disaster planning, 369, 370f
    drowsy driving, 364–365
    falls, 367
    fires and burns, 367–368
    home accidents, 367–368
    motorcycles, 366
    public accidents, 368
    work accidents, 368
Accidental death, causes of, 365f
Acquaintance rape, 376–377
ACSM; *see* American College of Sports Medicine
Actinic keratosis, 400
Active resistance, 375
Activity, 66; *see also* Physical activity
Activity nervosa, 36
Activity pyramid, 60f
Acupressure, 425
Acupuncture, 425–426, 425f
Adderall, 333
Addictive behavior, 357–358
Adoption, 279
Adrenaline, 24
Aerobic exercise, 58, 62–63, 67
    benefits of, 59–60, 62
    and cardiovascular fitness, 59–62
    defined, 62
Aging, 131–133
    and creativity, 132
AHA; *see* American Heart Association
AIDS, 288–290, 289t, 291t, 388; *see also* HIV
Air displacement method, 199
Alcohol, 334–336
    absorption and elimination, 337f
    binge drinking, 340
    drinking and driving, 337–339
    drinking problems, 342–343
    influence of, 338t
    intoxication, 336
    physiological effects, 336
    poisoning, 341–342
    prevalence, 334
    screening, 359–360
    societal problems, 337
    tolerance, 336
    use in college, 340, 341f
Alcohol abuse, 342–344
    long-term risks, 344f
Alcohol cirrhosis, 345
Alcoholic beverages, 150
Alcoholic hepatitis, 345
Alcoholism, 343–344
    chronic effects, 344–345
    organizations, 345
    signs and symptoms, 343
Alcohol laws, 336–337
    Driving Under the Influence (DUI), 336
    Minor in Possession (MIP), 336
    Zero Tolerance Law, 336
Alcohol pellagra, 345
Alternative healthcare systems, 424
    acupressure, 425
    acupuncture, 425–426, 425f
    ayurveda, 424
    homeopathy, 425
    naturopathy, 425
    Shiatsu, 426
Alternative medicine, 421
American College of Sports Medicine (ACSM), 55, 59, 107
American Heart Association (AHA), 55, 59, 107
American Red Cross, 369
Amino acids, 156
    essential, 158
    non-essential, 156
Amphetamines, 322–323
Anabolic steroids, 332–333
Anaerobic exercise, 62–63
    defined, 62
Anatomy
    female sexual anatomy, 256–258, 256f, 257f
    male sexual anatomy, 258–260, 259f
Anemia, 411
Aneurysm, 112
Angina pectoris, 61
Animal-assisted therapy, 435
Annals of Internal Medicine, 426
Anorexia nervosa, 34–35, 37
Anterograde amnesia, 330
Antioxidants, 162–163
    food sources, 162t
Aplastic anemia, 411
Appetite suppressants, 205–206
Applegate, Elizabeth, 212–214
Applied psycho-neuro-immunology, 433–434
Arteriosclerosis, 111–112
    defined, 111
Asthma, 407
Atherosclerosis, 112–113, 112f
Athlete triad, female, 36, 37f
Athletic shoes; *see* Footwear
Ayurveda, 424

B

BAC; *see* Blood alcohol concentration
Back muscles, 71
Bacterial meningitis, 393
Ballistic stretching, 78
Barbiturates, 327
Bars; *see* Energy bars
Basal cell carcinoma, 398
Beans, 168
Behavior change, 6–11, 19
    factors influencing on, 7f
Behavior modification planning, 28f, 30f
Belcher, Steve, 430
Benzodiazepines, 326
Bicycle safety, 366–367, 366f
Binge drinking, 340
Binge-eating disorder, 36
    recovery from, 38
Bioenergy, 435
Biological age, 131
Biological-based therapies, 428–431
    functional foods, 430, 431t
    herbals and dietary supplements, 428–430
    macrobiotics, 428
    vitamins and minerals, 430
Birth control; *see* Pregnancy prevention
Bisphenol A (BPA), 371
Blood
    route during gas transport, 61f
    testing, 287, 299

457

Blood alcohol concentration (BAC), 335, 338, 339f, 339t
Blood pressure classification, 115t
BMI; *see* Body Mass Index
Body composition, 199
    changes in, 76f
Body image, 197
Body mass index (BMI), 125, 198, 198t
    formula for, 199, 219
Body weight, healthy, 198–200
BPA; *see* Bisphenol A
Brain attack, 119
Brain dominance, 234t
Breast cancer, 126, 402–404, 403t
Breast self-exam (BSE), 402
Bulimia nervosa, 35–37

C

Caffeine, 324
    sources of, 325t
Caloric balance, 195f
Calorie needs
    determining, 199, 200t
    nutrients within, 147
Calories, 178–179
    consumed fat, 153t
    expenditure *vs.* death, 106
    percentage of fat in foods, 154t
    requirements, 200t
CAM; *see* Complementary and alternative medicine
Cancer, 125–126, 345, 396–407, 397t
    breast, 126, 402–404, 403t
    carcinoma, 396
    causing agents, 315
    cervical, 404–406
    colon and rectum, 407
    and exercise, 125–126
    leukemia, 396
    and lifestyle, 125
    lung, 319f, 402
    oral, 407
    and physical activity, 126t
    prevention of, 125, 398t
    risk factors, 396
    sarcomas, 396
    screening guidelines for detection, 405f
    skin, 398–402
    testicular, 406–407
    treatment, 396
Cannabis, 328
Cannabis sativa, 328
Carbohydrates, 149, 151
    complex, 151
    simple, 151
Carbon monoxide, 315, 317
    poisoning, 367
Carcinoma, 396
Cardiorespiratory endurance, 95
Cardiovascular disease (CVD), 108
    contributing risk factors for, 121
    controlled risk factors for, 120–121
    measuring health risk, 109–111
    prevention of, 109
    risk factor for, 113
    uncontrolled risk factors for, 121
Cardiovascular endurance, 58, 69
Cardiovascular fitness, 58–62
    assessing, 101
    defined, 58
    evaluating, 68–71
    measure of, 68
    self-assessment, 137
Carpal tunnel syndrome (CTS), 368
Casual friendships, 226
2C-B, 332
CDC; *see* Centers for Disease Control and Prevention
Cell phone usage, 364
Centers for Disease Control and Prevention (CDC), 59, 107
Cervical cancer, 404–406
Chewing tobacco; *see* Smokeless tobacco; Tobacco
Childhood obesity, 123–124, 195
    causes of, 124–125
Chiropractic treatment, 426–427
Chlamydia, 281, 282f
Chlamydia trachomati, 281
Cholesterol, 114t, 120–121
Chronic Obstructive Pulmonary Diseases (COPD), 316
Chronological age, 131
Cigarettes, 314–322
    clove, 317
Cigarette smoking, 120, 314–322; *see also* Smoking; Tobacco
    vs. water pipe smoking, 318f
Circulatory system, 61
Cirrhosis, 345
CLE; *see* Cutaneous lupus erythematosus
Clery, Jeanne, 374
Clery Act, 374
Clothing and exercise, 79
Clove cigarettes, 317
Club drugs
    2C-B, 332
    gamma hydroxybutyrate (GHB), 330, 332
    ketamine hydrochloride, 332
    MDMA, 330
    rohypnol, 330
CMV; *see* Cytomegalovirus
Cocaine, 323–324
Codeine, 327
Cold; *see* Common cold
Collateral arteries, 113
College campuses, 373–374
    sexual assault, 375–376
    stalking, 374–375
College students, 373
Colon and rectum cancer, 407
Common cold, 394, 395t
Communicable diseases, 388–395
    common cold, 394, 395t
    hepatitis; *see* Hepatitis
    HIV/AIDS, 388
    meningitis, 393–394, 394f
    mononucleosis, 389–390
    TB, 388–389
Communication
    nonverbal, 224
    open, 224–225
    verbal, 224
Complementary and alternative medicine (CAM), 420, 422f
Condom, 262, 269–270
Consumer Product Safety Commission (CPSC), 366
Contraceptives; *see* Pregnancy prevention
Conventional medicine, 420
COPD; *see* Chronic Obstructive Pulmonary Diseases
Core musculature in functional movement, 71
Coronary artery disease, 113
Crack cocaine; *see* Cocaine
Craniosacral therapy, 427–428
Creeping obesity, 200
Crime Awareness and Campus Security Act of 1990, 374–375
Crimes, 372
    on college campuses, 373–374
CTS; *see* Carpal tunnel syndrome
Cutaneous lupus erythematosus (CLE), 411
CVD; *see* Cardiovascular disease

D

Date rape, 233, 376
    drug, 330
Dating, 230–231
    activities, 232
Death
    and caloric expenditure, 106f
    leading causes of, 10f, 105f
Dehydration, 82, 83, 164
    adverse effect of, 84t
    progressive effect of, 164
Delayed-onset muscle soreness, 74
Department of Health and Human Services (DHHS), 107, 146
Depo-Provera, 274
Depressants, 326
    barbiturates, 327
    benzodiazepines, 326
Depression
    and exercise, 31–32
    and stress, 31–32
Destructive Emotions (Goleman), 432
DHHS; *see* Department of Health and Human Services
Diabetes, 121, 126–127, 408–411, 408f, 409f
    exercise and, 127
    gestational, 409
    prevention of, 127
    risk for, 410, 417–418
    Type I, 408
    Type II, 127, 408, 409
Diaphragm, 274–275
Diastolic blood pressure, 59

Diet
  choosing, 155
  daily recommendations, 156f
  fad, 202, 207, 208
  liquid, 207
  low-carbohydrate, 206
  vegetarian, 171
Dietary analysis, 183–185
Dietary fiber, 151, 165, 178
  insoluble, 151
  soluble, 151
  sources of, 152t
Dietary Guidelines for Americans,
    recommendations of, 146
  adequate nutrients within calorie
    needs, 147
  alcoholic beverages, 150
  carbohydrates, 149
  fats, 149
  food groups, 148–149
  food safety, 150
  physical activity, 148
  sodium and potassium, 149–150
  weight management, 147
Dietary habits, 146
Dietary reference intakes (DRIs),
    163t
Dietary supplements, 77, 204–205,
    428–430
Diet books, guide to ratings of,
    208f–209f
Dieting
  reasons to give up, 204
  yo-yo, 202
Diet plans, guide to ratings of,
    210f–211f
Disaster planning, 369, 370f
Diseases
  communicable; *see*
    Communicable diseases
  non-communicable; *see* Non-
    communicable diseases
  prevention of, 11
Distress, 24
Domestic violence, 377
Dowager's hump; *see* Kyphosis
Drinking and driving; *see* Alcohol;
    Driving Under the Influence
    (DUI)
Driving Under the Influence (DUI),
    336, 338t
Drowsy driving, 364–365
Drug-induced lupus, 411
Drug Induced Rape Prevention and
    Punishment Act of 1996, 332
Drugs; *see also* Club drugs
  alcohol, 334–345
  prescription, 333–334
  psychoactive; *see* Psychoactive
    drugs
  tobacco, 314–322
Drunk driving, 338, 339f, 339t, 365
Dual energy X-ray absorptiometry
    (DEXA), 199
DUI; *see* Driving Under the
    Influence
Duodenal ulcers, 412

E

Eating disorders
  activity nervosa, 36
  anorexia nervosa, 34–35, 37
  binge-eating disorder, 36
  bulimia nervosa, 35–37
  causes of, 37–38
  fear of obesity, 36
  helping with, 39, 40
  risk factors for, 34f
  and stress, 33–34
EBV; *see* Epstein-Barr virus
Ecstasy; *see* MDMA
Egg and fertilization, 264f, 265f
Emergency contraception (EC),
    morning after pill, 278
Emotional dimensions of wellness,
    2–3
Endometrial cycle, 264–265
Energy bars, 212–215
  40-30-30 bars, 213–214
  high-carb bars, 212–213
  high-protein bars, 214
  supplement bars, 214–215
Energy therapies, 435–436
  qi gong, 435
  reiki, 435
  therapeutic touch, 435
Environmental conditions
  and exercise, 82–83
  heat exhaustion, 82
Environmental dimension of
    wellness, 4
Environmental Protection Agency
    (EPA), 370
Environmental safety, 369–370
Environmental tobacco smoke
    (ETS), 318, 398
EPA; *see* Environmental Protection
    Agency
Ephedrine, 326
Epstein-Barr virus (EBV), 389
Essential amino acids, 158
Essential nutrients, 151
  antioxidants, 162–163
  carbohydrates, 151
  fats, 151–156
  minerals, 160–162
  protein, 156–158
  vitamins, 158–160
  water, 164
Ethyl alcohol, 334
ETS; *see* Environmental tobacco
    smoke
Eugenol, 317
Eustress, 24
Excedrin®, 324
Exercise, 196, 421
  aerobic; *see* Aerobic exercise
  anaerobic; *see* Anaerobic exercise
  benefits of, 108, 109
  cancer and, 125–126
  and clothing, 79
  and depression, 31–32
  and diabetes, 127
  and environmental conditions,
    82–83
  guide for related problems, 80t
  in heat, 82
  and low back pain, 128
  meditation, 432
  and osteoporosis, 130
  safety of, 89
  stretching; *see* Stretching
    exercises
  and weight loss, 201, 202
Exercise prescription
  frequency, 63
  intensity, 63
  time, 64
  type, 65
Exercise session, 65–66
  activity, 66
  cooldown and stretch, 66
  pre-stretch, 66
  warm-up, 65–66

F

Fad diets, 202, 207–208
Fast foods, 196, 215
Fatness, 125, 215–216
Fats, 149, 151–156
  calories in foods, 154t
  composition in oils, 153t
  essential functions, 152
  excess distribution of, 122f
  monounsaturated, 153
  polyunsaturated, 153
  saturated, 152
  trans, 153, 178, 195
  unsaturated, 153
  upper limit on consuming, 153t
Fat-soluble vitamins, 158
Fear of obesity eating disorder, 36
Federal Emergency Management
    Agency (FEMA), 369
Federal Trade Commission (FTC), 428
Feldenkrais method, 434
Female athlete triad, 36, 37f
Female sexual anatomy, 256–258,
    256f, 257f
  anal canal, 257
  clitoral hood, 256
  clitoris, 256
  fallopian tube, 257
  hymen, 257
  labia majora, 256
  labia minora, 256
  mons pubis, 256
  perineum, 257
  urethra, 256
  vagina, 257
  vulva, 256
Female sexual response, 258
Femcap, 274–275
Fertility awareness-based methods
    (FAMs), 268–269
Fertilization, 264f, 265, 265f
Fetal alcohol syndrome, 345
Fetal development, 266f
Fiber
  dietary, 151, 152t, 165, 178
  insoluble, 151
  soluble, 151

Financial wellness, 4–5
Fires and burns, 367–368
Fitness, 125, 215–216
 cardiovascular; *see* Cardiovascular fitness
 health-related, 58
 muscular, 58, 69
 skill-related, 58
Fitness training, principles of, 66–68
 individual differences, 67–68
 overload and adaptation, 66–67
 reversibility, 68
 specificity, 67
FITT (frequency, intensity, time, type), 63–65
Flexibility, 58, 77–79
 defined, 78
 training, 67
Flu; *see* Influenza
Flunitrazepam, 330
Food
 eating out, 215
 fast foods, 196, 215
 fat calories in, percentage of, 154t
 functional, 171
 functional components, 172t–174t
 junk food, 123, 215
 labels, 176, 177f
 organic, 170–171
 safety, 150
 shopping, 210–211
Food and Drug Administration (FDA), 315, 326, 333, 334, 426
Food groups
 recommendation, 148–149
 servings, 169t
Food Guide Pyramid, 157t, 165
 daily activity, 168
 "fat" group, 168–169
 fruits, 167
 grains, 165
 meats and beans, 168
 milk, 168
 oils, 168
 serving sizes, 175t
 vegetables, 167
Footwear, 81–82
 purchase, 81
 sport-specific, 81
Friendships, levels of, 226
Fruits, 167
FTC; *see* Federal Trade Commission
Functional foods, 171, 430, 431t
 components, 172t–174t
Functional movement, core musculature in, 71
Functional strength, 78

G

Gamma hydroxybutyrate (GHB), 330, 332
Gas transport, blood route during, 61f
Gastric ulcers, 412

Gastrointestinal disorders, 412
Genital herpes, 288
Gestational diabetes, 409
Glutes, 71
Glycogen, 62
Gonorrhea, 283–284, 284f
Grains, 165
 of wheat, 167f
Guided imagery, 434

H

Hallucinogens, 328
 lysergic acid diethylamide, 328
 phencyclidine hydrochloride, 329
HCG; *see* Human chorionic gonadotropin
HDL; *see* High-density lipoprotein
Health
 behaviors, 12
 defined, 2
 factors influencing on, 5f, 11
Health-related fitness, 58
Healthy dining, tips for, 216
Healthy habits
 food shopping, 210–211
 weight gain, 209
Healthy People 2010, 11–12, 107
 focus areas, 12–13
Healthy relationships, 224
Heart, blood flow in, 61
Heart attack, 115–119
 narrowed or blocked arteries, 116f
 risk reduction in, 118f
 symptoms and warning signs, 117
Heart disease, risk of, 114t
Heart rate range, target, 63, 64f
Heat exhaustion, 82
Heat-humidity chart, 83f
Heat injuries, 82
Helicobacter pylori, 412
Helmet laws, 366
Hepatitis
 hepatitis A, 390–392
 hepatitis B, 292–293, 392
 hepatitis C, 392–393
 hepatitis D, E, and G, 393
 risk assessment, 311
 viral, 390, 391t, 392f
Hepatotoxic trauma, 344
Herbals and dietary supplements, 428–430
Heroin, 327
Herpes simplex virus (HSV), 288
High blood pressure; *see* Hypertension
High-density lipoprotein (HDL), 195, 332
High-protein diets, 207
Hip muscles, 71
HIV, 288–290, 388; *see also* AIDS
Holistic self-care, 421
Home accidents, 367–368
Homeopathy, 425

Homeostasis, 24
Homophobia, 260
Homosexual orientation, 260
HPV; *see* Human papilloma viruses
HSV; *see* Herpes simplex virus
Human chorionic gonadotropin (HCG), 267
Human papilloma viruses (HPV), 290–292
Hydrocodone, 333
Hydrostatic weighing, 199
Hypertension, 113, 115f, 120
Hypokinetic conditions, 85, 103–134
 arteriosclerosis, 111–112
 atherosclerosis, 112–113
 cardiovascular disease (CVD), 108
 heart attack, 115–119
 hypertension, 113
 peripheral vascular disease, 113
 prevention of, 133–134
 stroke, 119
 types of, 108–119
Hyponatremia, 83–84

I

IDU; *see* Injecting drug use
Illness, 84
Inactivity, 121
 effects on older men, 132t
Individual differences principle, 67–68
Influenza, 395
Inhalants, 329–330
Injecting drug use (IDU), 292
Injuries, 79
 heat, 82
 unintentional, 364
Insoluble fiber, 151
Intellectual dimension of wellness, 3
Intimate violence, 377
Intoxication, 336, 337
 assault, 337
 manslaughter, 337
Intrauterine device (IUD), 275–276
Iron-deficiency anemia, 411
Irritable bowel syndrome (IBS), 412
IUD; *see* Intrauterine device

J

Junk food, 123, 215

K

Karvonen formula, 93
Kernel, 165
Ketamine hydrochloride, 332
Kinsey, Alfred, 260
Kinsey scale of sexual behavior, 261f
Korsakoff's syndrome, 345
Kyphosis, 129

L

Lactovegetarians, 171
Last menstrual period (LMP), 267, 279
Lats, 71
LDL; *see* Low-density lipoproteins
Leukemia, 396
Leukoplakia, 316
Life expectancy, 9f, 104
Lifestyle
    activity, 104
    assessment, 17
    change in habits, 202, 203
    choices, 103–134
Liquid diets, 207
Liver disease, 344
LMP; *see* Last menstrual period
Love
    defined, 230, 236
    types of, 236
Low back pain, 128
    exercise and, 128
    prevention of, 128
Low-carbohydrate diets, 206
Low-density lipoproteins (LDL), 152, 153, 195
Lung cancer, 402
    risks, 319f
Lupus, 411–412
Lysergic acid diethylamide (LSD), 328

M

Macrobiotics, 428
Macrominerals, 160
Macronutrients, 146
Male sexual anatomy, 258–260, 259f
    Cowper's glands, 259
    epididymis, 258, 259
    foreskin, 258
    glans penis, 258
    penis, 258
    scrotum, 258
    seminal vesicle, 259
    testes, 258
    vas deferens, 259
Male sexual response, 260
Malignant melanoma, 398
Malnutrition, 345
Manipulative and body-based therapies, 426–428
    chiropractic treatment, 426–427
    craniosacral therapy, 427–428
    massage, 427, 427f
    reflexology, 427
Marijuana; *see* Cannabis
Marriage
    characteristics of happy, 237
    tips for successful, 237
Massage, 427, 427f
Maximum oxygen uptake, 68
MDMA, 330
Meats, 168
Medical information, using internet for, 437

Meditation, 431–433, 431f
    exercise, 432
Melanomas, 400, 401; *see also* Skin cancer
Meningitis, 394f
    bacterial, 393
    diagnosis of, 394
    viral, 393
Menstrual cycle, 263–264, 263f
Mental health, 421
Mental health disorder, 30; *see also* Depression
Metabolic syndrome, 127–128
Metabolism boosters, 206–207
Methamphetamine, 323
Microbial foodborne illness, 150
Microminerals, 160, 162
Micronutrients, 146
Milk, 168
Mind-body medicine, 431–435
    animal-assisted therapy, 435
    applied psycho-neuro-immunology, 433–434
    Feldenkrais method, 434
    guided imagery, 434
    meditation, 431–433, 431f
    mindfulness, 436
    prayer and spirituality, 433, 434
    somatic movement, 435
    spiritual health, 433
    yoga, 434
Mindfulness, 436
Minerals, 160–162, 430
    facts about selected, 161t
    macrominerals, 160
    microminerals, 160, 162
Minor In Possession (MIP), 336
Moles, 401
Mononucleosis, 389–390
Monospot agglutination test, 389
Monounsaturated fats, 153
Morphine, 327
Motorcycle safety, 366
Motor vehicle accidents, 364, 368
Muscles
    major anterior, 72–73
    pelvic floor, 71
Muscle soreness
    delayed-onset, 74
    prevention of, 74
    weight training, 74
Muscular endurance, assessing, 97
Muscular fitness, 58, 69
    benefits of, 70–71
Muscular strength, 69
Mycobacterium tuberculosis, 388
Myocardial infarction, 61; *see also* Heart attack
My Pyramid, 166f, 168, 176f, 190–192; *see also* Food Guide Pyramid

N

Narcotics
    codeine, 327
    heroin, 327

    morphine, 327
    opium, 327
National Climatic Data Center (NCDC), 368
National Crime Prevention Council (NCPC), 372
National Health Interview Study (NHIS), 421
National Heart, Lung, and Blood Institute Obesity Guidelines, 210
National Highway Traffic Safety Administration (NHTSA), 364
National Institute on Alcohol Abuse and Alcoholism (NIAAA), 334, 340, 342, 345, 375
National Institute on Drug Abuse (NIDA), 333
National Safety Council (NSC), 364
National Sleep Foundation (NSF), 364
National Sports and Physical Education (NASPE), 55
Nature and spirituality, 433
Naturopathy, 425
Neisseria gonorrhea, 283
Neonatal lupus, 411
NIAAA; *see* National Institute on Alcohol Abuse and Alcoholism
Nicotine, 314, 315, 318
Non-communicable diseases, 396–412
    anemia, 411
    asthma, 407
    cancer, 396–407, 397t
    gastrointestinal disorders, 412
    lupus, 411–412
Non-essential amino acids, 156
Non-melanoma skin cancers, 400
Nutrients
    adequate intakes for, 163t
    within calorie needs, 147
    essential; *see* Essential nutrients
    recommended daily allowance (RDA) for, 163t
Nutrition facts label, 176–179, 177f
    accuracy requirements, 178
    daily values (DVs), 178

O

Obesity, 121–122, 200
    causes of, 124–125, 194–196
    childhood, 123, 195
    creeping, 200
    fear of, 36
    by gender, 58
    health risks, 121, 196
    medical cost associated with, 201f
    overweight, 194–196, 200
    physiological response to, 125
    prevention, 200–201
    by race, 58f
Occlusion, 112
Occupational dimension of wellness, 3

Occupational illnesses, 368
Oils, 168
    fat composition in, 153t
Omega-3 fatty acids, 171
O'Neil, Patrick, 194, 195
Open communication, 224–225
Opium, 327
Oral cancer, 407
Organic foods, 170–171
Osteoporosis, 129–131
    bone loss, 131
    and exercise, 130
    prevention of, 130
    risk of, 129
Ovarian cycle, 264
Ovaries, 258
Over-hydration; see Hyponatremia
Overload and adaptation principle, 66–67
Over-the-counter drugs (OTC), 428
Overweight, 194–196, 200
    children and adolescents, 122t, 123f
Ovolactovegetarians, 171
Oxycodone, 333

P

Pap smear, 406
Parenthood, 278–279
Passive resistance, 376
Pelvic floor muscles, 71
Pelvic inflammatory disease (PID), 281, 284–286
    causes of, 284
Peripheral vascular disease, 113
Pernicious anemia, 411
Personal safety, 372
    tips for, 372–373
Personal watercraft (PWC), 368
Phencyclidine hydrochloride, 329
Physical activity, 54–58, 108, 196f, 203t
    cancer and, 126t
    effects on older men, 132t
    guidelines, 56f
    health benefits of, 57f
    program, 67
    recommendation, 148
Physical dimension of wellness, 3
The "pill," 270–271
Pipe smoking, 317
PMS; see Premenstrual syndrome
PNF; see Proprioceptive neuromuscular facilitation
Poisoning
    alcohol, 341–342
    carbon monoxide, 367
Polyneuritis, 345
Polyunsaturated fats, 153
Portion size, 195, 197
Positive self-worth, 224
Potassium, 149–150
Prayer and spirituality, 433, 434
Pregnancy, 265–267, 266f
    and sexually transmitted infections, 267, 277t
    unplanned, 278

Pregnancy prevention, 277t
    abstinence, 268
    contraceptive implants, 276
    contraceptive patch, 272–274
    Depo-Provera, 274
    diaphragm, 274–275
    femcap, 274–275
    fertility awareness-based methods (FAMs), 268–269
    intrauterine device (IUD), 275–276
    male condom, 269–270
    over-the-counter contraceptives, 275
    the pill, 270–271
    sterilization, 276–277
    vaginal ring, 271–272
    withdrawal method, 268
Premenstrual syndrome (PMS), 264, 324
Prescription drugs, 333–334
Pre-stretch, 66
Proprioceptive neuromuscular facilitation (PNF), 79
Protein, 156–158
    essential amino acids, 158
    non-essential amino acids, 156
Protein bars, 214
Psychedelics; see Hallucinogens
Psychiatric disorders, 34
Psychoactive drugs, 322–327, 331t
    anabolic steroids, 332–333
    cannabis, 328
    club drugs, 330, 332
    depressants, 326–327
    hallucinogens, 328
    inhalants, 329–330
    narcotics, 327
    prescription drugs, 333–334
    stimulants, 322–326
Pubic lice, 293, 298
Public accidents, 368

Q

Qi, 426
Qi gong, 435

R

Rape
    acquaintance rape, 376–377
    active resistance, 375
    date rape, 233, 376
    passive resistance, 376
    prevention strategies, 383–386
Rating of perceived exertion scale (RPE), 63
Recommended daily allowance (RDA) for selected nutrients, 163t
Recovery heart rate, 68
Reflexology, 427
Reiki, 435
Relationships
    abusive, 238–239, 253
    arguing fairly, 235
    communication and affection in, 245

    compromise in, 225
    ending, 235–237
    healthy, 224
    interactive, 251
    jealous partner, 234
    marriage, 237
    readiness assessment, 243–244
    report card, 247–248
    stages, 229–237
    trust in, 226
    types of, 226–227
    unhealthy, 238
Repetitive strain injury (RSI), 368
Reproduction, 263–265
Reproductive cycle, 263f
Reproductive system
    female, 256f, 257f
    male, 259f
Resistance training, 76, 77; see also Weight training
Reversibility principle, 68
RICE (rest, ice, compression and elevation), 79
Ritalin, 333
Rockport fitness test, 68, 69t
Rohypnol, 330
RPE; see Rating of perceived exertion scale
RSI; see Repetitive strain injury

S

Safety awareness
    college campuses, 373–374
    domestic violence, 377
    personal safety, 372
    sexual assault, 375–376
Sarcomas, 396
Saturated fats, 152
Scabies, 293, 298
SCM; see Stages of change model
Secondhand smoke; see Environmental tobacco smoke (ETS)
Self-talk, 28
    negative, 29
    positive, 29
Selye, Hans, 24
Seminiferous tubules, 258
Semivegetarian, 171
Set-point theory, 198
Sexual activity, 233
    readiness for, 261–262
    risks of, 233, 261
    safe, 233
    unsafe, 233
Sexual anatomy; see Female sexual anatomy; Male sexual anatomy
Sexual arousal, 260
Sexual assault, 375–376
    rape, 375
Sexual behavior, 261
Sexual contact, safety, 280t
Sexual health, rules about, 230b
Sexuality
    and pregnancy, 265–267
    reproduction, 263–265

Sexually transmitted infections
    (STIs), 261, 280, 285f
  bacterial, 281–287
  common types, 294t–297t
  levels of risk, 281
  parasitic, 293–298
  and pregnancy, 267, 277t
  prevention of, 277t,
    298–300
  rates of, 285f
  risk sheet, 283f
  test for, 298
  viral, 288–293
Sexual orientation, 260–261
  bisexual, 260
  heterosexual, 260
  homosexual, 260
Sexual response
  female, 258
  male, 260
Sexual sensitivity, 260
Shiatsu, 432
Sickle-cell anemia, 411
Skill-related fitness, 58
Skin cancer, 398–402
  basal cell carcinoma, 398
  examining skin for, 400
  non-melanoma, 400
  skin self-exam (SSE), 402
  squamous cell carcinoma, 398
Skinfold calipers, 199
Skin self-exam (SSE), 402
Smokeless tobacco, 315–317
Smoking, 314–322
  benefits of quitting, 314f,
    319–320
  cessation, 318
  health effects of, 315–318, 316f
  pipe, 317
  water pipe, 317, 318t
  and women, 317
  and young people, 317
Snuff; *see* Smokeless tobacco;
    Tobacco
Social dimension of wellness, 3
Sodium, 149–150
Soluble fiber, 151
Somatic movement, 435
Specificity principle, 67
Sperm, 258–260
Spiritual dimension of wellness, 3
Spiritual health, 421
Squamous cell carcinoma, 398
Stages of change model (SCM)
  action, 6–7
  contemplation, 6
  maintenance, 8
  precontemplation, 6
  preparation, 6
Stalking, 374–375
Static stretching, 78
Sterilization, 276–277
Steroids, anabolic, 332–333
Stimulants
  amphetamines, 322–323
  caffeine, 324, 325t
  cocaine, 323–324

ephedrine, 326
methamphetamine, 323
STIs; *see* Sexually transmitted
    infections
Strength training, 67; *see also*
    Weight training
  guidelines, 75
Stress
  and cardiovascular disease, 121
  defined, 24
  and depression, 31–32
  distress, 24
  and eating disorders, 33–34
  eustress, 24
  impact on mental health, 30–40
  manifestations of, 25–26
  and suicidal behavior, 32–33
  and wellness, 24–28
Stress journal, 45
Stress managers, characteristics of,
    30f
Stressors
  in college students, 26f
  managing, 26–27
Stretching exercises, 78–79
  ballistic, 78
  PNF, 79
  static, 78–79
Stroke, 119
  causes of, 119f
  risk factors for, 119
  symptoms and warning signs,
    120
Stroke volume, 59
Student Stress Scale, 28, 29f
Suicidal behavior and stress, 32–33
Sun protection factor (SPF), 402
Surgeon General's Report (1996),
    59f, 107, 108
Syphilis, 286–287, 286f, 287f
Systemic lupus erythematosus
    (SLE), 411
Systolic blood pressure, 59

T

Tai chi, 78
Talk test, 64
Tar, 314
Target heart rate range, 63, 64f
TB; *see* Tuberculosis
TCM; *see* Traditional Chinese
    medicine
Testicular cancer, 406–407
Testicular self-exam (TSE), 407
Testosterone, 258
Tetrahydrocannabinol (THC), 328
Therapeutic touch, 435
Time budget, 43
Tobacco; *see also* Smoking
  components of, 314–315
  environmental tobacco smoke,
    318
  smokeless, 315–317
  smoking, 318–322
  types of use, 315–318
TOM; *see* Traditional oriental
    medicine

Toxoplasma gondii, 389
Traditional Chinese medicine
    (TCM), 425
Traditional oriental medicine
    (TOM), 425
Trans fats, 153, 178, 195
Treponema pallidum, 286
Trichomonas vaginalis, 298
Trichomoniasis, 298
Triglyceride, 114t, 121
Tuberculosis (TB), 388–389
Type I diabetes, 408
Type II diabetes, 408, 409

U

Ulcers, 412
Unhealthy relationships, 238
  abusive, 238–239
Unintentional injuries, classes of,
    364
Unsaturated fats, 153
U.S. Department of Agriculture
    (USDA), 146, 150, 165

V

Vasectomy, 276
Vegans, 171
Vegetables, 167
Vegetarianism, 171
Violence, domestic, 377
Viral hepatitis, 390, 391t, 392f
Viral meningitis, 393
Vitamins, 158, 162, 430
  facts about, 159t–160t
  fat-soluble, 158
  water-soluble, 158
VO_2 Max, 68

W

Wagener, Michael, 342
Waist-to-hip circumference ratio,
    109, 112, 121
  calculating, 110
Warm-up, 65–66
Water, 164
Water pipe smoking, 317, 318f
Water-soluble vitamins, 158
Weight gain, 147, 201, 202
  healthy, 209
Weight loss, 201–204, 207
  clinical and nonclinical
    programs, 206
  and exercise, 201, 202
  guidelines, 204, 205
  with walking and caloric
    restriction program, 202t
Weight loss products
  appetite suppressants,
    205–206
  fad diets, 202, 207, 208
  metabolism boosters, 206–207
Weight management, 147,
    193–216
Weight training, 74–79
  muscle soreness, 74
  myths, 76–77

Wellness
    defined, 2
    dimensions of, 2–4, 2f
    emotional, 2–3
    environmental, 4
    factors influencing on, 5f
    financial, 4–5
    intellectual, 3
    occupational, 3
    physical, 3
    profile, 5
    social, 3
    spiritual, 3
    and stress, 24–28
Wernickes disease, 345
Wheat, 167f
Whole grains
    defined, 165
    serving, 165
Withdrawal method, 268
Work accidents, 368
World Health Organization (WHO), 121, 196, 317, 425

Y
Yoga, 77, 434
Yo-yo dieting, 202

Z
Zero Tolerance Law, 336